Field and Laboratory Methods in Animal Cognition

A Comparative Guide

Would you ask a honeybee to point at a screen and recognize a facial expression? Or ask an elephant to climb a tree? While humans and non-human species may inhabit the same world, it's likely that our perceptual worlds differ significantly. Emphasizing Uexküll's concept of 'Umwelt', this volume offers practical advice on how animal cognition can be successfully tested while avoiding anthropomorphic conclusions.

The chapters describe the capabilities of a range of animals – from ants to lizards to chimpanzees – revealing how to successfully investigate animal cognition across a variety of taxa. The book features contributions from leading cognition researchers, each offering a series of examples and practical tips drawn from their own experience. Together, the authors synthesize information on current field and laboratory methods, providing researchers and graduate students with methodological advice on how to formulate research questions, design experiments and adapt studies to different taxa.

Nereida Bueno-Guerra is an Assistant Professor in the Department of Psychology at Comillas Pontifical University, Spain. With a background in Psychology and Criminology, as well as Ethology and Education, her research focuses on the topics of morality and revenge. Her interest in animal cognition began while conducting comparative studies of chimpanzees and humans at the Max Planck Institute for Evolutionary Anthropology (MPI).

Federica Amici is a Post-Doctoral Researcher in the Primate Kin Selection Group at the University of Leipzig and at the MPI. Her main research interests lie in the evolutionary forces shaping the distribution of cognitive skills across vertebrates, combining behavioural observations and controlled experimental procedures, both in the wild and in captivity.

Field and Laboratory Methods in Animal Cognition

A Comparative Guide

Edited by

NEREIDA BUENO-GUERRA
Comillas Pontifical University

FEDERICA AMICI
University of Leipzig

CAMBRIDGE
UNIVERSITY PRESS

CAMBRIDGE
UNIVERSITY PRESS

University Printing House, Cambridge CB2 8BS, United Kingdom

One Liberty Plaza, 20th Floor, New York, NY 10006, USA

477 Williamstown Road, Port Melbourne, VIC 3207, Australia

314–321, 3rd Floor, Plot 3, Splendor Forum, Jasola District Centre, New Delhi – 110025, India

79 Anson Road, #06–04/06, Singapore 079906

Cambridge University Press is part of the University of Cambridge.

It furthers the University's mission by disseminating knowledge in the pursuit of education, learning, and research at the highest international levels of excellence.

www.cambridge.org
Information on this title: www.cambridge.org/9781108420327
DOI: 10.1017/9781108333191

First published 2018

Printed in the United Kingdom by TJ International Ltd. Padstow Cornwall

A catalogue record for this publication is available from the British Library.

Library of Congress Cataloging-in-Publication Data
Names: Bueno-Guerra, Nereida, 1988- editor.
Title: Field and laboratory methods in animal cognition : a comparative guide / edited by Nereida Bueno-Guerra, Comillas Pontifical University, Federica Amici, Universitat Leipzig.
Description: Cambridge, United Kingdom ; New York, NY : Cambridge University Press, 2018. | Includes bibliographical references and index.
Identifiers: LCCN 2018016876| ISBN 9781108420327 (hardback : alk. paper) | ISBN 9781108413947 (paperback : alk. paper)
Subjects: LCSH: Cognition in animals–Research–Methodology.
Classification: LCC QL785 .F49 2018 | DDC 591.5/13–dc23
LC record available at https://lccn.loc.gov/2018016876

ISBN 978-1-108-42032-7 Hardback
ISBN 978-1-108-41394-7 Paperback

To my parents, Mercedes and Santiago, and to all those who dare to see the world from a different perspective.

To Zahir, Nivola, Juri, Amelie and Giorgio – my perfect Umwelt. To my mother, for her love, and to my father, living in our hearts.

> Yet I exist in the hope that these memoirs, in some manner (. . .) may find their way to the minds of humanity in Some Dimension, and may stir up a race of rebels who shall refuse to be confined to limited Dimensionality.
>
> (Abbot, 1884)

Contents

Contributors

Federica Amici
Junior Research Group 'Primate Kin Selection', Institute of Biology, University of Leipzig, Leipzig, Germany
Department of Primatology, Max Planck Institute for Evolutionary Anthropology, Leipzig, Germany

Lucy Aplin
Max Planck Institute for Ornithology, Radolfzell, Germany

Jean-Nicolas Audet
Department of Biology, McGill University, Montréal, Canada
Field Research Center, Rockefeller University, Millbrook, NY, USA

Filippo Aureli
Instituto de Neuroetología, Universidad Veracruzana, Veracruz, México
Research Centre in Evolutionary Anthropology and Paleoecology, Liverpool John Moores University, Liverpool, UK

Luigi Baciadonna
Queen Mary University of London, Biological and Experimental Psychology, School of Biological and Chemical Sciences, London, UK

Sigal Balshine
Department of Psychology, Neuroscience & Behaviour, McMaster University, Ontario, Canada

Lucy A. Bates
School of Psychology, University of Sussex, Falmer, UK

Marine Battesti
Department of Biology, McGill University, Montréal, Canada

Culum Brown
Department of Biological Sciences, Macquarie University, Sydney, Australia

Margaret Bruce
Graduate Program in Organismal and Evolutionary Biology, University of Massachusetts Amherst, Amherst, MA, USA

Nereida Bueno-Guerra
Departamento de Psicología, Universidad Pontificia Comillas, Madrid, Spain

Gordon M. Burghardt
Department of Psychology, University of Tennessee, Knoxville, USA
Department of Ecology and Evolutionary Biology, University of Tennessee, Knoxville, TN, USA

Judith M. Burkart
Department of Anthropology, University of Zurich, Zurich, Switzerland

Cinzia Chiandetti
Department of Life Sciences, University of Trieste, Trieste, Italy

Chuan-Chin Chiao
Department of Life Science, National Tsing Hua University, Hsinchu, Taiwan

Catherine Crockford
Department of Primatology, Max Planck Institute for Evolutionary Anthropology, Leipzig, Germany

Fiona Cross
School of Biological Sciences, University of Canterbury, Christchurch, New Zealand
International Centre of Insect Physiology and Ecology, Mbita Point, Kenya

Jonathon D. Crystal
Department of Psychological and Brain Sciences, Indiana University, Bloomington, IN, USA

Volker B. Deecke
Department of Science, Natural Resources and Outdoor Studies, University of Cumbria, Ambleside, UK
Cetacean Research Lab, Vancouver Aquarium Marine Science Centre, Vancouver, Canada

Simon Ducatez
Department of Biology, McGill University, Montréal, Canada
School of Biological Sciences, University of Sydney, Sydney, Australia

Robert W. Elwood
School of Biological Sciences, Queen's University, Belfast, Northern Ireland, UK

Chris G. Faulkes
School of Biological and Chemical Sciences, Queen Mary University of London, London, UK

Julia Fischer
Cognitive Ethology Laboratory, German Primate Center and Georg-August-University, Göttingen, Germany

Manfred Gahr
Max Planck Institute for Ornithology, Behavioural Neurobiology, Seewiesen, Germany

Cole Gilbert
Department of Entomology, Cornell University, Ithaca, USA

Ewen Glass
Lincoln School of Film and Media, University of Lincoln, Lincoln, UK

Michael S. Grace
Department of Biological Sciences, Florida Institute of Technology, Melbourne, FL, USA

Stefan Greif
School of Zoology, Faculty of Life Sciences, Tel-Aviv University, Tel-Aviv, Israel

Tristan L. Guttridge
Bimini Biological Field Station Foundation, South Bimini, Bahamas

Kay E. Holekamp
Department of Integrative Biology, Michigan State University, East Lansing, MI, USA

David M. P. Jacoby
Institute of Zoology, Zoological Society of London, London, UK

Elizabeth M. Jakob
Department of Biology, University of Massachusetts Amherst, Amherst, MA, USA

Frants Havmand Jensen
Aarhus Institute of Advanced Studies, Aarhus University, Aarhus, Denmark

Lily Johnson-Ulrich
Department of Integrative Biology, Michigan State University, East Lansing, MI, USA

Stephanie King
Centre for Evolutionary Biology, University of Western Australia, Crawley, Australia

Aaron R. Krochmal
Department of Biology, Washington College, Chestertown, MD, USA

Michael J. Kuba
Physics and Biology Unit, Okinawa Institute of Science and Technology Graduate University, Okinawa, Japan

Mark E. Laidre
Department of Biological Sciences, University of Dartmouth, Hanover, NH, USA

Manuel Leal
Division of Biological Sciences, University of Missouri, Columbia, USA

Phyllis Lee
Behaviour and Evolution Research Group, University of Stirling, Stirling, UK

Louis Lefebvre
Department of Biology, McGill University, Montréal, Canada

Kenna D. S. Lehman
Department of Integrative Biology, Michigan State University, East Lansing, MI, USA

Skye M. Long
Department of Biology, University of Massachusetts Amherst, Amherst, MA, USA

Evan L. MacLean
School of Anthropology, University of Arizona, Tuczon, AZ, USA

Marta Manser
Department of Evolutionary Biology and Environmental Studies, University of Zurich, Zurich, Switzerland

Jennifer A. Mather
Department of Psychology, University of Lethbridge, Lethbridge, Canada

Erin S. McCallum
Department of Psychology, Neuroscience & Behaviour, McMaster University, Ontario, Canada

Alan G. McElligott
Department of Life Sciences, University of Roehampton, London, UK

Richard McElreath
Department of Human Behavior, Ecology, and Culture, Max Planck Institute for Evolutionary Anthropology, Leipzig, Germany

Randolf Menzel
Department of Neurobiology, Freie Universität Berlin, Berlin, Germany

Noam Miller
Departments of Psychology & Biology, Wilfrid Laurier University, Waterloo, Canada

Felicity Muth
Department of Biology, University of Nevada, Reno, NV, USA

Stewart Nicol
School of Natural Sciences, University of Tasmania, South Hobart, Tasmania, Australia

Daniel W. A. Noble
School of Biological, Earth and Environmental Sciences, Ecology and Evolution Research Centre, University of New South Wales, Sydney, Australia

Sarah E. Overington
Department of Biology, McGill University, Montréal, Canada

Rachel A. Page
Smithsonian Tropical Research Institute, Ancón, Panama

Irene M. Pepperberg
Department of Psychology, Harvard University, Cambridge, MA, USA

Friederike Range
Wolf Science Center and Comparative Cognition, Messerli Research Institute, University of Veterinary Medicine, Vienna, Austria

Zhanna Reznikova
Institute of Systematics and Ecology of Animals, Siberian Branch RAS, Novosibirsk, Russia
Novosibirsk State University, Novosibirsk, Russia

Timothy C. Roth II
Department of Psychology, Franklin & Marshall College, Lancaster, PA, USA

Christian Rutz
Centre for Biological Diversity, School of Biology, University of St Andrews, St Andrews, UK

Colleen M. Schaffner
Instituto de Neuroetología, Universidad Veracruzana, Veracruz, México

Vera Schluessel
University of Bonn, Bonn, Germany

Carolynn K-lynn Smith
Department of Brain, Behaviour and Evolution, Macquarie University, Sydney, Australia

David S. Steinberg
Department of Biology, University of North Carolina, Chapel Hill, NC, USA

Barbara Taborsky
Behavioural Ecology Division, University of Bern, Bern, Switzerland

Michael Taborsky
Behavioural Ecology Division, University of Bern, Bern, Switzerland

Alex Thornton
Centre for Ecology and Conservation, University of Exeter, Exeter, UK

Neil D. Tsutsui
Department of Environmental Science, Policy, and Management, University of California, Berkeley, CA, USA

Julie W. Turner
Department of Integrative Biology, Michigan State University, East Lansing, MI, USA

Giorgio Vallortigara
Center for Mind/Brain Sciences, University of Trento, Trento, Italy

Catarina Vila Pouca
Department of Biological Sciences, Macquarie University, Sydney, Australia

Martin J. Whiting
Department of Biological Sciences, Macquarie University, Sydney, Australia

Anna Wilkinson
School of Life Sciences, University of Lincoln, Lincoln, UK
Wildlife Research Center, Kyoto University, Kyoto, Japan

Roman M. Wittig
Department of Primatology, Max Planck Institute for Evolutionary Anthropology, Leipzig, Germany
Taï Chimpanzee Project, Centre Suisse de Recherches Scientifiques, Abidjan, Côte d'Ivoire

Kara E. Yopak
Department of Biology and Marine Biology, University of North Carolina Wilmington, Wilmington, NC, USA

Yossi Yovel
School of Zoology, Faculty of Life Sciences, Tel-Aviv University, Tel-Aviv, Israel
'Sagol' School of Neuroscience, Tel-Aviv University, Tel-Aviv, Israel

Foreword

Superpowers are one of the defining features of superheroes. Unlike common humans, superheroes can see and hear beyond our normal perceptual range, they can run, swim or fly faster than even our fastest vehicles, and can even use electrical discharges to defeat villains. Animals do not have superpowers, but just like superheroes, some of their perceptual and motor skills often outstrip our own. The humble honeybee is capable of perceiving part of the visible spectrum down to 300 nm, well into the ultraviolet zone, an ability that they use to individuate flowers that look identical to us. Another 290 nm down the scale and bees would be within Superman's zone of X-ray vision. On the other side of the electromagnetic spectrum, next to the visible zone, one finds infrared radiation, which snakes use quite effectively to track and identify warm-blooded prey. Other species like the electric eel use powerful electrical discharges to stun not villains but prey, and some research suggests that they also use it to communicate with conspecifics.

The above examples are not aimed at unleashing a furious competition between non-humans and humans (or superheroes) for the crown of the most perceptive beast in the animal kingdom. Instead, they seek to illustrate that while humans and non-human species inhabit the same spatio-temporal coordinates, their perceptual and action worlds may differ in very significant ways. This was Jacob von Uexküll's great insight. Each species is adapted to a particular niche that includes the particular types of information that it extracts from it and the actions that it applies to it.

From a comparative perspective, the phenomenon of species-specific Umwelten is both fascinating and frustrating. On the one hand, it is fascinating because it illustrates the diversity of solutions in the animal kingdom to the problem of processing and using information available in the environment. On the other hand, it is frustrating because it makes the task of comparing species much more difficult, precisely at a time when behavioural ecologists, ethologists and comparative psychologists are showing a renewed interest for interspecific comparisons focused on elucidating how cognition evolves.

One major approach in this endeavour has been to investigate closely related species on a particular ability, for instance food caching in parids, transitive inference in corvids or inhibitory control in primates. Although these comparisons are fine-grained and precise, and often based on ecologically relevant tasks, they are limited in scope because they are typically restricted to one ability and one taxa. The other major approach to elucidate cognitive evolution is much more ambitious, encompassing both closely and distantly related species, but it is fraught with peril as soon as researchers abandon the comfort zone provided by ecologically relevant settings and venture into the territory of the 'one-size-fits-all' tasks.

A compromise between the two approaches might be possible – one that compares multiple closely and distantly related species, using multiple functionally equivalent tasks. Multiple tasks, not just one or two, are required because one cannot expect to capture the diversity of intelligences with one or two tasks. Crucially, each of these tasks is adapted to a particular species, but their functional equivalence makes them comparable across species. In other words, tasks may differ in the form that they might take, provided they still measure the same construct.

An essential ingredient for designing functionally equivalent tasks is precisely a good appreciation of the animals' Umwelt: not just how they perceive the world, but also how they respond to it. This volume represents a timely and valuable contribution to alleviate some of the frustration created by the need to embark on broad-ranging interspecific comparisons. The contributors to this volume provide the reader with valuable insights about how to tackle the study of various species with vastly different Umwelten. In keeping with the spirit of the volume, each of the chapters is written with a strong applied orientation by experts in a particular species or taxon. They combine a succinct state-of-the-art overview of what is known about each species with practical knowledge and sage advice about how to study their perceptual and cognitive abilities. This combination makes this book both unique and very practical – a first port of call for anybody wanting to begin investigating any of the species presented in the volume, or any new species in general.

Josep Call
School of Psychology and Neuroscience, University of St Andrews, Scotland, UK

Acknowledgements

Nereida Bueno-Guerra and Federica Amici would like to thank the Cambridge University Press (especially Megan Keirnan and Jenny van der Meijden) and all the contributors of this book for trusting and supporting the idea to disseminate the concept of Umwelt in animal cognition research.

Nereida Bueno-Guerra also thanks the University of Bern for organizing the workshop 'Minds of Animals: Reflections of the human–non-human continuum' in 2016, where as a junior researcher she could introduce the underlying idea of this book with senior researchers for the first time. In particular, she is very grateful to Josep Call, whose uplifting supervision has been inspirational across her career, broadening her understanding of animal cognition and encouraging her to go beyond the data under the strictest bioethical procedures. Five years after his dedication on a book, here is hers in return. In this regard, she also thanks the Max Planck Institute for Evolutionary Anthropology and the Wolfgang Köhler Research Primate Center in Leipzig (Germany) for allowing her to enjoy a fruitful research environment. It was there where this idea germinated. That is why she also thanks all the zookeepers, zoo managers and research assistants for their patience and understanding, as well as all the animals she shared time with (they were the true inspiration for this book). Many thanks go also to the University of Barcelona and Montserrat Colell, because there she could teach what she felt most passionate about during her PhD training. Many colleagues, students, family and friends also collaborated with their feedback and support in making this book real. Finally, as a posthumous tribute, she needs to mention the three readings that became the cornerstone of this project: *Cartas biológicas a una dama* (Jakob von Uexküll); *Los tónicos de la voluntad* (Santiago Ramón y Cajal); and *El origen de las especies* (Charles Darwin).

Federica Amici would like to thank the Humboldt Foundation and the Deutsche Forschungsgemeinschaft (DFG) for generously providing research funding across several years. She is further grateful to Filippo Aureli and Josep Call, for having been the best supervisors one could ever dream of, to Trix Cacchione, Anna Albiach-Serrano, Carla Sebastian-Enesco, Bino Majolo and Barbara Tiddi, for being much more than wonderful colleagues. She would also like to thank Juliane Braeuer, Lucas Bietti, Giulia Sirianni, Lorenzo von Fersen, Montserrat Colell Mimo, Anja Widdig and all the enthusiastic students and colleagues who have generously provided her with help and ideas throughout all these years, including Alex Sanchez Amaro, Alvaro Lopez Caicoya, Alba Castellano Navarro, Fabrizio dell'Anna, Simone Anzà, Laura Cancino, Maria Jose Alvarez,

Luisa Rebecchini, Lisa-Marie Kießling and Karimullah Karimullah – a living proof that science and knowledge can only advance when people and ideas are free to move across countries, in the face of borders and walls. Finally, thanks to her children and husband, for love and patience, and to her parents and family, for letting her study.

Zhanna Reznikova would further like to thank the Russian Fund for Basic Research (No. 17–04–00702) and the Federal Fundamental Scientific Research Program for 2013–2020 (AAAA-A16-116121410120-0) for support. Yossi Yovel and Stefan Greif are grateful to M. Taub for preparing the figures in this chapter. The Lefebvre Lab is grateful to the Natural Sciences and Engineering Research Council of Canada, the Foundation Fyssen of France and the staff of the Bellairs Research Institute of McGill University, St James, Barbados. Giorgio Vallortigara is thankful to the Caritro Foundation for providing support. Roman Wittig and Cathy Crockford conducted their research with the Sonso community in the Budongo Forest, Uganda, and the Taï chimpanzees in the Taï National Park, Ivory Coast. They are grateful to Uganda Wildlife Authority and Uganda National Council for Science and Technology for permission to conduct research with the Budongo chimpanzees, and to Ministers of Research and Environment of Côte d'Ivoire and the Office Ivorien des Parcs et Resaerves for permitting research with the chimpanzees of Taï. They want to thank the Budongo Conservation Field Station in Uganda and the Centre Suisse de Recherches Scientifique in Ivory Coast for their support. Finally, they are most grateful to the staff members of Budongo Conservation Field Station and the Taï Chimpanzee Project, without whom the research at both sites would not have been possible. The fieldwork described by Volker Deecke was conducted in collaboration with Michael de Roos, Graeme M. Ellis, Ari P. Shapiro, Jared Towers and Brianna M. Wright and funded by the Species at Risk Program, Fisheries and Oceans Canada, the University of Cumbria's Research and Scholarship Development Fund and a Marie Curie Inter-European Fellowship. He also thanks A. Ceschi, B. Weeks and the staff of God's Pocket Resort, and B. Falconer and the crew of the S/V 'Achiever' for logistic support; Laetitia Legat for help with data analysis; and the Editors and Stephanie King for valuable comments on a previous draft of the chapter. Lucy Bates would like to thank the Daphne Jackson Trust and the University of Sussex for her Fellowship. Robert Elwood is grateful to Mark Laidre for comments on an earlier version of his chapter, and to Gill Riddell for technical help over many years. The hyena team lead by Kay Holekamp are very grateful to Arjun Tekalur for measuring the force required to crack open cow femurs. They also thank the Kenyan National Council for Science and Technology, the Narok County Council, and the Kenya Wildlife Service for permission to conduct field research with hyenas. They want to thank also all those who assisted with long-term data collection in the field. Their fieldwork was supported by NSF Grants IOS 1121474, OISE 1556407 and DEB 1353110 to Kay E. Holekamp, by NSF Graduate Research Fellowships to Lily Johnson-Ulrich and Kenna D. S. Lehman, by a SICB Grants-In-Aid of Research to Lily Johnson-Ulrich, an Animal Behavior Society student research grant to Julie W. Turner, an American Society of Mammalogists grants-in-aid of research to Julie W. Turner, and by Fellowships from Michigan State University, the College of Natural Science and the programme in Ecology, Evolutionary Biology and Behavior at Michigan State

University to Lily Johnson-Ulrich, Julie W. Turner and Kenna D. S. Lehman. Their work was made possible by support from the BEACON Center for the Study of Evolution in Action, funded by NSF grant OIA 0939454. Martin Whiting and Daniel Nobel want to thank their students and collaborators that have spent many hours testing lizards and scoring videos, including Ben Clark, Fonti Kar, Julia Riley, Birgit Szabo, Pau Carazo, Dick Byrne, Yin Qi and Feng Xu. Their cognition work has been funded by the Australian Research Council (DP130102998 to M.J. Whiting and R.W. Byrne; DE150101774 DECRA to D.W.A. Noble). Marta Manser wants to thank the editors for the invitation to write her chapter and also for their impressive editing efforts. Also, she is very grateful to Megan Wyman and a referee on their helpful comments on an earlier draft of the chapter. The studies on meerkats were conducted at the Kalahari Meerkat Project (KMP) in collaboration with Tim Clutton-Brock and all the project managers, the hundreds of volunteers maintaining habituation and collecting the basic data, as well as the many PhD, MSc students and postdocs since 1993. The University of Zurich has funded writing Marta Manser's chapter and together with Cambridge University also the long-term research at KMP. The Swiss National Science Foundation has financed her specific projects since 1996. The Mammal Research Institute of the University of Pretoria has provided logistic support since the very beginning of the KMP. Michael Kuba's work was supported in part by funding from the Physics and Biology Unit, Okinawa Institute of Science and Technology Graduate University, which he wants to thank. Irene Pepperberg is very grateful to the donors to *The Alex Foundation*, who have supported her work for many years, and for the undergraduates and lab managers who have assisted with the studies. Tristan Guttridge would like to acknowledge Annie Guttridge for her never-ending guidance, support and inspiration. Kara E. Yopak would like to thank members of her lab, particularly E. Peele, and funding from the University of North Carolina Wilmington during the writing of this chapter. Thanks to S. P. Collin and T. Lisney, whose many years of collaboration have contributed to advancing the field of comparative neuroanatomy of elasmobranchs. Vera was funded by the German Science Foundation and would like to thank Horst Bleckmann for all his help and support throughout the last 10 years, and all of her enthusiastic students. The spider team led by Elizabeth M. Jakob want to thank A. H. Porter, C. Gilbert, the editors and anonymous reviewers for very helpful comments on their manuscript. Their work was supported by NSF IOS 0952822 and IOS 1656714 to Elizabeth M. Jakob. Anna Wilkinson and Ewen Glass would like to thank past and current members of the cold-blooded cognition research group, particularly Geoff Hall and Ludwig Huber. They think that without them their chapter would not exist. They also thank Sophie A. Moszuti for kindly providing some photos. Gordon Burghardt wants to thank Enrique Font for comments and suggestions in preparing his box.

Finally, the editors and the contributors are very grateful to all the reviewers who altruistically provided comments to help improve earlier versions of the chapters of this book, including Rachel Page, Sabine Tebbich, Lori Marino, Stephanie King, Mark Laidre, Oliver Höner, Alex Thornton, Daniel Osorio, Christian Schloegl, David Jacoby, Damian Elias, Tim Roth and Aaron Krochmal.

Introduction. The Concept of Umwelt in Experimental Animal Cognition

Nereida Bueno-Guerra and Federica Amici

Yes, the ant says again,
I've seen the stars (. . .)
The snail asks:
But, what are stars?
They're lights we carry
Over our heads.
We can't see them,
The ants say.
(. . .)
We'll kill you, you're
Lazy and perverse.
The Encounters of an Adventurous Snail
(Federico García Lorca, 1918)

Living in the world mostly consists of receiving perceptual information and performing actions according to this information. This combination of what we can perceive ('Merkwelt') and what we can do ('Wirkwelt') was defined as 'Umwelt' by Jakob Johann von Uexküll (1934/2010). According to Uexküll, the concept of Umwelt comprises the extent of every being's existence: there is no more external information than what we can perceive through our senses, and there is no more capacity of action than what we can actually do with our anatomy. Indeed, imagining the world with a different perspective from the one we daily live in is particularly challenging. Although all individuals and species live in the same objective reality (Kant's 'noumenon': Kant, 1781/1998), perceptual limitations only allow species to perceive part of this reality ('phenomenon') through their senses. Species' (and individuals') reality is therefore subjective and limited by their perceptual and factional characteristics – their Umwelt. In Uexküll's (1920/2014, pp. 92–93) words: 'The real thing is that there is no real world but as many worlds as species – and individuals'.

As humans, we are no exception to this rule: our perception of reality is also limited by our Umwelt, and it is no easy task for us to put ourselves in other animals' shoes. This limitation is especially relevant for comparative psychologists, ethologists and researchers interested in animal cognition. First, understanding the different Umwelt of other species is necessary to come up with socio-ecologically relevant tests of cognition and avoid anthropocentrism. Although interspecific comparisons can be highly informative on the evolution of human cognition (i.e. which specific cognitive skills are uniquely human, and why), studying cognition in species other than humans is also highly rewarding per se. In this respect, behavioural observations can tell us a lot about the socio-ecological challenges that different animals face in their everyday life, and on the cognitive skills that may be linked to these challenges, which can be very different from our own. As Ramón y Cajal (1897/2016) noted, 'our appreciation of what is important and what is accessory; what is big and what is small; lie on a false judgment, namely a truly anthropomorphic error'.

Second, considering the species' merkwelt is essential to design experimental set-ups best framed to the species' perceptual systems. Some species, for instance, rely on different senses (e.g. electroreception) or perceive stimuli with different thresholds (e.g. infrared light). Failing to take this into account may not only lead researchers to use stimuli with little relevance for the study species (e.g. colour stimuli that cannot be easily discriminated in a learning task), but also to inadvertently provide cues to the study subjects (e.g. odour cues when testing object permanence in species largely relying on olfaction).

Third, taking into account the species' wirkwelt is crucial to implement experimental set-ups that only require actions belonging to the species' natural repertoire. If we ignore interspecific differences in terms of wirkwelt, we may end up concluding that some species fall short of certain cognitive skills simply because their anatomical characteristics make the required action unnatural to the species. Adapting to the species' wirkwelt, therefore, often implies modifying our set-ups across taxa (e.g. requiring individuals to 'choose' by grabbing, approaching, touching with the nose or swimming around one of several objects), balancing the need to maintain experimental procedures both comparable across species and 'fair' to each different wirkwelt.

Consequently, the purpose of this book is to bring together leading researchers with extensive experience in the study of animal behaviour and cognition, to highlight the importance of the Umwelt concept and provide useful practical advice on how to take it into account when conducting cognitive experiments. First, researchers will introduce their study taxon, providing us with essential information on its anatomical, perceptual and socio-ecological characteristics. Then, they will explain how these characteristics may be linked to specific cognitive skills and how they may affect the choice of experimental procedures during cognitive tests. Finally, they will provide us with a series of examples and practical tips drawn by their everyday experience, to introduce the methodological tools most apt to work with their taxon.

To foster dialogue and open up to the study of novel species and methods across research areas, other scientists working with different taxa and/or methods will complement this information with small boxes within chapters. In these boxes, the authors will briefly comment (1) on the possibility to extend methods across taxa, introducing a different species with similar socio-ecological or physical characteristics, which may be tested in analogous ways ('All for one and one for all' boxes); (2) on the need to adapt methods across closely related taxa, as some socio-ecological or physical characteristics may differ deeply even across phylogenetically close taxa ('The devil is in the details' boxes); and (3) on the methodological differences and issues raised when testing wild and/or captive conspecific populations ('Wild vs. lab' boxes). This combination of chapters and boxes not only aims to help researchers to carefully plan experiments and interpret data, but also to open up to the use of new methodologies and taxa in animal cognition.

In this book, we have included species which have attracted much attention in the study of animal cognition, and others whose cognitive skills have just started being investigated. It is therefore a first attempt to highlight the need and urge to consider each animal's Umwelt when testing cognition, and a first proposal to dive in, explore and enjoy different ways of living the same world. However, the selection of taxa is necessarily partial and arbitrary, as every single species lives in a particular Umwelt and would be worth a chapter on its own. As no taxon is more relevant or interesting than others per se, and in contrast with the idea of a *scala naturae*, we have ordered the chapters in a strict alphabetical order.

In the first chapter, Zhanna Reznikova introduces us to the extraordinary world of ANTS – eusocial insects including around 12,000 species, with highly sophisticated communication and a variety of socio-ecological characteristics. She describes original methodological approaches to study cognition in individual ants, with a special focus on social learning, problem-solving and communication. Within her chapter, Felicity Muth draws interesting theoretical and practical parallels between ants and other eusocial species, like honeybees and bumblebees (Box 1.1). Moreover, Neil Tsutsui highlights the importance of combining field and laboratory studies, providing useful suggestions on how to practically investigate cognition in wild ants (Box 1.2).

In the second chapter, Yossi Yovel and Stefan Greif introduce us to one of the most diverse groups within the mammalian order – BATS. With their immense range of foraging strategies, social behaviours and sensory systems, bats constitute an intriguing model for studying cognition. The authors provide detailed information on how to implement innovative tasks, and explain how technology can help us overcome most of the challenges related to the study of bat cognition. In their chapter, Manfred Gahr fruitfully discusses the advantages and disadvantages of different telemetric and logging devices used to work with both bats and birds (Box 2.1). Further, Rachel Page provides suggestive examples of bat species with a very different Umwelt, and warns us about the risks of ignoring these differences in comparative cognition (Box 2.2).

In the third chapter, Randolf Menzel makes us acquainted with the fascinating taxon of HONEYBEES, revealing how the study of cognition can best thrive by individually testing honeybees foraging outside their colonies. Further, he discusses how different experiments can be conducted in the lab and in the wild, with a special focus on discrimination, memory, learning and navigation. Within this chapter, Chris Faulkes explains how eusocial naked mole rats have all the characteristics (e.g. longevity, complex socio-ecological environment) to probably bear comparison with other eusocial species in terms of cognition (Box 3.1).

In the fourth chapter, Simon Ducatez, Sarah Overington, Jean-Nicolas Audet, Marine Battesti and Louis Lefebvre discuss why CARIB GRACKLES, a blackbird species successfully adapted to a highly anthropogenic environment, are a valuable model to study cognition. Moreover, they extensively explain how to test wild individuals in controlled experimental set-ups, with a special focus on innovation, personality and interindividual variation in cognition. In this chapter, Noam Miller describes a further approach to investigate bird cognition – the study of collective movement and decision-making, which has been successfully used across a variety of taxa (Box 4.1). Finally, Lucy Aplin discusses the importance of testing cognition in even more natural set-ups and provides a series of elegant examples on how to do that (Box 4.2).

In the fifth chapter, Cinzia Chiandetti and Giorgio Vallortigara introduce us to the Umwelt of CHICKEN – a domestic species which has proven an excellent model for the study of early learning, memory consolidation and core knowledge, including understanding of numbers, space and objects. The authors describe a series of methodological approaches that can be used to successfully test cognition in chicks and discuss how they can crucially complement studies carried out with mammalian models. Within their chapter, Luigi Baciadonna and Alan McElligott draw unexpected parallels between cognition in chicks and goats, focusing on the role played by domestication on the evolution of cognitive skills (Box 5.1). In her Box 5.2, Carolynn K-lynn Smith familiarizes us with the wild counterpart of chicken, red jungle fowls, and stresses the socio-ecological and cognitive differences between the two subspecies.

In the sixth chapter, Roman Wittig and Catherine Crockford make us acquainted with our closest living relatives – CHIMPANZEES. Starting from chimpanzees' complex ecological and social system, they guide us through the amazing behaviour of this species in the wild and back to the evolutionary roots of human cognition. By focusing on this species' spatial skills, tool use and social cognition, the authors introduce readers to different possible experimental set-ups, including play-back experiments and object presentations. Within this chapter, Christian Rutz explains how a phylogenetically distant taxon, corvids, underwent convergent evolution, and how methods can be creatively extended from chimpanzees to corvids, and vice versa (Box 6.1). Finally, Julia Fischer convincingly discusses the importance of fostering dialogue between lab- and wild-based studies of primate cognition, trying to bring together both approaches (Box 6.2).

In the seventh chapter, Volker Deecke brings us over the ocean to observe DOLPHINS AND WHALES in their natural environment. While describing the variety of socio-ecological characteristics of these mammals, their sensory systems and cognitively skills uniquely adapted to the underwater world, he provides practical solutions to the multiple challenges of studying cognition in the wild, with a special focus on social behaviour, foraging and navigation. Moreover, Filippo Aureli and Colleen Schaffner draw our attention to one crucial aspect of social complexity, and remind us of the possible cognitive challenges faced by taxa characterized by high levels of fission–fusion (Box 7.1). In Box 7.2, Frants Havmand Jensen describes the peculiar Umwelt of deep-water whales, which likely posits special cognitive challenges not only to these cetaceans, but also to the researchers aiming to test them.

In the eighth chapter, Lucy Bates introduces us to one of the most long-living, large-brained and socially complex taxa we know – ELEPHANTS. She provides us with practical recommendations on how to implement socio-ecologically relevant cognitive studies in the wild and suggests possible future directions for cognitive research, in line with the elephants' Umwelt. Within this chapter, Phyllis Lee draws further attention to elephants' social cognition and complex social strategies, drawing interesting parallels with other taxa (Box 8.1).

In the ninth chapter, Catarina Vila Pouca and Culum Brown successfully condense our current knowledge on perception, socio-ecology and cognition in the group of vertebrates with the largest radiation – FISH. Although fish possess many anatomical and perceptual adaptations to the aquatic environment, the authors describe how most experimental procedures used to study cognition in other species (including spatial and social learning) are readily adaptable to fish. In this line, Jonathon Crystal takes things further and discusses different approaches to study memory across taxa, including fish (Box 9.1). Finally, Michael and Barbara Taborsky highlight the peculiarities of Cichlids, a group of fish with very unusual perceptual, social and cognitive characteristics (Box 9.2).

In the tenth chapter, Robert Elwood brings us inside the fascinating world of HERMIT CRABS, whose cognitive skills are still at an incipient stage of research. He describes a series of studies on shell investigation and shell preferences, to provide us with a socio-ecologically relevant approach to the study of cognition in this taxon, with a special focus on decision-making and planning. In Box 10.1, Erin McCallum and Sigal Balshine draw interesting parallels between hermit crabs and a small territorial fish, the round goby, which also competes for access to shelters. Finally, Mark Laidre discusses important differences across hermit crab species and meets the challenge of proposing possible experimental approaches to study hermit crabs in the wild (Box 10.2).

In the eleventh chapter, Lily Johnson-Ulrich, Kenna Lehman, Julie Turner and Kay Holekamp bring us to sub-Saharan Africa to study spotted HYENAS – scavengers with extended juvenile periods and complex societies. Especially focusing on their social cognitive skills and innovation abilities, they effectively explain how to conduct controlled experiments in wild and captive settings, using a variety of methodological approaches. In her Box 11.1, Friederike Range complements this information by discussing similarities and differences between hyenas, dogs and wolves, both in terms of cognition and experimental approaches required.

In the twelfth chapter, Martin Whiting and Daniel Noble introduce us to the mesmerizing Umwelt of LIZARDS, especially focusing on inter- and intraspecific differences in cognition. By providing us with useful practical examples, they explain how to test their cognition, including social learning and behavioural flexibility, according to the lizards' Umwelt. In his Box 12.1, Michael S. Grace further discusses the challenges of testing cognition in reptiles, with a series of suggestive examples from the study of snake cognition. Finally, David Steinberg and Manuel Leal explain why the unique Umwelt of lizards may posit special constraints when testing them in captive settings and propose possible approaches to the study of wild populations (Box 12.2).

In the thirteenth chapter, Marta Manser makes us acquainted with a cooperative breeding mongoose species – MEERKATS. She extensively discusses examples of successful research approaches to study the cognitive mechanisms involved in their complex social systems, elaborate vocal and olfactory communication and social learning, with a further focus on the pervasive effect of hormones on their social behaviour. Judith Burkart starts from the meerkats' cooperative breeding system to discuss the cognitive challenges they may face, and the possibility to successfully extend methodological approaches across different cooperative breeders (Box 13.1). Finally, Alex Thornton draws interesting parallels between meerkats and other closely related mongoose species, providing unique research opportunities to understand the selective pressures driving cognitive evolution (Box 13.2).

In the fourteenth chapter, Jennifer Mather and Michael Kuba bring us deep into the water to observe cognitive skills in OCTOPUSES. They explain how to investigate their personalities, play behaviour and learning skills, taking into account the striking peculiarities of their neural and behavioural systems. Within their chapter, Chuan-Chin Chiao discusses how, despite socio-ecological differences and phylogenetic distance, squids and cuttlefish share with octopuses similar body patterns for camouflage and communication, fostering interspecific comparisons by creative researchers in animal cognition (Box 14.1).

In the fifteenth chapter, Irene Pepperberg highlights the peculiar Umwelt characterizing her study species – grey PARROTS. She especially focuses on their vocal skills, which have proved a valuable way to implement unique methodological approaches to the study of cognition and language in this taxon. In Box 15.1, Stephanie King discusses some striking similarities between cognition (including vocal labelling) in parrots and bottlenose dolphins, and the similar methodological approaches that can be used in both taxa.

In the sixteenth chapter, Tristan Guttridge, Kara Yopak and Vera Schluessel describe SHARKS – a group of cartilaginous fishes with an incredible range of anatomical, foraging and social characteristics. The authors describe how technological advances (including biotelemetry and bio-logging techniques) have allowed researchers to broaden experimental investigations of cognition in these species. In Box 16.1, Stewart Nicol draws an unexpected parallel between sharks, which are 'atypical fishes', and monotremes, which are 'atypical mammals', providing inspiring inputs to test cognition in the latter. Finally, David Jacoby proposes interesting methodological approaches to study cognition in wild sharks and rays (Box 16.2).

In the seventeenth chapter, Elizabeth Jakob, Skye Long and Margaret Bruce discuss how the peculiar perceptual system of jumping SPIDERS makes them an ideal taxon to test cognition. The authors explain how their Umwelt posits specific challenges to researchers, and how these challenges can be easily met by carefully planning experiments. Within this chapter, Cole Gilbert highlights significant differences and similarities with tiger beetles and other species (Box 17.1). Furthermore, Fiona Cross provides convincing evidence that different species of spiders, even if belonging to the same family, may call for essential changes in experimental procedures (Box 17.2).

Finally, in the eighteenth chapter, Anna Wilkinson and Ewen Glass guide us through the amazing world of cold-blooded cognition to discover TORTOISES – a taxon which has long been ignored in the study of animal cognition. They provide useful tricks and original methodological approaches to successfully study visual and spatial cognition, social learning and memory. In his Box 18.1, Gordon Burghardt draws fascinating comparisons among tortoises and other reptiles, and draws attention to potential terminological caveats. Finally, Timothy C. Roth II and Aaron Krochmal stress the importance of testing tortoises in the wild, thoroughly discussing the advantages of such an approach (Box 18.2).

In its form, this book is therefore the result of a huge cooperation among experienced researchers, who have agreed to 'open the doors' of their laboratories and field sites, and to share with us their extensive first-hand knowledge about their study species. Through this book, we hope that readers will not only be fostered to reflect on the key role played by the Umwelt in animal cognition, but also stimulated to consider possible ways to work with novel species and methods.

The study of animal cognition is thrilling and provides creative minds with endless opportunities to come up with relevant research questions and novel methods to address them. We hope that this book will be successful in further fostering this development, facilitating interdisciplinary dialogue and inspiring new and old scholars to enthusiastically approach the study of different taxa, embrace new methodological approaches and generously share their knowledge. The immense diversity of different worlds inside the same world is our richness: to admire, protect and investigate.

References

García Lorca, F. (1918). *Obras completas* (Ed. Arturo del Hoyo). Aguilar.

Kant, I. (1781/1998). *Critique of pure reason*. Cambridge: Cambridge University Press.

Ramón y Cajal, S. (1897/2016). *Los tónicos de la voluntad: reglas y consejos sobre investigación científica*. Madrid: Gadir.

von Uexküll, J. (1920/2014). *Cartas biológicas a una dama*. Buenos Aires: Cactus.

von Uexküll, J. (1934/2010). *A foray into the worlds of animals and humans with a theory of meaning*. Minneapolis, MN: University of Minnesota Press.

1 Ants – Individual and Social Cognition

Zhanna Reznikova

Species Description

The total number of ants is estimated to be between one and ten million billion, which makes them a very successful life form (Hölldobler and Wilson, 1990). Ants are characterized by a very specific social evolution, perennial life cycle, unusual genetic method of sex determination and exceptional forms of collective decision-making.

Brain

Perhaps the first question about ants' individual cognition is whether their tiny brains are sufficient for solving intellectual problems. Darwin (1981) recognized this and considered the brain of an ant as 'one of the most marvellous atoms of matter in the world, perhaps more so than the brain of man'. Like some other animals with small brains, ants express behaviours and sensory capacities comparable to large-brained animals, despite the high energetic costs for maintaining a relatively large brain in small-bodied animals (e.g. Seid *et al.*, 2011). Unlike social vertebrates, which have larger brains and cerebral cortices than solitary species, ant brains are not larger than those of solitary insects, but they are more specialized (Gronenberg, 2008).

The central brain structures in insects are the mushroom bodies (Strausfeld *et al.*, 1998). Ant brains are equipped with structures and mechanisms that allow advanced learning and memory, including learning landmarks, odours and changes in their environment (Gronenberg, 2008). However, neural network analyses made by Chittka and Niven (2009) have shown that cognitive features found in ants and bees, such as numerosity, attention and categorization-like processes, may require only very limited neuron numbers. Moreover, there is no strong correlation between the volume of the mushroom body and cognitive abilities. A recent study (Groh *et al.*, 2014) revealed that in the highly polymorphic leaf-cutting ant *Atta vollenweideri*, mini workers have significantly larger mushroom bodies to total brain ratios, and synaptic densities play a much more important role than the relative size of the brain.

Perception

Antennae and compound eyes are the main sensory organs, with representations in the optic and the antennal lobes of the ant brain. Most ant species are guided mainly by smell and touch, and some species rely mainly on visual navigation, including the polarization pattern of the skylight and landmarks, and possibly magnetic cues (Hölldobler and Wilson, 1990). The demand on different sensory systems varies among species with different foraging strategies. For example, members of the *Cataglyphis* genus and bull ants of the genus *Myrmecia* forage individually and do not use odour trails, whereas fungi-growing ants of the tribe Attini have a highly developed olfactory system, necessary to meet the demands of complex olfactory-guided tasks such as pheromone communication or substrate selection.

Even within one ant colony, members of physical subcastes differ in their tasks and, correspondingly, in their sensory equipment (e.g. numbers of ommatidia in their eyes and sensilla on their antennae). In the desert ant *Cataglyphis bicolor*, the larger workers with 1200 ommatidia show better visual orientation abilities and serve as foragers, whereas the smaller workers (600 ommatidia) remain inside the nest (Menzel and Wehner, 1970). Despite the modest visual capabilities of ants in general, even ants with small eyes (e.g. *Leptothorax albipennis*; 60 ommatidia) are able to use bold landmarks as beacons (McLeman *et al.*, 2002). For visual navigation, ants can use not only landmarks but also stars, including sun and moon at night, and sky polarization (Wehner and Müller, 2006). They also have visual snapshots of what the area looks like, taken from some distance away and from several positions. This path integrator is more or less fixed and does not improve with training (Merkle and Wehner, 2009). Forest ants can memorize the entire canopy structure above them (Ehmer, 1999) and landmarks of different sizes, from grass and bushes to trees (Rosengren and Fortelius, 1986). The neotropical rainforest ant *Gigantiops destructor*, the ant species with the largest eyes (Gronenberg and Hölldobler, 1999), can travel individually through 20 m of rainforest – with all the trees and other objects in the scenery – without using any chemicals (Beugnon *et al.*, 2001). Ants have long been considered unique among Hymenopterans for having only two spectral classes of photoreceptors, while most bees and wasps have three (Briscoe and Chittka, 2001). A recent electrophysiological study (Ogawa *et al.*, 2015), however, demonstrated that the diurnal *Myrmecia croslandi* and the nocturnal *Myrmecia vindex* also enjoy trichromatic colour vision.

As in other insects, antennae are complex sensory arrays studded with different types of sensilla, which process a range of inputs in different modalities, including mechanical, odour and chemical stimuli, which can be referred to as taste, signals of humidity, temperature and CO_2 level. The majority of sensilla on the antenna contains olfactory neurons that respond to particular subsets of odorants or chemical compounds (Gronenberg, 2008; Ramirez-Esquivel *et al.*, 2014). In social Hymenoptera, individual olfactory sensilla on the antennae are generally equipped with a higher number of olfactory neurons and glomeruli as compared to other insects, possibly reflecting the rich diversity of olfactory-guided behaviours and the complexity of a social organization based on olfactory communication and chemical recognition (see Kelber *et al.*, 2009).

Social Characteristics

There are more than 12,000 ant species in the world, with different colony sizes (from tens to millions of individuals), social life and styles of cooperation, from single foraging to mass recruiting. All known ant species are eusocial, meeting the following criteria: reproductive division of labour and cooperative alloparental brood care, overlap of adult generations and lifelong philopatry. Like other members of the order Hymenoptera, including wasps and bees (from which not all are eusocial), ants are haplodiploid. Ant colonies consist of one or more reproductive females (queens) and a large number of female workers, which are either permanently or temporarily sterile and share the same diploid genome with queens. Males develop from unfertilized eggs, making them haploid. Haplodiploidy has important consequences that affect social behaviour and derive from different levels of relatedness among fertilized females (which can mate more than once), their daughters and sons. For instance, haplodiploidy opens the way for the evolution of a worker caste, devoted to helping their mother, although conflicts between the queen and the workers over who lays the male eggs in a nest are common (Walter and Heinze, 2015).

Caste polyphenism is rather expressive in some ant species, which harbour special castes of particularly large workers, 'soldiers' or 'majors', which play the main roles in colony defence, cutting up or carrying large objects. Morphology, physiology and behaviour thus differ profoundly between subcastes of workers. In leaf-cutting ants, for instance, tiny 'mini workers' cultivate fungi in the subterranean nest to feed the larvae. Other workers have an up to 200-fold increased body weight, leaving the nest for long foraging trips and bringing back leaves which are used as substrate for the fungi (Wilson, 1980). Remarkably, however, each female embryo has the potential to become either a queen or a major or a minor worker – all can be moulded from the same genome and regulated by epigenetic and nutritional factors (Chittka *et al.*, 2012).

Ant reproductive females may live hundreds of times longer than non-social insects of similar body size. Queens in some ant species live for up to three decades, whereas winged males are quite short-lived and survive only a few weeks, and workers live from a few days to 3 years (see Kramer *et al.*, 2015). Many researchers consider a colony of social Hymenopterans a 'superorganism', where workers represent the soma and the queen the germ line of the colony. However, cognitive responsibilities, if any, are distributed among relatively short-living sterile workers. One can hardly imagine a multicellular organism in which cells (unfertilized workers in an ant case) possess their own intelligence, and there is no central control of behaviour from a supreme brain.

In many ant species, complex dominance hierarchies and high levels of intracolonial aggression have been demonstrated. For example, in the Indian jumping ant *Harpegnathos saltator*, colonies are founded by a single queen, but after queen senescence, workers compete in a ritualized dominance tournament to establish the new group of reproductives, the gamergates. After mating with their brothers, gamergates display dominant behaviour and serve as the sole egg-layers in the colony (Peeters *et al.*, 2000). They also undergo extreme internal changes triggered by changes in dopamine levels: their brains shrink, their ovaries expand and their life expectancy jumps from about 6 months to several years (Penick *et al.*, 2014).

Many ant species are highly territorial animals (Adams, 2016). Hölldobler and Lumsden (1980) distinguished three types of ant territories: (1) absolute territories, in which the entire foraging space is defended regardless of food location; (2) trunk trail territories, in which defence is concentrated around long-lasting trails; and (3) spatio-temporal territories, in which defended regions shift from day to day according to where the ants are foraging. Territorial behaviour in ants includes recognition, avoidance, vigilance, demonstrations of aggression and fighting. Ants use odour cues to mark boundaries and ritual displays to solve conflicts (van Wilgenburg *et al.*, 2005). For instance, colonies of meat ants *Iridomyrmex purpureus* establish territories in which the boundaries are lined by workers engaged in pairwise ritual displays, sweeping legs and heads (Ettershank and Ettershank, 1982). While all these behaviours need not necessarily be cognitive, they are complex and flexible, and amazingly similar to territorial demonstrations in highly intelligent mammals and birds.

Interspecific hierarchies also emerge among ant communities of different species (Reznikova, 1980; Vepsäläinen and Pisarski, 1982; Savolainen *et al.*,1989; Stuble *et al.*, 2017). Interrelations between dominating *Formica* and subdominating *Serviformica* species, for instance, are behaviourally flexible, being directly related to both trophic competition and sophisticated 'cooperation' (Stebaev and Reznikova, 1972; Reznikova, 1975, 1982, 2007a). Dominant ants use members of the subdominant species as 'guides' while searching for prey, stealing their 'know-how'. At the same time, subdominants scrounge the prey from dominants and use their aphid colonies to obtain honeydew. Thus, 'cooperation' between dominant and subdominant ant species is based on reciprocal kleptoparasitic relations, which may require cognitive resources.

Ant colonies also interact through 'interspecific social control': dominant species actively regulate the level of the dynamic density of the subdominant species, exterminating 'superfluous' individuals or whole populations (Reznikova, 1999, 2003). In a manipulation experiment, for example, a sharp increase in the size of three *Formica picea* (subdominant) families was caused by adding 300 conspecific pupae in each family during 3 days and additional food sources only accessible to this species. Despite no decrease in food availability for the dominant species, *Formica uralensis* responded to an increase in the abundance of the subdominant species by killing and bringing into their nest about 250 *Formica picea* ants. Importantly, the number of subdominants killed by the dominant ants was close to the number of extra pupae added by the researchers to the subdominant species. This suggests that members of the dominant species can estimate number of encounters with subdominants quite precisely.

State of the Art

The majority of models consider cognitive skills and individual interactions in social insects redundant, and assume that their behaviour is based on what is called 'swarm intelligence', that is, it is only governed by collective decision-making (Miller *et al.*, 2013). These models are used to describe reactions of large groups as a whole to relatively simple stimuli from the environment. Indeed, there are many specific behaviours performed by ants collectively, such as nest architecture and nest climate control, consensus building, slave-making, agriculture and well-coordinated territorial wars (Hölldobler and Wilson, 2009). However, ants and bees are known to combine highly integrative colony organization with sophisticated cognitive skills implemented by individual tiny brains.

To date, ant ethograms are still scarce and mainly refer to few behavioural domains (e.g. within-nest behaviour, hunting, recruitment to food sources). Moreover, most cognitive studies have been conducted in laboratories and not in the wild (but see Reznikova and Bogatyreva, 1984). The number of behaviours recorded in ants (38 in Wilson, 1976; 40 in Villet, 1990), however, is comparable to that of other species (e.g. 22 in American moose, *Alces alces*; 44 in De Brazza monkeys, *Cercopithecus neglectus*; 123 in bottlenose dolphins, *Tursiops truncatus*: Changizi, 2003; 59 in honeybees, *Apis mellifera*: Chittka and Niven, 2009) and can largely vary across casts of workers (Brown and Traniello, 1998; but see Sempo and Detrain, 2010).

Social hymenopterans are capable of abstraction, extrapolation and simple arithmetic, and can solve rather sophisticated discrimination tasks, in a way comparable to dogs and monkeys (Reznikova, 2007a, 2017; Dornhaus and Franks, 2008; Loukola *et al.*, 2017; Perry *et al.*, 2017). These studies have mainly been carried out on just ants (Reznikova and Ryabko, 1994, 2011) and bees (see Chapter 3). In particular, there is evidence that ants are good at maze learning (Cammaerts Tricot, 2012), complex route learning (Rosengren and Fortelius, 1986; Czaczkes *et al.*, 2013) and visual discrimination of shapes (Cammaerts and Cammaerts, 2015). Moreover, highly social ant species possess sophisticated intelligent communication (*sensu* Reznikova, 2017; see below). With such a variety of ant species differing in social and foraging styles, however, it is clear that cognitive abilities may differ enormously across species, and also across colonies and individuals, due to task allocation and 'professional specialization' of individuals.

Individual Recognition

Ants use hydrocarbon labels to distinguish between members of their own and alien colonies at the inter- and intraspecific level, and between members of different casts and ages. Ants evolved a 'gestalt' organ (the postpharyngeal gland, Soroker *et al.*, 1995), which helps to homogenize recognition cues among colony members, through grooming and trophallaxis (mouth-to-mouth food sharing), shaping an internal representation of their own colony odour (Lenoir *et al.*, 2009; Bos and d'Ettorre, 2012). In *Myrmica rubra*, newly hatched ants attract adults via 'cuticular chemical insignificance' determined by underdeveloped postpharyngeal glands and ovaries (Lenoir *et al.*, 2009; Atsarkina *et al.*, 2017). However, these behaviours are fixed and do not require cognitive skills. Moreover, invertebrates are usually thought to be incapable of individually identifying conspecifics (but see Tibbetts, 2002). Field experiments with *Formica pratensis* ants showed that permanent units of ants patrolling the boundaries of their feeding territories differentiate at least between members of their own family, acquainted guards from neighbouring families and individuals from more remote areas (Reznikova, 1974, 2007a). This system of individual or at least group identification is cognitively demanding, and allows personally acquainted neighbours to establish boundaries, share resources and form a temporal society in which informative signals are shared (Fox and Baird, 1992; Godard, 1993).

Recognition of Competitors and Symbionts

One of the vital tasks faced by animals is to recognize, categorize and appropriately react to the stimuli encountered: whether it is prey, a dangerous predator, a competitor which should be driven away or a possible symbiotic organism. Red wood ants (*Formica aquilonia*), for instance, can recognize images of competitors, such as ground beetles (Dorosheva *et al.*, 2011; Reznikova and Dorosheva, 2013). By using live beetles and mock models in field and laboratory experiments, we showed that ants respond selectively to features of competitors like dark coloration, the presence of 'outgrowths' (legs, antennae), body symmetry, rate of movement and scent, even without previous experience. This suggests that red wood ants possess an innate template for recognition of potential competitors, although the ability to single out the key features, complete the integral image and display the behavioural patterns of guarding and defence appears to increase with experience, and thus requires learning and memory.

Recognition of symbionts, instead, is especially important in ants suckling Hemiptera species (e.g. aphids). The ants look after the symbionts, protect them from adverse conditions, carry them to new feeding sites and take care of their eggs. In return, the ants 'milk' the aphids, whose sweet excretions are one of their main sources of carbohydrates (Addicott, 1978; Novgorodova, 2015). Our experiments revealed that naïve red wood ants encountering aphids for the first time perceive aphids as any other unknown object, until they accidentally touch a drop of the aphid's excretion, which triggers the whole pattern of aphid milking: the ant gradually stops tapping at the aphids and begins to stroke them with folded antennae to obtain its excretion, then stopping and milking other aphids in the colony (Reznikova and Novgorodova, 1998; Reznikova, 2007a). Interestingly, this trophobiotic behaviour becomes more efficient with experience, completely developing in 60–90 minutes after the first contact with aphids. This can be considered a form of guided learning (*sensu* Gould and Marler, 1984), which requires the ability to integrate wired behaviours and acquired experience.

Communication

Ants largely communicate to recruit others, in the following contexts (Jackson and Ratnieks, 2006; Reznikova, 2007b, 2017; Leonhardt *et al.*, 2016): (1) tandem running, where a successful forager leads a recruit; (2) mass recruitment, by which recruiters returning from a food source to the nest lay a chemical trail that guides their nestmates to the source; (3) group recruitment, where the scout first lays a chemical trail upon return to the nest and subsequently leads a small group of recruits along this trail to the source; and (4) group-retrieving mode of foraging, based on distant homing (i.e. transferring messages about remote events from a scouting individual to foragers, without other cues such as a scent trail or direct guiding; see: Reznikova, 2008, 2017). The most striking examples of distant homing are the honeybee dance language (see Chapter 3) and the symbolic 'language' of highly social ant species (Reznikova 2007a, 2007b, 2017). In these species, distant homing confers productivity (i.e. the ability to generate a potentially unlimited number of messages on the basis of a finite number of signals) and flexibility (i.e. interlocutors grasp regularities in their environment and use them to optimize messages). Ant 'language' has been explained through information theory (Ryabko and Reznikova, 1996, 2009), which allows investigating the very process of information transmission, by measuring the time which animals spend on transmitting messages of definite length and complexity. The main point of this approach is that it is not necessary to 'decipher' ants' messages and understand how they represent information. As we show, analysing the duration of information transmission – provided the information content is (precisely) known to us – is sufficient to uncover many facts about ants' 'language' and their intellectual abilities (see below).

Red wood ants (*Formica rufa* group) are possibly the most promising and underestimated group for studying cognitive aspects of communication. They have hundreds of times more individuals per colony than other sympatric species, more spacious feeding territories, and face more complex vital problems (e.g. finding and possibly memorizing locations of thousands of aphid colonies in a three-dimensional space). Members of this group of species are able to transfer messages about the exact coordinates of a food source (Reznikova and Ryabko, 1990, 1994, 2012), and use distant homing to transfer exact information about remote events, like honeybees do (Reznikova, 2007a, 2007b, 2017; Tautz, 2008). Observing them solving complex search problems may be revealing to understand the processes of information transmission and task allocation between members of the ant society.

Cognitive Differences between Mass Foraging and Solitary Foraging Species

In many ant species, fairly simple interactions among individuals generate complicated group behaviour. For instance, many species of the subfamily Myrmicinae show *mass foraging*, that is, they broadcast guidance information to potentially all foragers, in the form of a trail network marked with varying amounts and types of pheromone (see Hölldobler and Wilson, 1990). However, as demonstrated in *Temnothorax albipennis* (Dornhaus, 2008), although workers differ in their ability to perform different tasks (e.g. foraging, collection of nest-building material, brood transporting), they are allocated to different tasks independently of their skills. Possibly, members of mass-foraging species, although they display variable capacities preceding 'professional specialization', have not further developed this system in their colonies, and so there may be no differences in cognitive responsibilities within families of mass-foraging ant species (Dornhaus and Franks, 2008). Members of *solitary foraging* species (e.g. desert *Cataglyphis* ants, solitary hunters of the genus *Myrmecia*, many species of the subgenus *Serviformica*), in contrast, are much more flexible than members of mass foraging

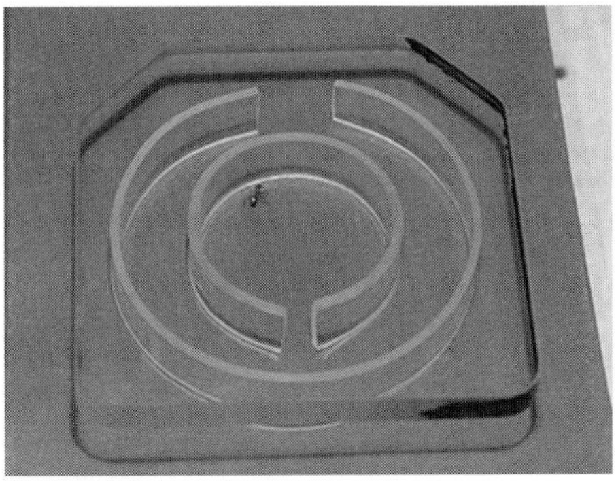

Figure 1.1. A round maze with three circles.
Photo by Ivan Iakovlev.

species, individually searching for food and making decisions. In field experiments with *Cataglyphis*, Wehner (2003) revealed that the same ant could flexibly learn different routes for the outward and homeward journeys and for journeys leading to different feeding sites.

A striking example of the difference between solitary foraging and mass foraging ant species lies in their ability to navigate 'round mazes'. In field experiments, ants were presented with mazes consisting of one to three concentric circles placed one inside the other in such a way that their entrances were placed on the opposite sides, and the inner circle contained food pellets (Figure 1.1): although in solitary foraging species (*Formica cunicularia*) nearly all foragers could successfully solve the maze, only 10 per cent of the mass-foraging ants (*Formica pratensis*) successfully navigated mazes (and only after observing *Formica cunicularia*). Interestingly, *Formica cunicularia* is also subdominant to *Formica pratensis*, and serves as a scout to the latter, being much more successful in learning new ways to search for food (see above; Reznikova, 1975, 1982, 2007a).

Cognitive Specialization within Colonies of Group-Retrieving Species

In group-retrieving species such as red wood ants, colonies include stable teams with one scout and four to eight foragers (Reznikova and Ryabko, 1994; Reznikova, 2007a, 2007b). Only scouts (but not foragers) are able to solve complex problems and pass information to other team members: they can memorize and transfer information about a sequence of turns toward a goal, grasp regularities in these sequences and also perform simple arithmetic operations (Reznikova and Ryabko, 2011). This cognitive specialization is based on the ability of some specific individuals to learn faster within specific domains, and it likely increases effectiveness at solving problems while searching for food (Reznikova, 2007a, 2012).

For instance, hungry ants can locate food on one of several 'leaves' in a 'binary tree' maze (Figure 1.2). In each trial, one scout was placed on a certain leaf of the binary tree, with food, and could then return to the foragers in the nest. The scout contacted one to

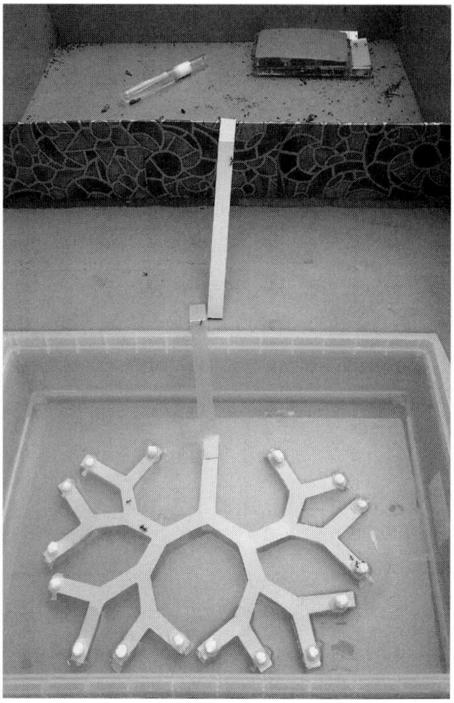

Figure 1.2. A laboratory arena divided into two parts, containing an artificial ant nest and a binary tree maze placed in a bath with water. This binary tree has four forks.
Photo by Nail Bikbaev.

four foragers, and the time the scout spent on 'informative contacts' was used as the main feature of ants' communicative means. All experiments were so devised as to eliminate all possible cues that could help the ants find the food (e.g. odour tracks), except for information contacts with the scout. If the group reached the correct point, they were immediately presented with the food. Crucially, scouts shared information about the discovered food only with members of their team (Reznikova and Ryabko, 1994, 2011; Reznikova, 2017).

Like honey bees, *Formica* scouting individuals do not bear any distinctive morphological traits. It is known that scouting bees constitute a very specific group in a hive, although, in contrast to *Formica* scouts, they transfer information not to the members of their own team but rather to anyone that is interested (see Chapter 3; Tautz, 2008). Some of the molecular underpinnings of their behaviour relative to foragers have been revealed (Liang *et al.*, 2012). Yet we know nothing about the peculiarities of the brains of scouting ants. For this reason, we designed the first battery of behavioural tests examining scouts' levels of aggression (estimating the variety of interactions with ground beetles), exploratory activities (recording ethograms of ants interacting with artificial models of natural objects) and spatial cognition (assessing the ability to memorize the path in a binary tree maze; Figure 1.3A–C), in comparison with members

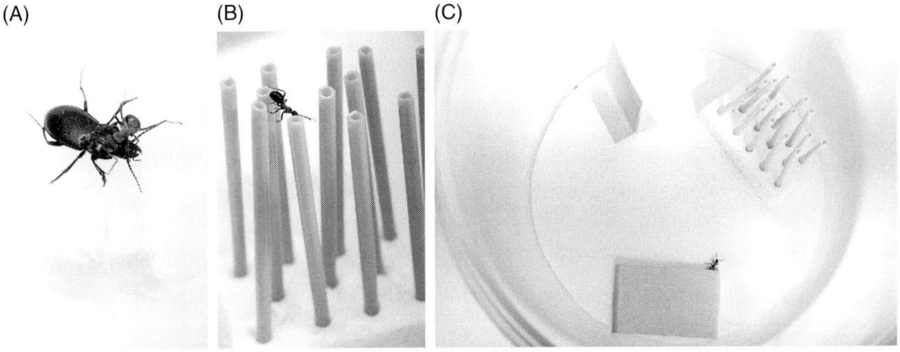

Figure 1.3. A piece of 'artificial world' designed for studying ants' exploratory activity and aggressiveness. (A) Test of aggressiveness: an ant is biting a beetle; (B) an ant is exploring 'grass'; (C) a shelter ('litter setup'), 'tree trunk' and grass stems imitated by 'brushes' made of plaster bars.
Photos by Nail Bikbaev.

of other task groups such as aphid milkers, guards and foragers. Both scouts and foragers were overall more exploratory than other out-nest workers, and scouts more than foragers. In unfamiliar situations, scouts more readily switched between different activities. Scouts and foragers displayed nearly equal levels of aggressiveness, more than aphid milkers and closer to guards, but never attacked beetles directly. The most distinctive feature of scouts was their high exploratory activity of novel items. Scouts also seem to form spatial memory faster and keep information longer and more precisely than foragers (Atsarkina *et al.*, 2014).

It is worth noting, however, that learning is costly for insect brains. Replicate *Drosophila* populations selected for improved learning lived on average 15 per cent shorter than the corresponding unselected control populations, and long-lived selected flies showed an almost 40 per cent reduction in learning ability early in life (Burger *et al.*, 2008). In our study (Reznikova and Ryabko, 1994, 2011), we observed scouts performing their tasks during up to 8–10 weeks, which is extremely long in comparison with, for example, *Cataglyphis* ants, having only about 6 days to perform feats of orientation (Schmid-Hempel, 1984). In ant species with a relatively low level of social organization, however, specialization does not predict individual efficiency. In our experiments with mass recruiting *Myrmica rubra* and solitary foraging *Formica cunicularia*, we did not find any evidence of distant homing (Reznikova and Ryabko, 1994). However, in *Myrmica* ants we found a system of distributed learning responsibilities, which possibly decreases the cost of learning at both individual and family levels (Reznikova and Panteleeva, 2008). In particular, the spreading of complex hunting behaviours towards jumping springtails appeared to be based on relatively simple forms of social learning, such as social facilitation, which triggers relevant behavioural patterns when these are encountered with sufficient frequency. This system of 'distributed social learning' can be considered alternative to individual cognition in ant societies.

All for One and One for All

Box 1.1 Cognition in Eusocial Species

Felicity Muth

Ants and bees are essentially cousins: they are both in the order Hymenoptera and are more closely related than ants are to social wasps like yellowjackets. While there are 20,000 species of bees, most of what we know about their cognition comes from three species: *Apis mellifera* (honeybees) and two bumblebee species: *Bombus impatiens* and *Bombus terrestris*. Given the intense interest in the cognitive abilities of these three eusocial species (most bee species are actually solitary), it is perhaps surprising that there has not been more investigation into the cognitive abilities of ants, which are all eusocial.

Working with species that live in colonies of tens to thousands of closely related individuals carries some common methodological challenges. For example, it is often important when studying cognition to be able to recognize individuals, to differentially manipulate their experiences. With ants, this is most often done through paint-marking individuals: each individual might have one colour mark on the head, one on the thorax and two on the abdomen: this allows for hundreds to thousands of individuals to be uniquely identifiable. More recently, ants have also been tagged using Radio-Frequency Identification (RFID) tags. In experiments on bee behaviour, both of these methods of tagging have been used, as well as thorax tags and more advanced tracking systems, such as transponders that allow radar tracking over much larger spatial scales (Riley *et al.*, 1996; Woodgate *et al.*, 2016).

Somewhat similar methods have also been used to address cognition in ants and bees: associative learning has long been studied in bees through the proboscis extension response (PER), where the bee is held in a harness and trained to learn an association through pairing a conditioned stimulus (e.g. a colour or scent) with a reward (sucrose, presented to the bee's proboscis; Bitterman *et al.*, 1983; see Chapter 3). An adaptation of this protocol has since been used for ants, where the ant's antennae are stimulated with sucrose, causing the ant to extend its maxilla-labium (Guerrieri and D'Ettorre, 2010). Many free-moving protocols also exist for testing bee and ant learning, although for bees this mostly consists of visiting artificial flowers, whereas for ants it often consists of learning about nest sites or landmarks. We recently designed a method to address learning in wild-caught bees (Muth *et al.*, 2018), which we believe could also be adapted for looking at learning in nectivorous ants.

Given the social structure of ants and social bees, individuals often explore and learn individually, but then share information with the colony. Ant behaviour is often studied in terms of how individual decisions lead to colony-level behaviour (Robinson *et al.*, 2011; Sasaki and Pratt, 2012). While similar questions have been asked in honeybees (Seeley, 2010), bee cognitive abilities are also often addressed on the individual rather than colony level (Perry *et al.*, 2017). Looking ahead, the large species diversity of ants and bees offers a useful opportunity for comparative

(*cont.*)

analyses: we could test hypotheses about which life-history traits favour particular cognitive abilities. Indeed, there are particular cognitive abilities that may be associated with sociality, diet breadth or resource specialization: for example, we might expect ant and bee species with a wider dietary breadth to be better at learning novel associations with food rewards.

References

Bitterman, M. E., Menzel, R., Fietz, A., and Schäfer, S. (1983). Classical conditioning of proboscis extension in honeybees (*Apis mellifera*). *Journal of Comparative Psychology*, **97**, 107–119.

Guerrieri, F. J., and D'Ettorre, P. (2010). Associative learning in ants: conditioning of the maxilla-labium extension response in Camponotus aethiops. *Journal of Insect Physiology*, **56**, 88–92.

Muth, F., Cooper, T. R., Bonilla, R. F., and Leonard, A. S. (2018). A novel protocol for studying bee cognition in the wild. *Methods in Ecology and Evolution*, **9**, 78–87.

Perry, C. J., Barron, A. B., and Chittka, L. (2017). The frontiers of insect cognition. *Current Opinion in Behavioral Sciences*, **16**, 111–118.

Riley, J., Smith, A., Reynolds, D., and Edwards, A. (1996). Tracking bees with harmonic radar. *Nature*, **379**, 29–30.

Robinson, E. J. H., Franks, N. R., Ellis, S., Okuda, S., and Marshall, J. A. R. (2011). A simple threshold rule is sufficient to explain sophisticated collective decision-making. *PLoS ONE*, **6**(5), e19981.

Sasaki, T., and Pratt, S. C. (2012). Groups have a larger cognitive capacity than individuals. *Current Biology*, **22**, 827–829.

Seeley, T. D. (2010). *Honeybee democracy*. Princeton, NJ: Princeton University Press.

Woodgate, J. L., Makinson, J. C., Lim, K. S., Reynolds, A. M., and Chittka, L. (2016). Life-long radar tracking of bumblebees. *PLoS ONE*, **11**(8), e0160333.

Field Guide

Depending on the research question, different ant species should be used. Although *Lasius, Temnothorax* or *Myrmica* species are easier to keep in the laboratory, species with distant homing (e.g. *Formica rufa, Formica sanguinea* and several *Camponotus*) should be preferred, for instance, when using communication as a tool for studying cognition.

To study communication and cognition, a laboratory should host at least 1000 specimens, although smaller groups can be used in complementary studies, such as deprivation experiments. Ideally, experiments should be performed with more laboratory groups on separate arenas. The laboratory groups should be taken from a typical colony in nature and hosted in one artificial nest (recommended size: 10 × 15 × 12 cm). Plain, transparent nests divided into several internal cameras should be preferred, as they allow observation of contacts among individuals. Ants should be gradually accustomed to light in the laboratory. Normal room temperature is suitable for ants (21–23°C), and a wet cotton tampon should be placed in one camera to give a certain moisture within the nest. The recommended size of the foraging arena is 150 × 50 cm, and its rims should be about 15 cm high and covered with a sticky substance (such as Vaseline) to prevent ants from escaping. The arena should be divided into two parts: a small living one and a part containing an experimental device (Figure 1.2). Laboratory mazes can be easily made from plastic folders and other materials at hand. Sugar syrup and immobilized small insects can be used to feed the ants in the living part of the arena. However, during the experiments, ants may be more strongly motivated by only receiving food in a certain point of a maze, once every 2–3 days.

The idea of using the natural communication of animals to study their cognitive capacities is based on an information-theoretic approach: experimenters force animals to transfer a predetermined quantity of information, and then measure the duration of the time spent by the subjects to transfer this information (Ryabko and Reznikova, 1996, 2009). Comparing time durations required for information transfer in different situations, one can reason about certain key characteristics of the communication system under study. This system may be potentially applied to other species such as bees (having a symbolic dance language) and possibly some highly social vertebrates, including those which have been language-trained (Savage-Rumbaugh and Lewin, 1994; Pepperberg, 2009; Herman, 2010), but could be tested using their natural signals rather than artificial intermediary languages. The crucial idea is that experimenters know exactly the quantity of information (in bits) to be transferred (for instance, the number and sequence of turns toward food). In ants, this system is based on two main experimental schemes: investigation of ants' ability to memorize and transfer sequences of turns in a binary tree maze, and of their ability to use the numbers of branches in the 'counting' mazes.

First, it is necessary to reveal the composition of the working teams (i.e. distinguishing between scouts and foragers: Reznikova, 2017; http://reznikova.net/research/ant-language), by administering preliminary familiarization trials lasting 2–3 weeks, in which ants have free access to the set-up and syrup. All active ants should be labelled individually by applying drops of paint to different parts of their bodies in different combinations of colours (Holbrook, 2009). In the course of the main experiments, then, one of the scouts actively moving on the living part of the arena can be placed in the maze with food, until it returns to the nest by itself. All contacts between the scout and its team should then be observed and measured in seconds. Usually, members of a team are waiting for 'their' scout on the living part of the arena (Figure 1.2) and their contacts can be easily video-recorded. However, recording contacts within a transparent nest is also possible. The experiments should be devised so as to eliminate all possible ways for the members of each foraging team to find the target, except for information contact with their scout. The set-up should be replaced with a fresh one, with all troughs filled

Table 1.1. Essential experimental tools required to study ants and their function.

Tool	Function
Forceps and a special trap to catch ants	To catch ants and manipulate them. I suggest to cut a hole in the bottom of a small retort and use it as a special trap to catch individual ants in the field (Reznikova, 2009), before labelling or manipulating them (e.g. releasing them in another part of their feeding territory for studying navigation and spatial memory)
Paint applicator (e.g. toothpick or bristle from paintbrush)	To mark individuals with a distinct colour code and track their movements in the field and laboratory. Recently, thin radio-trackers have been suggested (www.york.ac.uk/news-and-events/features/ant-behaviour/); however, in many cases researchers use simpler equipment
Sandwich boxes (24 × 30 × 1 cm, or so)	To keep live ants in the field and transport them to the lab or into alien territories
Field round mazes	To compare individual characteristics such as searching activity and ability to find a way across different colonies and species. Mazes can be easily made from plastic folders and other materials at hand
Field troughs	To study searching activity, navigation and memory in ants in the field. Round disposable plastic dishes (diameter from 2 to 4 cm) are recommended. Use 3 ml of 30% sucrose solution as carbohydrate food and pieces of tuna baits as protein food
Numbered pins or toothpicks	To track the route and record time and length of each foraging path, in order to investigate individual foraging strategies and spatial memory. As the ant walks, a numbered pin can be placed on the ground along its route, each 60 seconds. Each path can then be converted into a smaller grid on paper, digitized and overlapped with the other paths (see Pie, 2004)
Digital voice recorder	To record behavioural data for later transcription
Video-camera	Any camera capable of recording high-quality video
Video analysis	Relevant tools for video analysis should be chosen, such as The Observer 10 XT (Noldus Information Technology) and VLC media player, reducing the playback speed when necessary to 1/8

with water, while the scout is in the nest; if the foraging team reaches the correct branch in a compact group, then the water-filled trough is replaced with one with syrup as a reward. Each scout can master up to three trials per day. When working with the 'binary tree' maze, it should be taken into account that even those ant species which do use distant homing only do so when confronted with complex mazes, and not with the T maze.

Tree-mazes can also be used to assess whether ants grasp regularities in the information available: if food can be reached by turning right and left four times (RLRLRLRL), and ants grasp regularities, they should transmit this information more quickly (4LR) than random sequences like LRRLRLLR. *Formica sanguinea* ants, for instance, spent less time transferring information about more regular sequences of turns (e.g. transferring LLLLLL was quicker than transferring LRLRLR, which was in turn

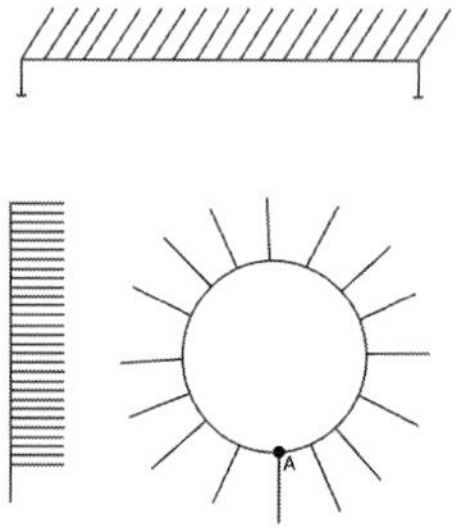

Figure 1.4. 'Counting mazes': a *horizontal trunk*, a *vertical trunk* and a *circle*.

quicker than transferring LRLLRL). This means that the ants are able to grasp regularities within these sequences, and the time spent transmitting information depends on its complexity (Ryabko and Reznikova, 1996, 2009; Reznikova, 2017). Interestingly, ants begin to use regularities to compress information only when sequences are rather long.

Given that ants can pass exact information about a target in a maze, in 'counting' experiments (Reznikova and Ryabko, 2011, 2012) scouting individuals can be required to transfer information to foragers about which branch of a special 'counting maze' they had to go to in order to obtain syrup (Figure 1.4): by estimating how much time individual ants spend on transferring information about index numbers of branches, experimenters can judge how ants represent numbers. The first variant of the counting maze is a comb-like set-up consisting of a long horizontal plastic trunk with 25–60 equally spaced plain plastic branches, each of them 6 cm in length. Each branch ends with an empty trough, except for one filled with syrup, and ants come to the initial point of the trunk over a small bridge. The second variant is a set-up with 60 vertically aligned branches. In order to test whether the time of transmission of information about the number of a branch depends on its length, as well as on the distance between the branches, a similar vertical trunk can be used, in which the distance between the branches is twice as large, and the branches themselves are three times and five times longer. The third variant is a circular trunk with 25-cm long branches. As before, all actively foraging ants are individually marked with coloured paint, strongly motivated scouts are placed directly on the trough and the time spent on 'informative contacts' with their teams once they are back in the nest is measured.

In red wood ants *Formica polyctena*, the teams left the nest after they were contacted by scouts and moved towards the trough by themselves on 152 trials. In 117 cases, the team immediately found the correct path to the trough, and in the remaining cases, ants came to the empty troughs and began looking for food by checking neighbouring branches, supporting the idea that scouts transmit information (Reznikova and Ryabko, 2011; Reznikova, 2017). The likely explanation of the results concerning ants' ability to find the 'right' branch is that they can evaluate the number of the branch in the sequence of branches in the maze and transmit this information to each other. Presumably, a scout can pass messages not about the number of the branch, but about the distance to it or about the number of steps. What is important is that even if ants operate with distance or with the number of steps, they are able to use quantitative values and pass on exact information about them. Moreover, scouts perform simple operations of addition and subtraction: as the 'special' branches can only be referred to by their numbers (i.e. as no other visual or olfactory cues are available), scouts placed on, say, branch 17 and heading to branch 20 have to correctly calculate that 17 is three branches away from 20. Similarly, when placed on the branch 23, the scout has to correctly compute that this branch is three branches away from branch 20, which, in the absence of any mark on the branch 20, requires addition. Overall, our studies show that ants can show impressive cognitive skills, although this may only be true for specific ant species with especially complex and flexible communication systems.

Wild vs. Lab

Box 1.2 Understanding the Nature of Ant Cognition by Studying Ant Cognition in Nature

Neil D. Tsutsui

Ants are fascinating and productive model systems for illuminating cognition and behaviour due to the sophisticated, coordinated behaviours they display. In addition, eusocial insects offer unparalleled opportunities to study systems that simultaneously display behaviour at multiple levels: individual organism (ant) and superorganism (colony).

Although field studies of ants are prominent in ecological research, behavioural studies tend to be more laboratory-oriented. This is due, in part, to the inherent challenges of studying ant behaviour in the field, which include small size (often minute), the anonymity of individual workers within the teeming masses of the colony, and the inordinate amount of time that ants spend in the inaccessible reaches of colonies underground or in fallen or standing deadwood. However, it is essential to complement laboratory-based studies of ants with corresponding data from the field. Important stimuli that occur in nature may be absent in the lab, or laboratory environments may introduce artificial variables or stressors that do not occur in the wild.

Ants are chemically oriented creatures, but studying chemical ecology in natural environments can be challenging, due to the abundance of confounding or contaminating natural odorants. At the same time, removing ants from their environment may produce stress and/or unnatural behaviours. In some cases, a hybrid approach may be fruitful. Youngsteadt and colleagues (2008), for example, combined olfaction experiments in the field with laboratory chemical analyses, to identify the specific chemicals that *Camponotus* ants use to locate and recognize seeds of their epiphyte mutualist.

Social interactions may also differ between the field and lab, both qualitatively and quantitatively, and these interactions shape the behaviours of both individuals and colonies. In Argentine ants (*Linepithema humile*), for example, a single fight with a worker from a different colony increases the likelihood of aggression in

(*cont.*)

subsequent encounters (van Wilgenburg *et al.*, 2010), and, in the wild, this significantly affects intercolony interactions (Thomas *et al.*, 2005). Because such sensitive responses to social stimuli can produce large-scale consequences, it is essential to complement laboratory-based assays with field studies.

In the future, chemical and genetic manipulations will be increasingly used in the field as powerful approaches for disentangling the determinants of behaviour and cognition. RNA interference (RNAi), for example, has been used for targeted gene silencing in a carpenter ant (*Camponotus floridanus*; Ratzka *et al.*, 2013) and the red imported fire ant (*Solenopsis invicta*; Cheng *et al.*, 2015), making it likely that such approaches will soon be taken outdoors to assess how the altered expression of candidate genes affects behaviour in the wild.

It is likely that many colony-level phenotypes are only expressed in natural substrates and foraging environments, which would be exceedingly difficult to replicate in the lab. The physical architecture of ant nests, for example, is an important determinant of harvester ant (*Veromessor andrei*) foraging behaviour (Pinter-Wollman, 2015). By combining cutting-edge imaging techniques for quantifying structural variation in the field with manipulative lab experiments, we will likely gain exciting new insights into how the built environment shapes the behaviour of social organisms, including ourselves (Pinter-Wollman *et al.*, 2017).

References

Cheng D., Lu, Y., Zeng, L., Liang, G., and He, X. (2015). Si-CSP9 regulates the integument and moulting process of larvae in the red imported fire ant, Solenopsis invicta. *Scientific Reports*, **5**, 9245.

Pinter-Wollman, N. (2015). Nest architecture shapes the collective behaviour of harvester ants. *Biology Letters*, **11**, 20150695.

Pinter-Wollman, N., Fiore, S. M., and Theraulaz, G. (2017). The impact of architecture on collective behaviour. *Nature Ecology & Evolution*, **1**, 111.

Ratzka, C., Gross, R., and Feldhaar, H. (2013). Systemic gene knockdown in *Camponotus floridanus* workers by feeding of dsRNA. *Insectes Sociaux*, **60**, 475–484.

Thomas, M. L., Tsutsui, N. D., and Holway, D. A. (2005). Intraspecific competition influences the symmetry and intensity of aggression in the Argentine ant. *Behavioral Ecology*, **16**, 472–481.

van Wilgenburg, E., Clemencet, J., and Tsutsui, N. D. (2010). Experience influences aggressive behaviour in the Argentine ant. *Biology Letters*, **6**, 152–155.

Youngsteadt, E., Nojima, S., Haberlein, C., Schulz, S., and Schal, C. (2008). Seed odor mediates an obligate ant–plant mutualism in Amazonian rainforests. *Proceedings of the National Academy of Sciences*, **105**, 4571–4575.

Resources

Popular books on ants:

- Hölldobler, B., and Wilson, E. O. (1994). *Journey to the ants: a story of scientific exploration*. Cambridge, MA: Harvard University Press.
- Hölldobler, B., and Wilson, E. O. (2009). *The superorganism: the beauty, elegance, and strangeness of insect societies*. New York, NY: W.W. Norton and Company.
- Reznikova, Z. (2017). *Studying animal languages without translation: an insight from ants*. Cham, Switzerland: Springer.

Popular books on individual and social cognition:

- Reznikova, Z. I. (2007). *Animal intelligence: from individual to social cognition*. Cambridge: Cambridge University Press.
- Shettleworth, S. J. (2010). *Cognition, evolution, and behavior*. Oxford: Oxford University Press.
- Menzel, R., and Fischer, J. (2011). *Animal thinking: contemporary issues in comparative cognition*. Cambridge, MA: MIT Press.
- Wynne, C. D. (2001). *Animal cognition: the mental lives of animals*. London: Macmillan.
- Bekoff, M., Colin, A., and Burghardt, G. M. (2002). *The cognitive animal: empirical and theoretical perspectives on animal cognition*. Cambridge, MA: MIT Press.

Some ant labs:

- www.uni-regensburg.de/biologie-vorklinische-medizin/evolutionsbiologie/
- www.bristol.ac.uk/biology/research/behaviour/antlab/
- http://en.nencki.gov.pl/laboratory-of-ethology
- http://reznikova.net/labs/
- http://icouzin.princeton.edu/
- https://web.stanford.edu/~dmgordon/
- www.schoolofants.net.au/our-team/
- http://sydney.edu.au/science/biology/socialinsects/
- http://ucanr.edu/sites/ucrurbanpest/Research/Ant/
- http://pratt.lab.asu.edu
- www.iiserkol.ac.in/~antlab/lab_members.html
- www.uibk.ac.at/ecology/forschung/molecular_ecology.html.en
- https://nature.berkeley.edu/tsutsuilab/
- www.rockefeller.edu/our-scientists/heads-of-laboratories/988-daniel-kronauer/
- https://wurmlab.github.io
- www.life.illinois.edu/suarez/

Profile

Zhanna decided to study ants as a first-year student at Novosibirsk State University. Ants allowed her to observe fragments of a 'civilization', asking questions through experiments, and getting answers, often for the first time in the world. Zhanna grew up in the Soviet Union behind the 'iron curtain' and was not allowed to go abroad until 1991 (for her first international conference in Kyoto, right after the 'August revolution', which she joined on her way to the conference). However, she always exchanged letters with researchers all over the world. The KGB only once gave her the approval to publish a paper outside the 'socialist camp' (in 1982, in *Behaviour*), so that many pioneering results remained long unknown to most scientists. Although she presently leads the laboratory of community ethology and develops comparative cognitive studies on rodents, birds and other wonderful creatures, ants remain her passion, being uniquely clever and enigmatic.

References

Adams, E. S. (2016). Territoriality in ants (Hymenoptera: Formicidae): a review. *Myrmecological News*, **23**, 101–118.

Addicott, J. F. (1978). Competition for mutualists: aphids and ants. *Canadian Journal of Zoology*, **56**, 2093–2096.

Atsarkina, N., Iakovlev, I., and Reznikova, Z. (2014). Individual behavioural features of scouts and recruits in red wood ants (Hymenoptera: Formicidae). *Euroasian Entomology Journal*, **13**, 209–218.

Atsarkina, N., Panteleeva, S., and Reznikova, Z. (2017). *Myrmica rubra* ants are more communicative when young: do they need experience? *Journal of Comparative Psychology*, **131**, 163.

Beugnon, G., Chagné, P., and Dejean, A. (2001). Colony structure and foraging behavior in the tropical formicine ant, *Gigantiops destructor. Insectes Sociaux*, **48**, 347–351.

Bos, N., and d'Ettorre, P. (2012). Recognition of social identity in ants. *Frontiers in Psychology*, **3**, 83.

Briscoe, A. D., and Chittka, L. (2001). The evolution of color vision in insects. *Annual Review of Entomology*, **46**, 471–510.

Brown, J. J., and Traniello, J. F. (1998). Regulation of brood-care behavior in the dimorphic castes of the ant *Pheidole morrisi* (Hymenoptera: Formicidae): effects of caste ratio, colony size, and colony needs. *Journal of Insect Behavior*, **11**, 209–219.

Burger, J., Kolss, M., Pont, J., and Kawecki, T. J. (2008). Learning ability and longevity: a symmetrical evolutionary trade-off in *Drosophila. Evolution*, **62**, 1294–1304.

Cammaerts, M. C., and Cammaerts, R. (2015). The acquisition of cognitive abilities by ants: a study on three *Myrmica* species (Hymenoptera, Formicidae). *Advanced Studies in Biology*, **7**, 335–348.

Cammaerts Tricot, M. C. (2012). Navigation system of the ant *Myrmica rubra* (Hymenoptera: Formicidae). *Myrmecological News*, **16**, 111–121.

Changizi, M. A. (2003). Relationship between number of muscles, behavioral repertoire size, and encephalization in mammals. *Journal of Theoretical Biology*, **220**, 157–168.

Chittka, L., and Niven, J. (2009). Are bigger brains better? *Current Biology*, **19**, 995–1008.

Chittka, A., Wurm, Y., and Chittka, L. (2012). Epigenetics: the making of ant castes. *Current Biology*, **22**, 835–838.

Czaczkes, T. J., Grüter, C., and Ratnieks, F. L. (2013). Negative feedback in ants: crowding results in less trail pheromone deposition. *Journal of the Royal Society Interface*, **10**, 20121009.

Darwin, C. (1981/1871). *The descent of man, and selection in relation to sex*. London: Penguin Classics.

Dornhaus, A. (2008). Specialization does not predict individual efficiency in an ant. *PLoS Biology*, **6**(11), e285.

Dornhaus, A., and Franks, N. R. (2008). Individual and collective cognition in ants and other insects (Hymenoptera: Formicidae). *Myrmecological News*, **11**, 215–226.

Dorosheva, E. A., Yakovlev, I. K., and Reznikova, Z. I. (2011). An innate template for enemy recognition in red wood ants. *Entomological Review*, **91**, 274–280.

Ehmer, B. (1999). Orientation in the ant *Paraponera clavata*. *Journal of Insect Behavior*, **12**, 711–722.

Ettershank, G., and Ettershank, J. A. (1982). Ritualised fighting in the meat ant *Iridomyrmex purpureus* (Smith) (Hymenoptera: Formicidae). *Australian Journal of Entomology*, **21**, 97–102.

Fox, S. F., and Baird, T. A. (1992). The dear enemy phenomenon in the collared lizard, *Crotaphytus collaris*, with a cautionary note on experimental methodology. *Animal Behaviour*, **44**, 780–782.

Godard, R. (1993). Tit for tat among neighboring hooded warblers. *Behavioral Ecology and Sociobiology*, **33**, 45–50.

Gould, J. L., and Marler, P. (1984). Ethology and the natural history of learning. In *The biology of learning* (pp. 47–74). Berlin: Springer.

Groh, C., Kelber, C., Grübel, K., and Rössler, W. (2014). Density of mushroom body synaptic complexes limits intraspecies brain miniaturization in highly polymorphic leaf-cutting ant workers. *Proceedings of the Royal Society of London B: Biological Sciences*, **281**, 20140432.

Gronenberg, W. (2008). Structure and function of ant (Hymenoptera: Formicidae) brains: strength in numbers. *Myrmecological News*, **11**, 25–36.

Gronenberg, W., and Hölldobler, B. (1999). Morphologic representation of visual and antennal information in the ant brain. *Journal of Comparative Neurology*, **412**, 229–240.

Herman, L. M. (2010). What laboratory research has told us about dolphin cognition. *International Journal of Comparative Psychology*, **23**, 310–330.

Holbrook, C. T. (2009). Marking individual ants for behavioral sampling in a laboratory colony. *Cold Spring Harbor Protocols*, **7**, pdb.prot5240.

Hölldobler, B., and Lumsden, C. J. (1980). Territorial strategies in ants. *Science*, **210**, 732–739.

Hölldobler, B., and Wilson, E. O. (1990). *The ants*. Berlin: Springer.

Hölldobler, B., and Wilson, E. O. (2009). *The superorganism: the beauty, elegance, and strangeness of insect societies*. New York, NY: W.W. Norton and Company.

Jackson, D. E., and Ratnieks, F. L. (2006). Communication in ants. *Current Biology*, **16**, 570–574.

Kelber, C., Rössler, W., Roces, F., and Kleineidam, C. J. (2009). The antennal lobes of fungus-growing ants (Attini): neuroanatomical traits and evolutionary trends. *Brain, Behavior and Evolution*, **73**, 273–284.

Kramer, B. H., Schrempf, A., Scheuerlein, A., and Heinze, J. (2015). Ant colonies do not trade-off reproduction against maintenance. *PLoS ONE*, **10**(9), e0137969.

Lenoir, A., Depickère, S., Devers, S., Christidès, J. P., and Detrain, C. (2009). Hydrocarbons in the ant *Lasius niger*: from the cuticle to the nest and home range marking. *Journal of Chemical Ecology*, **35**, 913–921.

Leonhardt, S. D., Menzel, F., Nehring, V., and Schmitt, T. (2016). Ecology and evolution of communication in social insects. *Cell*, **164**, 1277–1287.

Liang, Z. S., Nguyen, T., Mattila, H. R., Rodriguez-Zas, S. L., Seeley, T. D., and Robinson, G. E. (2012). Molecular determinants of scouting behavior in honey bees. *Science*, **335**, 1225–1228.

Loukola, O. J., Perry, C. J., Coscos, L., and Chittka, L. (2017). Bumblebees show cognitive flexibility by improving on an observed complex behavior. *Science*, **355**, 833–836.

McLeman, M. A., Pratt, S. C., and Franks, N. R. (2002). Navigation using visual landmarks by the ant *Leptothorax albipennis*. *Insectes Sociaux*, **49**, 203–208.

Menzel, R., and Wehner, R. (1970). Augenstrukturen bei verschieden groβen Arbeiterinnen von *Cataglyphis bicolor* Fabr. (Formicidae, Hymenoptera). *Zeitschrift für Vergleichende Physiologie*, **68**, 446–449.

Merkle, T., and Wehner, R. (2009). Repeated training does not improve the path integrator in desert ants. *Behavioral Ecology and Sociobiology*, **63**, 391.

Miller, N., Garnier, S., Hartnett, A. T., and Couzin, I. D. (2013). Both information and social cohesion determine collective decisions in animal groups. *Proceedings of the National Academy of Sciences*, **110**, 5263–5268.

Novgorodova, T. A. (2015). Organization of honeydew collection by foragers of different species of ants (Hymenoptera: Formicidae): effect of colony size and species specificity. *European Journal of Entomology*, **112**, 688.

Ogawa, Y., Falkowski, M., Narendra, A., Zeil, J., and Hemmi, J. M. (2015). Three spectrally distinct photoreceptors in diurnal and nocturnal Australian ants. *Proceedings of the Royal Society of London B: Biological Sciences*, **282**, 20150673.

Peeters, C., Liebig, J., and Hölldobler, B. (2000). Sexual reproduction by both queens and workers in the ponerine ant *Harpegnathos saltator*. *Insectes Sociaux*, **47**, 325–332.

Penick, C. A., Brent, C. S., Dolezal, K., and Liebig, J. (2014). Neurohormonal changes associated with ritualized combat and the formation of a reproductive hierarchy in the ant *Harpegnathos saltator*. *Journal of Experimental Biology*, **217**, 1496–1503.

Pepperberg, I. (2009). *Alex and me: how a scientist and a parrot discovered a hidden world of animal intelligence and formed a deep bond in the process*. London: Harper Collins.

Perry, C. J., Barron, A. B., and Chittka, L. (2017). The frontiers of insect cognition. *Current Opinion in Behavioral Sciences*, **16**, 111–118.

Pie, M. R. (2004). Foraging ecology and behaviour of the ponerine ant *Ectatomma opaciventre* Roger in a Brazilian savannah. *Journal of Natural History*, 38, 717–729.

Ramirez-Esquivel, F., Zeil, J., and Narendra, A. (2014). The antennal sensory array of the nocturnal bull ant *Myrmecia pyriformis*. *Arthropod Structure and Development*, **43**, 543–558.

Reznikova, J. I. (1982). Interspecific communication between ants. *Behaviour*, **80**, 84–95.

Reznikova, Z. (1974). Mechanism of territorial interaction of colonies in *Formica pratensis* (Hymenoptera, Formicidae). *Zoologicheskii Zhurnal*, **53**, 212–223 (in Russian with English summary).

Reznikova, Z. (1975). Non-antagonistic relationships of ants occupying similar ecological niches. *Zoologicheskii Zhurnal*, **54**, 1020–1031 (in Russian with English summary).

Reznikova, Z. (1980). Interspecific hierarchy in ants. *Zoologicheskii Zhurnal*, **59**, 1168–1176 (in Russian with English summary).

Reznikova, Z. (1999). Ethological mechanisms of population density control in coadaptive complexes of ants. *Russian Journal of Ecology*, **30**, 187–192.

Reznikova, Z. (2003). A new form of interspecies relations in ants: hypothesis of interspecies social control. *Zoologicheskii Zhurnal*, **82**, 816–824 (in Russian with English summary).

Reznikova Z. (2007a). *Animal intelligence: from individual to social cognition*. Cambridge: Cambridge University Press.
Reznikova, Z. (2007b). Dialog with black box: using Information Theory to study animal language behaviour. *Acta Ethologica*, **10**, 1–12.
Reznikova, Z. (2008). Experimental paradigms for studying cognition and communication in ants (Hymenoptera: Formicidae). *Myrmecological News*, **11**, 201–214.
Reznikova, Zh. I. (2009). Methods for field studies of behaviour and interspecies relations in ants. *Euroasian Entomological Journal*, **8**, 265–278 (in Russian with English summary).
Reznikova, Z. (2012). Altruistic behavior and cognitive specialization in animal communities. In *Encyclopedia of the Sciences of Learning* (pp. 205–208). New York, NY: Springer US.
Reznikova, Z. (2017). *Studying animal languages without translation: an insight from ants*. Berlin: Springer.
Reznikova, Z., and Bogatyreva, O. (1984). Individual behavior of ants of different species in the feeding habitat. *Zoologicheskii Zhurnal*, **63**, 1494–1503 (in Russian with English summary).
Reznikova, Z., and Dorosheva, E. (2013). Catalog learning: Carabid beetles learn to manipulate with innate coherent behavioral patterns. *Evolutionary Psychology*, **11**, 513–537.
Reznikova, Z., and Novgorodova, T. (1998). The importance of individual and social experience for interaction between ants and symbiotic aphids. *Doklady Biological Sciences*, **359**, 173–175.
Reznikova, Z., and Panteleeva, S. (2008). An ant's eye view of culture: propagation of new traditions through triggering dormant behavioural patterns. *Acta Ethologica*, **11**, 73–80.
Reznikova, Z., and Ryabko, B. (1990). Information Theory approach to communication in ants. In *Sensory Systems and Communication in Arthropods* (pp. 305–307). Basel: Birkhäuser.
Reznikova, Z., and Ryabko, B. (1994). Experimental study of the ants' communication system with the application of the Information Theory approach. *Memorabilia Zoologica*, **48**, 219–236.
Reznikova, Z., and Ryabko, B. (2011). Numerical competence in animals, with an insight from ants. *Behaviour*, **148**, 405–434.
Reznikova, Z., and Ryabko, B. (2012). Ants and bits. *IEEE Information Theory Society Newsletter*, **62**, 17–20.
Rosengren, R., and Fortelius, W. (1986). Ortstreue in foraging ants of the *Formica rufa* group – hierarchy of orienting cues and long-term memory. *Insectes Sociaux*, **33**, 306–337.
Ryabko, B., and Reznikova, Z. (1996). Using Shannon entropy and Kolmogorov complexity to study the communicative system and cognitive capacities in ants. *Complexity*, **2**, 37–42.
Ryabko, B., and Reznikova, Z. (2009). The use of ideas of information theory for studying 'language' and intelligence in ants. *Entropy*, **11**, 836–853.
Savage-Rumbaugh, E. S., and Lewin, R. (1994). *Kanzi: the ape at the brink of the human mind*. New York, NY: John Wiley & Sons.
Savolainen, R., Vepsäläinen, K., and Wuorenrinne, H. (1989). Ant assemblages in the taiga biome: testing the role of territorial wood ants. *Oecologia*, **81**, 481–486.
Schmid-Hempel, P. (1984). Individually different foraging methods in the desert ant *Cataglyphis bicolor* (Hymenoptera, Formicidae). *Behavioral Ecology and Sociobiology*, **14**, 263–271.
Seid, M. A., Castillo, A., and Wcislo, W. T. (2011). The allometry of brain miniaturization in ants. *Brain, Behavior and Evolution*, **77**, 5–13.
Sempo, G., and Detrain, C. (2010). Social task regulation in the dimorphic ant, *Pheidole pallidula*: the influence of caste ratio. *Journal of Insect Science*, **10**, 3.
Soroker, V., Vienne, C., and Hefetz, A. (1995). Hydrocarbon dynamics within and between nestmates in *Cataglyphis niger* (Hymenoptera: Formicidae). *Journal of Chemical Ecology*, **21**, 365–378.

Stebaev, I. V., and Reznikova, J. I. (1972). Two interaction types of ants living in steppe ecosystem in South Siberia, USSR. *Ecologia Polska*, **20**, 103–109.

Strausfeld, N. J., Hansen, L., Li, Y., Gomez, R. S., and Ito, K. (1998). Evolution, discovery, and interpretations of arthropod mushroom bodies. *Learning and Memory*, **5**, 11–37.

Stuble, K. L., Jurić, I., Cerda, X., and Sanders, N. (2017). Dominance hierarchies are a dominant paradigm in ant ecology (Hymenoptera: Formicidae), but should they be? And what is a dominance hierarchy anyways? *Myrmecological News*, **24**, 71–81.

Tautz, J. (2008). *The buzz about bees: biology of a superorganism*. Berlin: Springer.

Tibbetts, E. A. (2002). Visual signals of individual identity in the wasp Polistes fuscatus. *Proceedings of the Royal Society of London B: Biological Sciences*, **269**, 1423–1428.

Vepsäläinen, K., and Pisarski, B. (1982). Assembly of island ant communities. In *Annales Zoologici Fennici* (pp. 327–335). Helsinki: Finnish Academy of Sciences, Societas Scientiarum Fennica, Societas pro Fauna et Flora Fennica and Societas Biologica Fennica Vanamo.

Villet, M. (1990). Qualitative relations of egg size, egg production and colony size in some ponerine ants (Hymenoptera: Formicidae). *Journal of Natural History*, **24**, 1321–1331.

Walter, B., and Heinze, J. (2015). Queen–worker ratio affects reproductive skew in a socially polymorphic ant. *Ecology and Evolution*, **5**, 5609–5615.

Wehner, R. (2003). Desert ant navigation: how miniature brains solve complex tasks. *Journal of Comparative Physiology A*, **189**, 579–588.

Wehner, R., and Müller, M. (2006). The significance of direct sunlight and polarized skylight in the ant's celestial system of navigation. *Proceedings of the National Academy of Sciences*, **103**, 12575–12579.

van Wilgenburg, E., Lieshout, E., and Elgar, M. A. (2005). Conflict resolution strategies in meat ants (*Iridomyrmex purpureus*): ritualised displays versus lethal fighting. *Behaviour*, **142**, 701–716.

Wilson, E. O. (1976). A social ethogram of the neotropical arboreal ant *Zacryptocerus varians* (Fr. Smith). *Animal Behaviour*, **24**, 354–363.

Wilson, E. O. (1980). Caste and division of labor in leaf-cutter ants. II. The ergonomic organization of leaf cutting. *Behavioral Ecology and Sociobiology*, **7**, 157–165.

2 Bats – Using Sound to Reveal Cognition

Yossi Yovel and Stefan Greif

Species Description

Bats, or Chiroptera, are the second largest group and the only actively flying members in the mammalian order. Unlike birds, their wings are composed of a very thin but impressively elastic membrane, which is spread between their fingers. Despite spending a great deal of their life on the wing, bats have often been used in experimental designs which require them to crawl or be stationary. Due to their diversity of lifestyles (which exceeds any other group of mammals), different species require different keeping conditions when held in captivity. These keeping conditions can be highly specific, especially when kept long-term. Some species like to roost in cavities (like many insectivorous bats), some prefer to hang freely (like horseshoe bats, Rhinolophidae), some need warm and humid conditions, and others can cope with colder temperatures.

Some species are easy to keep in captivity, to train on behavioural tasks or to encourage to interact socially, while others are nearly impossible to keep. It is often a good starting point to consider the foraging ecology of a species in order to find the right one for your research question (see reference to the American Society of Mammalogists). In this chapter we will introduce the reader not to a single or a few model species, but to the possibilities of over 1300 model species and what they offer with their immensely wide variety of morphological, sensorial and behavioural adaptations (Fenton and Simmons, 2014; Tsang *et al.*, 2016; Figure 2.1).

Perception

Approximately 90 per cent of all bat species rely on echolocation for orientation and foraging. These bats sense their environment acoustically by emitting biosonar sound signals and analysing the returning echoes. This unique sensory system (shared with dolphins and two groups of birds) has fascinated scientists since its discovery, driving research in many different directions, such as the psychophysics of echolocation, its theoretic basis, its evolution and its underlying neural correlates (Kunz and Fenton, 2003; Altringham, 2011; Surlykke *et al.*, 2014).

Bats use echolocation for object detection, localization and even classification (Schnitzler and Kalko, 2001; Figure 2.2), and much research has focused on these abilities. However, echolocation can also serve as a great tool for studying animal cognition (Griffin, 1988). Cognitive scientists always want to know what their animal is

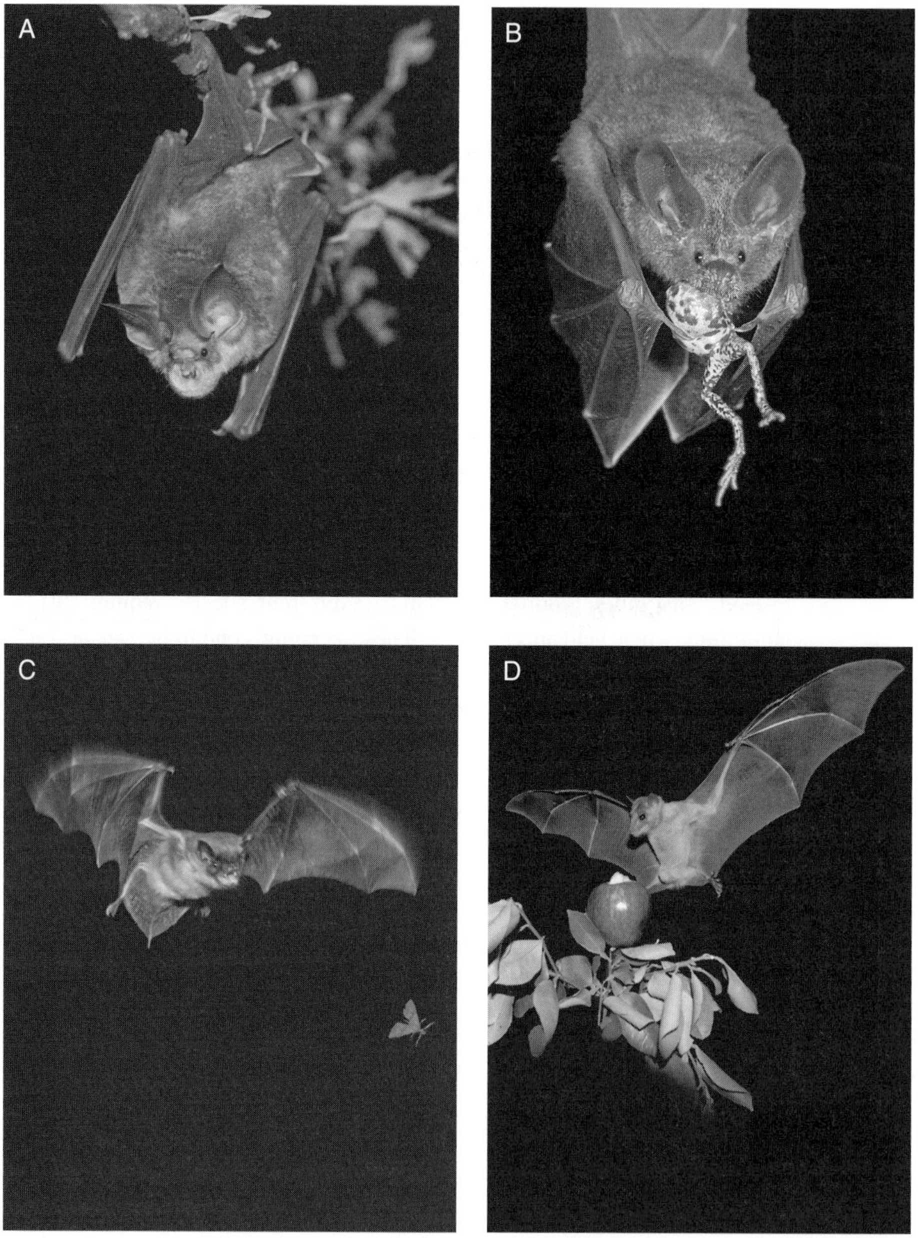

Figure 2.1. Four species (representing different families) used as animal models. (A) *Rhinolophus ferrumequinum*, family Rhinolophidae. (B) *Trachops cirrhosus*, family Phyllostomidae. (C) *Eptesicus fuscus*, family Vespertilionidae. (D) *Rousettus aegyptiacus*, family Pteropodidae. Photos were taken by S. Greif, A. Baugh, J. Nelson and Y. Yovel, respectively.

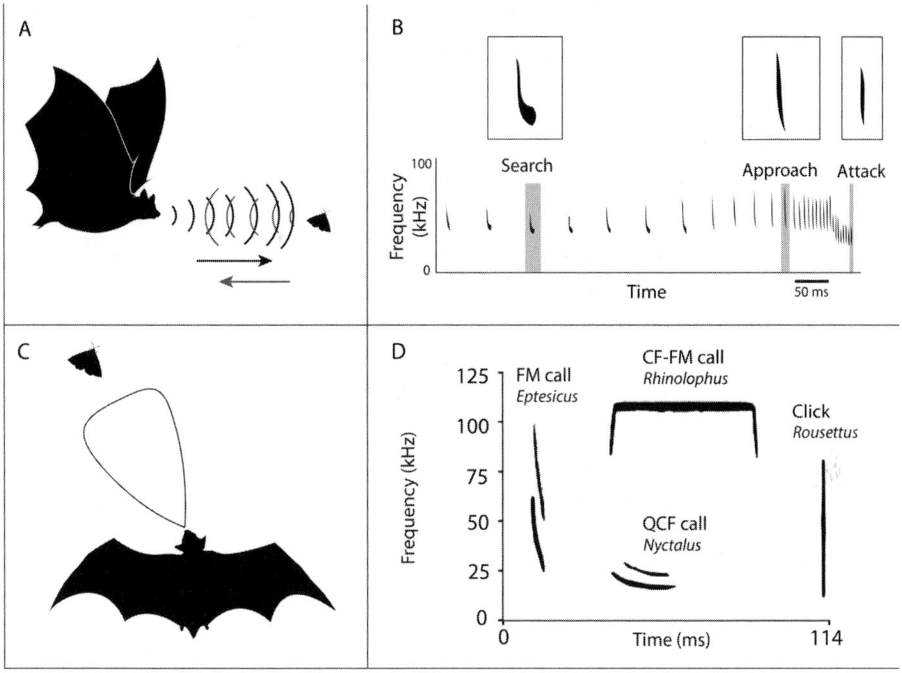

Figure 2.2. Principles of echolocation. (A) Bats emit sound signals and analyse the returning echoes to perceive their environment. (B) Spectrogram – frequency over time representation, showing a sequence of signals emitted by a bat that is approaching a prey item. Echolocation signals change their characteristics during the approach: they become shorter in duration and wider in frequency bandwidth (but not at the very end), and the intervals between them become shorter. This information can be acquired by researchers using a single microphone. Modified with permission from Geva-Sagiv *et al.* (2015). (C) Bats can steer their echolocation beam in space and thus control their sensory acoustic gaze. When using a microphone array, researchers can monitor this behaviour. (D) Bats that forage in different habitats or use different foraging strategies will rely on different echolocation signals. Image shows examples of three very different types of signals, representing most echolocation signals used by bats.
Modified with permission from Ulanovsky and Moss (2008).

doing during an experiment: where is it focusing its sensory attention? Did it attend a certain stimulus, and if so, for how long? The fact that bats emit sound in order to perceive their environment makes it possible to answer all these questions by simply recording their echolocation signals (Simmons, 1989). Moreover, as bats rapidly adapt their echolocation to the task they are performing, changes in behaviour can be registered with an accuracy of milliseconds (Geberl *et al.*, 2015; Luo *et al.*, 2017). For example, bats will rapidly increase emission rate when approaching a target (Schnitzler *et al.*, 2003; Moss and Surlykke, 2010; Figure 2.2B) and they will direct their acoustic gaze (i.e. the echolocation beam, see below; Figure 2.2C) towards an object of interest within dozens of milliseconds, all of which can be documented by researchers recording ultrasound (Surlykke *et al.*, 2009b; Yamada *et al.*, 2016). To date, however, the advantages of echolocation have hardly been used to address cognitive questions.

In addition to echolocation, bats possess all other well-known mammalian sensory systems, such as vision (Altringham, 2011; Eklöf *et al.*, 2014) and olfaction (Altringham and Fenton, 2003), and probably also a few less-common sensory abilities, such as magnetic sensing (Holland *et al.*, 2006) and thermoreception (Kürten and Schmidt, 1982). In comparison to acoustics, studies in other sensory modalities are underrepresented in bats and call for much more research. How bats integrate vision with echolocation is especially interesting, as these two sensory modalities potentially provide complementary information (Ratcliffe *et al.*, 2005) – vision allows long-range detection of larger objects (e.g. vegetation or other landscape elements) and high angular resolution, while echolocation allows detection of small objects (e.g. insects) and very high ranging accuracy. Likely, many bat species integrate information from these two modalities to simultaneously perform different tasks, such as obstacle avoidance and food detection (Boonman *et al.*, 2013; Danilovich *et al.*, 2015; Kong *et al.*, 2016), while others might rely solely on echolocation.

Life Cycle

Bats are extremely long-lived animals, especially considering their size, with proven records of more than 41 years for a species (*Myotis brandtii*) as small as 6 g (Podlutsky *et al.*, 2005). They reproduce very slowly, with most species rearing only one pup per year. In temperate zones, they typically mate in autumn, but females store the sperm until spring, when fertilization occurs. On the other hand, some species exhibit delayed implantation of the fertilized egg or even embryonic diapause. Tropical bats often mate (and rear pups) twice a year (Chrichton and Krutzsch, 2000; Altringham, 2011). Some bat species are nearly impossible to breed in the lab, while others will reproduce regularly. Juveniles reach adult morphometrics (and probably also behaviour) relatively quickly, within a few months after birth. For many species, the age of sexual maturity is not clearly known. Most mature within 1 year, but extremes of several months to 3 years can be observed (Kunz and Fenton, 2003; Altringham, 2011). Bats' extreme longevity opens exciting possibilities to conduct longitudinal cognitive studies, touching on questions such as memory retention or adaptations of behavioural strategies with experience.

With very few exceptions, bats are active during the night. For long-term experiments in captivity, the bats' circadian rhythm can be switched, by gradually reversing their light/dark cycle. This should be done slowly, with a shift of maximum 2 hours per day, and it requires the bats to be shifted back to a natural rhythm before being released again (Siemers and Page, 2009). For short-term experiments, it is better if the experiment takes place during the natural activity hours of the species, mostly at night, although data can also be acquired during dusk and dawn (and sometimes even day, depending on the question and species). Apart from their daily rhythms, it is also important to keep circannual rhythms in mind. In temperate-zone bats, these rhythms are characterized by winter hibernation, parturition in late spring–early summer, raising young in the summer and mating and preparing for hibernation in late summer–autumn. For tropical bats, these life stages are more flexible and often linked to food availability and climate seasons (dry and wet; Neuweiler, 2000; Altringham, 2011). The knowledge of hormonal control of bat physiology is fragmentary and restricted to selected species, demonstrating a variety of strategies (Krishna and Bhatnagar, 2011).

Individual Identification

Bats rely mostly on acoustic and olfactory cues for social and sexual communication, which is why they are generally rather inconspicuously coloured (with a few stunning exceptions, like *Kerivoula picta* or *Euderma maculatum*). Apart from random features like scars or aberrant colouration, they also offer very few visual cues to distinguish individuals. In some species, a small sexual size dimorphism is observed, but distinguishing sexes morphologically is generally easier through their apparent reproductive organs. Subadults often have fur of a different colour in comparison with adults, and this coloration will change within a few months. In addition, young subadults are recognizable through an apparent 'gap' in the joints of their fingers, which can be viewed by shining a torch from one side of the wing and observing from the other. This gap will narrow within the first few months of their life, with the ossification of the epiphyseal plates (Kunz and Parsons, 2009). Little information is available on differing foraging strategies between sexes, but in some species they seem to forage in separate regions (Senior *et al.*, 2005; Istvanko *et al.*, 2016). Sexual segregation in roosts is observed in some species, and it is most obvious in so-called maternity colonies, where females gather seasonally to raise their young in spring–summer (Altringham, 2011).

To overcome the lack of distinct individual characteristics, researchers can use a range of techniques to mark and recognize bats (Kerth and Dechmann, 2009). Most common in the field are bands that bats can carry on their wings long-term. The bands are typically made of metal or coloured plastic, and they each have a distinct number. They are different from bird-rings, as they should not be fully connected, to ensure that the wings are not injured (Kunz and Parsons, 2009). Moreover, some species are more sensitive to bands than others, so the literature or experienced researchers should be consulted before banding. For some years now, PIT (Passive Integrated Transponder) tags are becoming more common in use. These tiny cylindrical transponders (about 2 × 10 mm) are easily injected under the skin (which is very loosely connected to the body in bats) and carry an individual code that can be read with a reader (see below). Finally, in species like bigger flying foxes, a collar carrying coloured flags can be used. In captivity or for temporary markings in the field, there is also the possibility to cut or bleach the fur with specific patterns.

Ecological Characteristics

Bats can be found everywhere on the globe (except for the poles) inhabiting a huge variety of ecological habitats and niches. Species are not uniformly distributed, however, with a concentration of species in the tropics. Panama and Thailand, for example, house more than 100 species each, whereas one can find 44 species in all of Europe. The majority of bat species are insectivorous, but many are frugivorous or nectarivorous, and some even prey on vertebrates (e.g. fish, frogs and even other bats) or on blood (Neuweiler, 2000; Kunz and Fenton, 2003; Altringham, 2011). Although they all rely on insects, insectivorous bats can differ greatly in their foraging strategies. Some bats (referred to as aerial hawkers) search for insects on the wing, while others glean insects from surfaces such as vegetation, water or even the ground. Other bats use a sit-and-wait strategy and lurk for prey while perching. These differences in foraging strategy are strongly reflected in a specific echolocation-signal design, which is optimized according to its specific task (Schnitzler and Kalko, 2001; Schnitzler *et al.*, 2003; Moss and Surlykke, 2010; Denzinger and Schnitzler, 2013; Figure 2.2D). For example, bats that specialize in searching for large insects at high altitudes (where few reflecting objects exist) will generally use longer-duration echolocation signals with lower frequencies, as these signals spread further and allow bats to detect (large) insects from longer ranges. In contrast, bats use very short calls with a broad-frequency bandwidth to catch prey close to vegetation, to avoid temporal overlap between the echo returning from the prey and the echo returning from the (vegetation) background (Siemers and Schnitzler, 2004). The habitat also greatly influences their movement and flight style. Bats in open space are often fast flyers and can cover great distances on their foraging trips. On the other hand, bats that hunt in and around vegetation can be extremely manoeuvrable and can frustrate researchers when patrolling up and down a monofilament mist net, instead of flying into it. These differences will also be expressed in very different wing morphologies (Norberg and Rayner, 1987; Hedenström and Johansson, 2015).

Interest in bats' navigation abilities has greatly increased in recent years (Holland, 2007; Popa-Lisseanu and Voigt, 2009; Adams and Pedersen, 2013). As the only flying mammals, bats exhibit extreme navigation capacities. Many bats commute nightly over dozens of kilometres from their roosting sites to the foraging areas, and some species seasonally migrate over hundreds to thousands of kilometres (Hutterer *et al.*, 2005; Guilbert *et al.*, 2007; Voigt *et al.*, 2014, 2016). Little is known about the sensory systems and the navigational strategies guiding these behaviours. Translocation experiments suggest that some bat species use the Earth's magnetic field, as their orientation in the field is shifted following a magnetic manipulation (Holland *et al.*, 2006, 2010). A recent study suggests that the calibration of this magnetic compass is possibly mediated by the sky polarization pattern at dusk (Greif *et al.*, 2014). However, even when polarization cues were manipulated, bats that were translocated from their roost managed to return home, implying that, like birds and other animals, bats can rely on multiple sensory and navigation systems that complement each other. Egyptian fruit bats (*Rousettus aegyptiacus*), for example, seem to use visual information to navigate, relying on distal visual landmarks that give them a sense of direction (Tsoar *et al.*, 2011). A recent study has shown their ability to home from an unknown location as far as 90 km away from their roost, suggesting that bats can use cognitive maps (Tsoar *et al.*, 2011). On a smaller scale, many bats have been shown to possess an extremely precise spatial memory, but again, we are only beginning to understand the exact underlying mechanisms and features of this capability (Jensen *et al.*, 2005; Carter *et al.*, 2010;

Barchi *et al.*, 2013; Hulgard and Ratcliffe, 2014). Nectarivorous bats offer an especially interesting study case, as they can also combine temporal features with their spatial memory, taking into account nectar refilling rates of already visited flowers or seasonal flowering times of individual trees (Winter, 2005).

Social Characteristics

Many bat species are social, roosting in large colonies of tens to thousands and sometimes even millions of individuals, exhibiting a diversity of social behaviours (Kerth, 2008). Social organization can vary greatly among species, including harem-like structures in some species, seasonally separated male and female colonies, and year-round mixed-sex colonies. Some bats species are solitary (Altringham, 2011; Ortega, 2016). Social hierarchy has been hardly studied in bats, but it seems that in most social bats there is no clear dominance hierarchy in the colony (except for perhaps the reproducing male of the harem) (Chrichton and Krutzsch, 2000; Ortega, 2016). Although little is known about social cognition in bats, several studies have indicated high social-cognitive abilities. Most renowned is the reciprocal altruism exhibited by non-kin vampire bats (Desmodontinae), which regurgitate blood to feed hungry colony-mates who failed to find food, as has been shown both in the lab and in the field (Wilkinson, 1984; Adams and Pedersen, 2013). Other examples of high cognitive abilities include group decision-making regarding roost quality in insectivorous bats (Kerth *et al.*, 2006, 2011), information transfers about new food sources between colony members in Neotropical frugivorous and nectarivorous bats (O'Mara *et al.*, 2014a; Rose *et al.*, 2018) and long-lasting foraging bonds in Egyptian fruit bats (Harten et al., under rev.)

Group foraging is found in bat species that must exhaustively search large areas for an ephemeral resource, such as transient swarms of insects. This trait is probably a result of the very limited (<10 m) sensory range of echolocation in air, making it difficult to search alone, along with the vast social information provided by echolocation – the echolocation attack signals emitted by bats can be picked up by eavesdropping conspecifics from a rather large distance (Dechmann *et al.*, 2009; Cvikel *et al.*, 2015). Interestingly, this public information is sometimes even gleaned by heterospecifics that forage on similar prey (Dorado-Correa *et al.*, 2013; Voigt-Heucke *et al.*, 2016). In addition to this sonar-based communication, most bat species exhibit acoustic social communication (Ortega, 2016; Smotherman *et al.*, 2016). There is some evidence supporting the fact that the acquisition of bat social communication has a learning component and that it contains rich information about the emitter and the context of emission, but much more work is necessary on these topics (Knörnschild *et al.*, 2010; Knörnschild, 2014; Prat *et al.*, 2016). The use of a single sensory modality (audition) for both echolocation and social vocalizations raises interesting questions about bats' abilities to simultaneously process multiple sensory streams, as is the case when bats both echolocate and emit social calls, for instance when flying amid a group of bats. Bats' extreme longevity is especially interesting in the social context. In some cases, the same individuals have been documented roosting together for 20–30 years, suggesting the possibility of evolving long-term social bonds, but very little is known about such bonds in bats (Kerth *et al.*, 2011).

State of the Art

For several decades, studies on bat cognition mainly concentrated on the psychophysics of echolocation. Because bats turned out to be very accurate, showing ranging accuracies of less than 1 cm (Moss and Schnitzler, 1989; Simmons, 1989), there was a need for a method to present acoustic stimuli with precise timing. This experimental need has driven the development of a virtual reality approach, long before this became fashionable in other fields. Typically, in echolocation virtual reality experiments (Firzlaff *et al.*, 2007; Genzel and Wiegrebe, 2013), the bat is placed on a Y-platform and has to choose the correct one of the two virtual objects presented (one on each side of the platform; Figure 2.3B), showing its decision by crawling to one of the platform arms. For example, if ranging accuracy is the focus of the study, the bat can be trained to crawl to the closer of the two (virtual) objects. Experimenters produce the stimuli to present, by recording the bats' echolocation signals with a nearby microphone (one on each side). An echo representing the virtual object is then broadcast through a loudspeaker positioned behind each arm of the platform. Unlike visual virtual reality (which entails using screens and stimuli that are hardly ever fully natural), acoustic virtual reality can convey more realistic stimuli, as the played-back sound is potentially identical to the real echo. The great appeal of virtual reality is the control it enables over the sensory input the bat receives. Echoes representing non-physical objects can be generated, such as a very loud object with a very small cross-section (there is no physical object that produces such an echo). This approach can therefore allow investigators a glimpse into bats' perception of the world – bats' unique Umwelt. Moving to virtual reality experiments in flying bats (Genzel *et al.*, 2012; Goerlitz *et al.*, 2012), therefore, has the potential of opening new directions of research on bat cognition. However, even after several decades of studying bat echolocation, many questions remain open. Some of the main ones include the following:

- Is learning involved in the acquisition of echolocation? Previous studies suggest that the ontogeny of echolocation signals is innate (Moss *et al.*, 1997; Hiryu and Riquimaroux, 2011), but no isolation or cross-fostering experiments have been performed. Moreover, even if the acquisition of sound production is innate, learning might still play a role in acquiring control over using this system (Jones and Ransome, 1993; Prat *et al.*, 2015). People having reared orphan bats claim that they learn to forage on their own, but new evidence suggests that in some species (for example, species that specialize on prey that is difficult to find) mothers present prey items to their pups in the roost (Geipel *et al.*, 2013). Whether the function of this (or similar) behaviour is sensory learning remains to be shown.
- The fusion of information acquired through echolocation with other sensory modalities, such as vision and passive hearing, has received increasing amounts

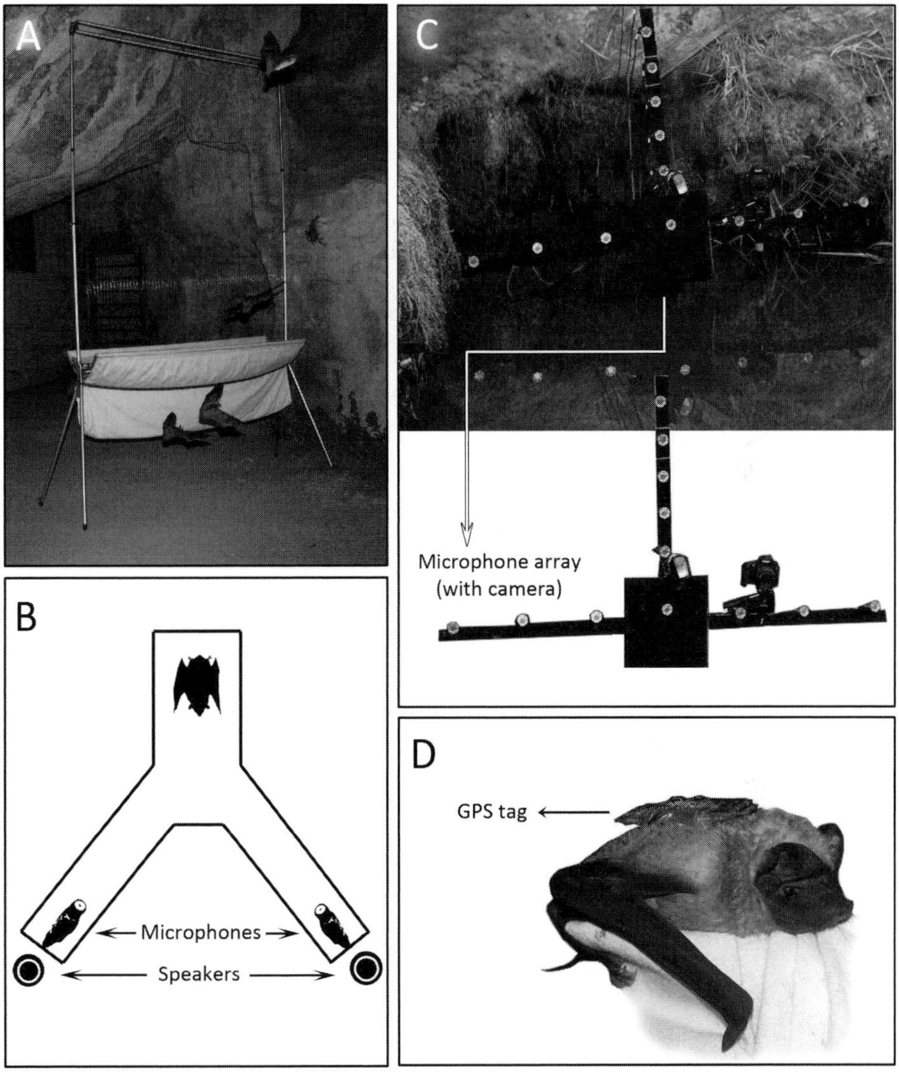

Figure 2.3. Methods for studying bats in the field and the lab. (A) A harp-trap can be used to catch bats when they exit a cave or fly along a known flightpath. (B) A Y-platform allows studying bats' psychophysics. Bats can be trained to sit on the platform and crawl towards one of two stimuli presented in each arm (a two-alternative forced-choice paradigm). In many studies, playbacks of echoes can replace the use of actual objects. This is done by recording the bat's signals with a microphone and playing back echoes through a speaker on each arm. (C) Microphone arrays (here positioned in a small pond) can be used to reconstruct the direction and width of the bats' echolocation beam, in the lab or in the field. (D) A bat carrying a tag that includes GPS tracking, acceleration and audio recordings.

Photos were taken by S. Greif (A), O. Eitan (C) and J. Koblitz (D).

of interest in recent years (Greif and Siemers, 2010; Danilovich *et al.*, 2015; Kong *et al.*, 2016), but it is still unknown how bats integrate visual and acoustic information, and to what degree they can translate the information acquired in one modality to the other one.

- The neural basis underlying echolocation also remains only partially understood. Despite the initial leap made by discovering delay-tuned neurons (which measure the time difference between the emitted echolocation signal and the returning echo, and thus convey range information), for many of the more complex aspects of echolocation we are just beginning to find neural explanations (Fenton *et al.*, 2016; Hoffmann *et al.*, 2016). The very strong bias of theoretic neuroscientists towards modelling the primate visual brain leaves a huge gap in fields such as echolocation, which are waiting for the first pioneers (Ulanovsky and Moss, 2008).

Echolocation could (and should) be used as a tool for addressing cognitive questions. Sensory decision-making is one example (Geberl *et al.*, 2015; Luo *et al.*, 2016). Currently, many studies follow eye saccades to quantify sensory attention when studying sensory decision-making (mostly in primates or in rodents). However, echolocation further allows estimating animals' allocation of sensory attention, with high precision and relatively little effort, without fixing the animal and without mounting it with instrumentations. As we will describe in the next section, using a microphone array (of multiple synchronized microphones; Figure 2.3C) allows monitoring the animal's instantaneous sensory gaze. The introduction of microphone arrays has already driven the use of bats for examining aspects of their behaviour, which have not been studied before, such as sensorimotor integration (i.e. how sensory inputs affect motor command and vice versa; Ghose *et al.*, 2006; Wohlgemuth *et al.*, 2016) and sensory negotiation of complex environments (Moss and Surlykke, 2010). Recording echolocation also provides information about the state of the animal. By analysing the momentary echolocation signals emitted by the bat, researchers can extract valuable behavioural information such as: is the bat still searching for an object, or is it preparing to land on or intercept it? Moreover, because of our good understanding of the physics of sound, given the emission of the bat and the objects in the environment, one can model the sensory input received by the bat rather accurately. In light of this, any cognitive question, which requires knowing the sensory input of the animal or its behaviour state with high time precision, could benefit from using bats as models, because echolocation opens a window into their sensory acquisition of the world. Here are a few examples of potentially promising aspects of cognition that could benefit from using bats as animal models.

- Social cognition. Several studies examined social cognition in bats, focusing on questions such as group decision-making (Fleischmann and Kerth, 2014), social information transfer (O'Mara *et al.*, 2014a; Ramakers *et al.*, 2016), social learning (Page and Ryan 2006; Wright *et al.*, 2011; Jones *et al.*, 2013) and reciprocal altruism (Wilkinson, 1984). Bats offer an interesting model to study sociality, as they live in communal colonies, use social vocal communication and in some species tend to forage in groups. The significant interspecific differences in sociality (e.g. in colony size, social structure and social foraging strategy) allow for a comparative approach. Because of the similarities in foraging strategy of some species, one interesting direction of research is interspecific social learning (interspecific eavesdropping has already been shown; Dorado-Correa *et al.*, 2013; Clarin *et al.*, 2014; Voigt-Heucke *et al.*, 2016).

- Navigation. Birds have traditionally served as models for studying navigation, even though bats have been shown to commute across many tens of kilometres even on a single night, and to seasonally migrate across thousands (Hutterer *et al.*, 2005; Voigt *et al.*, 2014, 2016). Bats' spatial abilities received some attention in the 1950s and 1960s, but due to technological limitations, research almost completely stopped for several decades. With the introduction of new miniature tracking technology, we are now witnessing a renaissance in this field (Holland *et al.*, 2006; Greif *et al.*, 2014; Cvikel *et al.*, 2015; Roeleke *et al.*, 2016). Some of the main navigation riddles include: which sensory modalities (e.g. echolocation, vision or magnetic sensing) facilitate spatial orientation, how they are combined and what are the navigation strategies (e.g. route following, path integration, map-based navigation). Connecting spatial with social cognition (i.e. navigating in a group) is another key question. Unlike birds, the bat brain is typically mammalian and human-like in many respects, so bats make much better models for human spatial cognition and spatial neural encoding (Geva-Sagiv *et al.*, 2015).
- Sensory perception. Despite decades of studying echolocation, many aspects of how bats acoustically perceive the world remain unclear. Some central open questions include: what are the important sensory dimensions of an echo (equivalent to the visual colour, shape and size), how is an acoustic image built and how detailed is it; and how are additional sensory modalities integrated with echolocation? A recent study on bats' sensory perception showed that they perceive water bodies acoustically, probably based on the unique acoustic signature of the echoes returning from such smooth horizontal surfaces (Greif and Siemers, 2010). The researchers also examined the importance of learning, and showed that acoustic-based water recognition is innate. On the other hand, they found that smooth vertical surfaces can constitute an acoustic illusion for bats, resulting in a sensory trap where bats collide with vertical smooth plates (Greif *et al.*, 2017). These studies therefore demonstrate both how intriguing bat sensory perception can be and how much there is still to learn about it.
- Studying the evolutionary traces of many basic aspects of cognition, such as learning (Page and Ryan, 2006; Page *et al.*, 2012; Jones *et al.*, 2013) and memory (Ruczynski and Siemers, 2011; Hulgard and Ratcliffe, 2014), can benefit from bats' immense diversity. Comparative studies looking at the cognitive capacities of closely related bat species, which inhabit different ecological niches, have the potential of teaching us about the evolution of cognition (Clarin *et al.*, 2013;

Hulgard and Ratcliffe, 2014). For example, it is intriguing to examine whether bats that inhabit more dynamic environments are also more flexible in their learning capacities, and if bats that rely on more predictable resources (such as fruit trees) have better spatial memories than bats that must search for ephemeral prey. These questions are of course oversimplified, but they demonstrate the kind of hypotheses that could be addressed. Finally, given the long life span of these animals, longitudinal studies might reveal how bats form long-term memories and build a knowledge that spans from food availability to spatial maps and social components. Intriguingly, it has already been shown that hibernation does not impair such long-term memory (Ruczynski and Siemers, 2011).

- Optimal foraging is another classic area of cognition research hardly touched by bat researchers. Can bats recognize and evaluate different prey types, and therefore be selective when going after it (Siemers and Güttinger, 2006; Goerlitz *et al.*, 2008; Koselj *et al.*, 2011)? This gets really interesting when the prey evolves countermeasures and leads to a classic predator–prey arms race, for example between bats and moths (Goerlitz *et al.*, 2010; Barber *et al.*, 2015; ter Hofstede and Ratcliffe, 2016).
- The neural correlates underlying the great majority of the behaviours described in this chapter are completely unknown, as most neural recordings have so far concentrated on the auditory regions of the bat brain (Neuweiler, 2000, 2003), or more recently on the hippocampus and entorhinal cortex (Yartsev *et al.*, 2011; Finkelstein *et al.*, 2014). Importantly, many of the past studies have been performed in anaesthetized bats, even though there is increasing evidence that the awake brain behaves differently from an anaesthetized one. New technology now allows recording the brains of freely flying bats (Geva-Sagiv *et al.*, 2016), opening a window into the bat's cognitive brain.

All for One, One for All

Box 2.1 Audiotelemetry of Vocal Behaviour

Manfred Gahr

The use of telemetric and logging devices to monitor the auditory environment and the own vocal output of behaving bats is a powerful strategy to study vocal behaviour and sensory capacities in (semi)natural settings (Hiryu *et al.*, 2007; Cvikel *et al.*, 2015). Similarly, such devices have been used in small birds to study song-based and call-based communication (ter Maat *et al.*, 2014; Gill *et al.*, 2015; D'Amelio *et al.*, 2017; Ma *et al.*, 2017). For both birds and bats, the devices are composed of small microphones and either an FM transmitter, which is connected to a transmitting antenna, or a data logger, which stores the data onboard. Audiotransmitters are the preferred devices for the study of vocal interactions, because they do not require external synchronization to allow time-stamped comparisons. Because

(*cont.*)

the weight of these devices is between 0.5 and 1.5 g, small flying animals (down to about 10–15 g) as well as smaller flightless animals could be equipped. Larger devices have also been used in vocal studies of small birds (e.g. Anisimov *et al.*, 2014), but they require highly unnatural environments, because they impair the flight of the animals and, therefore, should be avoided. In general, the impact of the weight and of the design of the devices on the movement performance and general behaviour of the study animals need to be evaluated under realistic conditions, in particular if the study aims are telemetric recordings in nature. For instance, audiotransmitter-equipped zebra finches needed 2–3 days to show normal vocal output after initial placement of the device on the animals using a backpack (Gill *et al.*, 2016). Thus, transmitter-based vocal studies are particularly valuable in case that the batteries are long-lasting, in particular if the battery lifetime considerably exceeds the time needed to adapt to the device. Thus, the essential feature of audiotransmitters is energy consumption and, in relation, transmission distance and working time. In each application, the user needs to trade off these features against the load the animals are able to carry, i.e. the weight of the experimental animal, and the goal of the study should determine the features of the transmitters (Gill *et al.*, 2016).

The advantages of carry-on audiotransmitters and loggers, as compared to microphone arrays and/or terrestrial microphones, is that these transmitters (1) facilitate the association of sound and emitter, (2) determine the hearing space of the receiver, while considering the noise, and (3) allow the study of several animals in synchrony (Gill *et al.*, 2016), which is essential for vocal communication such as male–female courtships, parent–offspring interactions and the vocal activities of social groups. Of course, audiotransmitters can be combined with transmitters that sense other modalities or neurophysiological activities (ter Maat *et al.*, 2014; Geva-Sagiv *et al.*, 2016), which opens up a broad range of possibilities in ecoacoustics, sensory physiology and behavioural neurobiology, among others.

References

Anisimov, V. N., Herbst, J. A., Abramchuk, A. N., Latanov, A.V., Hahnloser, R. H., and Vyssotski, A. L. (2014). Reconstruction of vocal interactions in a group of small songbirds. *Nature Methods*, **11**, 1135–1137.

Cvikel, N., Berg, K. E., Levin, E., *et al.* (2015). Bats aggregate to improve prey search but might be impaired when their density becomes too high. *Current Biology*, **25**, 206–211.

D'Amelio, P. B., Trost, L., and ter Maat, A. (2017). Vocal exchanges during pair formation and maintenance in the zebra finch (*Taeniopygia guttata*). *Frontiers in Zoology*, **14**, 13.

Geva-Sagiv, M., Romani, S., Las, L., and Ulanovsky, N. (2016). Hippocampal global remapping for different sensory modalities in flying bats. *Nature Neuroscience*, **19**, 952–958.

(cont.)

Gill, L. F., D'Amelio, P. B., Adreani, N. M., Sagunsky, H., Gahr, M., and ter Maat, A. (2016). A minimum-impact, flexible tool to study vocal communication of small animals with precise individual-level resolution. *Methods in Ecology and Evolution*, **7**, 1349–1358.

Gill, L. F., Goymann, W., ter Maat, A., and Gahr, M. (2015). Patterns of call communication between group-housed zebra finches change during the breeding cycle. *eLife*, **4**, 07770.

Hiryu, S., Hagino, T., Riquimaroux, H., and Watanabe, Y. (2007). Echo-intensity compensation in echolocating bats (*Pipistrellus abramus*) during flight measured by telemetry microphone. *Journal of the Acoustical Society of America*, **121**, 1749–1757.

Ma, S., Maat, A. T., and Gahr, M. (2017). Power-law scaling of calling dynamics in zebra finches. *Scientific Reports*, **7**, 8397.

ter Maat, A., Trost, L., Sagunsky, H., Seltmann, S., and Gahr, M. (2014). Zebra finch mates use their forebrain song system in unlearned call communication. *PLoS ONE*, **9**(10), e109334.

Field Guide

Catching bats in the field can be done (with the right permits) using a hand net, a mist net or a harp-trap (Figure 2.3A), either in the roost or at foraging sites and flightpaths, depending on the behaviour of the species of interest. One of the advantages of working with bats is that usually they readily take food in captivity. For insectivorous bats, this would often be mealworms, while frugivorous and nectarivorous bats will do a lot to get some fruit juice or a piece of fruit. This characteristic can be used to train them in experiments and reward them in small amounts, to increase the number of trials that can be obtained per session. Set-ups for experiments will vary depending on the research question and should take into account the needs of the species. Unlike with rodents, there are not many off-the-shelf behavioural tests for bats. Creative set-ups must therefore be developed for the specific experiment. Developing set-ups that test bats while they are flying freely are the golden route. Nevertheless, for some studies this might not (yet) be technically feasible. Luckily, bats have been very successfully tested in crawling or stationary experiments as well (Simmons, 1989; Siemers and Page, 2009; Aytekin *et al.*, 2010; Page *et al.*, 2012).

Acoustic Recordings

The most important method for studying bat echolocation or cognition is audio recording. For simple single microphone recordings, all that is needed is a microphone with sensitivity in the ultrasonic range (the exact range will strongly depend on the species), an amplifier and an analogue-to-digital (AD) converter, which can be connected to a storage unit (such as a laptop). There are many off-the-shelf products that offer a complete system suitable for ultrasonic recordings (e.g. Avisoft, Germany or

Wildlife Acoustics, USA), and it is also not too difficult to assemble such a system by buying the parts separately and connecting them. A single microphone is sufficient for detecting changes in the echolocation emission rate and signal design, which can be used to infer changes in sensory behaviour. For example, these parameters can detect when a bat switches from searching to attacking (Schnitzler *et al.*, 2003; Surlykke *et al.*, 2009b; Figure 2.2B), how noisy the environment in which it is flying is (Hage *et al.*, 2013; Luo *et al.*, 2016) and even how far a bat perceives a target to be (Stilz and Schnitzler, 2012; Figure 2.2B). If the absolute intensity or frequency content of the echolocation signals is important for the study, a calibrated microphone must be used (e.g. a GRAS or Bruel & Kjaer microphone). Note that the sensitivity of non-calibrated microphones might be different at different frequencies, and thus the spectrum of the recorded signal will differ from that actually emitted by the bat. This error can be compensated for by measuring the frequency response of the microphone. When choosing a microphone, one should remember the trade-off between sensitivity and directionality: a large microphone (e.g. 1/4 inch diameter) will usually be more sensitive, but it will only record sound from a narrow sector, and vice versa. This means that a large microphone will provide high-quality recordings when the bat is in front of its main axis, but it might miss the bat completely when it is to the side of the microphone, similar to using a very powerful, but very narrow-beam torch.

The main bottleneck of most ultrasonic recoding systems is the sampling rate allowed by the AD converter. To properly record a certain frequency, a signal must be sampled with a frequency that is at least twice as high. Many bat signals contain energy around 40 kHz, and therefore a sampling rate higher than 80 kHz is almost always necessary, while a typical computer only samples audio at a rate of up to 44 kHz. Many bat species use frequencies as high as 100 kHz (and some even reach 200 kHz), and thus researchers commonly use systems that allow sampling at 250–500 kHz. The miniaturization of technology in recent years now also allows mounting tiny microphones onboard bats (Hiryu *et al.*, 2008; Cvikel *et al.*, 2015), recording the acoustic scene from the tagged bat's point of view. Recordings with stationary microphones might be spectrally biased by Doppler shifts (when the bat is moving relative to the microphone), and by the directionality properties of the microphone (when the bat is not in front of the main axis of the microphone). These biases usually emphasize the lower frequencies of the signals and they are hard to compensate for because they depend on the exact velocity (speed and angle) of the bat relative to the microphone, which is usually unknown, unless multiple microphones are used (see below).

Many studies will benefit from sound recordings with an array of microphones (Figure 2.3C). For example, in order to study questions related to sensory attention, the echolocation beam must be reconstructed, and this cannot be done with a single microphone. Qualitatively, the biosonar beam can be thought of as the equivalent of the light beam of a flashlight, which is more intense in the centre and decays to the sides. Just like a human using a flashlight, the bat can only receive sensory information from the region within its beam. Because of the beam's two-dimensional nature, reconstructing it necessitates recordings with multiple synchronized microphones: the more microphones are used, the better the reconstruction will be.

Bats control the width of their beam determining how much of the world they sense (Surlykke *et al.*, 2009a; Jakobsen and Surlykke, 2010; Jakobsen *et al.*, 2015; Kounitsky *et al.*, 2015) and the direction of their beam in space (Figure 2.2C), determining which part of the scene they acquire information from (Ghose *et al.*, 2006, 2009; Yovel *et al.*, 2011a). By monitoring beam width and direction, researchers can reveal how a bat focuses its sensory attention in space. For example, it is possible to examine if a bat is scanning objects sequentially or in parallel (Surlykke *et al.*, 2009b) and which objects in a room have been attended by a flying bat. There are very few off-the-shelf products (e.g. Avisoft) that allow synchronized recording of multiple microphones at high sampling rates. When recording with multiple microphones, the sampling rate becomes an even more challenging bottleneck, because each of the channels must be sampled sufficiently fast.

Sound playbacks are complementary to sound recordings in many studies. They can be used to produce noise to study behavioural performance under noise (Schaub *et al.*, 2008; Hage *et al.*, 2013; Luo *et al.*, 2016), to mimic conspecifics (Dorado-Correa *et al.*, 2013), to mimic prey (Page and Ryan, 2006; Siemers *et al.*, 2012), to record echoes (Yovel *et al.*, 2008, 2011b), to create virtual auditory scenes and more (Weißenbacher and Wiegrebe, 2003; Genzel and Wiegrebe, 2013). The requirements of a playback system are similar to those of the recording system, except the microphone must be replaced by a speaker (some of the companies mentioned above offer playback systems as well). The frequency response of the speaker is extremely important when trying to mimic a real stimulus. Ultrasonic speakers with a flat frequency response (i.e. broadcasting the same intensity in all frequencies) are not easy to find, and it can be tricky to perfectly compensate for a non-flat response by amplifying certain frequencies and attenuating others. Also, when playing back signals via a speaker, one must crucially remember that the sound-beam of the speaker will usually be much narrower than that of a bat, because even the smallest speaker has an aperture that is much wider than a bat's mouth.

Many bat species are extremely social, exhibiting vast vocal communication (Ortega, 2016; Smotherman *et al.*, 2016; Prat *et al.*, 2017). The interest in bat vocal communication has increased in recent years, as more evidence has accumulated that bats can serve as a mammalian animal model for studying vocal learning (Knörnschild *et al.*, 2010; Knörnschild, 2014), a cognitive ability so far mainly studied in song birds. Because the vocal repertoire of many bats includes vocalizations within the audible range (i.e. < 20,000 Hz), standard microphones and recording systems used to record humans suffice for studying them. Some bats, however, include ultrasonic vocalizations in their social repertoire and will thus require higher sampling rates.

Tracking in the Field

One of the best methods to track bats in the field is using multiple-microphone recordings (Seibert *et al.*, 2013; Surlykke *et al.*, 2013; Gaudette *et al.*, 2014; Fujioka *et al.*, 2016). The position of the bat can be determined every time it emits sound (typically every 150 ms or less), based on the time difference between the arrival of the echolocation signals at the different microphones. A minimum of four microphones is required for obtaining 3D positioning, and more microphones can improve accuracy.

Table 2.1. Essential experimental tools required to study bats and their function.

Tool	Function
Mist net, harp-trap, hand net	To catch bats in their natural environments and in laboratory settings (hand net). Mist nets are similar to bird trapping nets and the most common way to capture bats. All methods can harm bats if applied incorrectly and should only be used after proper introduction by an experienced person. Small tip: use your capture bag to calm the bat and isolate it from the net when extracting it
Rings, PIT tags (+ reader)	Split metal rings and subcutaneously implanted PIT tags are used for individual recognition of bats over long times
Calliper, balance, fine scissors	Used to measure bats, remove glued tags or take hair samples. If there is a choice, use plastic callipers instead of metal ones to avoid light injuries
Capture bags	Cotton bags for keeping bats short-term. The seam should be on the outside, so that bats do not get entangled with their thumbs. Some bats have sensitive wrists; therefore, a softer fabric (like fluffy fleece) should be used
Radio/GPS tags	Tags are used to track movement or detect the presence of bats in natural environments. Tracking can be a tricky business, so it is highly advised to talk to experienced researchers before you venture out
Ultrasonic recording equipment	Microphones and recorders that can record high up in the ultrasonic range (e.g. Avisoft Bioacoustics, GRAS or Bruel & Kjaer). The recordings can then be analysed by software, like Avisoft SASLab, Matlab or other acoustic programs
Acoustic Monitoring Box	These devices allow you to conduct long-term monitoring of bat activity. Currently good recorders are e.g. Batcorder, BatLogger, SM3/4BAT (Wildlife Acoustics), Echo Meter Touch (Wildlife Acoustics), Pettersson D500X, Anabat Swift, Anabat Express
IR video-camera, IR lightning	IR light cannot be seen by bats, and it is therefore the standard equipment to record behavioural data
Sturdy gloves	Gloves are used for handling bats. They should not be thin latex gloves from the lab, but sturdy ones (although thick leather work gloves will not work either, as you will not have enough feeling to handle the bat properly). Often, gardening gloves are flexible, but prevent penetration of the bat teeth. Small tip: if you let the bat chew on a piece of the cotton bag while handling, it will be busy and refrain from biting your fingers
Food, water	This depends very much on the specific bat species. Many insectivorous bats will be very happy to take mealworms, once they discover their juicy guts. Frugivorous bats can go crazy for some banana, mango, etc., whereas nectarivorous bats need some sugar water to keep energy levels up and running (concentration depending on species, e.g. 30% for *Leptonycteris* sp.). And always remember to give them as much water as they want to drink using small pipettes

Data processing might be challenging, and there is currently no software that is available for purchasing. The best advice would be to contact someone who has already applied the methods successfully. The great advantage of acoustic tracking is that it does not require catching the bat or mounting markers on it (Holderied and von Helversen, 2003; Koblitz *et al.*, 2010; Kounitsky *et al.*, 2015). However, it does not allow individual recognition (so there is no way to know if the same individual has been recorded twice), and it is range-limited – the recording range does not normally exceed dozens of meters. This method is thus typically used at foraging and drinking sites or at flight paths where much bat activity can be expected (Seibert *et al.*, 2013; Fujioka *et al.*, 2016). Microphone array recordings are useful for studying sensorimotor aspects of prey capture and interactions between foraging bats, including competition over prey, sensory interference and predation strategies (Fujioka *et al.*, 2011, 2016). Moreover, when a suitable array is used, the biosonar beam can sometimes be computed to address questions related to sensory attention in the field (see above).

Another common approach for tracking bats without catching them is to use two or more thermal or IR cameras, but this method requires calibrating the volume covered by the cameras, which is a difficult task when done outdoors (Corcoran and Conner, 2014). Unlike acoustic tracking, which only provides trajectories, videoing allows visual scrutiny of the scene and the behaviour. However, videos will usually be accompanied by (acoustic) array recordings as well, in order to monitor the echolocation behaviour.

All other methods for tracking bats in the field require catching the bat and attaching some device. The most widely used method, radiotelemetry, includes mounting radio transmitters on the bat's back (O'Mara *et al.*, 2014b). Transmitters can be as light as 0.1 g, and they are connected either by a neck-collar or by surgical glue somewhere on the back. The transmitters emit radiofrequency pulses with some constant interval, which can be picked up by a suitable receiver. Each individual transmitter can have its own frequency, so that multiple bats (typically up to dozens) can be distinguished. The method can thus be used to study social aspects of foraging behaviour in the field (Ripperger *et al.*, 2016). The range of detection varies greatly from several kilometres in open space to dozens of metres in an environment with much occlusion (e.g. in the forest). The range will also depend on the power of the transmitter. In order to determine the position of the bat (and not only its presence), several antennae (at least two for 2D localization) at different locations around the bat must be used simultaneously. The method often requires tedious tracking (if the bat moves far) and offers varying degrees of accuracy, which are highly dependent on distance and environmental factors (Kenward, 2001; Withey *et al.*, 2001). However, modern systems are emerging that allow automatic triangulation of the position of the transmitter and are much more accurate (e.g. ATLAS – High-Throughput Wildlife Tracking; MOTUS – Wildlife Tracking System; Ripperger *et al.*, 2016). Alternatively, a single antenna can be used to determine the presence and the direction of the animal carrying the tag by pointing the antenna in different directions and determining the direction of maximum intensity. This approach is often used to study sensory navigation, for example by translocating animals to an unknown location and releasing them after some sensory manipulation (e.g. a shift in the experienced magnetic field). The animal's initial flight direction from the release site can then be monitored using radiotelemetry to determine the importance of the manipulated sensory system in navigation (Holland *et al.*, 2006, 2010; Greif *et al.*, 2014).

When only monitoring the presence/absence of bats at specific locations, automatic loggers registering the presence of the transmitter can be placed in strategic locations (e.g. the roost), to monitor when a bat has visited this location. Alternatively, RFID technology can be used: tiny tags (usually termed PIT tags) are easily implanted subcutaneously in even the smallest bat species, registering whenever the bat comes near a suitable tag-reader. However, the tag must be within a range of up to ~0.5 m from the reader to be read, so the method is only useful when there is accurate prior knowledge on the expected location of the bat. It has been applied at cave entrances and bat-box entrances, to monitor the bats going in and out of their roost. Because the tags do not require a battery (they are powered by the reader), they do not need replacement, although in reality they typically do not last for more than a few years. PIT tags can also be used to cleverly manipulate specific individuals in the field. For example, a system can be developed to respond only to the presence of specific individual bats, so that only some bats gain information about the roost or get access to some food source (Kerth *et al.*, 2001, 2006; Winter, 2005). Further development of such ideas should enable testing cognition in wild bats under natural conditions.

The increasing interest in bat navigation has driven the development of more accurate tracking technologies, such as miniature GPS devices (as small as 1 g, from companies like Biotrack, ecotone and ASD technologies; Figure 2.3D). Devices can either store the bat's locations onboard a memory card, which thus requires retrieval of the tag, or they can use some transmission mechanism (e.g. GSM or satellite). The trade-off is clear: retrieving the GPS device might be extremely difficult, especially when the bat does not return to its roost, while transmission is very costly in terms of energy, so that much less data can be collected. Increased use of GPS will advance our understanding of wild bats, providing essential information on their flights, nightly routines and migration routes (Weller *et al.*, 2016). Satellite tags have been used on bigger flying foxes and will soon become small enough to tag small bats (ICARUS Initiative – International Cooperation for Animal Research Using Space), although the number of calculated positions is still limited. An important technological direction, which will definitely become more important in future years, combines GPS with additional onboard sensors. Some relevant sensors include microphones to record echolocation behaviour or social communication, accelerometers to monitor wingbeat and behaviour, environmental sensors such as light and ambient temperature sensors, and physiological sensors to monitor electrocardiography (ECG) or electroencephalography (EEG).

The Devil Is in the Details

Box 2.2 Levelling the Playing Field: Comparative Cognition Studies in Bats

Rachel A. Page

Bats show extraordinary diversity and are in many ways ideal subjects for studies of comparative cognition. Arguably the most diverse order of mammals, bats occupy a vast array of foraging niches, with species that specialize on fruit, nectar, insects, fish, frogs and blood (Simmons, 2005). Likewise, bats encompass a broad range of social strategies, from species that roost alone to those that are highly social, relying on one another to compensate for missed meals and for group foraging (Ortega, 2016). As such, bats are well suited to comparative tests investigating the degree to

(cont.)

which cognitive skills reflect socio-ecological niche. However, there are significant pitfalls associated with comparative cognition in bats. I outline these below.

The very specializations that make bats so fascinating pose challenges to researchers attempting to design 'species-fair' tests (Siemers and Page, 2009). The frog-eating bat, *Trachops cirrhosus*, for example, is a highly flexible predator that locates its prey by eavesdropping on frog mating calls (Tuttle and Ryan, 1981; Page and Ryan, 2005). It learns acoustic cues rapidly and excels at acoustic tests in captivity (Page and Jones, 2016). In contrast, the fig-eating specialist, *Artibeus lituratus*, relies heavily on olfactory cues to find its food (Parolin *et al.*, 2015). If we want to compare learning and memory in these two species, and we choose an acoustic task to do so, *T. cirrhosus* would clearly come out ahead. In contrast, if we presented bats with an olfactory test, *A. lituratus* would probably excel. If we are interested in comparative cognition, we need to carefully design experiments to test cognitive ability per se, not the sensory adaptations bats use to forage in nature.

Differences in motor adaptations can also impede comparative work. Crawling mazes, for example, are an efficient way to test spatial learning, but some animals are inherently more comfortable moving through tight spaces than others. Bats that tend to roost in crevices or those that access their roosts at least in part by crawling tend to perform well in maze tests (e.g. Clarin *et al.*, 2013). In contrast, bat species that rarely crawl in nature may panic when placed inside an enclosed maze. Maze modifications can help; for example, a bat that is disinclined to crawl on all fours can be coaxed to navigate a vertical, flying maze (Ammersdörfer *et al.*, 2012). New technologies, such as touch screens and walking platforms, may also open new doors in the types of tests that can be used to compare cognition across species (Winter *et al.*, 2005).

Another motor constraint that can impede comparative tests is variation in flight manoeuvrability. The common big-eared bat, *Micronycteris microtis*, for example, can nimbly navigate densely cluttered rainforest understory, hovering in front of individual leaves to investigate potential prey (Geipel *et al.*, 2013). Not surprisingly, *M. microtis* excels at foraging tasks in small spaces (e.g. in a flight arena of $1.4 \times 1.0 \times 0.8$ m; Geipel *et al.*, 2013). The fishing bat, *Noctilio leporinus*, in contrast, requires a much larger arena to forage in captivity (e.g. $12 \times 5 \times 2$ m; Übernickel *et al.*, 2013). While these are two extreme examples, even closely related bat species can differ substantially in their flight manoeuvrability (Stockwell, 2001). Keeping in mind species-specific flight abilities and scaling the testing arena accordingly may enable researchers to keep variation in motor ability from masking differences in cognitive ability.

In sum, comparing different species on similar tasks can be a powerful tool to understand variation in cognition, but only if tests are not biased toward one species over another. By modifying the task and the testing arena, one can level the playing field, reducing the influences of sensory and motor constraints on species' performance. Employing species-fair tests, researchers can gain fascinating insights into cognitive variation across species.

(*cont.*)

References

Ammersdörfer, S., Galinski, S., and Esser, K. H. (2012). Effects of aversive experience on the behavior within a custom-made plus maze in the short-tailed fruit bat, Carollia perspicillata. *Journal of Comparative Physiology A*, **198**, 733–739.

Clarin, T. M. A., Ruczyński, I., Page, R. A., and Siemers, B. M. (2013). Foraging ecology predicts learning performance in insectivorous bats. *PLoS ONE*, **8**, e64823.

Geipel, I., Jung, K., and Kalko, E. K. V. (2013). Perception of silent and motionless prey on vegetation by echolocation in the gleaning bat Micronycteris microtis. *Proceedings of the Royal Society of London B: Biological Sciences*, **280**, 20122830.

Ortega, J. (2016). *Sociality in bats*. Berlin: Springer.

Page, R. A., and Jones, P. L. (2016). Overcoming sensory uncertainty: factors affecting foraging decisions in frog-eating bats. In *Perception and cognition in animal communication* (pp. 285–312). New York, NY: Springer.

Page, R. A., and Ryan, M. J. (2005). Flexibility in assessment of prey cues: frog-eating bats and frog calls. *Proceedings of the Royal Society of London B: Biological Sciences*, **272**, 841–847.

Parolin, L. C., Mikich, S. B., and Bianconi, G. V. (2015). Olfaction in the fruit-eating bats *Artibeus lituratus* and *Carollia perspicillata*: an experimental analysis. *Anais da Academia Brasileira de Ciências*, **87**, 2047–2053.

Siemers, B. M., and Page, R. A. (2009). Behavioral studies of bats in captivity: methodology, training, and experimental design. In *Ecological and behavioral methods for the study of bats* (pp. 373–392). Baltimore, MD: Johns Hopkins University Press.

Simmons, N. B. (2005). Chiroptera. In *Mammal species of the world: a taxonomic and geographic reference* (pp. 312–529). Baltimore, MD: Johns Hopkins University Press.

Stockwell, E. F. (2001). Morphology and flight manoeuvrability in New World leaf-nosed bats (Chiroptera: Phyllostomidae). *Journal of Zoology*, **254**, 505–514.

Tuttle, M. D., and Ryan, M. J. (1981). Bat predation and the evolution of frog vocalizations in the Neotropics. *Science*, **214**, 677–678.

Übernickel, K., Tschapka, M. T., and Kalko, E. K. V. (2013). Flexible echolocation behavior of trawling bats during approach of continuous or transient prey cues. *Frontiers in Physiology*, **4**, 96.

Winter, Y., von Merten, S., and Kleindienst, H. U. (2005). Visual landmark orientation by flying bats at a large-scale touch and walk screen for bats, birds and rodents. *Journal of Neuroscience Methods*, **141**, 283–290.

Resources

- Adams, R. A., and Pedersen, S. C. (2013). *Bat evolution, ecology, and conservation*. New York, NY: Springer Nature.
- Altringham, J. D. (2011). *Bats from evolution to conservation*. Oxford: Oxford University Press.
- Dietz, C., von Helversen, O., and Nill, D. (2009). *Bats of Britain, Europe and Northwest Africa*. London: A&C Black.

- Fenton, M. B., Grinnell, D. A., Popper, N. A., and Fay, R. R. (2016). *Bat bioacoustics*. New York, NY: Springer Nature.
- Griffin, D. (1958). *Listening in the dark. The acoustic orientation of bats and men*. Ithaca, NY: Cornell University Press.
- Kunz, T. H., and Fenton, M. B. (2003). *Bat ecology*. Chicago, IL: The Johns Hopkins University Press.
- Kunz, T. H. and Parsons, S. (2009). *Ecological and behavioral methods for the study of bats*. Baltimore, MD: The Johns Hopkins University Press.
- Neuweiler, G. (2000). *The biology of bats*. Oxford: Oxford University Press.
- Ortega, J. (2016). *Sociality in bats*. Berlin: Springer Nature.
- Surlykke, A., Nachtigall, E. P., Fay, R. R., and Popper, N. A. (2014). *Biosonar*. New York, NY: Springer Nature.
- Thomas, J. A., Moss, C. F., and Vater, F. (2004). *Echolocation in bats and dolphins*. Chicago, IL: The University of Chicago Press.
- www.batecho.eu
- www.batcon.org
- Bat Worker Manual: http://jncc.defra.gov.uk/page-2861
- Bat Catcher Manual: http://vleermuizenvangen.nl/attachments/article/28/2008%20%20Manual_Bats_sept2008_AJHaarsma_small.pdf

Profile

Yossi completed his studies in Physics and Biology at Tel-Aviv University. He worked on bat echolocation during his PhD in Tuebingen, Germany, and as a Post-doc in the Weizmann Institute, Israel. In 2011 he established the laboratory for NeuroEcology at Tel-Aviv University, developing miniature technologies to conduct controlled experiments with animals in their natural environment. The lab focuses on echolocating bats and on a range of fundamental behaviours, including navigation, social networks and collective behaviour, sensory decision-making, intersensory integration and vocal communication.

Stefan studied biology at the University of Tuebingen, Germany, where he first started working on bats. He then conducted his PhD on bat sensory ecology at the Max Planck Institute for Ornithology in Seewiesen, Germany. After a position at Queens University Belfast, UK, he joined Yossi at Tel-Aviv University, Israel. He did most of his field work at the Siemers Bat Research Station in Bulgaria, but also conducted studies in Germany, Panama, Mexico and Thailand. His main interests lie in (multi)sensory ecology, animal physiology and movement ecology.

References

Adams, R. A., and Pedersen, S. C. (eds.) (2013). *Bat evolution, ecology, and conservation*. New York, NY: Springer.

Altringham, J. D. (2011). *Bats – from evolution to conservation*. Oxford: Oxford University Press.

Altringham, J. D., and Fenton, M. B. (2003). Sensory ecology and communication in the Chiroptera. In *Bat ecology* (pp. 90–127). Chicago, IL: The John Hopkins University Press.

American Society of Mammalogists. Mammalian species. Available from https://academic.oup.com/mspecies.

ATLAS – High-throughput wildlife tracking. Available from www.tau.ac.il/~stoledo/tags.

Aytekin, M., Mao, B., and Moss, C. F. (2010). Spatial perception and adaptive sonar behavior. *The Journal of the Acoustical Society of America*, **128**, 3788–3798.

Barber, J. R., Leavell, B. C., Keener, A. L., *et al.* (2015). Moth tails divert bat attack: evolution of acoustic deflection. *Proceedings of the National Academy of Sciences*, **112**, 2812–2816.

Barchi, J. R., Knowles, J. M., and Simmons, J. A. (2013). Spatial memory and stereotypy of flight paths by big brown bats in cluttered surroundings. *Journal of Experimental Biology*, **216**, 1053–1063.

Boonman, A., Bar-On, Y., Cvikel, N., and Yovel, Y. (2013). It's not black or white – on the range of vision and echolocation in echolocating bats. *Frontiers in Physiology*, **4**, 248.

Carter, G. G., Ratcliffe, J. M., and Galef, B. G. (2010). Flower bats (*Glossophaga soricina*) and fruit bats (*Carollia perspicillata*) rely on spatial cues over shapes and scents when relocating food. *PLoS ONE*, **5**(5), 1–6.

Chrichton, E. G., and Krutzsch, P. H. (2000). *Reproductive biology of bats*. London: Academic Press.

Clarin, T. M. A., Ruczyński, I., Page, R. A., and Siemers, B. M. (2013). Foraging ecology predicts learning performance in insectivorous bats. *PLoS ONE*, **8**(6), e64823.

Clarin, T. M. A., Borissov, I., Page, R. A., Ratcliffe, J. M., and Siemers, B. M. (2014). Social learning within and across species: information transfer in mouse-eared bats. *Canadian Journal of Zoology*, **92**, 129–139.

Corcoran, A. J., and Conner, W. E. (2014). Bats jamming bats: food competition through sonar interference. *Science*, **346**, 745–747.

Cvikel, N., Egert Berg, K., Levin, E., *et al.* (2015). Bats aggregate to improve prey search but might be impaired when their density becomes too high. *Current Biology*, **25**, 206–211.

Danilovich, S., Krishnan, A., Lee, W. J., *et al.* (2015). Bats regulate biosonar based on the availability of visual information. *Current Biology*, **25**, 1124–1125.

Dechmann, D. K. N., Heucke, S. L., Giuggioli, L., Safi, K., Voigt, C. C., and Wikelski, M. (2009). Experimental evidence for group hunting via eavesdropping in echolocating bats. *Proceedings of the Royal Society of London B: Biological Sciences*, **276**, 2721–2728.

Denzinger, A., and Schnitzler, H. U. (2013). Bat guilds, a concept to classify the highly diverse foraging and echolocation behaviors of microchiropteran bats. *Frontiers in Physiology*, **4**, 164.

Dorado-Correa, A. M., Goerlitz, H. R., and Siemers, B. M. (2013). Interspecific acoustic recognition in two European bat communities. *Frontiers in Physiology*, **4**, 192.

Eklöf, J., Šuba, J., Petersons, G., and Rydell, J. (2014). Visual acuity and eye size in five European bat species in relation to foraging and migration strategies. *Environmental and Experimental Biology*, **12**, 1–6.

Fenton, M. B., and Simmons, N. B. (2014). *Bats – A world of science and mystery*. Chicago, IL: The University of Chicago Press.

Fenton, M. B., Grinnell, D. A., Popper, N. A., and Fay, R. R. (2016). *Bat bioacoustics*. New York, NY: Springer.

Finkelstein, A., Derdikman, D., Rubin, A., Foerster, J. N., Las, L., and Ulanovsky, N. (2014). Three-dimensional head-direction coding in the bat brain. *Nature*, **517**, 159–164.

Firzlaff, U., Schuchmann, M., Grunwald, J. E., Schuller, G., and Wiegrebe, L. (2007). Object-oriented echo perception and cortical representation in echolocating bats. *PLoS Biology*, **5**, 1174–1183.

Fleischmann, D., and Kerth, G. (2014). Roosting behavior and group decision making in 2 syntopic bat species with fission-fusion societies. *Behavioral Ecology*, **25**, 1240–1247.

Fujioka, E., Mantani, S., Hiryu, S., Riquimaroux, H., and Watanabe, Y. (2011). Echolocation and flight strategy of Japanese house bats during natural foraging, revealed by a microphone array system. *The Journal of the Acoustical Society of America*, **129**, 1081–1088.

Fujioka, E., Aihara, I., Sumiya, M., Aihara, K., and Hiryu, S. (2016). Echolocating bats use future-target information for optimal foraging. *Proceedings of the National Academy of Sciences*, **113**, 4848–4852.

Gaudette, J. E., Kloepper, L. N., Warnecke, M., and Simmons, J. A. (2014). High resolution acoustic measurement system and beam pattern reconstruction method for bat echolocation emissions. *The Journal of the Acoustical Society of America*, **135**, 513–520.

Geberl, C., Brinkløv, S., Wiegrebe, L., and Surlykke, A. (2015). Fast sensory–motor reactions in echolocating bats to sudden changes during the final buzz and prey intercept. *Proceedings of the National Academy of Sciences*, **112**, 4122–4127.

Geipel, I., Kalko, E. K. V., Wallmeyer, K., and Knörnschild, M. (2013). Postweaning maternal food provisioning in a bat with a complex hunting strategy. *Animal Behaviour*, **85**, 1435–1441.

Genzel, D., and Wiegrebe, L. (2013). Size does not matter: size-invariant echo-acoustic object classification. *Journal of Comparative Physiology A*, **199**, 159–168.

Genzel, D., Gebert, C., Dera, T., and Wiegrebe, L. (2012). Coordination of bat sonar activity and flight for the exploitation of three-dimensional objects. *Journal of Experimental Biology*, **215**, 2226–2235.

Geva-Sagiv, M., Las, L., Yovel, Y., and Ulanovsky, N. (2015). Spatial cognition in bats and rats: from sensory acquisition to multiscale maps and navigation. *Nature Reviews Neuroscience*, **16**, 94–108.

Geva-Sagiv, M., Romani, S., Las, L., and Ulanovsky, N. (2016). Hippocampal global remapping for different sensory modalities in flying bats. *Nature Neuroscience*, **19**, 952–958.

Ghose, K., Horiuchi, T. K., Krishnaprasad, P. S., and Moss, C. F. (2006). Echolocating bats use a nearly time-optimal strategy to intercept prey. *PLoS Biology*, **4**, 865–873.

Ghose, K., Triblehorn, J. D., Bohn, K., Yager, D. D., and Moss, C. F. (2009). Behavioral responses of big brown bats to dives by praying mantises. *Journal of Experimental Biology*, **212**, 693–703.

Goerlitz, H. R., Greif, S., and Siemers, B. M. (2008). Cues for acoustic detection of prey: insect rustling sounds and the influence of walking substrate. *Journal of Experimental Biology*, **211**, 2799–2806.

Goerlitz, H. R., ter Hofstede, H. M., Zeale, M. R. K., Jones, G., and Holderied, M. W. (2010). An aerial-hawking bat uses stealth echolocation to counter moth hearing. *Current Biology*, **20**, 1568–1572.

Goerlitz, H. R., Genzel, D., and Wiegrebe, L. (2012). Bats' avoidance of real and virtual objects: implications for the sonar coding of object size. *Behavioural Processes*, **89**, 61–67.

Greif, S., and Siemers, B. M. (2010). Innate recognition of water bodies in echolocating bats. *Nature Communications*, **1**, 107.

Greif, S., Borissov, I., Yovel, Y., and Holland, R. A. (2014). A functional role of the sky's polarization pattern for orientation in the greater mouse-eared bat. *Nature Communications*, **5**, 5488.

Greif, S., Zsebők, S., Schmieder, D., and Siemens, B. M. (2017). Acoustic mirrors as sensory traps for bats. *Science*, **1047**, 1045–1047.

Griffin, D. R. (1988). Cognitive aspects of echolocation. In *Animal sonar* (pp. 683–690). New York, NY: Plenum Press.

Guilbert, J. M., Walker, M. M., Greif, S., and Parsons, S. (2007). Evidence of homing following translocation of long-tailed bats (*Chalinolobus tuberculatus*) at Grand Canyon Cave, New Zealand. *New Zealand Journal of Zoology*, **34**, 239.

Hage, S. R., Jiang, T., Berquist, S. W., Feng, J., and Metzner, W. (2013). Ambient noise induces independent shifts in call frequency and amplitude within the Lombard effect in echolocating bats. *Proceedings of the National Academy of Sciences*, **110**, 4063–4068.

Harten, L., Matalon, Y., Galli, N., Navon, H., Dor, R., and Yovel, Y. (2018). Persistent producer-scrounger relationships in bats. *Science Advances*, **4**, e1603293.

Hedenström, A., and Johansson, L. C. (2015). Bat flight: aerodynamics, kinematics and flight morphology. *Journal of Experimental Biology*, **218**, 653–663.

Hiryu, S., and Riquimaroux, H. (2011). Developmental changes in ultrasonic vocalizations by infant Japanese echolocating bats, *Pipistrellus abramus*. *The Journal of the Acoustical Society of America*, **130**, 147–153.

Hiryu, S., Shiori, Y., Hosokawa, T., Riquimaroux, H., and Watanabe, Y. (2008). On-board telemetry of emitted sounds from free-flying bats: compensation for velocity and distance stabilizes echo frequency and amplitude. *Journal of Comparative Physiology A*, **194**, 841–851.

Hoffmann, S., Vega-Zuniga, T., Greiter, W., *et al.* (2016). Congruent representation of visual and acoustic space in the superior colliculus of the echolocating bat phyllostomus discolor. *European Journal of Neuroscience*, **44**, 2685–2697.

ter Hofstede, H. M., and Ratcliffe, J. M. (2016). Evolutionary escalation: the bat–moth arms race. *The Journal of Experimental Biology*, **219**, 1589–1602.

Holderied, M. W., and von Helversen, O. (2003). Echolocation range and wingbeat period match in aerial-hawking bats. *Proceedings of the Royal Society of London B: Biological Sciences*, **270**, 2293–2299.

Holland, R. A. (2007). Orientation and navigation in bats: known unknowns or unknown unknowns? *Behavioral Ecology and Sociobiology*, **61**, 653–660.

Holland, R. A., Thorup, K., Vonhof, M. J., Cochran, W. W., and Wikelski, M. (2006). Bat orientation using earth's magnetic field. *Nature*, **444**, 702.

Holland, R. A., Borissov, I., and Siemers, B. M. (2010). A nocturnal mammal, the greater mouse-eared bat, calibrates a magnetic compass by the sun. *Proceedings of the National Academy of Sciences*, **107**, 6941–6945.

Hulgard, K., and Ratcliffe, J. M. (2014). Niche-specific cognitive strategies: object memory interferes with spatial memory in the predatory bat *Myotis nattereri*. *Journal of Experimental Biology*, **217**, 3293–3300.

Hutterer, R., Ivanova, T., Meyer-Cords, C., and Rodrigues, L. (2005). *Bat migrations in Europe – a review of banding data and literature*. Bonn: Federal Agency for Nature Conservation.

ICARUS Initiative – International Cooperation for Animal Research Using Space. Available from http://icarusinitiative.org

Istvanko, D. R., Risch, T. S., and Rolland, V. (2016). Sex-specific foraging habits and roost characteristics of *Nycticeius humeralis* in North-Central Arkansas. *Journal of Mammalogy*, **97**, 1336–1344.

Jakobsen, L., and Surlykke, A. (2010). Vespertilionid bats control the width of their biosonar sound beam dynamically during prey pursuit. *Proceedings of the National Academy of Sciences*, **107**, 13930–13935.

Jakobsen, L., Olsen, M. N., and Surlykke, A. (2015). Dynamics of the echolocation beam during prey pursuit in aerial hawking bats. *Proceedings of the National Academy of Sciences*, **112**, 8118–8123.

Jensen, M. E., Moss, C. F., and Surlykke, A. (2005). Echolocating bats can use acoustic landmarks for spatial orientation. *Journal of Experimental Biology*, **208**, 4399–4410.

Jones, G., and Ransome, R. (1993). Echolocation calls of bats are influenced by maternal effects and change over a lifetime. *Proceedings of the Royal Society of London B: Biological Sciences*, **252**, 125–128.

Jones, P. L., Ryan, M. J., Flores, V., and Page, R. A. (2013). When to approach novel prey cues? Social learning strategies in frog-eating bats. *Proceedings of the Royal Society of London B: Biological Sciences*, **280**, 20132330.

Kenward, R. E. (2001). *A manual for wildlife radio tagging*. San Diego, CA: Academic Press.

Kerth, G. (2008). Causes and consequences of sociality in bats. *BioScience*, **58**, 737–746.

Kerth, G., and Dechmann, D. K. N. (2009). Field-based observations and experimental studies of bat behavior. In *Ecological and behavioral methods for the study of bats* (pp. 393–406). Baltimore, MD: The Johns Hopkins University Press.

Kerth, G., Ebert, C., and Schmidtke, C. (2006). Group decision making in fission-fusion societies: evidence from two-field experiments in Bechstein's bats. *Proceedings of the Royal Society of London B: Biological Sciences*, **273**, 2785–2790.

Kerth, G., Wagner, M., and König, B. (2001). Roosting together, foraging apart: information transfer about food is unlikely to explain sociality in female Bechstein's bats (*Myotis bechsteinii*). *Behavioral Ecology and Sociobiology*, **50**, 283–291.

Kerth, G., Perony, N., and Schweitzer, F. (2011). Bats are able to maintain long-term social relationships despite the high fission–fusion dynamics of their groups. *Proceedings of the Royal Society of London B: Biological Sciences*, **278**, 2761–2767.

Knörnschild, M. (2014). Vocal production learning in bats. *Current Opinion in Neurobiology*, **28**, 80–85.

Knörnschild, M., Nagy, M., Metz, M., Mayer, F., and von Helversen, O. (2010). Complex vocal imitation during ontogeny in a bat. *Biology Letters*, **6**, 156–159.

Koblitz, J. C., Stilz, P., and Schnitzler, H. V. (2010). Source levels of echolocation signals vary in correlation with wingbeat cycle in landing big brown bats (*Eptesicus fuscus*). *Journal of Experimental Biology*, **213**, 3263–3268.

Kong, Z., Fuller, N., Wang, S., *et al.* (2016). Perceptual modalities guiding bat flight in a native habitat. *Scientific Reports*, **6**, 27252.

Koselj, K., Schnitzler, H. U., and Siemers, B. M. (2011). Horseshoe bats make adaptive prey-selection decisions, informed by echo cues. *Proceedings of the Royal Society of London B: Biological Sciences*, **278**, 3034–3041.

Kounitsky, P., Rydell, J., Amichai, E., *et al.* (2015). Bats adjust their mouth gape to zoom their biosonar field of view. *Proceedings of the National Academy of Sciences*, **112**, 6724–6729.

Krishna, A., and Bhatnagar, K. P. (2011). Hormones and reproductive cycles in bats. In *Hormones and reproduction of vertebrates* (pp. 241–289). London: Elsevier.

Kunz, T. H., and Fenton, M. B. (2003). *Bat ecology*. Chicago, IL: The University of Chicago Press.

Kunz, T. H., and Parsons, S. (2009). *Ecological and behavioral methods for the study of bats*. Baltimore, MD: The Johns Hopkins University Press.

Kürten, L., and Schmidt, U. (1982). Thermoperception in the common vampire bat (*Desmodus rotundus*). *Journal of Comparative Physiology A*, **146**, 223–228.

Luo, J., Goerlitz, H. R., Brumm, H., and Wiegrebe, L. (2016). Linking the sender to the receiver: vocal adjustments by bats to maintain signal detection in noise. *Scientific Reports*, **5**, 18556.

Luo, J., Kothari, N. B., and Moss, C. F. (2017). Sensorimotor integration on a rapid time scale. *Proceedings of the National Academy of Sciences*, **114**, 6605–6610.

Moss, C. F., and Schnitzler, H. U. (1989). Accuracy of target ranging in echolocating bats: acoustic information processing. *Journal of Comparative Physiology A*, **165**, 383–393.

Moss, C. F., and Surlykke, A. (2010). Probing the natural scene by echolocation in bats. *Frontiers in Behavioral Neuroscience*, **4**, 33.

Moss, C. F., Redish, D., Gounden, C., and Kunz, T. H. (1997). Ontogeny of vocal signals in the little brown bat, *Myotis lucifugus*. *Animal Behaviour*, **54**, 131–141.

MOTUS – Wildlife Tracking System. Available from https://motus.org.

Neuweiler, G. (2000). *The biology of bats*. Oxford: Oxford University Press.

Neuweiler, G. (2003). Evolutionary aspects of bat echolocation. *Journal of Comparative Physiology A*, **189**, 245–256.

Norberg, U. M., and Rayner, J. M. V. (1987). Ecological morphology and flight in bats (Mammalia; Chiroptera): wing adaptations, flight performance, foraging strategy and echolocation. *Philosophical Transactions of the Royal Society B*, **316**, 335–427.

O'Mara, T. M., Dechmann, D. K. N., and Page, R. A. (2014a). Frugivorous bats evaluate the quality of social information when choosing novel foods. *Behavioral Ecology*, **25**, 1233–1239.

O'Mara, T. M., Wikelski, M., and Dechmann, D. K. N. (2014b). 50 years of bat tracking: device attachment and future directions. *Methods in Ecology and Evolution*, **5**, 311–319.

Ortega, J. (ed.) (2016). *Sociality in bats*. Berlin: Springer.

Page, R. A., and Ryan, M. J. (2006). Social transmission of novel foraging behavior in bats: frog calls and their referents. *Current Biology*, **16**, 1201–1205.

Page, R. A., von Merten, S., and Siemers, B. M. (2012). Associative memory or algorithmic search: a comparative study on learning strategies of bats and shrews. *Animal Cognition*, **15**, 495–504.

Podlutsky, A. J., Khritankov, A. M., Ovodov, N. D., and Austad, S. N. (2005). A new field record for bat longevity. *The Journals of Gerontology Series A*, **60**, 1366–1368.

Popa-Lisseanu, A. G., and Voigt, C. C. (2009). Bats on the move. *Journal of Mammalogy*, **90**, 1283–1289.

Prat, Y., Taub, M., and Yovel, Y. (2015). Vocal learning in a social mammal: demonstrated by isolation and playback experiments in bats. *Science Advances*, **1**, e1500019.

Prat, Y., Taub, M., and Yovel, Y. (2016). Everyday bat vocalizations contain information about emitter, addressee, context, and behavior. *Scientific Reports*, **6**, 39419.

Prat, Y., Azoulay, L., Dor, R., and Yovel, Y. (2017). Crowd vocal learning induces vocal dialects in bats: playback of conspecifics shapes fundamental frequency usage by pups. *PLoS Biology*, **15**, e2002556.

Ramakers, J. J. C., Dechmann, D. K. N., Page, R. A., and O'Mara, M. T. (2016). Frugivorous bats prefer information from novel social partners. *Animal Behaviour*, **116**, 83–87.

Ratcliffe, J. M., Raghuram, H., Marimuthu, G., Fullard, J. H., and Fenton, M. B. (2005). Hunting in unfamiliar space: echolocation in the Indian false vampire bat, *Megaderma lyra*, when gleaning prey. *Behavioral Ecology and Sociobiology*, **58**, 157–164.

Ripperger, S., Josic, D., Hierold, M., *et al.* (2016). Automated proximity sensing in small vertebrates: design of miniaturized sensor nodes and first field tests in bats. *Ecology and Evolution*, **6**, 2179–2189.

Roeleke, M., Blohm, T., Kramer-Schadt, S., Yovel, Y., and Voigt, C. C. (2016). Habitat use of bats in relation to wind turbines revealed by GPS tracking. *Scientific Reports*, **6**, 28961.

Rose, A., Kolar, M., Tschapka, M., and Knörnschild, M. (2016). Learning where to feed: the use of social information in flower-visiting Pallas' long-tongued bats (*Glossophaga soricina*). *Animal Cognition*, **19**, 251–262.

Ruczynski, I., and Siemers, B. M. (2011). Hibernation does not affect memory retention in bats. *Biology Letters*, **7**, 153–155.

Schaub, A., Ostwald, J., and Siemers, B. M. (2008). Foraging bats avoid noise. *Journal of Experimental Biology*, **211**, 3174–3180.

Schnitzler, H. U., and Kalko, E. K. V. (2001). Echolocation by insect-eating bats. *BioScience*, **51**, 557–569.

Schnitzler, H. U., Moss, C. F., and Denzinger, A. (2003). From spatial orientation to food acquisition in echolocating bats. *Trends in Ecology and Evolution*, **18**, 386–394.

Seibert, A. M., Koblitz, J. C., Denzinger, A., and Schnitzler, H. U. (2013). Scanning behavior in echolocating common pipistrelle bats (*Pipistrellus pipistrellus*). *PLoS ONE*, **8**(4), e60752.

Senior, P., Butlin, R. K., and Altringham, J. D. (2005). Sex and segregation in temperate bats. *Proceedings of the Royal Society of London B: Biological Sciences*, **272**, 2467–2473.

Siemers, B. M., and Güttinger, R. (2006). Prey conspicuousness can explain apparent prey selectivity. *Current Biology*, **16**, 157–159.

Siemers, B. M., and Page, R. A. (2009). Behavioral studies of bats in captivity: methodology, training, and experimental design. In *Ecological and behavioral methods for the study of bats* (pp. 373–392). Baltimore, MD: The Johns Hopkins University Press.

Siemers, B. M., and Schnitzler, H. U. (2004). Echolocation signals reflect niche differentiation in five sympatric congeneric bat species. *Nature*, **429**, 657–661.

Siemers, B. M., Kriner, E., Kaipf, I., Simon, M., and Greif, S. (2012). Bats eavesdrop on the sound of copulating flies. *Current Biology*, **22**, 563–564.

Simmons, J. A. (1989). A view of the world through the bat's ear: the formation of acoustic images in echolocation. *Cognition*, **33**, 155–199.

Smotherman, M., Knörnschild, M., Smarsh, G., and Bohn, K. (2016). The origins and diversity of bat songs. *Journal of Comparative Physiology A*, **202**, 535–554.

Stilz, W. P., and Schnitzler, H. U. (2012). Estimation of the acoustic range of bat echolocation for extended targets. *The Journal of the Acoustical Society of America*, **132**, 1765–1775.

Surlykke, A., Boel Pedersen, S., and Jakobsen, L. (2009a). Echolocating bats emit a highly directional sonar sound beam in the field. *Proceedings of the Royal Society of London B: Biological Sciences*, **276**, 853–860.

Surlykke, A., Ghose, K., and Moss, C. F. (2009b). Acoustic scanning of natural scenes by echolocation in the big brown bat, *Eptesicus fuscus*. *Journal of Experimental Biology*, **212**, 1011–1020.

Surlykke, A., Jakobsen, L., Kalko, E. K. V., and Page, R. A. (2013). Echolocation intensity and directionality of perching and flying fringe-lipped bats, *Trachops cirrhosus* (Phyllostomidae). *Frontiers in Physiology*, **4**, 143.

Surlykke, A., Nachtigall, E. P., Fay, R. R., and Popper, N. A. (2014). *Biosonar*. New York, NY: Springer.

Tsang, S. M., Cirranello, A. L., Bates, P. J. J., and Simmons, N. B. (2016). The roles of taxonomy and systematics in bat conservation. In *Bats in the Anthropocene* (pp. 503–538). Cham: Springer.

Tsoar, A., Nathan, R., Bartan, Y., Vyssotski, A., Dell'Omo, G., and Ulanovsky, N. (2011). Large-scale navigational map in a mammal. *Proceedings of the National Academy of Sciences*, **108**, 718–724.

Ulanovsky, N., and Moss, C. F. (2008). What the bat's voice tells the bat's brain. *Proceedings of the National Academy of Sciences*, **105**, 8491–8498.

Voigt, C. C., Lehnert, L. S., Popa-Lisseanu, A. G., *et al.* (2014). The trans-boundary importance of artificial bat hibernacula in managed European forests. *Biodiversity and Conservation*, **23**, 617–631.

Voigt, C. C., Lindecke, O., Schönborn, S., Kramer-Schadt, S., and Lehmann, D. (2016). Habitat use of migratory bats killed during autumn at wind turbines. *Ecological Applications*, **26**, 771–783.

Voigt-Heucke, S. L., Zimmer, S., and Kipper, S. (2016). Does interspecific eavesdropping promote aerial aggregations in European pipistrelle bats during autumn? *Ethology*, **122**, 745–757.

Weißenbacher, P., and Wiegrebe, L. (2003). Classification of virtual objects in the echolocating bat, *Megaderma lyra*. *Behavioral Neuroscience*, **117**, 833–839.

Weller, T. J., Castle, K. T., Liechti, F., Hein, C. D., Schirmacher, M. R., and Cryan, P. M. (2016). First direct evidence of long-distance seasonal movements and hibernation in a migratory bat. *Scientific Reports*, **6**, 34585.

Wilkinson, G. S. (1984). Reciprocal food sharing in the vampire bat. *Nature*, **312**, 181–184.

Winter, Y. (2005). Foraging in a complex naturalistic environment: capacity of spatial working memory in flower bats. *Journal of Experimental Biology*, **208**, 539–548.

Withey, J. C., Bloxton, T. D., and Marzluff, J. M. (2001). Effects of tagging and location error in wildlife radiotelemetry studies. In *Radio tracking and animal populations* (pp. 43–75). San Diego, CA: Academic Press.

Wohlgemuth, M. J., Kothari, N. B., and Moss, C. F. (2016). Action enhances acoustic cues for 3-D target localization by echolocating bats. *PLoS Biology*, **14**, e1002544.

Wright, G. S., Wilkinson, G. S., and Moss, C. F. (2011). Social learning of a novel foraging task by big brown bats, *Eptesicus fuscus*. *Animal Behaviour*, **82**, 1075–1083.

Yamada, Y., Hiryu, S., and Watanabe, Y. (2016). Species-specific control of acoustic gaze by echolocating bats, *Rhinolophus ferrumequinum nippon* and *Pipistrellus abramus*, during flight. *Journal of Comparative Physiology A*, **202**, 791–801.

Yartsev, M. M., Witter, M. P., and Ulanovsky, N. (2011). Grid cells without theta oscillations in the entorhinal cortex of bats. *Nature*, **479**, 103–107.

Yovel, Y., Franz, M. O., Stilz, P., and Schnitzler, H. U. (2008). Plant classification from bat-like echolocation signals. *PLoS Computational Biology*, **4**, e1000032.

Yovel, Y., Falk, B., Moss, C. F., and Ulanovsky, N. (2011a). Active control of acoustic field-of-view in a biosonar system. *PLoS Biology*, **9**, e1001150.

Yovel, Y., Franz, M. O., Stilz, P., and Schnitzler, H. U. (2011b). Complex echo classification by echo-locating bats: a review. *Journal of Comparative Physiology A*, **197**, 475–490.

3 Bees – The Experimental Umwelt of Honeybees

Randolf Menzel

Species Description

Life Cycle and Social Characteristics

Honeybees are middle-sized flying insects of the order Hymenoptera. A colony usually consists of 10,000–50,000 workers (sterile females) and a queen. Queens mate with several male bees (drones) in consecutive mating flights. Drones' life is limited to a few weeks in spring, and they contribute little to the social life of the colony. Colonies multiply by a process called swarming, during which some of the workers leave the colony with the old queen, and the remaining workers raise a new queen. Multiple swarms may be formed in rather short intervals, depending on the size of the colony and the space available.

Workers proceed through a sequence of age-dependent behaviours. The indoor life lasts usually for 2–3 weeks, during which they start caring for the queen, then feeding the larvae, cleaning the colony, and finally receiving incoming foragers (providing them with feedback on the colony's needs) and defending the colony at the hive entrance (Robinson and Page, 1989). Worker bees live two lives, as a social animal inside the colony (whose behaviour is highly controlled by innate age-dependent mechanisms, largely based on pheromones) and as individual animals exploring and foraging outside the colony. As foragers, workers differ with respect to their experience, as they have to constantly adapt to the changing conditions of the environment, optimize their foraging trips by learning to navigate efficiently in time and space, and gather the necessary information for the reproduction of the whole colony during swarming.

Ecological Characteristics

Honeybees are most efficient pollinators of flowers. Their flower fidelity results from their perfect discrimination of colours and patterns, their fast sensory and motor learning and their stable memories (see below). Because their colonies survive even long winter periods, many worker bees are available when spring flowering starts. Several products of the colony can be produced at a very large scale (honey, pollen, resin, royal jelly) and are commercially exploited by humans. However, commercial bee keeping is under pressure, due to both parasites and the uptake of pesticides such as neonicotinoids, which act on the nicotinic acetylcholine receptors of high-order interneurons in the bee brain, compromising learning and memory, and even killing bees at higher doses.

Individual Identification

A major step in the study of cognition in honeybees was von Frisch's move to individualize foraging bees by marking them with coloured dots on the thorax, representing a numbering system (von Frisch, 1967; Figure 3.1). Meanwhile, we use number tags or computer-read black/white patterns. This allows researchers to keep track of an individual during its life history and better study bee cognition and social behaviour. Wilson (1971) stated that 'insect societies are, for the most part, impersonal. The sheer number of colony members and the short life of the members appears to make it inefficient, if not impossible, to establish individual bonds'. However, olfaction in bees is so powerful that it might allow distinguishing among body odours of colony members, providing the potential for discriminating a very large number of group constellations, even to the level of individual recognition. Members of kin groups (i.e. bees with the same drone as father), for example, can be identified by their hydrocarbon composition of cuticular odours (Getz *et al.*, 1986), and as a honeybee queen usually mates with several drones, kin groups provide an intrinsic structure of the colony.

Age groups also differ with respect to the pheromones they produce (Plettner *et al.*, 1993; Bloch *et al.*, 2003) and to their behaviour, including different dance forms (e.g. whether they produce a shaking dance, a waggle dance or a stop signal; Gahl, 1975). Working with a group of foraging bees over several days often allows experimenters to recognize

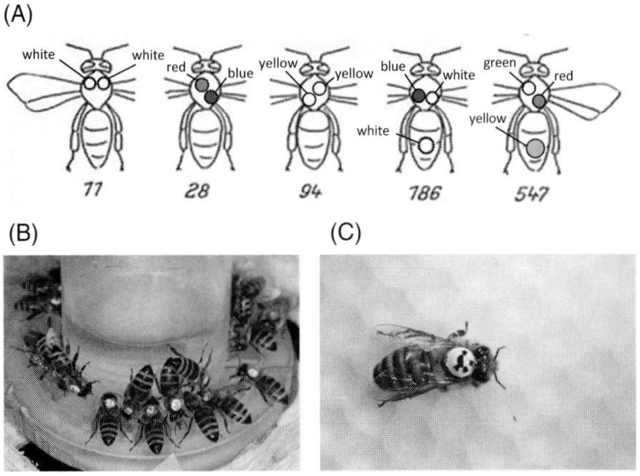

Figure 3.1. Honeybees become individuals by marking them with numbers. (A) Von Frisch used a system in which five coloured dots at four different positions on the thorax code the numbers from 1 to 99. A single colour dot on the abdomen codes the 100 numbers (white), the 200 numbers (red), the 300 numbers (blue), the 400 numbers (yellow) and the 500 numbers (green). (B) We use number tags for our experiments that are produced for marking queens. Five different colours and four different directions of the number tag allow marking of up to 1900 bees (some numbers are usually excluded, because orientations cannot be distinguished, e.g. 66 and 99). Together with coloured dots on the abdomen, more than 5000 bees can be marked individually. (C) A black pattern on a white background allows marking of more than 100,000 bees and can be used for automatic detection of bees inside the colony.
Right lower figure: courtesy of Dr Tim Landgraf.

individuals according to their particular behaviour, e.g. how quickly they settle at a feeder, whether they are more prepared to recruit other bees, whether they mark the feeder with a scent, whether they specialize on pollen/nectar foraging or on scouting (collecting information about productive flowers or new nest sites). However, it is so far unknown whether differences in odours and behavioural patterns allow recognition up to the individual level. Individual recognition is documented in the small, relatively primitive colonies of *Polistes* wasps, partially based on the visual patterns of their faces (Tibbetts, 2002; Tibbetts and Dale, 2004). However, in other kinds of social insects (particularly in colonies with many members), personalized relationships may play little to no role.

Perception

Bees have a trichromatic colour vision with UV, blue and green receptors, discriminate a large range of odours (resolving the temporal structure of the odour plume in the millisecond range) and are very sensitive to substrate vibration. Bees do not perceive sound as changes in air pressure, but rather by detecting the velocity changes in sound waves. Moreover, they can perceive linearly polarized light and can detect, learn and discriminate electrostatic fields. In flying bees, the wax-covered body charges up by friction in air and does not discharge when landing, due to the high electrical resistance of the body surface. Therefore, movements of the charged body (e.g. during waggle dances) emanate electrostatic fields, which couple via Coulomb forces to the charged appendages (antennae, mechanosensory hairs) of neighbouring bees.

State of the Art

Learning

Bees easily learn to go for the colour associated with a reward (e.g. Werner *et al.*, 1988) and also for the pattern (Hempel de Ibarra *et al.*, 2002; Avargues-Weber *et al.*, 2011). Prolonged training to multiple symmetrical versus asymmetrical shapes, for instance, showed that bees develop a concept of symmetry (Giurfa *et al.*, 1996). Moreover, bees trained with delayed matching to sample or non-sample tasks (DMTS and DMTNS) in the visual domain (colours, patterns) can also transfer the rules within the visual domain and to the olfactory domain. Bees can further learn context-dependent cue rewarding (Gerber and Smith, 1998). Interestingly, bees do not learn to respond with proboscis extension to the visual stimulus alone, but neural responses are predictive for the learned visual context (Filla and Menzel, 2015). Bees also solve transwitching and cue-context reversal tasks (Hussaini and Menzel, 2013). In these problems, bees are differentially trained with two olfactory stimuli, A and B, and with two different visual contexts, C1 and C2. When C1 is available, stimulus A (but not stimulus B) is rewarded, while the opposite is true with C2. Focusing on the elements alone, therefore, would not allow solving the problem, as each element (A, B) appears equally rewarded, and bees have to learn that C1 and C2 define the valid contingency. In addition, bees

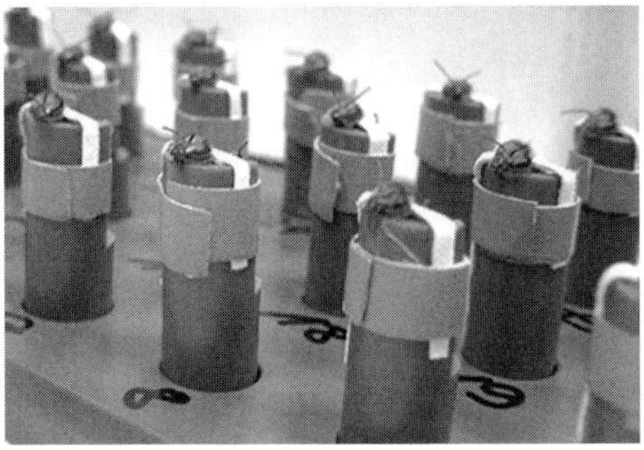

Figure 3.2. Honeybees prepared for proboscis extension response (PER) conditioning. Usually, 30–80 bees are harnessed in tubes, in such a way that the antennae, mandibles and proboscis are free to move. The bees survive in the tube for several days, if fed at least once every day. The movements of the antennae and the proboscis can be quantified with video techniques.

can be trained in the lab to odours using reward conditioning of the proboscis extension response (see below; Figure 3.2).

Memory

Reward learning in honeybees initiates a sequence of at least four memory phases, which lead to long-lasting memory (Menzel and Müller, 1996; Menzel, 1999). An associative-learning trial induces an early form of short-term memory (eSTM) in the second range, which is rather unspecific and quickly converted into a late short-term memory (STM). The transition to mid-term memory (MTM) takes hours and makes the memory trace unsusceptible to retrograde amnesic treatments. Single and multiple learning trials lead to different long-term forms of memory (LTM) depending on whether they are administered in massed or spaced trials (Menzel, 2001).

Foraging in pollinating insects is a behaviour with a highly regular sequential structure of events, ranging from actions within seconds to those separated by months, so that different memories are consulted during the sequence of events while foraging (Menzel, 1999). In the bee, the time courses of successive behaviours during foraging match the temporal dynamics of memory stages. Choices between flowers within the same patch quickly succeed each other and are performed during early STM. Choices between flowers of different patches occur after transition to late STM. Successive bouts are interrupted by the return to the hive, such that flower choices in a subsequent bout require retrieving information from MTM. The separation between the two forms of LTM may be related to the periods when flower patches are blooming.

The capacity and time span of working memory (i.e. the active memory guiding ongoing behaviour) has been estimated in invertebrates only for honeybees, during nectar foraging. In a natural foraging setting, short intervals (<1 min) between a learning and a test trial lead to high but rather unspecific responses, while long intervals lead to more specific responses (Menzel, 1999). Chittka and colleagues (1997) recorded the frequency of intervals between stay and shift flights made by bumblebees foraging on more than two plant species. Stay flights appeared at shorter intervals (around 2 s) than shift flights, indicating that immediate choices were dominated by the most recent and effective STM, but reference to more remote memories needed more time. In other words, longer intervals released working memory from the dominant memory of the last visit, allowing contributions from an earlier memory that had meanwhile been consolidated. Greggers and Menzel (1993) tested honeybees while foraging in a patch of four feeders, which delivered different flow rates of sucrose solution: bees stored the reward properties of these feeders in working memory. Similar results were found for eight feeders, indicating that the reward properties of up to eight feeders can be stored in working memory, with the time range of these specific working memories lying around 6 min. In DMTS, instead, the duration of working memories (to match the testing stimuli to the sample) are much shorter, around 5 s (Zhang *et al.*, 2005).

Exploratory Learning and Navigational Skills

Exploration is an elementary and fundamental form of learning about the structure of the world (Birke and Archer, 1983), training sensory and perceptual capacities, enhancing motor performance and learning about the guiding structures of the environment. However, exploration does not lead directly to the reduction of physical needs; it requires energy and time, and exposes bees to hazards and predators. As social animals, bees may also improve their perceptual and motor performances, and develop new behaviours by observation. Many forms of social learning (imitation, acoustic and visual communication, traditions in the social context) are based on observation, without obvious external reinforcing stimuli as in associative learning.

Honeybees exhibit multiple forms of exploratory learning, both for local navigation and for way-finding over greater distances. A characteristic behaviour close to the hive entrance (i.e. within 5 m) and feeding sites is 'turn-back-and-look' (TBL), with the bee turning around immediately after takeoff, hovering close to the location and performing half-circles in slow motion. Interestingly, bees prevented from performing TBL at a novel feeding site do not return to the hive, in contrast to the bees performing TBL (Opfinger, 1931; Lehrer, 1993). On returning to the goal, foragers tend to repeat the TBL, suggesting that they follow an optimization process by reducing the mismatch between current and stored views (Stürzl *et al.*, 2016). Experienced foragers trained to a feeding place, which is characterized by its spatial relation to surrounding landmarks, apply a similar matching strategy, suggesting that an egocentric reference frame may partially explain navigation also for way-finding over further distances (Collett and Graham, 2004; Zeil, 2012).

If foragers only relied on egocentric navigation, however, they would not need to explore the environment, carrying with them their path integration and the memory of the views established by TBL at the hive or the feeding place. Indeed, bees also need to relate landscape features to their sun compass, through exploratory orientation flights (i.e. within 30 m), which help them become familiar with the surroundings of their hive, and calibrate their sun compass and visual distance estimation: only after performing at least one exploratory orientation flight, can bees start their foraging activity (Becker, 1958; Vollbehr, 1975). Harmonic radar tracking has further allowed examination of whether these exploratory flights follow a systematic strategy of exploration and whether the structure of the environment induces specific exploratory flight patterns (Degen *et al.*, 2015). Moreover, exploratory flights further from the hive entrance increase in effectiveness through time, as bees reduce the time spent inspecting the immediate environment of the hive to explore different portions of the landscape. During these flights, bees learn landmark features: if displaced to directions explored after their first orientation flight, they return to the hive faster and with higher flight straightness, as compared to bees displaced to unexplored directions, even when egocentric navigation is excluded (Degen *et al.*, 2016). Possibly, bees return to the hive after localizing themselves according to learned spatial relations of ground structures to the hive (see Cheeseman *et al.*, 2014 for a controversial discussion).

Bees trained to a distant feeder return home not only by direct flights to the hive, but also via the feeder (Figure 3.3). The ability to decide between the hive and the feeder as the destination for a homing flight requires some form of relational representation of the two locations: given that neither of these two locations can be approached with the help of a beacon or the panorama, it is tempting to conclude that bees make decisions between potential goals, eventually taking novel shortcuts, by referring to a map-like structure of their spatial memory (Cheeseman *et al.*, 2014). Moreover, learned and dance-communicated locations are embedded in the same spatial memory structure, and their respective locations are taken into account when bees take decisions on the foraging route to follow (Menzel *et al.*, 2011). Experienced foragers, for instance, received food at the location FT, but only for 2–3 days (Figure 3.4). After several unsuccessful visits to the location, these bees started following dancers indicating another food location (FD): bees observing more than 15 waggle runs flew first to FD, the others to FT. Crucially, if the distance between the locations FD and FT was the

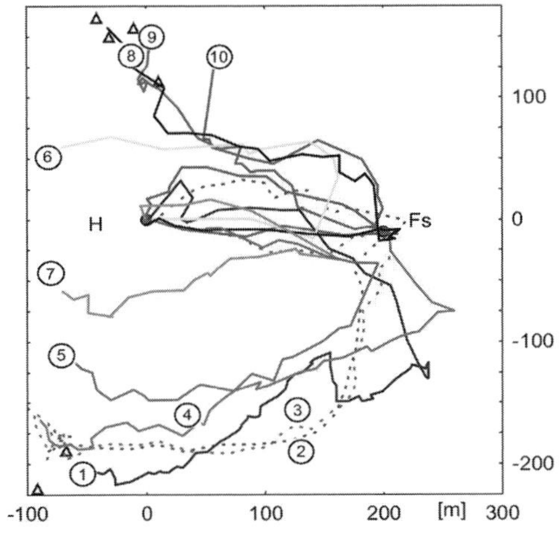

Figure 3.3. Homing flights of trained bees via the feeder F. Bees were trained from the hive to F, 200 m east of the hive. They were transported and released as described in the text. About a third of these bees directed their homing flights first to the area close to F, and then back to the hive. Only one of the 10 bees shown here landed at F (after Menzel *et al.*, 2005).

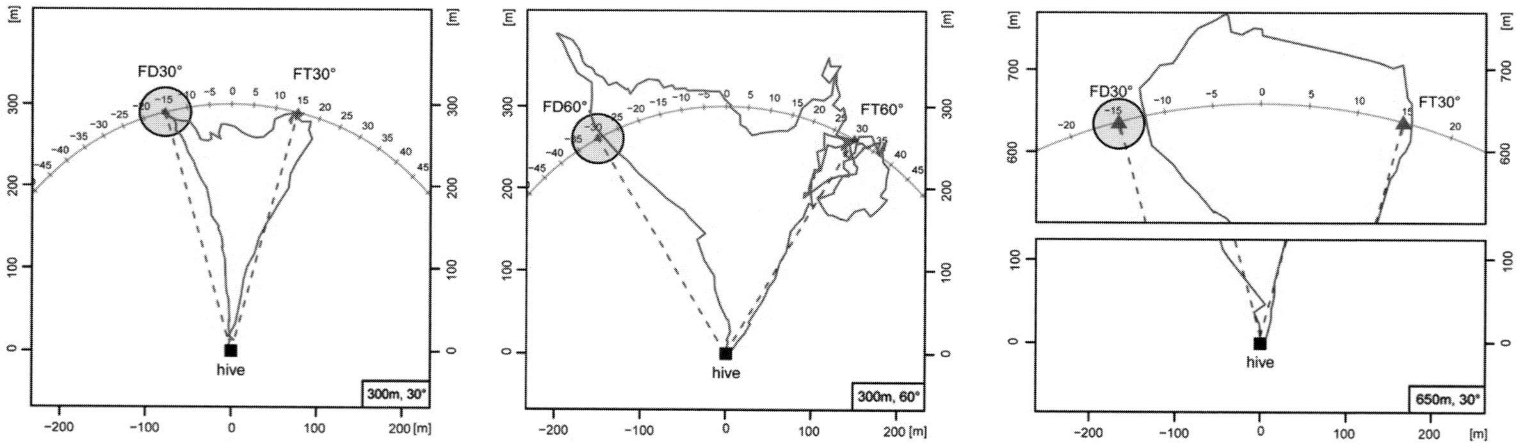

Figure 3.4. Novel short-cut flights of bees that were trained to the location FT (FT30° or FT60°) and afterwards followed a dancing bee that indicated a location FD (FD30° or FD60°; see text).
Modified after Menzel *et al.*, 2011.

same as the distance back to the hive, the bees also flew to the other location, taking a novel short cut (i.e. one which bees had not previously flown, nor had been communicated in the dance) when the hive was relatively close (i.e. 300 m), but not when it was further (i.e. 600 m). The information for the dance-indicated location FD was sufficient for the decision to aim for it when the animal was out in the field (having experienced that there was no more food available at FT), but not to fly directly to FD. The decision to steer towards one of the two locations obviously depended on the expected value at the respective locations: initially, this value was high for FT, but then it was degraded by experience and became lower than that for FD, if many dance rounds took place. Taken together, these data indicate a form of spatial memory that can be best conceptualized as cognitive map *sensu* Tolman (Tolman, 1948; Wiener *et al.*, 2011; see Cheeseman *et al.*, 2014; Cheung *et al.*, 2014, for the current state of the controversial debate about the concepts of a cognitive map in honeybees).

Social Communication

Bees perform a waggle dance to communicate to other bees the direct flight path to the indicated goal (a feeding site or a new nesting site), and the other bees (the recruits) perform their outbound flights according to the vector component of the dance message (von Frisch, 1967; Riley *et al.*, 2005). Thus, the waggle dance encodes the direct flight path in a symbolically communicated vector. The flight direction in relation to the current azimuth of the sun is given by the angle of the waggle phase relative to gravity on the vertical comb in the dark hive. The distance from the hive to the indicated location is measured visually and encoded in the number of waggle movements (and possibly other associated parameters such as waggle time, length of waggle run and time taken to complete a rotation). Remarkably, this kind of symbolic communication of locations is not known to exist in any other animal.

To date, it is still debated whether bees communicate the outbound flight vector as a flight instruction or rather the location of the indicated goal (food source, nest site), meaning that the recruits may use the encoded vector information to retrieve from their memory the spatial location of the goal – a series of landscape characteristics stored in the navigational memory. In the first case, the recruit uses only the information about the direct flight path from the hive to the communicated goal and follows this instruction without referring to its own memory of the landscape. In the second case, the recruit would interpret the communicated vector as being embedded in its navigation memory, and recall the flight along the reported vector and its end point, from a memory landscape. If the attending bee has gained experience about the indicated location (e.g. how rich the feeding site is, what odour it has, how the flower is to be manipulated, whether nectar or pollen is to be collected), then she will make her decision about whether she will reach the location depending on that experience, and will have certain expectations not only regarding the place, but also regarding its properties and the landscape characteristics she can expect to encounter. Therefore, different assumptions can be made about the cognitive processes involved in the communication process, decision-making and subsequent navigation during the waggle dance. Currently, no convincing evidence has been published supporting the higher-order cognitive components of the waggle dance communication process.

Nevertheless, it is difficult to avoid an assumption of intentionality involved in this communication process, because practically all the signals attached to the flight performance are not accessible during the communication process inside the dark hive, and they need to be interpreted on the base of the navigation memory of the receiving bee (Menzel, 2017). A striking example of message evaluation by receiving bees is the stop signal produced by scouts in a swarm. Scouts that have discovered a superior nest side inhibit another scout bee's efforts to continue advertising an inferior nest site, without actually inspecting the inferior nest site (Seeley *et al.*, 2012). This evaluation is based merely on the symbolic communication process, suggesting a mental state in which a comparison is made between transformed own experience and information provided by other animals.

All for One and One for All

Box 3.1 Cognition in Eusocial Naked Mole-Rats (*Heterocephalus glaber*)

Chris G. Faulkes

Naked mole-rats (NMRs), *Heterocephalus glaber*, have gained widespread attention since the 1980s, when they were the first vertebrate to be described to exhibit social insect-like behaviour (Jarvis, 1981). NMRs fit the classic definition of eusociality originally applied, for example, to bees, ants, wasps and termites, and their social system is at the extreme end of a continuum of cooperative breeding vertebrates. Living in colonies that commonly number around 100 individuals (but can exceed 290), with burrows that can total 3–4 km in total length, reproduction is restricted to a single 'queen' and 1–3 males. The rest of the colony of both sexes is reproductively suppressed by behavioural cues from the dominant queen – more than 99 per cent of NMRs will never breed directly, but gain indirect (inclusive) fitness benefits by aiding the queen, who is usually closely related. While much research has focused on the ultimate and proximate causes of sociality in NMRs (see Faulkes and Bennett, 2013), and more recently on their longevity, lack of senescence and extreme adaptations to the subterranean niche, surprisingly little work has been done on cognition. This is despite the fact that they live in an environment being both socially and spatially complex (i.e. with many individuals within their labyrinthine burrow).

It is clear even from a brief observation of a colony of NMRs that they recognize other individuals within their social group. This is manifest in dominance-related passing behaviour. On meeting face-to-face in a tunnel, and following a bout of sniffing, the dominant individual in the encounter will normally pass over the top of the subordinate (Clarke and Faulkes, 1997). The role of odour in this social decision-making has recently been supported in a study by Toora and colleagues (2015), where ablation of the primary olfactory epithelium affected dominance scores – although auditory cues may also be implicated (NMRs have more than 18

(*cont.*)

context-specific vocalizations). Odour is also important in colony-level recognition. NMRs are known to be highly xenophobic and will attack 'foreign' conspecifics. Indeed, in captivity it can be difficult to reintroduce animals back into their parent colonies after just a few days of removal. These individual- and colony-level discriminatory behaviours potentially imply establishing and maintaining a very large olfactory memory of individuals, at least for some days. The neural substrates of any such memory remain to be investigated.

Another cognitive challenge for NMRs is navigation through a complex network of tunnels. Could they perhaps exhibit a 'taxi driver effect', with increased development of the hippocampus associated with spatial learning? A preliminary study has indicated that the hippocampus in NMRs is relatively small for a rodent, although there are some structural distinctions (Amrein *et al.*, 2014). Intriguingly, Judd and Sherman (1996) found that NMRs returning from foraging vocalise and then follow each other's odour trails to food, paralleling the foraging recruitment system of some social insects.

Clearly, there exists a wealth of possibilities for studies of NMR cognition. The challenges of working on NMR colonies in the wild are considerable, given their habitat and subterranean lifestyle. However, they are relatively easily studied in captivity, in artificial burrow systems composed of clear Perspex boxes and interconnecting tubes that facilitate behavioural observation. Animals can also be easily identified individually with RFID tags, commonly used for laboratory animals and pets. With increasing numbers of captive colonies and many fascinating questions, cognitive studies of NMRs are certain to increase in the future.

References

Amrein, I., Becker A. S., Engler S., *et al.* (2014). Adult neurogenesis and its anatomical context in the hippocampus of three mole-rat species. *Frontiers in Neuroanatomy*, **8**, 39.

Clarke, F. M., and Faulkes C. G. (1997). Dominance and queen succession in captive colonies of the eusocial naked mole-rat, *Heterocephalus glaber*. *Proceedings of the Royal Society of London B*, **264**, 993–1000.

Faulkes, C. G., and Bennett, N. C. (2013). Plasticity and constraints on social evolution in African mole-rats: ultimate and proximate factors. *Philosophical Transactions of the Royal Society B*, **368**, 1618.

Jarvis, J. U. M. (1981). Eusociality in a mammal: cooperative breeding in naked mole-rat colonies. *Science*, **212**, 571–573.

Judd, T. M., and Sherman, P. W. (1996). Naked mole-rats recruit colony mates to food sources. *Animal Behaviour*, **52**, 957–969.

Toora, I., Clement, D., Carlson, E. N., and Holmes, M. M. (2015). Olfaction and social cognition in eusocial naked mole-rats, *Heterocephalus glaber*. *Animal Behaviour*, **107**, 175–181.

Field Guide

Testing in the Wild

Foraging bees learn the features of their food sources (flowers) by exploratory and operant forms of learning. This natural behaviour can be easily transferred into an experimental paradigm under natural conditions by offering droplets of sucrose solution at the hive entrance. Bees will be quickly attracted and will follow the droplets when these are gradually moved further away from the entrance, up to several hundred metres away within a few hours. Foragers will return to the feeding place every few minutes with high motivation to search for food, and because a practically unlimited number of potentially fast-learning animals are available in the hive, these experiments are very efficient.

Discrimination tests are performed by displaying two or more alternatives on a horizontal or vertical plate, rewarding only one with sucrose solution, and then testing the individually marked animal without reward (extinction tests). Sucrose solutions are obtained by mixing commercial sugar with water. Extinction tests are usually performed with only one bee approaching the testing place and video recording its choices. Tests usually run for up to 4–6-minute sessions for each bee and day. If new bees are required, highly concentrated sucrose solution is offered to the already trained bees: their waggle dances inside the colony will recruit new bees, which will be marked individually and exposed to a new training and testing session. Multiple perceptual tests can be performed with this simple set-up. Von Frisch (1914, 1921, 1922), for instance, discovered that bees distinguish colours, patterns and odours. Sophisticated test procedures can be combined with this operant form of training and have been successfully used to test colour constancy (with bees entering a box with two coloured plates, one having been previously associated with a reward), pattern recognition (using black/white and coloured patterns) and odour discrimination. These data can be used to interpret data from neurophysiological recordings of first- or higher-order sensory integration centres in the bee brain (colour vision: Vorobyev *et al.*, 2001; odour discrimination: Guerrieri *et al.*, 2005).

This simple set-up can also be used with Y-mazes examining delayed matching to sample or non-sample tasks (DMTS, DMTNS) to assess whether bees can extract and generalize rules, for instance (Giurfa, 2003). In these tasks, bees see a stimulus (the sample) through which they have to fly, and then have to choose (or not choose) the one out of two targets which resembles the sample by entering the arm of the Y-maze where the similar target has been positioned. If the bee matches her choice to the sample, she is rewarded with sucrose solution. DMTS have also been used to test working memory in foraging honeybees (Giurfa *et al.*, 2001) by delaying the bee's choice to estimate the duration of the working memory for the visual sample (Zhang *et al.*, 2005).

The structure of the navigation memory has been studied with catch-and-release experiments. Performing experiments under natural conditions makes it difficult to address some questions, but resorting to the lab or to simpler test conditions reduces the environment and may not allow animals to apply their real cognitive capacities. It is

Table 3.1. Essential tools to study cognition in honey bees and their function.

Tool	Function
Tags	Number tags are used to mark bees individually. These number tags are commercially available and are used by beekeepers for marking queens. Using two digit numbers, 5 different colours and 4 different orientations on the thorax, 2000 bees in a colony can be marked individually
Sucrose solution	Sucrose solution made of household sugar is used to reward bees both during natural training experiments and laboratory reward conditioning. Different concentrations lead to different reward effects
Neurophysiology of the honeybee brain	Usual intra- and extracellular recording techniques are used in neurobiological studies of the honeybee brain. The methods applied are more difficult than in insects with larger brains and require quite some sophistication
Radar tracking	Freely flying bees can be tracked over distances of up to 2 km using harmonic radar tracking. The bees tracked carry a transponder that converts the radar pulse (9 GHz) into its first harmonic (18 GHz). The harmonic signal is received by a custom-made amplifier and filter. The technique requires rather sophisticated instrumentation and can only be used in flat, horizontal and open areas
Patience	Bees defend themselves by stinging. Anybody working with bees needs to know whether they are insensitive to the bee venom

still possible to control landscape features by selecting appropriate study areas, e.g. those that exclude beacon orientation and image matching for close and distant cues as a navigation strategy. Animals familiar with the landscape surrounding the hive are trained stepwise to a feeding place. An animal is caught in a defined motivational state (e.g. when leaving a feeding place to return to the hive, or when leaving the hive after following a waggle dance) and then transported to an unexpected release site within its explored area. Because all experimental animals are individually marked by number tags, it is easy to select the respective animal for the current test situation. The animal is transferred to a small glass vial, kept in the dark during transfer, and released within 10 minutes at the indicated release site. In order to record the flight of the test animal, a radar transposer is attached to its number tag, as described in Menzel and colleagues (2005). Because the motivational state at the moment of capture changes during the time in the dark glass vial, it is important to release the animal as soon as possible. In our experiments, in which the test animal needed to be transferred to a release site several hundred metres away from the capture site, we usually required up to 10 minutes. Control tests showed that such an interval between capture and release did not affect the motivation of the animal. It is particularly impressive that recruits (i.e. bees that had just followed a waggle dance) still perform according to the information they gathered from the dancing bee (Riley *et al.*, 2005).

Flight trajectories are recorded by a custom-made harmonic radar system (Osborne *et al.*, 1997; Menzel *et al.*, 2012). Because the transponders attached to the bee emanate a very low energy of the first harmonic (18 GHz) of the radar pulse (9 GHz), special care has to be taken that no radar-reflecting objects are within the vicinity of the radar which would reflect the high energy of the primary wave. Furthermore, the area within the range of the radar (usually up to a 1-km radius) has to be horizontal in order to avoid any reflection of the transmitted primary wave from the ground. Because the custom-made radar requires expert maintenance and care, it is not a simple system to use. The transponders are also custom-made and require special training in how the miniature diode is fixed to the coil of the silver wire. Taken together, the harmonic radar system offers a range of potentials to study the navigation of middle-sized insects in the range of 1–2 km.

Testing in the Lab

Classical conditioning of restrained bees is a highly useful method to test the relation between learning and memory and brain structures (Matsumoto *et al.*, 2012; Menzel, 2012, 2014; Figure 3.2). Foraging bees are caught at the hive entrance, cooled as single bees on ice until they stop moving, and then fixed in a tube with a sticky tape in the neck region, such that the mouth parts and antennae are free to move. In winter time, bees are collected from a hive that is kept in a greenhouse, within a cage of approximately 1 m^3. Under these conditions, care is taken that bees collecting sucrose syrup or pollen are selected for the conditioning experiment. The bees are fed until satiation and kept overnight in a moist and cool place (18°C) until the next morning. These harnessed hungry animals rarely respond to an odour presentation with an extension of their mouthparts (proboscis), whereas they will almost invariably do so if a sugar solution touches their antennae (as unconditioned stimulus). Pairing odour presentation (as conditioned stimulus) with a sucrose reward will lead to a stable memory of this association after only a few pairing trials, and the bee will exhibit the conditioned proboscis extension to future presentations of the odour alone (Menzel and Bitterman, 1983). One particularly exciting result using this conditioning method combined with intracellular recording, staining and stimulation was that a single neuron, the neuromodulator octopamine VUMmx1 (ventral unpaired median neuron number 1 of the maxillary neuromere), represents the neural substrate of the rewarding stimulus and exhibits neural activity paralleling the animal's expectations, responding to unexpected sucrose presentations, but not to expected ones (Hammer, 1997).

Resources

Basic books:

- Menzel, R., and Eckoldt, M. (2016). *Die Intelligenz der Bienen*. KNAUS.
- Menzel, R., and Eckoldt, M. (2017). *L'intelligenzo del api*. Raphaello Cortina Editore.

Some labs working on bee cognition:

- My lab: www.bcp.fu-berlin.de/biologie/arbeitsgruppen/neurobiologie/ag_menzel/index.html
- The Robinson Lab: www.life.illinois.edu/robinson/
- The Seeley Lab: http://nbb.cornell.edu/thomas-seeley

Profile

Randolf studied biology, chemistry and zoology in Germany, and prepared his dissertation on colour learning in bees in 1967. Since 1976, he has been directing the Neurobiology Institute at the Freie Universität Berlin, where he investigates neurobiology, behaviour and cognition in honeybees, with a special focus on the neurobiology of learning and memory in a comparative perspective, and navigation.

References

Avargues-Weber, A., Deisig, N., and Giurfa, M. (2011). Visual cognition in social insects. *Annual Review of Entomology*, **56**, 423–443.

Becker, L. (1958). Untersuchungen über das Heimfindevermögen der Bienen. *Zeitschrift für Vergleichende Physiologie*, **41**, 1–25.

Birke, L. I., and Archer, J. (1983). Some issues and problems in the study of animal exploration. In *Exploration in animals and humans* (pp. 1–21). London: Van Nostrand Reinhold Co. Ltd.

Bloch, G., Solomon, S. M., Robinson, G. E., and Fahrbach, S. E. (2003). Patterns of PERIOD and pigment-dispersing hormone immunoreactivity in the brain of the European honeybee (*Apis mellifera*): age- and time-related plasticity. *Journal of Comparative Neurology*, **464**, 269–284.

Cheeseman, J. F., Millar, C. D., Greggers, U., *et al.* (2014). Way-finding in displaced clock-shifted bees proves bees use a cognitive map. *Proceedings of the National Academy of Sciences*, **111**, 8949–8954.

Cheung, A., Collett, M., Collett, T. S., *et al.* (2014). Still no convincing evidence for cognitive map use by honeybees. *Proceedings of the National Academy of Sciences*, **111**, 4396–4397.

Chittka, L., Gumbert, A., and Kunze, J. (1997). Foraging dynamics of bumble bees: correlates of movements within and between plant species. *Behavioral Ecology*, **8**, 239–249.

Collett, T. S., and Graham, P. (2004). Animal navigation: path integration, visual landmarks and cognitive maps. *Current Biology*, **14**, 475–477.

Degen, J., Kirbach, A., Reiter, L., *et al.* (2015). Exploratory behaviour of honeybees during orientation flights. *Animal Behaviour*, **102**, 45–57.

Degen, J., Kirbach, A., Reiter, L., *et al.* (2016). Honeybees learn landscape features during exploratory orientation flights. *Current Biology*, **26**, 2800–2804.

Filla, I., and Menzel, R. (2015). Mushroom body extrinsic neurons in the honeybee (*Apis mellifera*) brain integrate context and cue values upon attentional stimulus selection. *Journal of Neurophysiology*, **114**, 2005–2014.

Gahl, R. A. (1975). The shaking dance of honey bee workers: evidence for age discrimination. *Animal Behaviour*, **23**, 230–232.

Gerber, B., and Smith, B. H. (1998). Visual modulation of olfactory learning in honeybees. *Journal of Experimental Biology*, **201**, 2213–2217.

Getz, W. M., Brückner, D., and Smith, K. B. (1986). Conditioning honeybees to discriminate between heritable odors from full and half-sisters. *Journal of Comparative Physiology A*, **159**, 251–256.

Giurfa, M. (2003). Cognitive neuroethology: dissecting non-elemental learning in a honeybee brain. *Current Opinion in Neurobiology*, **13**, 726–735.

Giurfa, M., Eichmann, B., and Menzel, R. (1996). Symmetry perception in an insect. *Nature*, **382**, 458–461.

Giurfa, M., Zhang, S. W., Jenett, A., Menzel, R., and Srinivasan, M. V. (2001). The concepts of 'sameness' and 'difference' in an insect. *Nature*, **410**, 930–933.

Greggers, U., and Menzel, R. (1993). Memory dynamics and foraging strategies of honeybees. *Behavioral Ecology and Sociobiology*, **32**, 17–29.

Guerrieri, F., Lachnit, H., Gerber, B., and Giurfa, M. (2005). Olfactory blocking and odorant similarity in the honeybee. *Learning & Memory*, **12**, 86–95.

Hammer, M. (1997). The neural basis of associative reward learning in honeybees. *Trends in Neurosciences*, **20**, 245–252.

Hempel de Ibarra, N., Giurfa, M., and Vorobyev, M. V. (2002). Discrimination of coloured patterns by honeybees through chromatic and achromatic cues. *Journal of Comparative Physiology A*, **188**, 503–512.

Hussaini, S. A., and Menzel, R. (2013). Mushroom body extrinsic neurons in the honeybee brain encode cues and context differently. *Journal of Neuroscience*, **33**, 7154–7164.

Lehrer, M. (1993). Why do bees turn back and look? *Journal of Comparative Physiology A*, **172**, 549–563.

Matsumoto, Y., Menzel, R., Sandoz, J. C., and Giurfa, M. (2012). Revisiting olfactory classical conditioning of the proboscis extension response in honey bees: a step toward standardized procedures. *Journal of Neuroscience Methods*, **211**, 159–167.

Menzel, R. (1999). Memory dynamics in the honeybee. *Journal of Comparative Physiology A*, **185**, 323–340.

Menzel, R. (2001). Searching for the memory trace in a mini-brain, the honeybee. *Learning & Memory*, **8**, 53–62.

Menzel, R. (2012). The honeybee as a model for understanding the basis of cognition. *Nature Reviews Neuroscience*, **13**, 758–768.

Menzel, R. (2014). The insect mushroom body, an experience-dependent recoding device. *Journal of Physiology*, **108**, 84–95.

Menzel, R. (2017). Navigation and communication in insects. In *Learning and memory: a comprehensive reference* (pp. 389–405). Elsevier.

Menzel, R., and Bitterman, M. E. (1983). Learning by honey bees in an unnatural situation. In *Neuroethology and behavioral physiology: roots and growing points* (pp. 206–215). Berlin: Springer.

Menzel, R., and Müller, U. (1996). Learning and memory in honeybees: from behavior to neural substrates. *Annual Review of Neuroscience*, **19**, 379–404.

Menzel, R., Greggers, U., Smith, A., *et al.* (2005). Honey bees navigate according to a map-like spatial memory. *Proceedings of the National Academy of Sciences*, **102**, 3040–3045.

Menzel, R., Kirbach, A., Haass, W. D., *et al.* (2011). A common frame of reference for learned and communicated vectors in honeybee navigation. *Current Biology*, **21**, 645–650.

Menzel, R., Lehmann, K., Manz, G., Fuchs, J., and Kobolofsky, M. G. (2012). Vector integration and novel shortcutting in honeybee navigation. *Apidologie*, **43**, 229–243.

Opfinger, E. (1931). Über die Orientierung der Biene an der Futterquelle. *Zeitschrift für Vergleichende Physiologie*, **15**, 432–487.

Osborne, J. L., Williams, I. H., Carreck, N. L., *et al.* (1997). Harmonic radar: a new technique for investigating bumblebee and honeybee foraging flight. *Proceedings of the International Symposium on Pollination, Acta Horticulturae*, **437**, 163.

Plettner, E., Slessor, K. N., Winston, M. L., Robinson, G. E., and Page, R. E., Jr. (1993). Mandibular gland components and ovarian development as measures of caste differentiation in the honey bee (*Apis mellifera*). *Journal of Insect Physiology*, **39**, 235–240.

Riley, J. R., Greggers, U., Smith, A. D., Reynolds, D. R., and Menzel, R. (2005). The flight paths of honeybees recruited by the waggle dance. *Nature*, **435**, 205–207.

Robinson, G. E., and Page, R. E., Jr. (1989). Genetic determination of nectar foraging, pollen foraging, and nest-site scouting in honey bee colonies. *Behavioral Ecology and Sociobiology*, **24**, 317–323.

Seeley, T. D., Visscher, P. K., Schlegel, T., Hogan, P. M., Franks, N. R., and Marshall, J. A. (2012). Stop signals provide cross inhibition in collective decision-making by honeybee swarms. *Science*, **335**, 108–111.

Stürzl, W., Zeil, J., Boeddeker, N., and Hemmi, J. M. (2016). How wasps acquire and use views for homing. *Current Biology*, **26**, 470–482.

Tibbetts, E. A. (2002). Visual signals of individual identity in the wasp *Polistes fuscatus*. *Proceedings of the Royal Society of London B: Biological Sciences*, **269**, 1423–1428.

Tibbetts, E. A., and Dale, J. (2004). A socially enforced signal of quality in a paper wasp. *Nature*, **432**, 218–222.

Tolman, E. C. (1948). Cognitive maps in rats and men. *Psychological Review*, **55**, 189–208.

Vollbehr, J. (1975). Zur Orientierung junger Honigbienen bei ihrem 1. Orientierungsflug. *Zoologische Jahrbücher Physiologie*, **79**, 33–69.

von Frisch, K. (1914). Der Farbensinn und Formensinn der Biene. *Zoologische Jahrbücher Physiologie*, **37**, 1–238.

von Frisch, K. (1921). Über den Sitz des Geruchssinnes bei Insekten. *Zoologische Jahrbücher Physiologie*, **38**, 1–68.

von Frisch, K. (1922). Methoden sinnesphysiologischer und psychologischer Untersuchungen an Bienen. In *Handbuch der biologischen Arbeitsmethoden* (Abt. VI, Teil D, E). Urban und Schwarzenberg.

von Frisch, K. (1967). *The dance language and orientation of bees*. Cambridge, MA: Harvard University Press.

Vorobyev, M., Brandt, R., Peitsch, D., Laughlin, S. B., and Menzel, R. (2001). Colour thresholds and receptor noise: behaviour and physiology compared. *Vision Research*, **41**, 639–653.

Werner, A., Menzel, R., and Wehrhahn, C. (1988). Color constancy in the honeybee. *Journal of Neuroscience*, **8**, 156–159.

Wiener, J., Shettleworth, S., Bingman, V. P., *et al.* (2011). Animal navigation: a synthesis. In *Animal thinking: contemporary issues in comparative cognition* (pp. 51–78). Cambridge, MA: MIT Press.

Wilson, E. O. (1971). *The insect societies*. Cambridge, MA: Harvard University Press.

Zeil, J. (2012). Visual homing: an insect perspective. *Current Opinion in Neurobiology*, **22**, 285–293.

Zhang, S. W., Bock, F., Si, A., Tautz, J., and Srinivasan, M. V. (2005). Visual working memory in decision making by honey bees. *Proceedings of the National Academy of Sciences*, **102**, 5250–5255.

4 Carib Grackles – Field and Lab Work on a Tame, Opportunistic Island Icterid

Simon Ducatez, Sarah E. Overington, Jean-Nicolas Audet, Marine Battesti and Louis Lefebvre

Species Description

Barbados is a relatively small island (432 km²) in the Lesser Antilles. Characterized by a dry and a wet season, the island is the geological result of an accretionary prism and is covered over most of its area by a series of coral reef limestone terraces, with very few freshwater streams. Largely anthropized and lacking any remnant of primary habitat, it is mostly covered with urban areas, tourism-related infrastructures and sugar cane plantations. Although the avian diversity is relatively low on the island (31 native and seven invasive breeding species; Buckley *et al.*, 2009), a handful of species are particularly abundant. The Carib grackle (*Quiscalus lugubris fortirostris*) is one of them, and the squeaky and metallic notes of its display song make up the background acoustic atmosphere almost everywhere on the island. From Bridgetown airport's car park to the cliffs of North Point, the Carib grackle's 'song-spread' display is likely the most easily observed avian behaviour on the island. While raising the head and lifting the beak towards the sky, the bird extends its wings and raises its tail (Figure 4.1), singing all the while.

Listed in the *Least Concern* category by the IUCN, with overall populations being stable, this grackle's ability to exploit and spread in anthropized and disturbed habitats (including urban areas) likely explains its success. Its distribution includes coastal Northern South America from Colombia to Brazil, and Trinidad and Tobago and the Lesser Antilles, from Grenada to Montserrat. In addition to its boldness and ease of observation in the field, the Carib grackle's ability to thrive throughout highly disturbed areas makes it an excellent candidate species to investigate how cognition may have shaped these birds' strategies to deal with major environmental changes.

Except for a few anecdotal observations, all investigations of Carib grackle behaviour and cognition have been conducted in Barbados. *Quiscalus lugubris fortirostris* is a subspecies endemic to Barbados, and contrary to many Barbadian species that came from the west in the Lesser Antilles, originated from the south in Trinidad (Lovette *et al.*, 1999).

Anatomy

Barbados grackles are unique in lacking the colour dimorphism that characterizes almost all other *Quiscalus lugubris* populations. The male is entirely black with violet

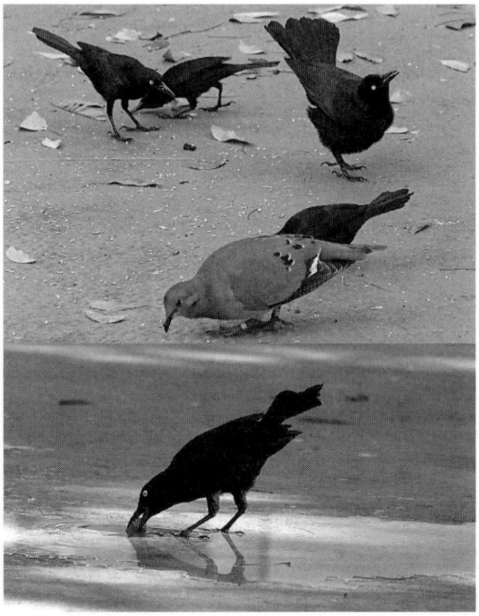

Figure 4.1. Carib grackles in the wild in Barbados. Top: typical group foraging on the ground, in association with a Zenaida dove. The individual on the upper right side is showing the 'song-spread' display. Bottom: a grackle dunking a dog pellet to soften it before swallowing it.

iridescence, with a medium-long keel-shaped tail. Its beak and feet are entirely black, whereas its iris is pale yellow. Females are almost as dark as males, although males (M) and females (F) can nevertheless be reliably distinguished by several morphological traits that differ between the sexes (all $p < 0.001$, $n = 94$; Overington *et al.*, 2010): weight (F = 49.6 g ± 0.96; M = 61.1 g ± 0.54), length of the tail (F = 83 mm ± 0.84; M = 93 mm ± 0.68), wing (F = 98.2 mm ± 0.86; M = 110.0 mm ± 0.43), tarsus (F = 29.6 mm ± 0.20; M = 32.2 mm ± 0.17) and bill (F = 17 mm ± 0.24; M = 19 mm ± 0.15; width: F = 5 mm ± 0.09; M = 6 mm ± 0.07). Carib grackles are noticeably smaller than closely related species such as *Q. major, Q. mexicanus* and *Q. quiscula.*

Grackles, including *Q. lugubris*, have a strong beak which they use for pecking, digging in the ground looking for food, turning over litter, and pulling, probing or prying with an open beak (Lefebvre *et al.*, 1997). The mobility of the head and beak contributes to the high motor diversity of this species (Griffin *et al.*, 2014), which is a trait likely favouring innovative problem-solving (Huber and Gajdon, 2006).

Grackles have residual (corrected by body size allometry) brain sizes that are approximately 0.5 standard deviations above the avian mean (Iwaniuk, 2003), suggesting natural or sexual selection on their brain processing capacities. Among grackles and their Icterid relatives, *Q. lugubris* are close to the larger-brained extreme of the phylogenetic distribution of residual brain sizes (Figure 4.2). Mean endocranial volume is 2.02 for males (± SD = 0.19, $n = 14$) and 1.81 for females (± 0.13, $n = 9$). Ancestral state reconstruction (Maddison and Maddison, 2008; see Figure 4.2) suggests that the residual brain size of *Q. lugubris* has increased over time.

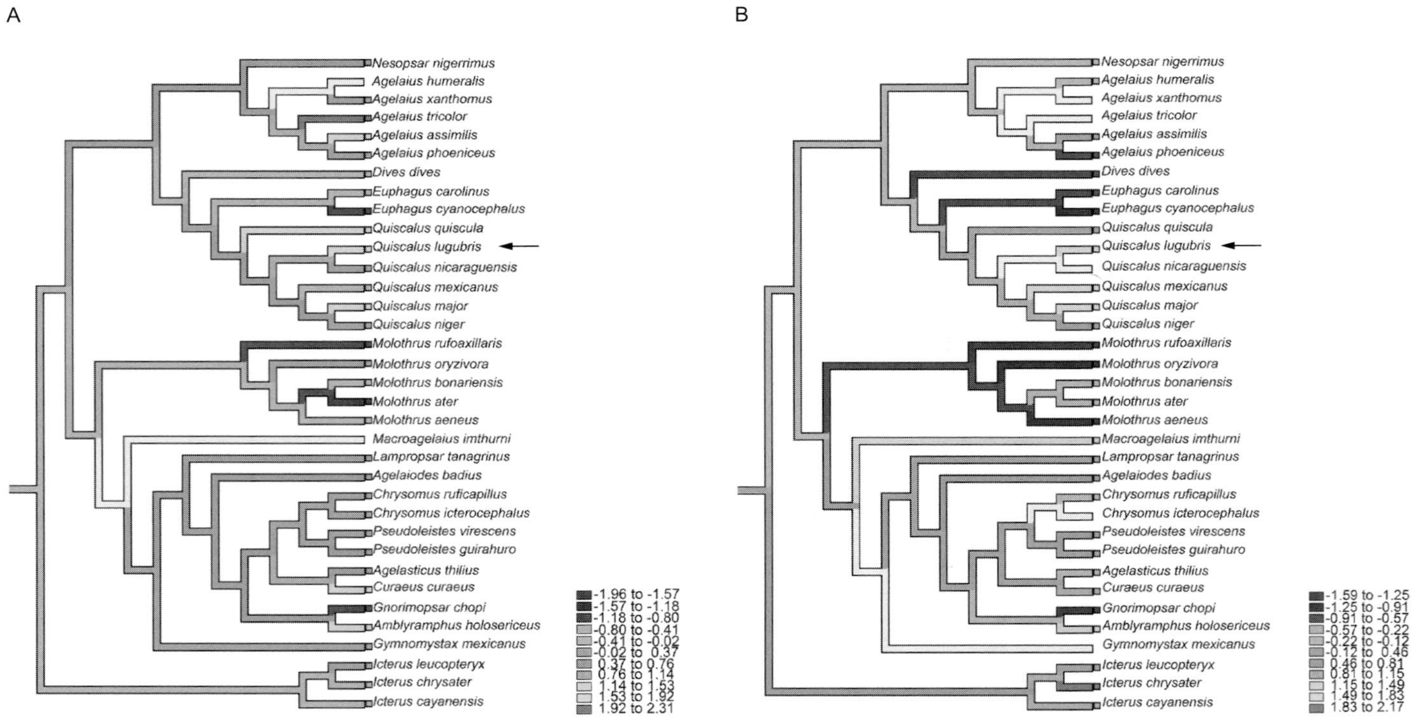

Figure 4.2. Parsimony ancestral state reconstruction of residual endocranial volume across grackles and allies (and three *Icterus* outgroup species), for male (A) and female (B) birds. A positive residual represents an endocranial volume that is larger than expected, given the slope of the log–log allometric relationship between endocranial volume and body mass in this clade. *Q. lugubris* is indicated by an arrow.
From Overington *et al*. (2010).

Perception

Like most birds, Carib grackles predominantly rely on sight. No specific information is available on how *Q. lugubris* might differ from other species, but some comparative information is available on the related common grackle *Q. quiscula* (McNeil *et al.*, 2005). Like most passerines, Carib grackles also have good acoustic perception. They emit a display song in social interactions, as well as a 'chuck'-like alarm call in threatening situations.

Life Cycle

The life cycle of Carib grackles has been investigated in detail in Trinidad and Venezuela, but to our knowledge not on the Barbados subspecies. Carib grackles normally nest in colonies that vary from a few to several dozens per tree, although solitary nests have also been found. The female builds the nest alone, before laying 2–4 eggs. She incubates for 12 days, and then both parents feed the chicks for a period of about 14 days. The exact period of post-fledging parental care has not been precisely studied, but immatures begging their parents for food and being fed far from the colonies are frequently observed in Barbados.

Because males and females play different roles during the breeding period (only females build the nest), sexual differences in cognition and behaviour might be expected. For instance, Griffin (pers. comm.) has observed that females in captivity tend to respond to conspecific alarm calls with more calls, but males with fewer. Although this species has a relatively short development time, its relatively long post-fledging parental care period and the relatively long lifetime for a bird of this size are consistent with the development of a larger brain and an innovative lifestyle (Sol *et al.*, 2016).

Identification

Individual identification requires banding, as different individuals are indistinguishable except for morphological abnormalities (some birds have deformed legs or feet). Combinations of coloured aluminium bands (size 3 or 3B) are particularly convenient to quickly and easily identify birds.

Ecological Characteristics

The Carib grackle is both a habitat and a dietary generalist. It occurs from open woodlands and scrubs to pastures, plantations, palm groves, parks and gardens, urban and suburban areas, covering pretty much every habitat type in Barbados. Omnivorous, it feeds on arthropods, small vertebrates, seeds and fruits. In urban areas, it mostly forages in flocks on the ground, and also feeds on food scraps, eventually entering restaurants and houses and opening garbage bags and food containers – all examples of its opportunistic behaviour. Breeding decisions are also opportunistic: birds can practically nest throughout the entire year, as long as the conditions are favourable, although in Trinidad and Venezuela, *Q. lugubris* mostly breed between May and September. This flexibility in terms of habitat use, diet and breeding season suggests that grackles may be able to respond opportunistically to different environmental conditions and to changes in their environment through plastic behavioural responses.

In Barbados, invasive species such as the feral cat and the small Asian mongoose (*Herpestes javanicus*) are likely the most important predators of Carib grackles. Alarm calls are also given to feral vervet monkeys, dogs and humans (Griffin, 2008). A recent blog post (http://100barbadosbirds.blogspot.com/2015/06/the-grackles-chronicle-other-side-of.html) has documented predation of grackle nestlings by a cattle egret (*Bubulcus ibis*), another invasive species. The apparent absence of predators before these invasions likely explains the boldness of the birds today, although the low species diversity (and thus limited number of competitors) and the anthropogenically modified nature of the island also likely contributed to the behavioural characteristics of these birds.

Social Characteristics

Carib grackles live in open social groups of up to a few dozens of individuals. The organization of this social system remains poorly studied, although fission–fusion dynamics, especially in response to changes in food aggregation, are expected. As a result, recapture rates at the same site are low. As a social forager, the Barbados Carib grackle is an excellent model species to investigate producer–scrounger interactions (Morand-Ferron *et al.*, 2007); like other *Quiscalus* species (Keeler, 1963), the Carib grackle shows frequent intraspecific kleptoparasitism.

As a communal rooster and a social breeder, relatively strong social bonds seem to associate parents and their fledglings. Adults, for instance, can often be observed passing bread and rice to begging juveniles through the wire mesh of their cage during captive experiments (Reader *et al.*, 2002). Finally, Carib grackles aggregate in mixed species groups with Shiny cowbirds (*Molothrus bonariensis*), Zenaida doves (*Zenaida aurita*; Figure 4.1), common ground doves (*Columbina passerin*) and Barbados bullfinches (*Loxigilla barbadensis*), especially around anthropogenic food sources.

A Model Species to Investigate Innovation, Problem-Solving and Learning in Wild Populations

The anatomical, life cycle, ecological and social characteristics of the Carib grackle suggest a potentially important role of cognition in shaping this opportunistic, generalist and social lifestyle. Supporting this idea, several innovative behaviours have been observed in Barbados. Carib grackles, like many *Quiscalus* species, will dunk dry food pellets in water before ingesting them (Figure 4.1). Barbados grackles have also been seen foraging for dead insects under the windshield wipers of parked cars (Reader *et al.*, 2002) and eating fish scraps at a fish market. On several islands, Carib grackles have been seen preying on lizards (Wunderle, 1981; Audet, pers. comm.), and in Venezuela catching small fish (Rodriguez-Ferraro, 2015). In Curaçao, *Q. lugubris* were seen foraging for scraps in a parking lot at night under artificial lights (Debrot, 2014). The whole genus *Quiscalus* is innovative, coming second only to *Corvus* among North

American passerines (Overington et al., 2009a), while the family to which the genus belongs, Icteridae, is only slightly less innovative than Thraupidae in the Neotropics, when research effort is taken into account (see figure 2 in Lefebvre *et al.*, 2016). Moreover, the behavioural characteristics of this species, such as tameness, exploratory behaviour and opportunism, make it relatively easy to work on it, because it quickly habituates to captivity and is easily motivated to participate in different tasks. Finally, the existence of a comprehensive phylogeny of the Icteridae family (Powell *et al.*, 2014) favours comparative studies across species of this family.

State of the Art

Field and aviary studies of Carib grackle cognition have focused on four main topics: (a) social learning of feeding and alarm behaviours; (b) innovation and problem-solving; (c) other cognitive measures, like string-pulling, associative and reversal learning; and (d) temperament.

Social Learning

In Barbados, Carib grackles are often the first avian species to discover a new food source. Because of their conspicuous plumage, vocalization and social behaviour, they attract other birds to the food. In particular, territorial Zenaida doves learn socially from grackles, with which they feed unaggressively in the field (Figure 4.1), in contrast to the aggressive interactions doves have with territorial neighbours (Dolman *et al.*, 1996). Grackles learn socially from other grackles and doves, copying the technique (i.e. open-beak or closed-beak pecks) shown by their tutor (Lefebvre *et al.*, 1997).

The alarm behaviour that Carib grackles show towards a predator can be socially transferred to a previously innocuous stimulus (a pigeon-like model), when alarm calls are presented after the innocuous stimulus (as in classical conditioning; Griffin, 2008), or even simultaneously (Griffin and Galef, 2005). In the field, grackle alarm calls are also used by Zenaida doves, which respond by interrupting feeding and showing flight preparation behaviour (Griffin *et al.*, 2005).

Innovation and Problem-Solving

Carib grackles (like other *Quiscalus* species, see table 1 in Morand-Ferron *et al.*, 2004) sometimes dunk dry food in the field. However, this might not be an example of spontaneous innovation. Most adult grackles are indeed capable of dunking in captivity (Morand-Ferron *et al.*, 2004) and the frequency with which they do so in the field varies extensively depending on social and environmental conditions. When food is rare, soft and far from a source of water, with numerous competitors and a barrier increasing dunking cost, dunking can be entirely absent or low (Morand-Ferron *et al.*, 2004, 2006, 2007; Morand-Ferron and Lefebvre, 2007). When food is abundant, hard and close to water, and potential conspecific thieves distant, dunking frequency increases. The rarity of dunking in most field contexts is thus a question of expression (depending on its costs and benefits) rather than a question of limited capacity in few individuals, and it is partially governed by the frequency-dependent relationship between dunkers and conspecific thieves of dunked food (Morand-Ferron *et al.*, 2007). Even in cages where potential thieves are on the other side of a wire mesh, grackles will dunk pellets in the water source that is farthest from the conspecific (Overington *et al.*, 2009b). However, they will not use a barrier to hide from the competitor, contrary to what some corvids have been shown to do (Bugnyar and Heinrich, 2005; Clayton *et al.*, 2007).

Most experiments on innovative problem-solving in *Quiscalus lugubris* require obstacle removal (Figure 4.3). Carib grackles are fast at solving such tasks, both in the field and in aviaries (Webster and Lefebvre, 2001; Overington *et al.*, 2009b, 2011; Ducatez *et al.*, 2015). When given visible food in a dish with a lid that needs to be removed by pulling, lifting or pecking at its edges, grackles will first peck at the part of the lid above the food, and then vary the location of their pecks until those directed near the edges cause the lid to move. Grackles that succeed at this task have a higher rate of pecking at the edges than individuals that fail, with the latter birds persisting more at ineffectual pecks at the lid centre under which the food is visible. Changing from centre to edge pecks is progressive, yielding no suggestion of an 'insightful' sudden shift in

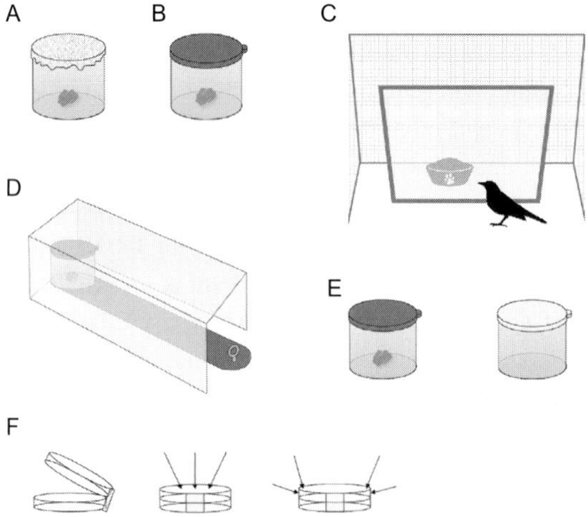

Figure 4.3. (A) Plastic cup with visible food reward covered with aluminium foil. The bird has to pierce the aluminium to access the reward. (B) Obstacle removal task used by Ducatez and colleagues (2015): transparent plastic cup with visible food reward covered with a plastic lid. The bird has to push or pry off the lid to access the reward. (C) Detour-reaching task made of a transparent Plexiglas sheet (25 × 55 × 3 cm) inserted in a wood frame; the reward is on the side opposite to the bird, so that it has to detour around the board to get the reward. (D) The 'tunnel' task, used by Ducatez and colleagues (2015): a transparent rectangular box opens on only one side. A transparent cylindrical tube containing food is inserted at the closed end of the tunnel and a wooden stick attached to it, so that the bird has to pull on the stick to get the tube out of the tunnel. (E) Associative learning task, made of two plastic cups covered with a plastic lid. The reward is shown for illustrative purposes, but it is not visible during the tests, as each cup is covered with a differently coloured tape. (F) Obstacle removal task used by Overington and colleagues (2011): a transparent, hinged dish. Left: the task is drawn from the experimenter's viewpoint; middle: incorrect probe locations, which can never lead to solving it; right: correct probe locations, which lead to solving it.

strategy. Gluing the lid so that it does not move when pecked, pulled or lifted near the edges reduces later success (Overington *et al.*, 2011). More complicated versions of obstacle removal (like the tunnel task, which first requires the bird to pull a lid-covered dish from an enclosure) are readily solved by Carib grackles. Individuals that solve this task faster also tend to solve the simpler lid removal task faster (Ducatez *et al.*, 2015), suggesting individual consistency in problem-solving.

Other Cognitive Measures: String-Pulling, Associative and Reversal Learning

String-pulling is a classic test often thought to require insight and causal reasoning. Carib grackles were capable of string-pulling, but only two of 31 individuals tested were successful (as compared to 17 of 42 Barbados bullfinches, in line with other studies comparing Icteridae and Thraupidae; Audet *et al.*, 2016).

Associative learning is also a learning mechanism often tested in animal cognition, especially in its reversal learning version, which is considered the standard paradigm for cognitive flexibility. Compared to their strong problem-solving and social learning performance, Carib grackles are surprisingly slow at discrimination and reversal learning. Fast problem-solvers are in fact slower in discrimination learning as compared to slow problem-solvers (Ducatez *et al.*, 2015). This might be due to a speed–accuracy trade-off, where the tendency to rapidly approach and interact with the novel apparatus in a problem-solving context, using a variety of motor acts, leads to many errors in two-choice learning tasks, where exploration of multiple options is penalized (Ducatez *et al.*, 2015). Whatever the case may be, obstacle removal problems and reversal learning trends appear to differ at all the scales where they are assessed, whether interindividual, interpopulation or interspecific, suggesting that they do not measure similar cognitive processes (Audet and Lefebvre, 2017).

Temperament: Boldness and Neophobia

In the field, Carib grackles are usually the first (or second, shortly after Barbados bullfinches) avian species to arrive at a novel food source or a novel testing apparatus (Webster and Lefebvre, 2001; Ducatez *et al.*, 2017). In captivity, exploration of a new cage, latency to feed after disturbance by a human and response to a novel object placed near food (neophobia) are associated with problem-solving in lid removal tasks (Overington *et al.*, 2011; Ducatez *et al.*, 2015).

All for One and One for All

Box 4.1 Collective Cognition

Noam Miller

Many animal species, including several birds, live in groups. Aggregating in groups provides benefits (from reduced predation to improved foraging), as well as costs

(cont.)

(due to competition and interference; Krause and Ruxton, 2002). For example, sparrows in larger flocks can spend less time on vigilance when foraging, because there are more pairs of eyes scanning for predators (Lima, 1995), but may also experience increased resource competition (Johnson *et al.*, 2001). Some raptors hunt collectively and many avian prey species collectively mob predators to drive them off. Being part of a group also shapes many cognitive processes, such as learning and decision-making. Individuals may have to compromise on their preferred behavioural choice in order to remain within a moving group. For example, pairs of pigeons homing together average their preferred individual routes, while larger pigeon flocks form navigational hierarchies (Nagy *et al.*, 2010).

Animals in groups often have to balance environmental information derived from their own past experiences with potentially conflicting information gleaned from the behaviours of conspecifics, all while maintaining the cohesion of the group. Studies that manipulate either or both these sources of information are gradually uncovering the rules by which such compromises are made (Hoppitt and Laland, 2011). Additional factors, such as consistent individual differences (sometimes referred to as animal 'personalities'), are increasingly seen to influence – and be influenced by – collective dynamics, in ways that have yet to be completely understood.

Studying the dynamics of collective behaviour presents several challenges. Group sizes can range from two (e.g. a breeding pair) to several thousands (e.g. starling flocks), groups may cover large distances (e.g. when migrating), and the interactions between individuals can range in complexity from maintaining a personal space to the organization of alloparental care. In species that form stable membership groups, individuals may recognize each other, form hierarchies and track lineages (e.g. in pigeons, Japanese quails, or chickens).

Traditional methods of studying collective behaviour mostly involved presenting a group with a task or stimulus, recording their resulting movement (often, of necessity, in a lab) and extracting some basic features of their spatial distribution, such as the mean nearest neighbour distance (i.e. the distance between each individual and the closest other member of the group) or group polarization (i.e. the degree to which individuals in the group are all facing the same direction). Given the complexity of social interactions noted above, these measures have recently been supplemented by network-based analyses (Krause *et al.*, 2015), sophisticated algorithms for determining group membership (replacing definitions based purely on between-individual distances; Rosenthal *et al.*, 2015) and social learning tasks that assess how information flows through animal groups (Hoppitt and Laland, 2011; Krause *et al.*, 2015).

Improvements in automated tracking technology and lighter GPS loggers have allowed researchers to collect detailed trajectories of flocks in the wild (Nagy *et al.*, 2010) and follow animals for longer periods of time and over greater distances. These advances and others are gradually shifting the kinds of questions that researchers ask about collective effects on cognition. Better tools and a growing understanding of the underlying principles of such effects have also helped increase

(cont.)

the diversity of species that are being studied. Researchers have observed coordination of behaviour within groups extending from parts of a single-celled slime mould (e.g. Reid *et al.*, 2016) to members of human crowds; collective decisions being shaped by (the lack of) consensus in ants, fish, birds and herding mammals (Sumpter, 2006); and local interactions driving large-scale behavioural correlations in everything, from flocks of starlings (Cavagna *et al.*, 2010) to Facebook networks (Goel *et al.*, 2010).

References

Cavagna, A., Cimarelli, A., Giardina, I., *et al.* (2010). Scale-free correlations in startling flocks. *Proceedings of the National Academy of Sciences*, **107**, 11865–11870.

Goel, S., Mason, W., and Watts, D. J. (2010). Real and perceived attitude agreement in social networks. *Journal of Personality and Social Psychology*, **99**, 611–621.

Hoppitt, W., and Laland, K. N. (2011). *Social learning: an introduction to mechanisms, methods, and models*. Princeton, NJ: Princeton University Press.

Johnson, C. A., Giraldeau, L. A., and Grant, J. W. A. (2001). The effect of handling time on interference among house sparrows foraging at different seed densities. *Behaviour*, **138**, 597–614.

Krause, J., and Ruxton, G. D. (2002). *Living in groups*. Oxford: Oxford University Press.

Krause, J., James, R., Franks, D. W., and Croft, D. P. (2015). *Animal social networks*. Oxford: Oxford University Press.

Lima, S. L. (1995). Back to the basics of anti-predatory vigilance: the group size effect. *Animal Behavior*, **49**, 11–20.

Nagy, M., Ákos, Z., Biro, D., and Vicsek, T. (2010). Hierarchical group dynamics in pigeon flocks. *Nature*, **464**, 890–894.

Reid, C. R., MacDonald, H., Mann, R. P., Marshall, J. A. R., Latty, T., and Garnier, S. (2016). Decision-making without a brain: how an amoeboid organism solves the two-armed bandit. *Interface*, **13**, 20160030.

Rosenthal, S. B., Twomey, C. R., Hartnett, A. T., Wu, H. S., and Couzin, I. D. (2015). Revealing the hidden networks of interaction in mobile animal groups allows prediction of complex behavioral contagion. *Proceedings of the National Academy of Sciences*, **112**, 4690–4695.

Sumpter, D. J. T. (2006). The principles of collective animal behaviour. *Philosophical Transactions of the Royal Society B*, **361**, 5–22.

Field Guide

To measure cognition in wild birds, two approaches are possible: direct observations in the wild, or capture and maintenance in captivity for short testing periods. An important limitation to working with wild birds, compared to birds raised in captivity, is the lack of knowledge of their age and previous experience, and thus of how these may shape response to cognitive tasks. In wild birds, it is also difficult to follow individuals across seasons and years, to assess consistency in cognitive performances, and associations between cognition and life history. However, working on wild birds has a range of advantages, including the greater ecological relevance of measuring cognition and behaviour on them, as compared to captive conspecifics.

The first approach relies on observations of wild individuals in their natural habitat, devising systems and protocols to manipulate the birds' environment, in order to record their response to this manipulation. Direct tests of problem-solving can be conducted in the field (e.g. Webster and Lefebvre, 2001), but indirect tests can also be devised, for example by manipulating foraging conditions that affect social interactions (e.g. Morand-Ferron *et al.*, 2007). Grackles are tame and used to anthropogenic food, making them ideal for field experiments. The downside is that the social behaviour of grackles makes it difficult to obtain independent measures of individual birds, as conspecifics will interfere with the test targeted for single birds. In contrast, territorial defence will keep conspecifics away from the testing site in species like *Zenaida aurita* (see Boogert *et al.*, 2010) or *Loxigilla barbadensis*. In the second approach, birds can be caught and maintained in captivity for a few days or weeks. After a period of habituation to captivity and to the presence of humans (during which individual differences in boldness can be assessed), a range of protocols can be used to test cognition in standardized conditions, controlling in particular the hunger levels that may strongly affect motivation to participate in tests rewarded with food.

Permits

Elaborating protocols that take into account animal welfare and ethical considerations is the key towards obtaining permits, in addition to the requirements of the competent authorities. To work with animals in Barbados, you need permission from the Heritage Department of the Barbados Ministry of Environment and Drainage (www.heritage.gov.bb/about_nhd.html). Permit requests need to be detailed and may take several months to be approved.

Where and How to Catch the Birds

Carib grackles occur virtually everywhere on the island of Barbados, which allows the capture of individuals from different habitats to test for environmental variation in cognition. We mostly caught birds around the Bellairs Research Institute, an urban area where grackles are particularly tame and used to anthropogenic food (the institute is next to a public park with picnic tables), making them easier to attract into traps and limiting stress during transportation. Transport, even if from a slightly farther site, can be done by putting the birds in individual fabric bags, where darkness and narrow space limit the possibility of movement and injury.

Several trapping methods can be used, although the use of walk-in traps on the ground, baited with seeds, bread and/or dog pellets, is the most effective one (Figure 4.4). This trapping method, however, may select the tamest individuals within a population, with shyer ones avoiding entering the trap. To limit this potential bias, leaving the trap open for several days allows birds to habituate to it. Alternatively, mist nets can be used, although the experimenter needs to know where the birds are likely to fly. Moreover, grackles are particularly skilled at escaping, limiting the efficiency of this method. Furthermore, predators such as mongooses and cats were commonly seen around the traps, attracted by the birds feeding around the bait or trapped in the net. Continuous surveillance of the traps and nets is thus needed to avoid predation of the targeted birds. Human disturbance is also an important factor to consider when deciding where to put the traps or nets, especially in urban areas.

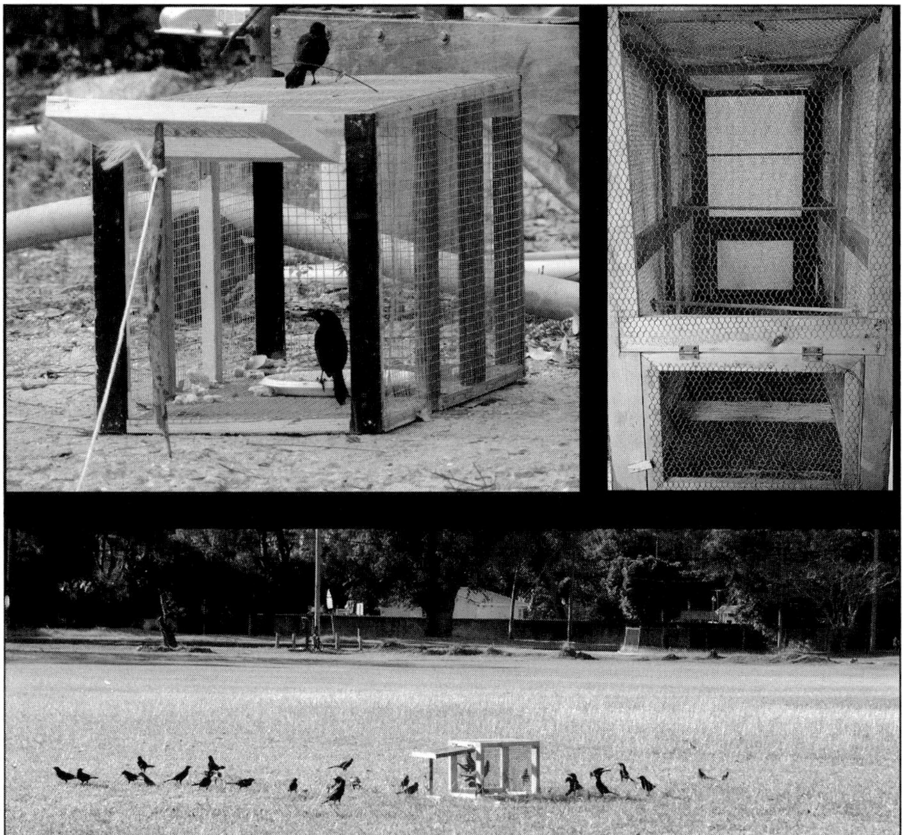

Figure 4.4. Top left: walk-in trap with a grackle inside. Top right: cage used when keeping individuals captive for a few days to measure cognition, including visual isolation curtains. Bottom: walk-in trap surrounded by Carib grackles and shiny cowbirds on a soccer field in an urban area of Holetown.

Once caught, a range of morphological measurements can be easily taken on the birds, and banding them is usually essential to avoid measuring the same individual several times. Body condition is likely one of the most important variables to consider, as it may affect both motivation to respond to behavioural tests and response to stress in captivity (see Peig and Green, 2009, 2010, for methodological advice on how to estimate body condition). Having the bird in hand makes it easy to collect other data, for example by sampling blood (to determine a range of physiological parameters or for DNA) or feathers (to estimate growth rate, stress hormone levels, colouration, measure isotopes to determine diet, stress layers during feather growth, external parasites; Grubb, 1989; Kelly, 2000; Bortolotti *et al.*, 2008; Biard *et al.*, 2015).

Captivity Conditions

To keep birds in captivity, it is essential to consider both the animals' well-being and the handiness of their maintenance. The birds' well-being is of course an ethical requirement, but it also favours birds' participation in behavioural tests. Adapting the cage size to the species (e.g. for grackles: 2.63 × 1.52 × 1.10 m; Figure 4.4) and arranging the cages to limit the bird's stress and make captive conditions as natural as possible (e.g. by adding some wooden perches per cage, as grackles spend a lot of time perched when they are not foraging) are key aspects. These details largely vary across species (e.g. some will need a nest box or elaborate leafy branches to hide in, others may require a grassy floor), but grackles are very easy to keep in captivity. Over the years, we have had near zero mortality in captivity, and we have routinely seen grackles come back near the aviaries after release. Visual isolation from the external environment, including other birds (e.g. through plastic shower curtains, easy to clean), is also essential to decrease stress, especially in outdoor cages. Food and water should always be available, except when deprivation periods are required for behavioural testing (see below). Carib grackles are omnivorous and easy to keep in good health, and a mix of dog pellets, meat scraps (e.g. chicken bones with some meat left on it), seeds, rice and bread largely meets their needs.

Cages should be positioned to observe the birds without being seen by them. The cage height and the position of the doors should also be thoroughly considered, as these will have to be opened and closed quite often during testing. You may also need to think about a good place for a camera and about introducing it early in the captive environment, to familiarize the birds with it. Cages will also need to be often cleaned and completely disinfected before new birds are introduced in order to limit disease transmission. Keeping cages in a shaded area and using white or clear material (e.g. to cover the cages) is also necessary to limit temperatures within the cages, a must in tropical countries.

Food Deprivation Protocol

Deprivation periods preceding testing phases may be necessary to standardize hunger levels. They should last long enough so that the birds are sufficiently hungry to respond to the tests, but should be kept as short as possible to preclude strong discomfort. In Carib grackles, 15 hours, starting at sunset and including nighttime (when grackles do not normally feed), yield a good level of motivation. Note that the deprivation period can vary according to a species' diet and digestion mode: for example, Columbids, which have a relatively large crop, are able to fast for longer periods. Importantly, the birds also need a period during which they can feed *ad libitum*, before being released, to make sure that they recover in case they did not have enough food during the tests. Maintaining similar levels of hunger across individuals can be particularly tricky as individuals may differ in the number of trials needed to succeed at a given task, so that some individuals will be rewarded over longer periods of time than others. Providing food on a regular basis to individuals that get fewer rewards is thus important to maintain similar hunger levels across individuals.

Temperament

How temperament relates to cognition is still not completely understood, but it is obvious that tamer individuals will be more prone to participate in tests, potentially increasing their chances of success at tasks for non-cognitive reasons. Both stress in reaction to captivity and temperament should thus be considered when measuring cognition. Although stress can be measured physiologically (e.g. via hormonal measurements or by measuring cardiac rhythm), behaviour can be an excellent cue. Observing bird behaviour in the cage (e.g. prostration, panic flight, alarm calls) is the first indicator of how stressed a bird is in response to captivity.

The most important temperament measures for cognition are probably the reaction to the observer's intrusion (i.e. measured as the latency to feed after disturbance) and neophobia, as the apparatus used in the tests will be new to the birds. To measure neophobia, objects should be chosen so that the birds have never been in contact with them. Measuring neophobia is not necessarily straightforward and should be considered carefully (Greenberg, 2003). Latency to feed near a new object (compared to feeding without the object) is one method. Standard tests of exploratory behaviour can also be conducted, measuring the time it takes a bird to visit a series of perches or zones in an unfamiliar cage, or the total number of zones visited (Overington *et al.*, 2011).

Habituation to Captive Conditions

A habituation period allows birds to accommodate to their captive conditions and to the intervention of humans. Both a period of calm and some contact with the experimenter (e.g. bringing food into the cage) will favour a more rapid habituation and increase birds' response to the different devices that will be introduced during the testing phase. In our studies, a 48-hour captivity period was sufficient to observe a clear decrease in the birds' stress. It is, however, important to note that we worked with urban birds used to interacting with humans and anthropogenic food, and that birds from other habitats may need more time. Notably, participation increases across time, while latency to feed after disturbance decreases. Some grackles are so tame at the end of the testing period that

Table 4.1. Essential tools to study cognition in Carib grackles and their function.

Tool	Function
Permits	Required to work in Barbados
Bands	To individually recognize birds
Traps	To catch the birds for testing (Figure 4.4)
Aviaries	To keep birds for a few days during testing (Figure 4.4)
Dog pellets	To reward birds for correctly solving a task; better given wet
Obstacle removal problems	The manipulative ability of the species makes it ideal to test obstacle removal problems (Figure 4.3)

they even come back around the cage area after being released. Differences in individual habituation to captivity (e.g. measured in terms of decreased activity and alarm call frequency) can also be a crucial parameter to take into account. In our experience, giving all individuals an identical sequence of tasks of increasing difficulty is the best way to reduce the effect of stress on performance. Varying task order between individuals can create a spurious negative relationship in performance, if individual 1 gets task A soon after capture (when stress is higher), and individual 2 gets it much later.

Measuring Problem-Solving Abilities

Designing problem-solving tasks can be more challenging than expected: the birds need to have the motor abilities to solve the task, but the task needs to be sufficiently challenging to cause interindividual variation in success. Depending on the apparatus, different motor and cognitive skills will be required for the bird to succeed at accessing the food. Important factors to consider when devising problem-solving tasks are: (1) the abilities that the experimenter aims at measuring and (2) the fact that the bird will aim at obtaining the food, not at performing the task. Whether the reward should be visible is an important aspect: starting a testing session with a device offering no visual reward is likely to be unsuccessful, as the bird has no reason to be motivated to access the reward. It can thus be of interest to start with transparent devices to increase birds' motivation, before testing performance on more challenging devices where the reward is not directly visible. The order in which tasks are presented to the birds is also of importance, as some tasks may be too difficult at the beginning of a testing session (as the birds are not yet used to interacting with new devices, or to providing some specific motor actions) or too easy at the end of it (as the birds are too used to interacting with new devices). After testing Carib grackles with two complex tasks, for instance, we exposed them to an easier task where the reward was visible and the birds had to pierce an aluminium foil to access it, and all individuals succeeded within their first trial. Starting with the easier task would have probably yielded more variation in individuals' performance. At the other end, we designed a complex three-step task with a hidden reward to test for social learning, such that birds could not succeed without being shaped or observing a demonstrator. However, it appeared that the task was far too difficult for a bird to succeed without intensive and time-consuming training. Although we could train demonstrators to solve the task, the observers would never be able to master more than two of the three steps needed to access the reward without losing motivation. Examples of problem-solving tasks that we designed successfully, balancing feasibility and easiness of the task, are provided in Figure 4.3.

String-Pulling Test

An anecdote that illustrates particularly well the fact that birds do not necessarily react to a new device the way we expect them to is the string-pulling test we conducted on grackles. The device we initially used was a simple reward attached to the end of a string tied to a wooden perch. The bird was expected to succeed by pulling the string with its beak and grab it with its foot, before pulling again with the beak, and so on until it got access to the reward. Some birds did succeed the way we anticipated, but a range of other methods were also tried, which eventually distracted the birds away from the technique we expected them to use. Some individuals tried to use a kind of hovering flight in front of the reward, pecking at it directly. Although we tried to limit the success of this strategy by inserting the reward within a cup, it sometimes worked, especially when birds shook the device strongly enough to spill the food. Other birds tried to shake the string from the wooden perch, to also spill the food at the bottom of the cage (which also eventually worked). We thus had to change our device, to make sure that there was only one way for the birds to access the reward (i.e. by using the classical string-pulling method described in the literature). To that aim, we surrounded the reward (and the lower part of the string) with a Plexiglas cylinder, so that the bird could not directly touch the reward or get access to fallen food, but could only pull the string to access the food. We concluded that only a small number of grackles could pass the standard version of the test (Audet *et al.*, 2016), but the diversity of alternate techniques tried by the birds was a testimony to their high level of innovativeness.

Measuring Discrimination and Reversal Learning

To test associative learning, birds are trained to associate a cue (usually a colour) with the presence of a reward and a second cue with its absence, and performance is measured as the time/number of trials needed to reach a success criterion (e.g. a given number of successive trials without mistakes). However, if there is almost no cost in opening the unrewarded device (e.g. if the bird can, on each trial, open both the rewarded and the unrewarded ones), there is no advantage for the bird in learning which colour is rewarded. An active, highly exploratory bird like the Carib grackle will very quickly go to the second stimulus if the first one is unrewarded – a behaviour that will strongly interfere with discrimination learning (see in contrast Audet *et al.*, 2018, on a shyer species). The best way to increase the cost is thus to prevent the bird from trying out more than one of the two options, and keep a fixed time lapse between two choices, so that an error causes an absence of reward for a given amount of time. Associative learning can be highly time-consuming (in Carib grackles, over 70 trials were needed for some individuals to reach success criterion), so that developing protocols that maximize the costs of errors is important. Devices that require a motor act to open an apparatus can also be favoured, as they are expected to increase the costs of errors. However, opening the device should be similarly difficult for all individuals, to maintain similar costs across them.

Another aspect to consider is the fact that birds may show innate biases towards the proposed cues. A way to limit this bias is to test birds' initial preference and then choose the non-preferred cue as the rewarded one. Spatial biases can also be avoided by randomly choosing the position of the rewarded and unrewarded colours on each trial, or by reversing it. Finally, the chosen success criterion will also play an important role (e.g. seven successive successful trials, or seven of eight trials): some individuals may have associated a colour with the reward, but still explore the other colour from time to time, whereas others may, once they have associated the colour with the reward, permanently focus on the rewarded colour. Depending on the exact question, different criteria may thus be used.

Wild vs. Lab

Box 4.2 Bringing Avian Cognition to the Wild

Lucy Aplin

The study of avian cognition is in an exciting growth period (ten Cate and Healey, 2017). In particular, technological advances in animal tracking are allowing for novel observational and experimental approaches, opening up new avenues for research in wild birds. The series of studies on grackles detailed in this chapter have been pioneering in this process of bringing cognition to the wild, using a 'hybrid' methodology. Here, wild birds are kept in aviaries for short periods of time, during which they are tested for cognitive abilities. This allows for larger sample sizes than is often possible in traditional laboratory experiments, and has thus been invaluable in describing interindividual differences in cognition (Ducatez *et al.*, 2015). However, while this may provide more ecological validity than previous methods, it has two major limitations. First, birds may not behave as they would in natural contexts. Second, aviary studies can rarely follow individuals over long periods of time, losing the opportunity to investigate how interindividual differences in cognition might relate to life history.

Recently, several projects in another model species, the great tit (*Parus major*), have gone some way to addressing these questions. This species has been the subject of several long-term studies, resulting in a great depth of knowledge of its behaviour and ecology. Over the last 10 years, there has also been a miniature revolution in the study of this species, with the extensive use of passive-integrated transponder (PIT) tags to track entire populations of individuals; when combined with sensing antennae (e.g. at feeders or nests), these can lead to detailed data sets of movement, breeding and foraging patterns. PIT tags can also be used to create an interactive interface between tagged birds and cognitive tasks, allowing studies to be conducted

(cont.)

in the wild. For example, Morand-Ferron and colleagues (2015) presented wild-tagged great tits with automated 'skinner boxes' that gave individuals personalized learning programmes to test associative and reversal learning. Similarly, Aplin and colleagues (2015) explored social learning using a series of 'puzzle-boxes', where subpopulations were seeded with demonstrators trained on one of two alternative solutions. The traditions that emerged through the transmission of this behaviour through social networks were then mapped.

Finally, an elegant series of studies has tested life-history correlates of individual differences in cognition by using a simple problem-solving task, whereby individuals could obtain food by pulling a lever to release a trapdoor (Morand-Ferron *et al.*, 2011). Larger flocks of tits were quicker to solve this task, suggesting a significant influence of the social context (Morand-Ferron and Quinn, 2011). However, even when tested in isolation, birds showed consistent individual differences in their ability to solve this problem (Cole *et al.*, 2011). Ultimately, researchers were able to follow birds over their subsequent breeding attempts, showing that differences in problem-solving performance were related to foraging efficiency and breeding success (Cole *et al.*, 2012). As such studies continue to produce increasingly detailed observations on large samples of wild birds, we can expect more exciting insights into the evolution and ecology of avian cognition.

References

Aplin, L. M., Farine, D. R., Morand-Ferron, J., Cockburn, A., Thornton, A., and Sheldon, B. C. (2015). Experimentally induced innovations lead to persistent culture via conformity in wild birds. *Nature*, **518**, 538–541.

Cole, E. F., Cram, D. L., and Quinn, J. L. (2011). Individual variation in spontaneous problem-solving performance among wild great tits. *Animal Behaviour*, **81**, 491–498.

Cole, E. F., Morand-Ferron, J., Hinks, A. E., and Quinn, J. L. (2012). Cognitive ability influences reproductive life history variation in the wild. *Current Biology*, **22**, 1808–1812.

Ducatez, S., Audet, J. N., and Lefebvre, L. (2015). Problem-solving and learning in Carib grackles: individuals show a consistent speed-accuracy trade-off. *Animal Cognition*, **18**, 495–496.

Morand-Ferron, J., and Quinn, J. L. (2011). Larger groups of passerines are more efficient problem solvers in the wild. *Proceedings of the National Academy of Sciences*, **108**, 15898–15903.

Morand-Ferron, J., Cole, E. F., Rawles, J. E. C., and Quinn, J. L. (2011). Who are the innovators? A field experiment with 2 passerine species. *Behavioral Ecology*, **22**, 1241–1248.

Morand-Ferron, J., Hamblin, S., Cole, E. F., Aplin, L. M., and Quinn, J. L. (2015). Taking the operant paradigm into the field: associative learning in wild great tits. *PLoS ONE*, **10**(8), e0133821.

ten Cate, C., and Healy, S. D. (2017) *Avian cognition*. Cambridge: Cambridge University Press.

Resources

- The website Xenocanto (www.xeno-canto.org/explore?query=Quiscalus+lugubris) includes several song recordings of *Q. lugubris* from South America and several islands of the Lesser Antilles, but none from Barbados.
- The Carib grackle page in the Handbook of the Birds of the World Alive provides information and references on the species: www.hbw.com/species/carib-grackle-quiscalus-lugubris (cf. Fraga, 2017).
- Jaramillo and Burke's monograph on Icteridae brings together information on grackles and their relatives: Jaramillo, A., and Burke, P. (1999). *New World blackbirds*. Princeton, NJ: Princeton University Press.

Profile

Taking advantage of the fact that McGill has a field station in Barbados, the Lefebvre lab started working several decades ago with Carib grackles as social learning tutors for Zenaida doves. The grackles soon proved to be so tame and innovative in the field and in captivity that we focused more and more on them. Over the years, Daniel Sol, Sarah Overington and Julie Morand-Ferron contributed important work on this species. More recently, Fyssen post-doctoral fellowships from France allowed Simon Ducatez and Marine Battesti to continue this tradition, while Jean-Nicolas Audet added grackles to his PhD research on Barbados bullfinches and black-faced grassquits.

References

Audet, J. N., Kayello, L., Ducatez, S., Perillo, S., *et al.* (2018). Divergence in problem-solving skills is associated with differential expression of glutamate receptors in wild finches. *Science Advances*, **4**, eaa063669.

Audet, J. N., and Lefebvre, L. (2017). What's flexible in behavioral flexibility? *Behavioral Ecology*, **28**, 943–947.

Audet, J. N., Ducatez, S., and Lefebvre, L. (2016). Bajan birds pull strings: two wild Antillean species enter the select club of string-pullers. *PLoS ONE*, **11**, e0156112.

Biard, C., Monceau, K., Motreuil, S., and Moreau, J. (2015). Interpreting immunological indices: the importance of taking parasite community into account. An example in blackbirds *Turdus merula*. *Methods in Ecology and Evolution*, **6**, 960–972.

Boogert, N. J., Monceau, K., and Lefebvre, L. (2010). A field test of behavioural flexibility in Zenaida doves (*Zenaida aurita*). *Behavioural Processes*, **85**, 135–141.

Bortolotti, G. R., Marchant, T. A., Blas, J., and German, T. (2008). Corticosterone in feathers is a long-term, integrated measure of avian stress physiology. *Functional Ecology*, **22**, 494–500.

Buckley, P. A., Massiah, E. B., Hutt, M. B., Buckley, F. G., and Hutt, H. F. (2009). The birds of Barbados. *BOU Checklist Series*, **24**. Retrieved from www.bou.org.uk/barbados-sample.pdf.

Bugnyar, T., and Heinrich, B. (2005). Ravens, *Corvus corax*, differentiate between knowledgeable and ignorant competitors. *Proceedings of the Royal Society of London B: Biological Sciences*, **272**, 1641–1646.

Clayton, N. S., Dally, J. M., and Emery, N. J. (2007). Social cognition by food-caching corvids. The western scrub-jay as a natural psychologist. *Philosophical Transactions of the Royal Society B: Biological Sciences*, **362**, 507–522.

Debrot, A. O. (2014). Nocturnal foraging by artificial light in three Caribbean bird species. *The Journal of Caribbean Ornithology*, **27**, 40–41.

Dolman, C. S., Templeton, J., and Lefebvre, L. (1996). Mode of foraging competition is related to tutor preference in *Zenaida aurita*. *Journal of Comparative Psychology*, **110**, 45–54.

Ducatez, S., Audet, J. N., and Lefebvre, L. (2015). Problem-solving and learning in Carib grackles: individuals show a consistent speed–accuracy trade-off. *Animal Cognition*, **18**, 485–496.

Ducatez, S., Audet, J.-N., Rodriguez, J. R., Kayello, L., and Lefebvre, L. (2017). Innovativeness and the effects of urbanization on risk-taking behaviors in wild Barbados birds. *Animal Cognition*, **20**, 33–42.

Fraga, R. (2017). Carib grackle (*Quiscalus lugubris*). In: *Handbook of the birds of the world alive*. Barcelona: Lynx Edicions.

Greenberg, R. (2003). The role of neophobia and neophilia in the development of innovative behaviour of birds. In *Animal innovation* (pp. 175–196). Oxford: Oxford University Press.

Griffin, A. S. (2008). Socially acquired predator avoidance: is it just classical conditioning? *Brain Research Bulletin*, **76**, 264–271.

Griffin, A. S., and Galef, B. G. (2005). Social learning about predators: does timing matter? *Animal Behaviour*, **69**, 669–678.

Griffin, A. S., Savani, R. S., Hausmanis, K., and Lefebvre, L. (2005). Mixed-species aggregations in birds: Zenaida doves, *Zenaida aurita*, respond to the alarm calls of Carib grackles, Quiscalus lugubris. *Animal Behaviour*, **70**, 507–515.

Griffin, A. S., Diquelou, M., and Perea, M. (2014). Innovative problem solving in birds: a key role of motor diversity. *Animal Behaviour*, **92**, 221–227.

Grubb, T. C. (1989). Ptilochronology: feather growth bars as indicators of nutritional status. *The Auk*, **106**, 314–320.

Huber, L., and Gajdon, G. K. (2006). Technical intelligence in animals: the kea model. *Animal Cognition*, **9**, 295–305.

Iwaniuk, A. N. (2003). *The evolution of brain size and structure in birds*. Clayton: Monash University.

Keeler, J. E. (1963). Common grackles catching live shad. *Alabama Birdlife*, **11**, 23–24.

Kelly, J. F. (2000). Stable isotopes of carbon and nitrogen in the study of avian and mammalian trophic ecology. *Canadian Journal of Zoology*, **78**, 1–27.

Lefebvre, L., Templeton, J., Brown, K., and Koelle, M. (1997). Carib grackles imitate conspecific and Zenaida dove tutors. *Behaviour*, **134**, 1003–1017.

Lefebvre, L., Ducatez, S., and Audet, J. N. (2016). Feeding innovations in a nested phylogeny of Neotropical passerines. *Philosophical Transactions of the Royal Society B: Biological Sciences*, **371**, 20150188.

Lovette, I. J., Seutin, G., Ricklefs, R. E., and Bermingham, E. (1999). The assembly of an island fauna by natural invasion: sources and temporal patterns in the avian colonization of Barbados. *Biological Invasions*, **1**, 33–41.

Maddison, W. P., and Maddison, D. R. (2008). Mesquite: a modular system for evolutionary analysis. Version 2.75. Available at http://mesquiteproject.org.

McNeil, R., McSween, A., and Lachapelle, P. (2005). Comparison of the retinal structure and function in four bird species as a function of the time they start singing in the morning. *Brain, Behavior and Evolution*, **65**, 202–214.

Morand-Ferron, J., and Lefebvre, L. (2007). Flexible expression of a food-processing behaviour: determinants of dunking rates in wild Carib grackles of Barbados. *Behavioural Processes*, **76**, 218–221.

Morand-Ferron, J., Lefebvre, L., Reader, S. M., Sol, D., and Elvin, S. (2004). Dunking behaviour in Carib grackles. *Animal Behaviour*, **68**, 1267–1274.

Morand-Ferron, J., Veillette, M., and Lefebvre, L. (2006). Stealing of dunked food in Carib grackles (*Quiscalus lugubris*). *Behavioural Processes*, **73**, 342–347.

Morand-Ferron, J., Giraldeau, L. A., and Lefebvre, L. (2007). Wild Carib grackles play a producer–scrounger game. *Behavioral Ecology*, **18**, 916–921.

Overington, S. E., Morand-Ferron, J., Boogert, N. J., and Lefebvre, L. (2009a). Technical innovations drive the relationship between innovativeness and residual brain size in birds. *Animal Behaviour*, **78**, 1001–1010.

Overington, S. E., Cauchard, L., Morand-Ferron, J., and Lefebvre, L. (2009b). Innovation in groups: does the proximity of others facilitate or inhibit performance? *Behaviour*, **146**, 1543–1564.

Overington, S. E., Wattier, R., Côté, K.-A., Cauchard, L., and Lefebvre, L. (2010). Behavioural, biometric and molecular sexing of *Quiscalus lugubris fortirostris* in Barbados. Behavioural innovation and the evolution of cognition in birds (pp. 262–276). PhD thesis, McGill University, Montréal, Canada.

Overington, S. E., Cauchard, L., Côté, K. A., and Lefebvre, L. (2011). Innovative foraging behaviour in birds: what characterizes an innovator? *Behavioural Processes*, **87**, 274–285.

Peig, J., and Green, A. J. (2009). New perspectives for estimating body condition from mass/length data: the scaled mass index as an alternative method. *Oikos*, **118**, 1883–1891.

Peig, J., and Green, A. J. (2010). The paradigm of body condition: a critical reappraisal of current methods based on mass and length. *Functional Ecology*, **24**, 1323–1332.

Powell, A. F. L. A., Barker, F. K., Lanyon, S. M., Burns, K. J., Klicka, J., and Lovette, I. J. (2014). A comprehensive species-level molecular phylogeny of the New World blackbirds (Icteridae). *Molecular Phylogenetics and Evolution*, **71**, 94–112.

Reader, S. M., Morand-Ferron, J., Côté, I., and Lefebvre, L. (2002). Unusual feeding behaviors in five species of Barbadian birds. *El Pitirre*, **15**, 117–123.

Rodriguez-Ferraro, A. (2015). Fishing behavior of the Carib grackle (*Quiscalus lugubris*) in Venezuela. *Ornitologia Neotropical*, **26**, 207–209.

Sol, D., Sayol, F., Ducatez, S., and Lefebvre, L. (2016). The life-history basis of behavioural innovations. *Philosophical Transactions of the Royal Society B: Biological Sciences*, **371**, 20150187.

Webster, S. J., and Lefebvre, L. (2001). Problem solving and neophobia in a columbiform–passeriform assemblage in Barbados. *Animal Behaviour*, **62**, 23–32.

Wunderle, J. M. (1981). Avian predation upon Anolis lizards on Grenada, West Indies. *Herpetologica*, **37**, 104–108.

5 Chicken – Cognition in the Poultry Yard

Cinzia Chiandetti and Giorgio Vallortigara

Species Description

Anatomy

The domestic chick (*Gallus gallus domesticus*) is a peculiar species of bird that neither flies, except for reaching fences or branches, nor sings, despite its nearly 30 distinguishable stereotyped calls (Collias and Joos, 1953). Chicks have laterally placed eyes that allow a 270° vision, with about 7–8° of overlapping binocular frontal field (see below). The use of these fields has been well characterized: chicks tend to view close objects (20–30 cm away) and fine elements for food consumption with the frontal field and distant objects with the lateral field (Rogers *et al.*, 2004); pecks at conspecifics involve the left visual hemi-field, showing a right-hemisphere enrolment for individual face recognition (Vallortigara *et al.*, 2011; Regolin *et al.*, 2012). Hens also show jerky head movements to compensate for the absence of saccades, and turn from side to side to view the object with different eyes and, in the same eye, with different parts of the retina (Dawkins, 2002).

Perception

Chicks rely especially on vision, and their colour discrimination, based on tetrachromatic colour vision, is quite sophisticated. They possess four types of single-cone photoreceptor sensitive to ultraviolet, short-, medium- or long-wavelength light, and when trained to small food containers of different shades, recognize the colour quickly and accurately (Osorio *et al.*, 1999). Their favourite colour falls in the range of orange and red, but preferences are also modelled by experience and genetic differences (Ham and Osorio, 2007).

Audition serves the discrimination of specific calls and the learning of the voice of different individuals (see below). On the first day of life, chicks exposed to the sound of a cluck, the typical hen's call, show an ear preference to attend the same call at test that depends on the length of exposure time (Miklósi *et al.*, 1996).

Olfaction has received only meagre interest, but recent evidence shows that, despite a relatively small size of the olfactory bulb, several olfactory receptor genes deserve further investigation (reviewed in Krause *et al.*, 2016). From a behavioural point of view, it is well attested that chicks can learn and remember odours of the nest, predators and different alarm contexts. Olfaction has also been studied in relation to imprinting and lateralization (e.g. Vallortigara and Andrew, 1994).

Life Cycle

The chick belongs to the so-called precocial species, walking around and exploring the environment immediately after hatching, thanks to a rapid sensory-motor development. Its natural life span ranges from 10 to 15 years. It hatches in autonomy by breaking the egg shell with a small tooth on the beak (that is lost in the first 2–3 days post-hatching). By devising specific tasks, a precocial animal can thus be tested immediately after hatching and hence inform about predispositions transmitted across generations, helping researchers to differentiate this knowledge from that learned through experience (reviewed in Johnson *et al.*, 1992; Versace and Vallortigara, 2015; Versace, 2017). Furthermore, a particular form of learning can be combined with the controlled rearing conditions: the filial imprinting. In a limited time-window, which closes at around 8 days of age, the chick displays affiliative responses to the first conspicuous object encountered in the surroundings (reviewed in McCabe, 2013; Vallortigara and Versace, 2017).

Individual Identification

Male chicks can be discriminated from females at the hatching moment by a simple inspection of the wing feathers' length in some breeds (other breeds show sex differences in the colour of plumage). Male chicks present primary feathers of about the same length or shorter than the coverts, whereas female chicks have longer primary feathers. On the second week, sexual dimorphism is more evident, especially on the wings and tail (with longer feathers in females). Chicks appear quite similar to one another, hence an individual code has to be assigned to identify each baby bird; individuals tested in pairs can be marked on the back with non-toxic colours. These markers also allow an automated track system to detect chicks' movements within an arena and to compute the measurements of the associated dependent variables.

Socio-Ecological Characteristics

Higher-ranking individuals dominate subordinate ones and can approach food first. Direct fighting between two individuals is the means through which hens and roosters determine the pecking order (Rushen, 1982). Chickens can individually recognize group members: they know and remember not only each individual face but also their typical call; by means of transitive inference, they can avoid a direct encounter with a dominant individual they have never directly fought with (Daisley *et al.*, 2010). The same linear hierarchy is maintained in the order that roosters follow to announce the break of the dawn (Shimmura *et al.*, 2015), so that the lower-ranking rooster always waits for the higher-ranking one to crow the 'cock-a-doodle-do', despite each rooster being potentially able to initiate the crow at the new dawn. Dominance hierarchy also applies to a single couple constituted by individuals of the same sex; this should be considered in experiments, because the performance of each individual cannot be scored as an independent data point (see Chiandetti *et al.*, 2005).

Optimal ecological composition of groups does not exceed 30 individuals, with only one dominant male. Single members alert to an approaching predator to defend conspecifics, informing whether the danger is travelling via land or via sky, thus allowing conspecifics to adopt the best defence strategy. If one finds food, it can signal its presence to conspecifics or it can choose to remain silent (Mench and Keeling, 2001; Nicol, 2004), because they have proved to be artful deceivers, especially to attract unfamiliar females for mating (Marler *et al.*, 1986).

There seem to be important differences between sexes in social behaviour. Female chicks lose sight of the mother hen less often than do males of the same age (Workman and Andrew, 1989), and they show stronger tendencies than males to reinstate social contact in open-field tests (Vallortigara and Zanforlin, 1988). Also, when trained in a runway with either food or the possibility to rejoin cage-mates as rewards, females ran faster than males with social reinforcement, whereas males ran faster than females with non-social reinforcement (see Cailotto *et al.*, 1989; Vallortigara *et al.*, 1990a). Social discrimination also reveals striking sex differences. In approach-response tests, females tend to show shorter latencies when tested with cage-mates than when tested with strangers, whereas males do the reverse. In simultaneous-choice tests, females tend to spend more time near a cage-mate, whereas males spend more time near a stranger chick. Finally, in aggressive-pecking tests, both sexes peck more at strangers than at cage-mates; aggressive pecking at strangers, however, is usually higher in males than in females (Vallortigara, 1992).

In natural populations of feral (as well as domesticated) animals, adult fowls exhibit territorial behaviour wherein single dominant cocks maintain and patrol a large territory within which a number of females live (McBride and Foenander, 1962; McBride *et al.*, 1969). This sort of social organization may have favoured the prevalence of gregarious and affiliative behaviours in females and of aggressive and exploratory behaviours in males. Sex differences have also been observed in the relative use of object-specific (such as colour) and spatial-specific cues in male and female chicks (Vallortigara, 1996), as well as in response to novel-coloured objects (Vallortigara *et al.*, 1994).

State of the Art

Predispositions (Two Alternatives Forced Choice)

A few hours after hatching, young fowls can be directly tested for their spontaneous preferences. Hence, a baby naïve chick can be taken out of the incubator and placed in the middle of a runway that presents two alternative stimuli at its ends. The chick's approaching behaviour will reveal its natural predispositions. By using this experimental design, inborn predispositions similar to human ones (Di Giorgio *et al.*, 2017) have been revealed in the social domain:

- *Faces.* Three dark blobs organized in a triangular shape and resembling a schematic face are preferable to a series of control stimuli with altered geometric relations between the three elements (Rosa Salva *et al.*, 2010, 2011).
- *Biological motion.* A point-light display of an animation reproducing a walking hen is interpreted as biological motion when being upright oriented (Vallortigara and Regolin, 2006), and is preferred to random or rigid motion of the same amount of points (Vallortigara *et al.*, 2005).
- *Animacy.* Stimuli spoiled of any resemblance to living organisms, such as simple circular shapes, are attractive to chicks because of the perceived animacy in the speed changes, during the linear motion of the stimulus itself. Naïve chicks prefer the 'speed-change stimulus' to an identical stimulus moving at a constant speed (Rosa Salva *et al.*, 2016; Lorenzi *et al.*, 2017).

As an alternative to letting the chick walk within a runway with the two testing stimuli placed at each end, the chick can operate a wheel positioned midway between the two stimuli. The number of revolutions will inform the preference for one of the two stimuli. For instance, this strategy has shown that different breeds of chicks differ in early social predispositions, with all breeds preferring a naturalistic hen over a scrambled one, but only Polverara chicks continuing to prefer the predisposed stimulus after some minutes (Versace *et al.*, 2017a).

Imprinting to Artificial Companion + Two Alternatives Forced Choice

The early exposure learning associated with filial imprinting co-occurs with the possibility to exert an accurate control of chicks' sensory experiences. By means of this manipulation, it is possible to expose visually naïve domestic chicks only to specific stimuli. Hence, chicks can observe in a controlled environment a certain stimulus for a time interval ranging from 1–2 hours to 7 days; next, the chicks are allowed to choose between two alternatives in a runway or by operating a running wheel such as the one described above. Assuming that chicks will associate with the object they prefer the most, we can explore chicks' sensitivity to different stimuli. Implementing this testing strategy, several studies support the conclusion that chicks perceptually organize the visual scene by means of rules that are functionally comparable to those humans use:

- *Amodal completion* (Figure 5.1). A triangle partially occluded by a horizontal rectangle is shown to the chick; at test, the chick goes for the entire triangle with a dislocated rectangle, rather than to an amputated triangle perceptually identical to the occluded one with a dislocated rectangle, seen during the imprinting phase (Regolin and Vallortigara, 1995; Regolin *et al.*, 2004); the same result is obtained when the occluded object is set in motion behind an occluding horizontal rod (Lea *et al.*, 1996). Mechanisms of interpolation among partly occluded objects operate even with chromatically homogeneous stimuli (Forkman and Vallortigara, 1999; Vallortigara and Tommasi, 2001), in a way that parallels human perception (e.g. Tommasi *et al.*, 1995).

- *Illusory contours*. After seeing a triangle, chicks also identify the same shape when it is produced by anomalous contours, as shown in Figure 5.2 (Zanforlin, 1981).
- *Stereokinetic effects*. A 2D shape is put in motion to create the stereokinetic illusion of a 3D shape. At test, chicks join the solid object identical to the one illusorily perceived before (Clara *et al.*, 2006).
- *Structure-from-motion*. 3D objects are used during exposure. At test, a random-dot display is used to produce the perception of a solid shape only when set in motion. Chicks peer with the corresponding 3D figure learned (Mascalzoni *et al.*, 2009).
- *Object invariance*. A specific object seen from a certain angle is presented during the imprinting phase. At test, chicks show shape recognition when the object is presented at different angles and in different contexts, despite viewpoint variability and independently from practice or experience (Wood, 2013).

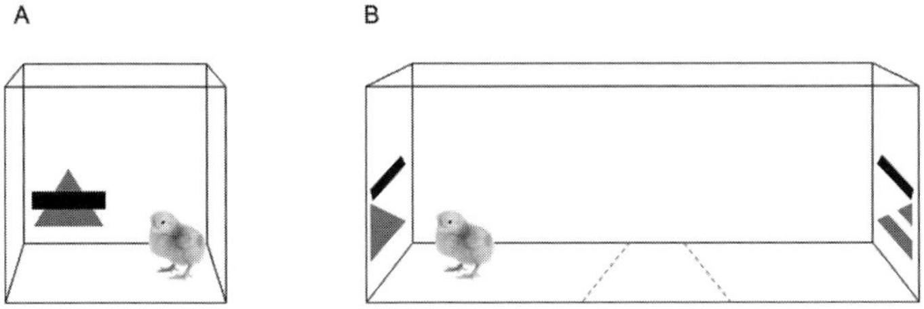

Figure 5.1. Example of imprinting + two alternative forced choice in a runway. The chick is exposed to a particular stimulus in the home-cage (an occluded triangle in the case of panel A) and then left free to choose between two alternatives (as represented in B: the stimuli provide the same distal stimulation, but only the one on the left corresponds to the triangle seen in A, in virtue of the amodal completion). The chick's starting point at the beginning of the test is represented by the area included within the two dotted lines.
Drawing by Cinzia Chiandetti.

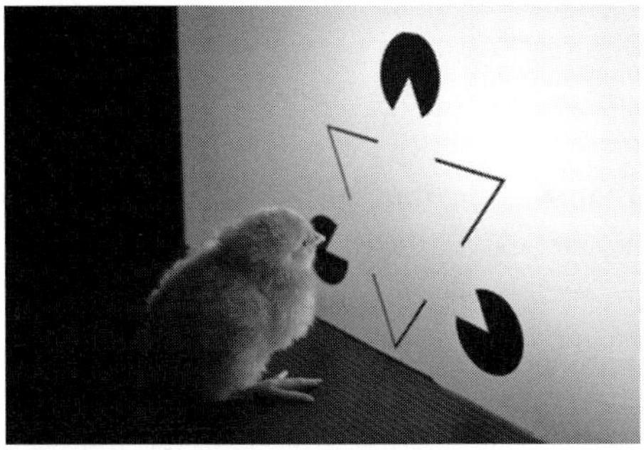

Figure 5.2. Example of a chick choosing an illusory figure. The entire triangle to which the chick was exposed during the imprinting phase is also recognized when it is only illusory present, due to the anomalous contours.
Picture by Cinzia Chiandetti.

Using the same procedure, it has been investigated whether imprinting modulates chicks' attention towards objects:

- *Biological motion*. Exposed to point-light animation sequences depicting either a walking hen or a rotating cylinder, chicks at test preferentially approach the novel stimulus (Regolin *et al.*, 2000).
- *Agency*. A shape is shown moving on a computer screen either by self-produced motion or by induced motion (i.e. by physical contact from another shape). Chicks prefer to associate with self-propelled objects (Mascalzoni *et al.*, 2010).
- *Hollow vs. filled objects*. A filled or hollow cylinder lives with the chick, whose preference for the two stimuli is then tested during a simultaneous presentation. Chicks seem to prefer hollow objects, which are also approached spontaneously in a version of the task without imprinting (Versace *et al.*, 2016).

Such a 'life-detector' pertains also to the acoustic modality. Chicks hatch with a predisposed raw model of maternal calls. Specific height, frequency and intensity of a hen's call may be preferable to others (Kent, 1993). Moreover, baby chicks like consonant sounds (Chiandetti and Vallortigara, 2011a; Baiocchi and Chiandetti, 2016), which are typical of vocal calls, and also complex rhythms defined by faster tempos and an alternation of pauses and accents (De Tommoso *et al.*, under rev.). These predispositions have been tested also by scoring chicks' propensity to operate a running wheel in response to the sounds, which were administered in two ways: either in a darkened environment where the chick ran towards the acoustic source, or with a visible imprinting object emitting the sounds and placed nearly 50 cm apart.

From the fourth day of life, the chick can distinguish its mother from the other hens on the basis of her personal clucks. When baby chicks cry out loud, the mother hen responds with her distinguishable cluck and the baby chicks diminish their distress calls (Bermant, 1963).

In a different domain, imprinting experiments clarify chicks' numerical abilities. Chicks reared with one or more identical objects, when tested for a free choice between the familiar stimulus and a novel stimulus differing in the number of elements, prefer to join the larger group of elements (Rugani *et al.*, 2010). Moreover, chicks imprinted with clearly discernible objects (i.e. different in shape, colour and dimension) could choose at task the one of two sets with the same number of elements as the imprinted object, when overall area and volume were identical (Rugani *et al.*, 2010). Chicks also seem to be capable of doing simple arithmetic on imprinting objects, taking into account addition and subtraction of them (see below).

Imprinting to an Artificial Companion + Complex Choice Task

Taking advantage of chicks' spontaneous responses to rejoin the imprinting object as soon as it is displaced, it has been possible to investigate further cognitive abilities. For instance, chicks placed in a cage in which they can see but not reach the imprinting object recede from the target, go around the barriers to find the object and delay the gratification to the moment after which the correct path will be found, showing that they represent the object itself even when it has disappeared from direct sensory perception (Regolin *et al.*, 1995).

In another case, chicks were initially confined behind a transparent partition, from where they could track an object disappearing behind one of two opaque screens. Chicks could maintain a memory trace of the concealment trajectory up to about 180 s, and if the partition was made opaque, thus impeding the chicks' view during the waiting time, chicks could still select the correct hiding position over 60 s (Vallortigara and Regolin, 1998). Similarly, chicks can maintain working memories of the location of an attractive food item for up to 180 s (Vallortigara *et al.*, 1998; Regolin *et al.*, 2005).

Chicks can also choose the barrier of the appropriate size for concealing a certain object behind it. In the experiments, different groups of chicks are reared with imprinting objects of different sizes (in height or width), and then they are shown their specific object hiding behind one or the other of two identical barriers. Chicks spontaneously keep track of the place where the object has gone and easily rejoin it. In the crucial situation, chicks could first see the imprinting object moving along a straight line towards the middle of the two barriers, but their view was then blocked by an opaque partition, while the experimenter changed the barriers, so that only one had the proper relative size or inclination to conceal the imprinting object behind it. When the chicks were finally released, they chose to explore the barrier with the adequate size or inclination. Preventing chicks touching or pecking at objects (i.e. avoiding any kind of experience about their solidity) does not compromise the performance at test; hence, this confirms that basic intuitive reasoning is possible from birth (Chiandetti and Vallortigara, 2011b).

In a rectangular room, an animal can reorient on the basis of the symmetry of the environment, which makes a corner and the one diagonally opposite identical in terms of wall length and left–right sense (pairs of corners are both defined by a long wall on the right and a short wall on the left, or vice versa; Vallortigara *et al.*, 1990c). Baby chicks hatched in darkness and exposed to the imprinting object directly in a rectangular testing environment (Figure 5.3) first observe the object moving in a particular corner.

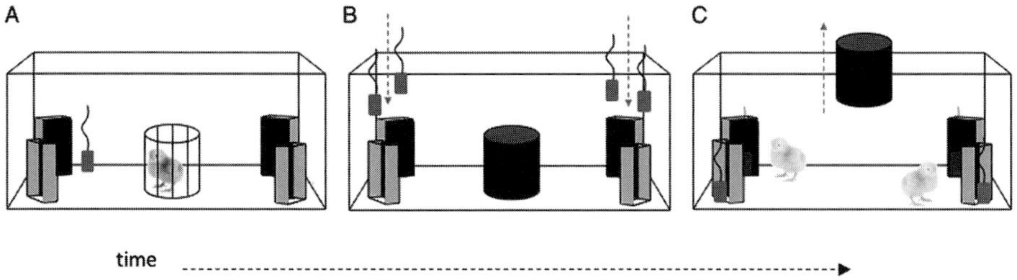

Figure 5.3. Example of complex choice task. The chick is exposed to the imprinting object hiding behind a panel placed in a certain corner (A). Then, the chick's view is occluded, while the experimenter places four identical replicas in each corner (B). When the chick is finally released for the choice, it visits the two diagonally opposite corners (C, chicks in light grey), which have the same arrangement of the long and short walls, with respect to its left and right directional sense, as the corner in A.
Drawing by Cinzia Chiandetti.

They are then disoriented in darkness under a black cylinder, while the experimenter places four identical replicas of the imprinting object at the four corners. When chicks are finally released for a reorientation choice, they show spontaneous recovery of their bearings by making use of distances between surfaces and directional left–right relations, to reorient themselves to the imprinting object (Chiandetti *et al.*, 2015). Chicks demonstrate that they can use the metric information in the absence of the experience of navigating in a geometrically structured environment.

Chicks reared with an imprinting object formed by a set of five elements are shown each single element hiding one at a time behind one or another of two identical barriers. Chicks that watched the displacement had no difficulty in exploring the barrier concealing the larger number of objects. In a more difficult situation, the elements could also be displaced from one to the next barrier so that the chick, which was still watching all the movements, had to summate and subtract the elements from the total hidden at the beginning of the trial in order to be able to peer with the larger number of elements. Chicks visited the screen hiding the larger number of elements, showing that they track the number of elements moved computing an exact result (Rugani *et al.*, 2009).

Observational Learning with Food

Chicks in their rearing cage can also be exposed to pictures or objects that will be encoded and memorized by mere exposure. This paradigm has been successfully used to test:

- *Ebbinghaus illusion*. Chicks find food in the proximity of either a big or a small circle, and then are presented with the Ebbinghaus stimuli (Figure 5.4A). In such a situation, chicks approach the corresponding illusory configuration (e.g. chicks reinforced on the small target choose the configuration with big inducers, in which the central target appears perceptually smaller; Rosa Salva *et al.*, 2013).
- *Impossible figures*. Chicks are fed from jars located below objects in which junctions are occluded (Figure 5.4B). At test, they choose the figure depicting the possible rather than the impossible object (Regolin *et al.*, 2011).
- *Symmetry*. Different chicks find food behind either a symmetrical or an asymmetrical abstract figure, and then can choose from new pairs of symmetrical and asymmetrical configurations. In this situation, chicks generalize to the reinforced pattern (Mascalzoni *et al.*, 2012).

(A) (B)

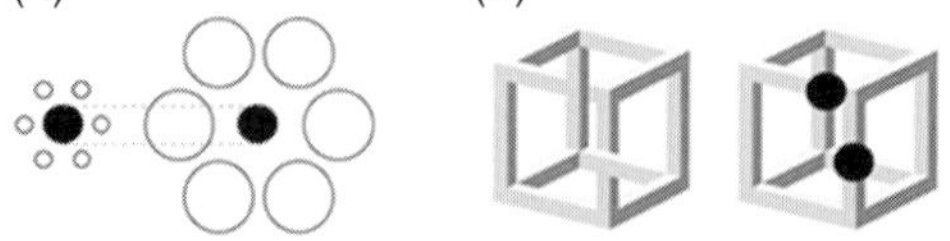

Figure 5.4. Example of experimental stimuli. In A, you have the impression that the left-most black circle, surrounded by small inducers, is larger than the right-most one, surrounded by larger inducers, despite their size being the same, as shown by dotted lines (Ebbinghaus illusion). In B, you perceive an impossible cube, unless two circles occlude the overlapping edges and make it coherent.
A, Drawing adapted from Regolin *et al.* (2011). B, Drawing by Cinzia Chiandetti.

Training with Canonical Associative Learning

Canonical training with associative methods can be used to understand how information is encoded and then retrieved and used to find a solution to a certain problem (Rosa Salva *et al.*, 2011). For instance, in the domain of spatial cognition, ground-scratching the sawdust is used to train the chick to obtain a food reinforcement buried in the centre of a large squared arena. The food is progressively made to disappear below the sawdust in subsequent trials, so that the chick spontaneously acts to extract the food. Even in the absence of any food, chicks were able to focus the ground-scratching to the central area and generalize the concept of 'centre' to arenas of different shapes, as a triangular or a circular one (Tommasi *et al.*, 1997).

A further chick's natural response is pecking, which is directed to all small elements available in the surroundings, especially if shining or sparkling. In a study, chicks had to protrude the head and the neck through a circular opening to sample the elements evenly spread on a plane in front of it. The chick spontaneously inserted the head through the window a few seconds after being placed within a small starting box, because the inside was darker than the outside, which was homogeneously illuminated (Diekamp *et al.*, 2005; Chiandetti, 2011).

Chicks' propensity to peck at small elements has also been used to investigate their perceptual organization. In so-called hierarchical or Navon stimuli, global shapes are created with a series of local identical elements that can be either a diminished version of the larger shape or a different one. When the two levels (global and local) are incongruent in shape, there is an attested delay in reporting the shape of the local element, because the global shape is processed first and it takes some time for the cognitive system to process and report the incongruence at the local level (Chiandetti *et al.*, 2014). Chicks can be trained to select a global shape in a concurrent discrimination task by progressively accustoming them to peck at a screen with an infrared frame scoring the peck coordinates (Figure 5.5). At the beginning of the training, in a shaping phase (Chiandetti, 2018), a single flickering element will attract a chick's attention, and

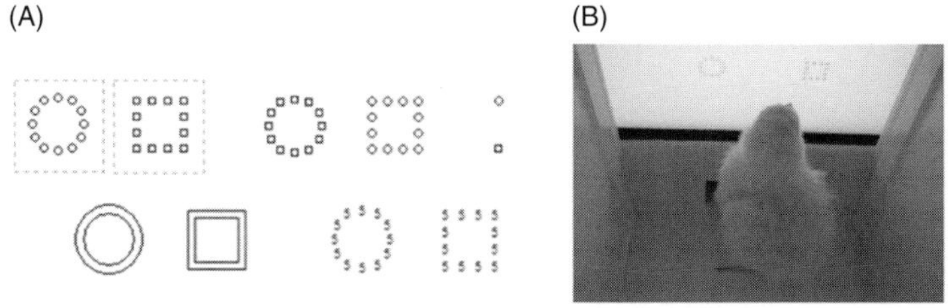

Figure 5.5. Example of training and testing with Navon stimuli. In A, you appreciate the training stimuli (a circle made of small circles and a square made of small squares), and several combinations of local- and global-level changes, used to test the chick's preference to attend to either the local or the global shape. In B, a chick is staring at the target stimulus (a square made of small squares), before pecking at it in order to open the drawer with the food reward (at the bottom, occluded by the chick). Picture by Tommaso Pecchia, adapted from Chiandetti and colleagues (2014).

the correct peck at it will open a drawer with food acting as reinforcer. The chick's response will be repeated onto progressively larger stimuli, up to the phase in which the Navon stimuli will be presented. After training, when chicks are tested with congruent–incongruent stimuli, they are prone to attend the smaller elements first, rather than the global shape.

Chicks can be trained for food to peck at a shape placed on a drawer (that opens if the shape is the one that has to be reinforced) in order to see whether the chick is learning a shape or a position (e.g. Vallortigara and Zanforlin, 1989; Vallortigara *et al.*, 1990b). Devaluation procedures can further be used to investigate some aspects of chicks' representational abilities, exploiting the observation that prior feeding with one type of food selectively reduces the value of that food for both chicks (see Cozzutti and Vallortigara, 2001) and adult hens (Forkman, 2000). This suggests that chicks can remember the contents of food caches other than their positions: conjoining 'where' and 'what' information, they would thus form 'declarative-like' representations.

Chickens can also be trained to choose an average human female/male face, and then tested with new stimuli to study their sexual preferences. Interestingly, chicks show the same preferences humans have, choosing the same stimuli rated as the most pleasant one by a human sample of university students (Ghirlanda *et al.*, 2002).

Chicks reinforced to discriminate small sets of identical dots were then required to choose between sets of similar numerousness, but with non-numerical variables (such as spatial distribution, contour length and overall surface area) being equalized (Rugani *et al.*, 2008). Basically, chicks from a very early age seem to possess an approximate number system, allowing them to perform simple arithmetic, like addition and subtraction (see above), and show a non-symbolic mental number line, in which magnitudes are orderly represented from left to right (Rugani *et al.*, 2015; see Vallortigara, 2014, 2017).

Training to locate a food reward in a particular corner is not facilitated by living in a geometrically structured environment, like a rectangular cage (Chiandetti and Vallortigara, 2008, 2010), showing that their ability to deal with the geometry of the environment is not modulated by experience (Vallortigara *et al.*, 2009).

Chicks are also capable of sophisticated context-dependent associative learning. Chicks' freezing response to a sudden loud noise (i.e. interruption of the wheel-running behaviour) habituates after repeated stimulation. However, recovery of the freezing response is observed again when chicks are exposed to the same sound, but in a different context (Chiandetti and Turatto, 2017).

Finally, chicks can learn regularities and apply them to subsequent choices. Chicks imprinted on coloured cylinders that followed the (AB)n, (A)n (B)n and (A(BB)A) patterns could recognize the familiar pattern irrespectively of its colour (Versace *et al.*, 2006; Santolin *et al.*, 2016a). Chicks also learn to discriminate triplets of shapes with alternating sequences of elements and are able to generalize the "pattern-following" vs. "pattern-violating" sequences in novel triplets, using statistical learning (Santolin *et al.*, 2016b). Rule-learning generalization is more effective after multimodal stimulation (i.e. acoustic other than visual), and gender explains differences in cognitive style, with males being especially attracted by unfamiliar patterns, and females by familiar ones (Versace *et al.*, 2017b).

All for One and One for All

Box 5.1 Cognitive and Social Skills in Goats: State of Art and Future Directions

Luigi Baciadonna and Alan G. McElligott

In the past, goats have not been regarded as an ideal species to investigate cognitive abilities in animals. However, recent research indicates that they have cognitive and social abilities comparable to those of species domesticated for human companionship, such as dogs and horses (Nawroth *et al.*, 2016a). Here, we present some examples of these abilities and propose areas for future research.

Goats are able to decode information cues from humans (i.e. head direction and body posture) to locate food successfully and to copy humans when learning how to go around an obstacle (Nawroth *et al.*, 2016b; Nawroth and McElligott, 2017). Moreover, they are able to request help when trying to get a small food reward from a closed box, by looking at a forward-facing versus an away-facing experimenter (Nawroth *et al.*, 2016a). This provides evidence to audience-dependent human-directed behaviour. Despite these promising findings, social learning in ungulates is still debated, because of conflicting results for different species (Briefer *et al.*, 2014). It is likely that confounding factors play a role in determining this inconsistency, and therefore further rigorous research is needed to shed light on this topic.

Goats show impressive communicative abilities, despite having a limited vocal repertoire. Their contact calls convey information about individuality, age, sex, body size and group membership (Briefer and McElligott, 2011). Vocalizations are used for recognition in mother–offspring relationships, and to distinguish individuals that are more and less familiar in combination with visual information (Briefer *et al.*, 2012; Pitcher *et al.*, 2017). Goat vocalizations also convey important information about the arousal and valence of the emotional state of the caller (Briefer *et al.*, 2015). An interesting research question is whether goats are able to decode emotional information in the call structure and/or in the body configuration of other goats or humans. Methods largely used in developmental psychology, such as the habituation–dishabituation paradigm, would enable researchers to test the hypothesis that they are able to discriminate and respond to the calls of other individuals based on arousal and valence. In addition, tasks based on simple choice preference, such as those used in dogs (Albuquerque *et al.*, 2016), would enable testing whether goats are also preferentially attracted to human faces displaying specific emotions (e.g. happy vs. sad).

Finally, goats are a social and gregarious species with a fission–fusion organization, which form dominance hierarchies and complex interindividual relationships (Barroso *et al.*, 2000; Stanley and Dunbar, 2013). Within a herd, they establish strong social bonds, are able to reconcile in post-conflict events, and form alliances during agonistic interactions (Schino, 1998). In light of this, two hypotheses worth testing are whether goats are able to use social connection to buffer the effects of negative events, and whether they are responsive to the distress of other individuals.

(cont.)

In poultry, hens are responsive to the distress of their chicks and listening to mother 'cluck' calls reduces the impact of a stressor, such as a puff of air (Edgar *et al.*, 2010, 2015). The use of similar research paradigms in goats is warranted to investigate their social skills.

To conclude, research in goats, and more in general in farm livestock, has the great potential to shed light on the complex interindividual and social abilities of these species within a comparative framework.

References

Albuquerque, N., Guo, K., Wilkinson, A., Savalli, C., Otta, E., and Mills, D. (2016). Dogs recognize dog and human emotions. *Biology Letters*, **12**, 20150883.

Barroso, F., Alados, C., and Boza, J. (2000). Social hierarchy in the domestic goat: effect on food habits and production. *Applied Animal Behaviour Science*, **69**, 35–53.

Briefer, E., and McElligott, A. G. (2011). Indicators of age, body size and sex in goat kid calls revealed using the source–filter theory. *Applied Animal Behaviour Science*, **133**, 175–185.

Briefer, E. F., Padilla de la Torre, M., and McElligott, A. G. (2012). Mother goats do not forget their kids' calls. *Proceedings of the Royal Society of London B: Biological Sciences*, **279**, 3749–3755.

Briefer, E. F., Haque, S., Baciadonna, L., and McElligott, A. G. (2014). Goats excel at learning and remembering a highly novel cognitive task. *Frontiers in Zoology*, **11**, 20.

Briefer, E. F., Tettamanti, F., and McElligott, A. G. (2015). Emotions in goats: mapping physiological, behavioural and vocal profiles. *Animal Behaviour*, **99**, 131–143.

Edgar, J. L., Lowe, J. C., Paul, E. S., and Nicol, C. J. (2010). Avian maternal response to chick distress. *Proceedings of the Royal Society of London B: Biological Sciences*, **278**, 3129–3143.

Edgar, J., Kelland, I., Held, S., Paul, E., and Nicol, C. (2015). Effects of maternal vocalisations on the domestic chick stress response. *Applied Animal Behaviour Science*, **171**, 121–127.

Nawroth, C., and McElligott., A. G. (2017). Human head orientation and eye visibility as indicators of attention for goats (*Capra hircus*). *PeerJ*, **5**, e3073.

Nawroth, C., Brett, J. M., and McElligott, A. G. (2016a). Goats display audience-dependent human-directed gazing behaviour in a problem-solving task. *Biology Letters*, **12**, 20160283.

Nawroth, C., Baciadonna, L., and McElligott, A. G. (2016b). Goats learn socially from humans in a spatial problem-solving task. *Animal Behaviour*, **121**, 123–129.

Pitcher, B. J., Briefer, E. F., Baciadonna, L., and McElligott, A. G. (2017). Cross-modal recognition of familiar conspecifics in goats. *Royal Society Open Science*, **4**, 160346.

Schino, G. (1998). Reconciliation in domestic goats. *Behaviour*, **135**, 343–356.

Stanley, C. R., and Dunbar, R. I. M. (2013). Consistent social structure and optimal clique size revealed by social network analysis of feral goats, *Capra hircus*. *Animal Behaviour*, **85**, 771–779.

Field Guide

According to the transposition of the Directive 2010/63/EU into national legislation, projects are submitted (depending on the various countries) through local ethics or institutional animal welfare bodies to the national competent authorities, and authorized as required for those that imply the use of live animals. A permit number has to be obtained before the research starts, and all the procedures must follow what described in the approved experimental design.

Here we describe in detail the protocols that are currently in use in our laboratories. Chicks arrive in the lab in the form of fertilized eggs collected weekly from a commercial hatchery and are kept under controlled conditions within automatic egg-turner incubators. The chicks are the Ross 308 breed from Aviagen. Eggs can be candled to control the embryonic development (see in Resources the atlas to individuate the developmental stages), but this procedure should be avoided if pre-natal light has to be avoided or only administered during certain time-windows (as, for instance, in studies on the development of lateralization; Rogers, 1982). Twenty-one days after their arrival at the laboratory, the chicks hatch and a few hours later, once completely dried, they enter the experimental manipulations (i.e. they are reared in cages with specific stimuli, are kept within the incubator until the moment of test, are directly tested in the runway, etc.).

For maintenance in single cages, metal boxes are used, opened on the upper part to let the light in and with a circular opening on the frontal wall, to allow the caregiver easy access for daily care. Light should follow the natural cycle, and temperature should be constant at 30–32°C during the first post-hatching days. Two separate jars provide the animal with water and crumbles. The caregiver should show the chicks how to drink water by gently dipping their beak into the water: this procedure can be done once; chicks will learn very fast how to drink autonomously and where to find water. Be sure that the chick has enough space to stretch the neck and swallow the water down, before deciding where to position the water jar. Chicks start eating crumbles a few hours after hatching, although the interest in food increases a few days after, when the nutrients contained in the yolk have been completely absorbed, nearly 3 days post-hatching (Rogers, 1995). The corresponding reward of a sweet for human participants is a *Tenebrio molitor* larvae for a chick, and it is used especially during training procedures. The natural habitat of the fowl is a forest with dim light (Wood-Gush, 1971), and a typical naturalistic situation has been successfully recreated in the laboratory to explore chicks' use of the visual fields, covering the ground with pebbles and grains of similar size and shape. Chicks will learn fast how to avoid pebbles and direct pecks at grains of food. A very effective way to record chicks' pecks at different elements is to record the behaviour by placing a camera below a transparent ground suspended from the floor: chicks are not afraid of stepping onto a transparent surface, provided that part of the depth cues are neutralized by white plastic material placed all around the camera, and they are accustomed to find crumbles on that surface from the first instances.

Chicks grow very rapidly; recent domestication and strong selective pressures to obtain industrial chickens have pushed their development to be completed in half of the

Table 5.1. Experimental tools to study chickens and their function.

Tool	Function
Incubator	Incubation and hatching of chicks under controlled lab conditions (i.e. with or without light or acoustic stimulation, etc.)
Cages	During experiments, small cages host up to two individuals, or a chick and the imprinting object. Each cage is furnished with two jars, one for water and one for food; a larger cage (1 m^2) hosts several chicks, while they wait to be donated to local farmers, and in any case from the second week of age onwards
Objects of different shape and size	An object hanging at about chick's head height serves as imprinting object. Different colours and shapes have been used in the literature, but large red cylinders (6 × 7.5 cm in diameter and height, respectively) seem very much appreciated
Food	Chicks' crumbles can be used for regular diet; mealworms (*Tenebrio molitor*) can be used as food rewards in training conditions
Material for apparatus	Plexiglas and polipack can be used to create the apparatus, the separations between animals, or animals and objects, providing the experimenter with a surface that is easy to clean
Computer	A desktop can be easily equipped with a graphic card supporting two identical screens and hence providing the possibility to administer two different stimuli with the very same visual features at the same time (for instance at the opposed ends of a runway, with or without a running-wheel placed centrally); a separate one is used to record the behaviour, for subsequent offline scoring and video analysis
Video-camera	A standard webcam is sufficient to record the chick's behaviour within the apparatus; specific cameras (for instance infrared ones) can be chosen for specific needs (for instance the recording of hatching time within a darkened incubator)

time needed by our grandfathers' chickens (Zuidhof *et al.*, 2011). Therefore, stimuli presentation for prolonged training requires continuous adjustments in the first and the second weeks of age (e.g. stimulus height on a computer screen has to be regulated to allow pecking, if stimuli are not administered on the ground).

In all experimental set-ups, a camera connected to a computer allows online observations from a distance that minimises disturbance. Furthermore, recording chicks' performance allows scoring offline by independent blind observers.

Simultaneous presentation of stimuli at the ends of a runway benefit from the use of two identical monitors connected to the same computer, in order to obtain an identical administration of the experimental material. Computers also allow an automated presentation and a reward schedule, as in the work depicted in Figure 5.5. The apparatus can be created with wooden material, and small compartments (e.g. starting boxes or separators) can be made out of plastic material. This last option makes the constant cleaning of the environment easier, so that every influence from the chick tested before is eliminated from the experimental area. The room in which the apparatus is placed is usually a dark and silent environment: the apparatus can be covered by a net working as a unidirectional screen, and the light illuminating the testing area (arriving either from the computer screens or from one or two symmetrical light bulbs) makes the environment uniform and attracts chicks' attention to the stimuli and cues available within it, rather than to outer cues. However, a careful randomization of the entrance site of the animal or of the starting point for each trial (within and between subjects) is always recommended. At the end of a trial and before another animal enters the same apparatus, the environment should be carefully cleaned using professional disinfectant to avoid biological samples acting as visual or olfactory cues.

By the end of the experiments, 1-week-old chicks are reared altogether in a large (1 m^2) cage with water (coming from a bottle waterer hanging from above or a round drinker with a plate on the ground) and food provided *ad libitum*: in this space, they have the possibility to run and move with no restraints; some slanted surfaces with a place to perch provide the chicks with an enriched condition for all the time they spend within this large cage, awaiting local farmers to collect them and bring them to the countryside.

Wild vs. Lab

Box 5.2 Chicken Challenges: Studying Fowl Behaviour in the Wild

Carolynn K-lynn Smith

Chickens have changed dramatically in the 8000 years since they were first domesticated (Storey *et al.*, 2012) from red jungle fowl (*Gallus gallus*; Xiang *et al.*, 2014). Domestic chickens have been bred for commercial purposes, such as fast growth in meat chickens and year-round egg production in egg-laying strains, and for appearances (e.g. size, feather colour and comb shape).

The process of domestication has brought about physiological and behavioural changes that may allow an animal to adapt to captive conditions, such as increased proximity to humans and confinement, as well as increased social interactions associated with higher stocking density. Some physiological differences between wild and domestic chickens include changes in brain size and structure (Agnvall *et al.*, 2017). For example, differences in the visual processing system structure suggest that domestic birds may have diminished vision compared to wild fowl (ICGSC, 2004). Furthermore, differences have been identified in stress-related genes in the brain, pituitary and adrenal glands. For example, white leghorns have a reduced stress response compared to red jungle fowl (Løtvedt *et al.*, 2017). Genetics also play a part in social motivation, and some studies have shown that red jungle fowl are better able to adjust to novel social environments (Väisänen and Jensen, 2004). Other studies found that red jungle fowl have better spatial learning when reared under unpredictable conditions, and are more exploratory when foraging (Andresson *et al.*, 2001). This suggests that red jungle fowl chicks are better adapted to unpredictable environments than domestic breeds (Lindqvist and Jensen, 2009).

Jungle fowl are known to hybridize with escaped domestic chickens and the purity of wild strains is often difficult to determine without genetic testing. Birds that have

(cont.)

gone feral (i.e. escaped from captivity to live in the wild) may also be different from wild birds and from the captive ones from which they arose (Gering *et al.*, 2015). These differences in behaviour and physiology mean that comparative studies of wild, feral and different breeds of domestic chickens may reveal selective pressures on behaviours and genetics.

Studying fowl in the wild can be accomplished, but has challenges. Many of the experiments presented in this chapter used controlled conditions, such as standardized lighting and digital representations of stimuli. It is possible to replicate these types of test conditions in the wild with weatherized equipment (e.g. Wilson and Evans, 2010). Because rearing conditions are known to affect behaviour (Håkansson *et al.*, 2007), studies of wild jungle fowl chicks may require the collection and incubation of eggs. In the wild, a group of jungle fowl live in a territory that is approximately 1 hectare. The individually distinctive crows of males can be used to identify territories. Birds typically use the same roost trees each night and are easier to catch in the roost (McBride *et al.*, 1969). Once captured, hens can be radio-tracked to locate nests.

Many of the cognitive abilities described in this chapter are likely to be conserved across breeds. However, given the differences between breeds, empirical tests are needed to confirm this assumption.

References

Agnvall, B., Bélteky, J., and Jensen, P. (2017). Brain size is reduced by selection for tameness in red junglefowl – correlated effects in vital organs. *Scientific Reports*, **7**, 3306.

Andresson, M., Nordin, E., and Jensen, P. (2001). Domestication effects on foraging strategies in fowl. *Applied Animal Behaviour Science*, **72**, 51–62.

Gering, E., Johnsson, M., Willis, P., Getty, T., and Wright, D. (2015). Mixed ancestry and admixture in Kauai's feral chickens: invasion of domestic genes into ancient red junglefowl reservoirs. *Molecular Ecology*, **24**, 2112–2124.

Håkansson, J., Bratt, C., and Jensen, P. (2007). Behavioural differences between two captive populations of red jungle fowl (*Gallus gallus*) with different genetic background, raised under identical conditions. *Applied Animal Behaviour Science*, **102**, 24–38.

International Chicken Genome Sequencing Consortium. (2004). Sequence and comparative analysis of the chicken genome provide unique perspectives on vertebrate evolution. *Nature*, **432**, 695–716.

Lindqvist, C., and Jensen, P. (2009). Domestication and stress effects on contrafreeloading and spatial learning performance in red jungle fowl (*Gallus gallus*) and white Leghorn layers. *Behavioral Processes*, **81**, 80–84.

Løtvedt, P., Fallahshahroudi, A., Bektic, L., Altimiras, J., and Jensen, P. (2017) Chicken domestication changes expression of stress-related genes in brain, pituitary and adrenals. *Neurobiology of Stress*, **7**, 113–121.

McBride, G., Parer, I. P., and Foenander, F. (1969). The social organization and behaviour of the feral domestic chicken. *Animal Behaviour Monographs*, **2**, 127–181.

(*cont.*)

Storey, A.A., Athens, J. S., Bryant, D., *et al.* (2012). Investigating the global dispersal of chickens in prehistory using ancient mitochondrial DNA signatures. *PLoS ONE*, **7**(7), e39171.

Väisänen, J., and Jensen, P. (2004). Responses of young red jungle fowl (*Gallus gallus*) and white leghorn layers to familiar and unfamiliar social stimuli. *Poultry Science*, **83**, 335–343.

Wilson, D., and Evans, C. (2010). Female fowl (*Gallus gallus*) do not prefer alarm-calling males. *Behaviour*, **147**, 525–552.

Xiang, H., Gao, J., Yu, B., *et al.* (2014). Early Holocene chicken domestication in northern China. *Proceedings of the National Academy of Sciences*, **111**, 17564–17569.

Resources

Basic literature:

- Andrew, R. J. (1991). *Neural and behavioural plasticity: the use of the domestic chick as a model*. Oxford: Oxford University Press.
- Lawler, A. (2014). *Why did the chicken cross the world? The epic saga of the bird that powers civilization*. New York, NY: Atria Books.
- Marino, L. (2017). Thinking chickens: a review of cognition, emotion, and behavior in the domestic chicken. *Animal Cognition*, **20**, 127–147.
- Nicol, C. J. (2015). *The behavioural biology of chickens*. Wallingford: CABI Publishing.
- Rogers, L. J. (1995). *The development of brain and behaviour in the chicken*. Wallingford: CABI Publishing.
- Wood-Gush, D. G. M. (1971). *The behaviour of the domestic fowl*. London: Heinemann Educational Books Ltd.

Websites:

- Our chicks' breed: http://en.aviagen.com/
- Chicken development: https://embryology.med.unsw.edu.au/embryology/index.php/Chicken_Development
- Thoughtful birds in action: www.youtube.com/watch?feature=player_embedded&v=zyceeJNiYwk

Profile

Cinzia had a grandfather with hens in his courtyard and an aunt with a hill myna repeating 'Avanti popolo!' when people walked by. At the University of Padova, Professor Zanforlin and Regolin's unforgettable lessons evoked infancy memories. She thus decided to discuss her master thesis on chickens under their supervision, before continuing at the University of Trieste, where she also investigates the biological roots of prosody and musical preferences.

Giorgio struggled as a student to decide whether to be a scientist of some sort or a philosopher, being fascinated by the way biological organisms acquire knowledge. After reading Lorenz's book *The other face of the mirror*, he opted for behavioural biology and ethology, entering a comparative psychology lab, studying visual perception and learning in newly hatched chicks. He then moved to the UK to study imprinting and brain asymmetry with chicks. His lab currently hosts a variety of other creatures (from fish to chimps, bees and dogs), but chicks remain his unforgettable first love.

References

Baiocchi, V., and Chiandetti, C. (2016). Chicks run harder toward a consonant over a dissonant clucking hen: biological roots for the appreciation of consonant sounds. In *Trieste Symposium on Perception and Cognition 2016*. Trieste: EUT, P03.

Bermant, G. (1963). Intensity and rate of distress calling in chicks as a function of social contact. *Animal Behaviour*, **11**, 514–517.

Cailotto, M., Vallortigara, G., and Zanforlin, M. (1989). Sex differences in the response to social stimuli in young chicks. *Ethology Ecology and Evolution*, **1**, 323–327.

Chiandetti, C. (2011). Pseudoneglect and embryonic light stimulation in the avian brain. *Behavioral Neuroscience*, **125**, 775–782.

Chiandetti, C. (2017). Shaping. In *Encyclopedia of animal cognition and behavior*. New York, NY: Springer.

Chiandetti, C., and Turatto, M. (2017). Context-specific habituation of the freezing response in newborn chicks. *Behavioral Neuroscience*, **131**, 437–446.

Chiandetti, C., and Vallortigara, G. (2008). Is there an innate geometric module? Effects of experience with angular geometric cues on spatial re-orientation based on the shape of the environment. *Animal Cognition*, **11**, 139–146.

Chiandetti, C., and Vallortigara, G. (2010). Experience and geometry: controlled-rearing studies with chicks. *Animal Cognition*, **13**, 463–470.

Chiandetti, C., and Vallortigara, G. (2011a). Chicks like consonant music. *Psychological Science*, **22**, 1270–1273.

Chiandetti, C., and Vallortigara, G. (2011b). Intuitive physical reasoning about occluded objects by inexperienced chicks. *Proceedings of the Royal Society of London B: Biological Sciences*, **278**, 2621–2627.

Chiandetti, C., Regolin, L., Rogers, L. J., and Vallortigara, G. (2005). Effects of light stimulation of embryos on the use of position-specific and object-specific cues in binocular and monocular domestic chicks (*Gallus gallus*). *Behavioural Brain Research*, **163**, 10–17.

Chiandetti, C., Pecchia, T., Patt, F., and Vallortigara, G. (2014). Visual hierarchical processing and lateralization of cognitive functions through domestic chicks' eyes. *PLoS ONE*, **9**(1), e84435.

Chiandetti, C., Spelke, E. S., and Vallortigara, G. (2015). Inexperienced newborn chicks use geometry to spontaneously reorient to an artificial social partner. *Developmental Science*, **6**, 972–978.

Clara, E., Regolin, L., Zanforlin, M., and Vallortigara, G. (2006). Domestic chicks perceive stereokinetic illusions. *Perception*, **35**, 983–992.

Collias, N., and Joos, M. (1953). The spectrographic analysis of sound signals of the domestic fowl. *Behaviour*, **5**, 175–188.

Cozzutti, C., and Vallortigara, G. (2001). Hemispheric memories for the content and position of food caches in the domestic chick. *Behavioral Neuroscience*, **115**, 305–313.

Daisley, J. N., Vallortigara, G., and Regolin, L. (2010). Logic in an asymmetrical (social) brain: transitive inference in the young domestic chick. *Social Neuroscience*, **5**, 309–319.

Dawkins, M. S. (2002). What are birds looking at ? Head movements and eye use in chickens. *Animal Behaviour*, **63**, 991–998.

De Tommaso, M., Kaplan, G., Chiandetti, C., and Vallortigara, G. (under rev.). Naive 3-day-old domestic chicks (*Gallus gallus*) are attracted to discrete acoustic patterns characterizing natural vocalizations.

Di Giorgio, E., Loveland, J. L., Mayer, U., Rosa-Salva, O., Versace, E., and Vallortigara, G. (2017). Filial responses as predisposed and learned preferences: early attachment in chicks and babies. *Behavioural Brain Research*, **325**, 90–104.

Diekamp, B., Regolin, L., Güntürkün, O., and Vallortigara, G. (2005). A left-sided visuospatial bias. *Current Biology*, **15**, 372–373.

Forkman, B. (2000). Domestic hens have declarative representations. *Animal Cognition*, **3**, 135–137.

Forkman, B., and Vallortigara, G. (1999). Minimization of modal contours: an essential cross-species strategy in disambiguating relative depth. *Animal Cognition*, **2**, 181–185.

Ghirlanda, S., Jansson, L., and Enquist, M. (2002). Chickens prefer beautiful humans. *Human Nature*, **13**, 383–389.

Ham, A. D., and Osorio, D. (2007). Colour preferences and colour vision in poultry chicks. *Proceedings of the Royal Society B: Biological Sciences*, **274**, 1941–1948.

Johnson, M. H., Bolhuis, J. J., and Horn, G. (1992). Predispositions and learning: behavioural dissociations in the chick. *Animal Behaviour*, **44**, 943–948.

Kent, J. (1993). The chick's preference for certain features of the maternal cluck vocalization in the domestic fowl (*Gallus gallus*). *Behaviour*, **125**, 177–187.

Krause, E. T., Schrader, L., and Caspers, B. A. (2016). Olfaction in chicken (*Gallus gallus*): a neglected mode of social communication? *Frontiers in Ecology and Evolution*, **4**, 94.

Lea, S. E. G., Stater, A. M., and Ryan, C. M. E. (1996). Perception of object unity in chicks: a comparison with human infant. *Infant Behavior and Development*, **19**, 501–504.

Lorenzi, E., Mayer, U., Rosa-Salva, O., and Vallortigara, G. (2017). Dynamic features of animate motion activate septal and preoptic areas in visually naïve chicks (*Gallus gallus*). *Neuroscience*, **354**, 54–68.

Marler, P. R., Dufty, A., and Pickert, R. (1986). Vocal communication in the domestic chicken: II. Is a sender sensitive to the presence and nature of a receiver? *Animal Behaviour*, **34**, 194–198.

Mascalzoni, E., Regolin, L., and Vallortigara, G. (2009). Mom's shadow: structure-from-motion in newly hatched chicks as revealed by an imprinting procedure. *Animal Cognition*, **12**, 389–400.

Mascalzoni, E., Regolin, L., and Vallortigara, G. (2010). Innate sensitivity for self-propelled causal agency in newly hatched chicks. *Proceedings of the National Academy of Sciences*, **107**, 4483–4485.

Mascalzoni, E., Osorio, D., Regolin, L., and Vallortigara, G. (2012). Symmetry perception by poultry chicks and its implications for three-dimensional object recognition. *Proceedings of the Royal Society B: Biological Sciences*, **279**, 841–846.

McBride, G., and Foenander, F. (1962). Territorial behaviour in flocks of domestic fowls. *Nature*, **102**, 4823.

McBride, G., Parer, I. P., and Foenander, G. (1969). The social organization and behaviour of the feral domestic fowl. *Animal Behaviour Monographs*, **2**, 125–181.

McCabe, B. J. (2013). Imprinting. *Wiley Interdisciplinary Reviews: Cognitive Science*, **4**, 375–390.

Mench, J., and Keeling, L. J. (2001). The social behaviour of domestic birds. In *Social behaviour in farm animals* (pp. 177–210). Wallingford: CABI Publishing.

Miklósi, A., Andrew, R. J., and Dharmaretnam, M. (1996). Auditory lateralisation: shifts in ear use during attachment in the domestic chick. *Laterality*, **1**, 215–225.

Nicol, C. J. (2004). Development, direction and damage limitation: social learning in domestic fowl. *Learning and Behavior*, **32**, 72–81.

Osorio, D., Vorobyev, M., and Jones, C. D. (1999). Colour vision of domestic chicks. *The Journal of Experimental Biology*, **202**, 2951–2959.

Regolin, L., and Vallortigara, G. (1995). Perception of partly occluded objects by young chicks. *Perception and Psychophysics*, **57**, 971–976.

Regolin, L., Vallortigara, G., and Zanforlin, M. (1995). Object and spatial representations in detour problems by chicks. *Animal Behaviour*, **49**, 195–199.

Regolin, L., Tommasi, L., and Vallortigara, G. (2000). Visual perception of biological motion in newly hatched chicks as revealed by an imprinting procedure. *Animal Cognition*, **3**, 53–60.

Regolin, L., Marconato, F., and Vallortigara, G. (2004). Hemispheric differences in the recognition of partly occluded objects by newly hatched domestic chicks (*Gallus gallus*). *Animal Cognition*, **7**, 162–170.

Regolin, L., Rugani, R., Pagni, P., and Vallortigara, G. (2005). Delayed search for social and nonsocial goals by young domestic chicks, *Gallus gallus domesticus*. *Animal Behaviour*, **70**, 855–864.

Regolin, L., Rugani, R., Stancher, G., and Vallortigara, G. (2011). Spontaneous discrimination of possible and impossible objects by newly hatched chicks. *Biology Letters*, **7**, 654–657.

Regolin, L., Daisley, J. N., Rosa-Salva, O., and Vallortigara, G. (2012). Advantages of a lateralised brain for reasoning about the social world in chicks. In *Behavioral lateralization in vertebrates* (pp. 39–54). Berlin: Springer.

Rogers, L. J. (1982). Light experience and asymmetry of brain function in chickens. *Nature*, **297**, 223–225.

Rogers, L. J. (1995). *The development of brain and behaviour in the chicken*. Wallingford: CAB International.

Rogers, L. J., Zucca, P., and Vallortigara, G. (2004). Advantages of having a lateralized brain. *Proceedings of the Royal Society B: Biological Sciences*, **271**, 420–422.

Rosa Salva, O., Regolin, L., and Vallortigara, G. (2010). Faces are special for newly hatched chicks: evidence for inborn domain-specific mechanisms underlying spontaneous preferences for face-like stimuli. *Developmental Science*, **13**, 565–577.

Rosa Salva, O., Farroni, T., Regolin, L., Vallortigara, G., and Johnson, M. H. (2011). The evolution of social orienting: evidence from chicks (*Gallus gallus*) and human newborns. *PLoS ONE*, **6**(4), e18802.

Rosa Salva, O., Regolin, L., Mascalzoni, E., and Vallortigara, G. (2012). Cerebral and behavioural asymmetries in animal social recognition. *Comparative Cognition and Behavior Reviews*, **7**, 110–138.

Rosa Salva, O., Rugani, R., Cavazzana, A., Regolin, L., and Vallortigara, G. (2013). Perception of the Ebbinghaus illusion in four-day-old domestic chicks (*Gallus gallus*). *Animal Cognition*, **16**, 895–906.

Rosa Salva, O., Grassi, M., Lorenzi, E., Regolin, L., and Vallortigara, G. (2016). Spontaneous preference for visual cues of animacy in naïve domestic chicks: the case of speed changes. *Cognition*, **157**, 49–60.

Rugani, R., Regolin, L., and Vallortigara, G. (2008). Discrimination of small numerosities in young chicks. *Journal of Experimental Psychology: Animal Behavior Processes*, **34**, 388–399.

Rugani, R., Fontanari, L., Simoni, E., Regolin, L., and Vallortigara, G. (2009). Arithmetic in newborn chicks. *Proceedings of the Royal Society B: Biological Sciences*, **276**, 2451–2460.

Rugani, R., Regolin, L., and Vallortigara, G. (2010). Imprinted numbers: newborn chicks' sensitivity to number vs. continuous extent of objects they have been reared with. *Developmental Science*, **13**, 790–797.

Rugani, R., Vallortigara, G., Priftis, K., and Regolin, L. (2015). Number-space mapping in the newborn chick resembles humans' mental number line. *Science*, **347**, 534–536.

Rushen, J. (1982). The peck orders of domestic chickens: how do they develop and why are they linear? *Animal Behaviour*, **30**, 1129–1137.

Santolin, C., Rosa-Salva, O., Regolin, L., and Vallortigara, G. (2016a). Generalization of visual regularities in newly hatched chicks (*Gallus gallus*). *Animal Cognition*, **19**, 1007–1017.

Santolin, C., Rosa Salva, O., Vallortigara, G., and Regolin, L. (2016b). Unsupervised statistical learning in newly hatched chicks. *Current Biology*, **26**, 1218–1220.

Shimmura, T., Ohashi, S., and Takashi, Y. (2015). The highest-ranking rooster has priority to announce the break of dawn. *Scientific Reports*, **5**, 11683.

Tommasi, L., Bressan, P., and Vallortigara, G. (1995). Solving occlusion indeterminacy in chromatically homogeneous patterns. *Perception*, **24**, 391–403.

Tommasi, L., Vallortigara, G., and Zanforlin, M. (1997). Young chickens learn to localize the centre of a spatial environment. *Journal of Comparative Physiology A*, **180**, 567–572.

Vallortigara, G. (1992). Affiliation and aggression as related to gender in domestic chicks (*Gallus gallus*). *Journal of Comparative Psychology*, **106**, 53–57.

Vallortigara, G. (1996). Learning of colour and position cues in domestic chicks: males are better at position, females at colour. *Behavioural Processes*, **36**, 289–296.

Vallortigara, G. (2014). Foundations of number and space representations in precocial species. In *Evolutionary origins and early development of number processing* (pp. 35–66). New York, NY: Elsevier.

Vallortigara, G. (2017). An animal's sense of number. In *The nature and development of mathematics. Cross disciplinary perspective on cognition, learning and culture* (pp. 43–65). New York, NY: Routledge.

Vallortigara, G., and Andrew, R. J. (1994). Olfactory lateralization in the chick. *Neuropsychologia*, **32**, 417–423.

Vallortigara, G., and Regolin, L. (1998). Delayed search for a concealed imprinted object in the domestic chick. *Animal Cognition*, **1**, 17–24.

Vallortigara, G., and Regolin, L. (2006). Gravity bias in the interpretation of biological motion by inexperienced chicks. *Current Biology*, **16**, 279–280.

Vallortigara, G., and Tommasi, L. (2001). Minimization of modal contours: an instance of an evolutionary internalized geometric regularity? *Brain and Behavioral Sciences*, **24**, 706–707.

Vallortigara, G., and Versace, E. (2017). Filial imprinting. In *Encyclopedia of animal cognition and behavior*. New York, NY: Springer.

Vallortigara, G., and Zanforlin, M. (1988). Open-field behavior of young chicks (*Gallus gallus*): antipredatory responses, social reinstatement motivation, and gender effects. *Animal Learning and Behavior*, **16**, 359–362.

Vallortigara, G., and Zanforlin, M. (1989). Place and object learning in chicks (*Gallus gallus domesticus*). *Journal of Comparative Psychology*, **103**, 201–209.

Vallortigara, G., Cailotto, M., and Zanforlin, M. (1990a). Sex differences in social reinstatement motivation of the domestic chick (*Gallus gallus*) revealed by runway tests with social and nonsocial reinforcement. *Journal of Comparative Psychology*, **104**, 361–367.

Vallortigara, G., Zanforlin, M., and Compostella, S. (1990b). Perceptual organization in animal learning: cues or objects? *Ethology*, **85**, 89–102.

Vallortigara, G., Zanforlin, M., and Pasti, G. (1990c). Geometric modules in animals' spatial representations: a test with chicks (*Gallus gallus domesticus*). *Journal of Comparative Psychology*, **104**, 248–254.

Vallortigara, G., Regolin, L., and Zanforlin, M. (1994). The development of responses to novel-coloured objects in male and female domestic chicks. *Behavioural Processes*, **31**, 219–229.

Vallortigara, G., Regolin, L., Rigoni, M., and Zanforlin, M. (1998). Delayed search for a concealed imprinted object in the domestic chick. *Animal Cognition*, **1**, 17–24.

Vallortigara, G., Regolin, L., and Marconato, F. (2005). Visually inexperienced chicks exhibit spontaneous preference for biological motion patterns. *PLoS Biology*, **3**, 3–7.

Vallortigara, G., Sovrano, V. A., and Chiandetti, C. (2009). Doing Socrates experiment right: controlled rearing studies of geometrical knowledge in animals. *Current Opinion in Neurobiology*, **19**, 20–26.

Vallortigara, G., Cozzutti, C., Tommasi, L., and Rogers, L. J. (2011). How birds use their eyes. Opposite left–right specialization for the lateral and frontal visual hemifield in the domestic chick. *Current Biology*, **11**, 29–33.

Versace, E. (2017). Precocial. In *Encyclopedia of animal cognition and behavior*. New York, NY: Springer.

Versace, E., and Vallortigara, G. (2015). Origins of knowledge: insights from precocial species. *Frontiers in Behavioral Neuroscience*, **9**, 338.

Versace, E., Regolin, L., and Vallortigara, G. (2006). Emergence of grammar as revealed by visual imprinting in newly-hatched chicks. In *The evolution of language. Proceedings of the 6th International Conference* (pp. 457–458). Singapore: World Scientific.

Versace, E., Schill, J., Nencini, A. M., and Vallortigara, G. (2016). Naïve chicks prefer hollow objects. *PLoS ONE*, **11**(11), e0166425.

Versace, E., Fracasso, I., Baldan, G., Zotte, A. D., and Vallortigara, G. (2017a). Newborn chicks show inherited variability in early social predispositions for hen-like stimuli. *Scientific Reports*, **7**, 40296.

Versace, E., Spierings, M. J., Caffini, M., ten Cate, C., and Vallortigara, G. (2017b). Spontaneous generalization of abstract multimodal patterns in young domestic chicks. *Animal Cognition*, **20**, 521–529.

Wood, J. N. (2013). Newborn chickens generate invariant object representations at the onset of visual object experience. *Proceedings of the National Academy of Sciences*, **110**, 14000–14005.

Wood-Gush, D. G. M. (1971). *The behaviour of the domestic fowl*. London: Heinemann.

Workman, L., and Andrew, R. J. (1989). Simultaneous changes in behaviour and in lateralization during the development of male and female domestic chicks. *Animal Behaviour*, **38**, 596–605.

Zanforlin, M. (1981). Visual perception of complex forms (anomalous surfaces) in chicks. *Italian Journal of Psychology*, **8**, 1–16.

Zuidhof, M. J., Schneider, B. L., Carney, V. L., Korver, D. R., and Robinson, F. E. (2011). Growth, efficiency, and yield of commercial broilers from 1957, 1978, and 2005. *Genetics*, **93**, 1–13.

6 Chimpanzees – Investigating Cognition in the Wild

Roman M. Wittig and Catherine Crockford

Species Description

Anatomy

Chimpanzees (*Pan troglodytes*) are a long-lived species with the oldest known individuals in the wild exceeding 50 years. Once becoming adult at the age of 15 years, chimpanzees have an average height of 1.20 m (Coolidge and Shea, 1982) and show sexual dimorphism, with males being slightly heavier in the wild than females (male weight $\pm$ SD = 40.9 kg $\pm$ 4.6, N = 18; female weight $\pm$ SD = 33.4 kg $\pm$ 4.7, N = 23; Uehara and Nishida, 1987). Although chimpanzees have longer arms than legs and are well adapted to life in the trees, they have a mainly terrestrial lifestyle. They move on all fours, clenching their hands and supporting themselves on their knuckles. Their hands consist of an opposed thumb, allowing easy manipulation of objects and the precision grip frequently used during such manipulations (Christel, 1993). Chimpanzees have a U-shaped jaw with 32 teeth (2, 1, 2, 3), a diastema between incisors and canine, and a set of deciduous and permanent teeth.

Perception

Chimpanzees are diurnal animals with colour vision and forward-facing eyes allowing for stereoscopic vision (Matsuno *et al.*, 2004), making vision one of their main senses, as with all other simians. Without relying on their visual sense, the large genital swellings of female chimpanzees would not be an effective indicator of their fertility, nor would social learning be able to create cultural variance or conformity of immigrants to existing cultures (Luncz *et al.*, 2015). Chimpanzees use their visual sense, among other things, to inspect fruit in the trees while remaining on the ground, to focus on and catch prey, while coordinating with several chimpanzees in a tree during a hunt (Boesch and Boesch, 1989), or to detect dangers and rival chimpanzee communities in the forest (Crockford *et al.*, 2012).

Living in a forest, however, hampers the visual range, making the chimpanzees' acoustic sense probably as important as the visual one. Chimpanzees have a similar hearing range to humans (20 Hz to 20 kHz), but they are less sensitive to lower and more sensitive to higher frequencies (Kojima, 1990). Calls can travel long distances, with pant-hoots having an approximate range of 1 km, and more quiet calls (e.g. hoos and grunts) still travelling several hundred metres through the forest. Because some calls convey information about context (e.g. Crockford and Boesch, 2003) and individual identity (Crockford *et al.*, 2004), chimpanzees can gain information about the presence of nearby individuals and the context associated with call production from listening to others' calls (Schel *et al.*, 2013a, 2013b; Wittig *et al.*, 2014a).

The olfactory sense may also play an important role in some contexts (Heymann, 2006; Matsumoto-Oda *et al.*, 2007). Through olfaction, chimpanzees can detect predators, pick up the identity of rival chimpanzees (Samuni *et al.*, 2017) and detect whether fruits are ripe or if females ovulate (Matsumoto-Oda *et al.*, 2007).

Ecological Characteristics

Chimpanzees are native to the tropical forests and woodlands of Africa. They range from Senegal in the west to Tanzania in the east, and are genetically and geographically distinguishable into four subspecies: West African chimpanzees (*Pan troglodytes verus*), Nigeria–Cameroon chimpanzees (*P. t. eliotti*), Central African chimpanzees (*P. t. troglodytes*) and East African chimpanzees (*P. t. schweinfurthii*; Figure 6.1). Chimpanzee behaviour varies across populations (Whiten *et al.*, 1999). Although some evidence suggests that genetic variation plays a role in explaining population differences in chimpanzee behaviour (Langergraber *et al.*, 2010), research has provided evidence that cultural underpinnings explain some of the variation of behaviour across chimpanzee groups and populations (Gruber *et al.*, 2009; Luncz *et al.*, 2012).

Chimpanzees are omnivorous and feed on a wide range of food items. They mostly consume ripe fruits, but also nuts, mushrooms and leaves. They also hunt mammals, mainly monkeys, eat insects, such as ants, termites and maggots, raid honey and fish for

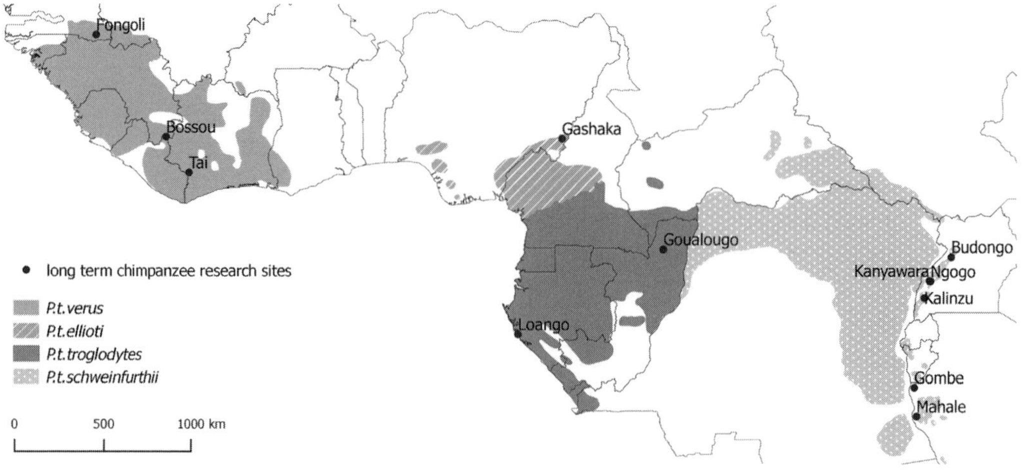

Figure 6.1. Distribution of chimpanzee subspecies across Africa, including the location of long-term research sites.

algae. Many of these foods require tools to extract the edible content. Chimpanzees, for example, use long grass blades to fish termites from termite mounds (Lonsdorf, 2006), they use sticks to dip for ants in ant nests (Humle and Matsuzawa, 2002), wooden or stone hammers to crack open nuts (Boesch and Boesch, 1982), leaves to sponge water out of treeholes (van Lawick-Goodall, 1968), complex stick tool sets to detect and extract underground bee nests (Boesch *et al.*, 2009), and they use wooden spears to extract prey out of treeholes (Pruetz and Bertolani, 2007). Many of these tool-using behaviours have been identified as traditions or cultures (Whiten *et al.*, 1999), and individuals acquire tool-using skills over several years during development. Observations in wild populations suggest that this process includes social learning (Matsuzawa *et al.*, 2008), involving watching others handling tools, or even teaching others how to handle a tool (Boesch, 1991). The tool use of juveniles develops over years, and migrants between groups may conform to local cultures (Luncz *et al.*, 2015).

Social Characteristics

Chimpanzees live in fission–fusion communities of multiple males and females (Nishida, 1968). A growing body of research at long-term study sites shows that community sizes of chimpanzees under natural conditions vary from 20 to 200 individuals (Wilson *et al.*, 2014), including all adults (> 15 years), subadults (10–15 years), juveniles (5–10 years) and infants (< 5 years). The central unit of the chimpanzee community is the mother with her offspring. Offspring are completely dependent on the mother until about 5 years of age, but they continue to stay with their mothers until they reach sexual maturity, at 12–15 years old. Emigrating from their natal community can be costly to the immigrating females (Kahlenberg *et al.*, 2008a), since they compete with the resident ones over adequate food sources (Wittig and Boesch, 2003a; Kahlenberg *et al.*, 2008b).

Chimpanzee males, in contrast, stay in their natal community. Once they reach adulthood, they start to compete with other males within their community over the dominance ranks. Indeed, there is considerable reproductive skew in favour of higher-ranking males (Boesch *et al.*, 2006; Wroblewski *et al.*, 2009). Males build 'revolutionary' coalitions, such that lower-rank males cooperate with each other to gain mating opportunities from dominant males (Duffy *et al.*, 2007) and to overpower dominants, increasing their dominance status (Nishida *et al.*, 1992; Mitani *et al.*, 2000). These in-group competitors, however, become strong cooperators once they are threatened by neighbours in rival communities. Male chimpanzees show group-level cooperation to compete with males of rival communities (Wilson and Wrangham, 2003; Samuni *et al.*, 2017). Males, and sometimes females, patrol into the rivals' territory (Watts and Mitani, 2001), take rival females hostage (Boesch *et al.*, 2008) and may kill rival males once they have them separated from the rival community (Mitani *et al.*, 2010; Wilson *et al.*, 2014).

Such a strong level of coalitionary support in chimpanzees is reflected in distinctive friendships, or bonds, formed mostly between non-kin (Langergraber *et al.*, 2007). Dyads that associate more frequently show above-average levels of cooperative behaviours and have lower aggression rates (Wittig *et al.*, 2014a, 2016; Surbeck *et al.*, 2017a, b). Therefore, if a researcher wants to investigate the cooperative abilities of chimpanzees, he or she needs to take the social relationships between potential cooperators into account.

Chimpanzees engage in group-level cooperation to defend their territory (Samuni *et al.*, 2017). Strong in-group cooperation is likely key to avoiding injuries (Mitani *et al.*, 2010; Wilson *et al.*, 2014). Coalitionary support by in-group cooperators probably reduces the likelihood of being injured or killed during intergroup encounters (Boesch *et al.*, 2008). Chimpanzees also share food, whether this is meat (Mitani and Watts, 2001), fruit (Hockings *et al.*, 2007) or even tools for extracting food (pers. obs.). Sharing may avoid harassment (Gilby, 2006) in some communities, whereas in others it may facilitate the formation and maintenance of social bonds (Wittig *et al.*, 2014b), coalitionary support (Nishida *et al.*, 1992) or access to mating partners (Gomes and Boesch, 2009). Finally, chimpanzees may adopt orphans (Goodall, 1986; Hobaiter *et al.*, 2014), even if genetically unrelated to them (Boesch *et al.*, 2010).

State of the Art

Genetic evidence suggests that the lineages of chimpanzees and humans diverged about 7–8 million years ago (Langergraber *et al.*, 2012), allowing us to peek several million years into the past, when comparing cognitive abilities of *Pan* and humans. This comparative approach has had considerable impact on our present knowledge of the evolution of human's unprecedented cognitive abilities (Tomasello and Call, 1997; Tomasello, 2009a). Chimpanzee cognition has been under intense investigation for over 100 years, when Wolfgang Köhler started testing chimpanzees with problem-solving tasks (Köhler, 2013). Since then, many scientists have followed in Köhler's footsteps, investigating different aspects of chimpanzee cognition to understand the evolutionary roots of human cognition (Tomasello and Call, 1997; Herrmann *et al.*, 2007, 2010).

For this reason, much research focuses on cognitive capacities considered to be uniquely human, in order to determine whether other animals share these capacities. One example in social cognition is the question of whether chimpanzees have a theory of mind (i.e. what individuals know about others' knowledge and beliefs; Premack and Woodruff, 1978). Despite many conflicting results (Povinelli and Vonk, 2003; cf. Hare *et al.*, 2001), new evidence suggests that chimpanzees have a fully developed theory of mind, understanding others' false beliefs (Krupenye *et al.*, 2016), but possibly lacking the motivation to share these psychological states with others (Call, 2009).

In physical cognition, memory tests revealed that chimpanzees have a working memory that outcompetes humans in the effectiveness and speed of numerical recollection (Inoue and Matsuzawa, 2007), and that chimpanzees even show some episodic-like memory, retaining information about the what, where and when of personal past events (Menzel, 1999; Martin-Ordas *et al.*, 2010). Bonobos and orangutans save appropriate tools to use them up to 14 hours later, suggesting that episodic-like memory provides apes with the ability to plan for the future (Mulcahy and Call, 2006). Further, problem-solving tasks showed that chimpanzees emulate the way others solve problems, but only once causal information is available (Horner and Whiten, 2005). All these results suggest that our own cognitive abilities are rooted in those of chimpanzees, in the social and physical domains. Interestingly, almost all this work has been conducted on captive chimpanzees, disengaged from their natural ecological and social environment, despite the fact that cognition is shaped by both (Zuberbühler and Byrne, 2006), and its development may be affected by unnatural captive conditions (Boesch, 2007; Ramsey *et al.*, 2007). Here, we will therefore focus on studies conducted on wild animals living in their natural socio-ecological environment.

Research on wild chimpanzees can only be conducted in two handfuls of long-term research sites across Africa (Figure 6.1), where chimpanzee identities are known and habituation to human presence permits researchers to follow them without altering their behaviour. Investigation of cognitive abilities requires detailed natural observations, which can be supplemented by remote camera recordings (e.g. in Budongo and Kanyawara: Gruber *et al.*, 2009; in Goualougo: Sanz and Morgan, 2007; in Loango: Estienne *et al.*, 2017) or through field experiments. Field experiments have so far only been conducted in few sites, including Bossou, Budongo, Kanyawara and Taï.

Social Cognition – Third-Party Knowledge

In a competitive situation, an individual's success may depend on his ability to know who are the friends and enemies of his opponent (Byrne and Whiten, 1989). While the opponent's friend will support the opponent, the opponent's enemy might support him against the opponent. In a chimpanzee society, friendships can also be formed between non-kin individuals (Wittig *et al.*, 2014a), allowing friends and enemies to change over time. Friendships can be deduced by observers through repeated observations of affiliative and aggressive behaviours among community members (Wittig *et al.*, 2014a), although this may require considerable computational power (Seyfarth and Cheney, 2012). In chimpanzees, moreover, the necessary observations that inform about others' relationships are hampered by fission–fusion dynamics (i.e. frequent splitting of group members into subgroups of varying size and composition), creating an additional challenge for individuals to stay well informed. Chimpanzees (and some monkeys), nonetheless, show awareness of third-party relationships, even without all players being present. Chimpanzees accept reconciliation mediated by a friend of the former opponent when direct contact between former opponents is risky (Wittig and Boesch, 2010) and are repelled by aggressive vocalizations from friends of the former opponent, even hours after an unreconciled aggression and even in the absence of the former opponent (Wittig *et al.*, 2014a).

Both studies show that chimpanzees use their knowledge of third-party relationships, among kin and non-kin, to navigate their social life to their own advantage. These results mirror those in baboon studies, where vocal support (Wittig *et al.*, 2007a) and bond-mediated reconciliation (Wittig *et al.*, 2007b) have similar effects as in chimpanzees, with one crucial difference: baboons form bonds mainly with kin, following the pattern of matrilinear societies, while chimpanzees also routinely form relationships with non-kin individuals, and as such relationships can change over time.

Finally, chimpanzees (like forest-living sooty mangabeys) show awareness of triadic relationships, when intervening in others' grooming bouts. Both species show a similar likelihood to intervene more in others' grooming bouts when the grooming between others could negatively impact them (e.g. when the interveners risked losing a key grooming partner or when grooming individuals could become allies; Mielke *et al.*, 2017). Mangabeys', but not chimpanzees', choices in grooming interventions were hampered by dominance rank, so that lower-ranking mangabeys rarely intervened in the grooming bouts between dominant individuals.

Social Cognition – Theory of Mind

When chimpanzees spot a hidden threat (e.g. a sedentary and venomous snake), it is advantageous to inform others about the snake's whereabouts, so that the others can also avoid the danger. Stumbling over a Gaboon viper, chimpanzees give alert-hoo vocalizations (Crockford *et al.*, 2012, 2015) that attract others' attention to the snake. Interestingly, alert-hoos are more likely to be emitted when receivers have been exposed to less snake-related cues (Crockford *et al.*, 2012, 2017). Therefore, chimpanzees seem more motivated to inform ignorant than knowledgeable group members about the presence of the snake. This result supports others suggesting that chimpanzees have intentional call production (i.e. socially and goal-directed; Schel *et al.*, 2013b), although more experiments are needed to better understand whether chimpanzees use full-blown mental state attribution.

Concepts of theory of mind are also related to empathy, teaching and self-recognition (Brüne and Brüne-Cohrs, 2006; Seyfarth and Cheney, 2013). Empathy may be a mechanism that facilitates adoptions or consolation. Adoptions are common in Taï (Boesch *et al.*, 2010) and occur in other chimpanzee communities (Wroblewski, 2008; Hobaiter *et al.*, 2014). Adopters are often not closely related to adoptees (Boesch *et al.*, 2010), making inclusive fitness an unlikely explanation. Research to examine the underlying mechanisms supporting adoption behaviour may help determine if empathy is involved. Consolation (e.g. when a bystander affiliates with a victim of aggression) also occurs in all human and chimpanzee populations (Arnold and Whiten, 2001; Wittig and Boesch, 2003b; Kutsukake and Castles, 2004). In humans, it is thought to be closely related to empathy (Carter *et al.*, 2011). Chimpanzee behaviour suggests the capacity for empathy; however, excluding alternative explanations in experimental tests is required (Fraser *et al.*, 2009; Wittig and Boesch, 2010).

Social Cognition – Cooperation between Unrelated Individuals

Unusually for species living in multimale, multifemale societies, chimpanzees use a wide range of cooperative behaviours. In reciprocal exchanges, they groom partners who will groom them back later in time (Watts, 2000; Gomes *et al.*, 2009; Newton-Fisher and Lee, 2011; Figure 6.2). Reciprocal exchanges happen between kin and non-kin, creating the question of how reciprocal exchange is maintained over longer periods

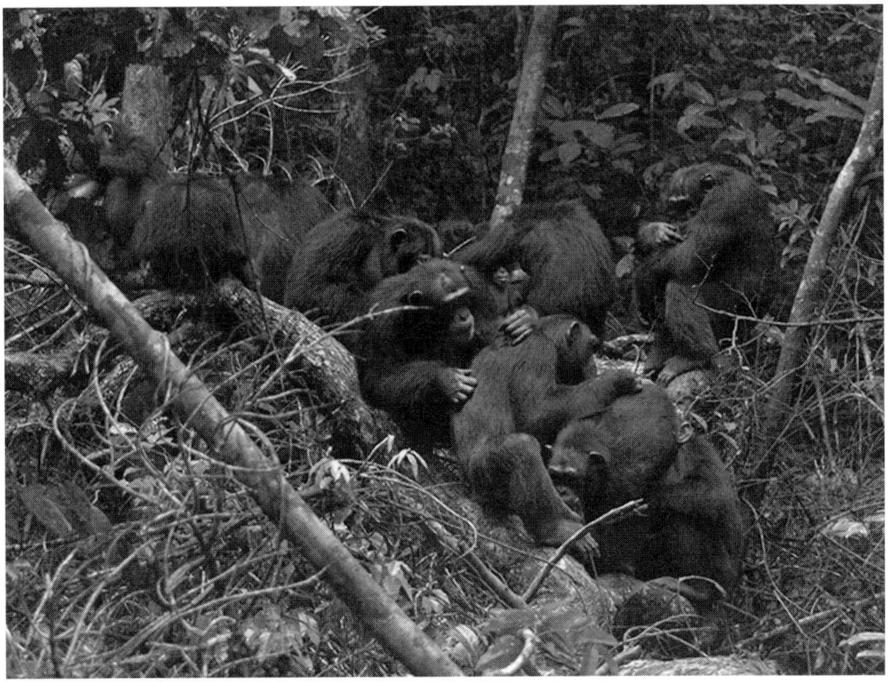

Figure 6.2. Members of the East-Group of the Taï Chimpanzee Project, resting and grooming each other.
Photo by Roman Wittig.

of time, despite the potential of exploitation by cheaters. Cognitive bookkeeping would be an option, if chimpanzees had the cognitive capacity to keep track of exchanges over time. Alternatively, reciprocal grooming exchanges could be mediated at an emotional rather than cognitive level (Crockford *et al.*, 2013), via emotional bookkeeping (Schino and Aureli, 2010). The neuropeptide oxytocin, which is a key facilitator in mammalian social bond formation and is active in the reward centres in the brain (Rilling and Young, 2014), is involved in grooming bouts between closely bonded chimpanzees. Thus, grooming with a bond partner may feel rewarding, and grooming between those two individuals may be more likely to happen again.

Chimpanzees also prey on monkey species, which they capture during group hunts. Although there is considerable variation in degree of cooperation across chimpanzee populations (Boesch, 1996; Gilby and Connor, 2010), chimpanzees usually gain more meat when being part of the hunting party (Boesch, 2002). In addition, once chimpanzees possess meat, they may share it to gain future support (Mitani and Watts, 2001) or to receive future copulations (Gomes and Boesch, 2009; cf. Gilby *et al.*, 2010). Although the reciprocity of these exchanges is likely based on emotional bookkeeping facilitated by oxytocin, some partner choices may be independent from emotions and may be tactically used (Wittig *et al.*, 2014a).

Chimpanzees also engage in other group-level cooperative actions. During patrols, they sometimes penetrate into neighbouring territories in search of rival communities

(Watts and Mitani, 2001), coordinate their activity and use coordinated ambush techniques to gain an advantage when attacking (see Samuni *et al.*, 2017). Once two rival communities detect each other, either fighting or fleeing ensues. Isolated individuals may be attacked and killed (Mitani *et al.*, 2010) and females taken hostage (Boesch *et al.*, 2008). The outcome of territorial conflicts seems to be dependent on the relative number of males in each community (Wilson *et al.*, 2012). How much cognition is involved in these group-level cooperative actions remains unclear (Tomasello, 2009b), although experience through age seems to be a good predictor of successful group-level cooperation (Boesch and Boesch-Achermann, 2000).

Physical Cognition – Ecological and Spatial Knowledge

Chimpanzees' main food sources are ripe, patchy ephemeral fruits with unpredictable fruiting patterns. Windows of access to ripe fruit are therefore short, with intense food competition within and between species (Janmaat *et al.*, 2014). Thus, there is likely selection pressure for chimpanzees to predict which fruits are ripe, when and where, to avoid unnecessary visits to areas without ripe fruits. In Taï, female chimpanzees inspected more trees of the same species once they had discovered ripe fruits in one tree (Janmaat *et al.*, 2013). Chimpanzees found the trees of the same species using their knowledge of their spatial distribution from former visits (Normand *et al.*, 2009) and travelled in straight lines between the feeding sites (Normand and Boesch, 2009). They chose their nest site for the night in relation to the location of the first feeding site in the morning, and they left earlier in the morning for highly contested ephemeral fruits, such as figs (Janmaat *et al.*, 2014). These results suggest that chimpanzees appear to have some knowledge about the phenology of food species, the location of trees in the forest and how to directly navigate to them.

Physical Cognition – Physical Properties of Tools

Tools need to have specific properties to function optimally. Chimpanzees in Loango use different sticks to pound a hole into underground bee hives and eat the honey afterwards (Boesch *et al.*, 2009). Indeed, sturdy sticks are better to poke a hole through hard mud, but more flexible and longer sticks are more efficient to extract the honey afterwards. Similarly, when cracking nuts, the optimal hammer properties are a combination of right material, right shape and right weight, which change according to the age of the nut. Chimpanzees approaching a nut-cracking site choose a hammer sometimes more than 100 m before they reach the anvil (Sirianni *et al.*, 2015a). Hammer choices vary according to whether they crack nuts in the tree or on the ground, with the latter showing a preference for larger, heavier hammers than the former. Chimpanzees also anticipate the weight of a wooden hammer: when lifting lighter hollow hammers, chimpanzees accelerate the hammer faster and adjust the lifting force, compared to solid hammers of the same size (Sirianni *et al.*, 2015b). This suggests that chimpanzees have some knowledge about object properties such as weight.

All for One and One for All

Box 6.1 Studying Corvids in Lab and Field

Christian Rutz

Members of the Corvidae family ('corvids') exhibit a wide range of 'primate-like' behaviours. Ravens, for example, form social relationships of notable complexity (Massen *et al.*, 2014), some food-caching jays have the ability to plan for the future (Raby *et al.*, 2007) and two tropical crow species use tools for extractive foraging (Hunt, 1996; Rutz *et al.*, 2016a). This striking evolutionary convergence has sparked considerable research interest, as it provides valuable opportunities for comparative research (Emery and Clayton, 2004).

The socio-ecology and cognition of corvids is being studied productively in both laboratory and field. Lab-based studies, which often use hand-reared subjects, offer a high degree of experimental control, good replication and opportunities to expose birds to food, materials or problems they would not normally encounter in nature (Taylor *et al.*, 2007; Bird and Emery, 2009; Wascher *et al.*, 2015; Kabadayi and Osvath, 2017). This said, some species do not tolerate permanent captivity well, or at least should not be held longer-term in social isolation or outside their natural climes, so expert advice must be sought before setting up new research colonies. Sometimes, it is possible to work with temporarily captive subjects: wild birds are trapped and housed in (field) aviaries for the brief duration of behavioural experiments (from a few hours up to several weeks), before being released again at the site of capture (Klump *et al.*, 2015; Hunt, 2016; Chapter 4). This approach can only be used with species that habituate well to novel environments, and requires carefully designed study protocols to ensure the welfare of birds both in captivity and after release, and to avoid the unintentional 'seeding' of novel behaviours in wild populations.

In field studies, corvid researchers have an arsenal of well-established ornithological techniques at their disposal, including straightforward methods for marking individuals (leg rings, wing-tags, radio-tags) and assessing their body condition (flight-muscle development, parasites) and reproductive performance (laying date, clutch and brood size). Free-ranging birds can often be enticed to engage with experimental set-ups (St Clair *et al.*, 2015; Swift and Marzluff, 2015; Greggor *et al.*, 2016), including naturalistic or artificial stimuli, or baited problem-solving tasks. This enables close-range observation of natural behaviours from hides or with camera traps, and/or controlled investigation of social interactions, foraging performance or cognitive capacities; again, care should be taken not to alter irreversibly the behavioural repertoire of wild populations. Finally, recent advances in cutting-edge 'bio-logging' technology offer exciting opportunities to remotely investigate the behaviour and social dynamics of free-ranging corvids. For example, GPS tags have been used to chart the movements of wide-ranging species (Loretto *et al.*, 2017), bird-mounted miniature video cameras can spy on completely undisturbed

(cont.)

behaviour (Rutz *et al.*, 2007) and so-called 'proximity loggers' are capable of recording – minute by minute – the social interactions of entire populations (St Clair *et al.*, 2015).

Two closely related 'common-sense' approaches have proved particularly useful for boosting the efficiency of corvid research programmes. First, a sound understanding of the study species' natural history is usually key to asking productive research questions (Balda *et al.*, 1996), and principal investigators should encourage their teams to spend time observing wild birds, especially if fieldwork is not a primary objective. Many corvid researchers have fascinating stories to tell of how anecdotal observations inspired some of their most important work. Second, combining lab- and field-based research often generates fruitful synergy, and as a result, exciting insights (Rutz *et al.*, 2016b). Sometimes, intriguing field observations (Hunt, 1996) inspire controlled laboratory experiments (Klump *et al.*, 2015), while on other occasions, interpretation of experimental results requires a sound understanding of species-typical behaviours (Rutz *et al.*, 2016b).

Corvid research is thriving, making critical contributions to comparative studies of social complexity, cognition and tool behaviour (Emery and Clayton, 2004). Research opportunities abound, and it is surprising just how little we still know about some of the most widespread and abundant species, such as carrion crows, American crows, ravens, house crows, jackdaws, rooks and various jays and magpies. In fact, many of us regularly encounter corvids where we live and work – willing participants, no doubt, for field experiments that offer interesting puzzles and some juicy morsels of meat.

References

Balda, R. P., Kamil, A. C., and Bednekoff, P. A. (1996). Predicting cognitive capacity from natural history: examples from four species of corvids. *Current Ornithology*, **13**, 33–66.

Bird, C. D., and Emery, N. J. (2009). Insightful problem solving and creative tool modification by captive nontool-using rooks. *Proceedings of the National Academy of Sciences*, **106**, 10370–10375.

Emery, N. J., and Clayton, N. S. (2004). The mentality of crows: convergent evolution of intelligence in corvids and apes. *Science*, **306**, 1903–1907.

Greggor, A. L., McIvor, G. E., Clayton, N. S., and Thornton, A. (2016). Contagious risk taking: social information and context influence wild jackdaws' responses to novelty and risk. *Scientific Reports*, **6**, 27764.

Hunt, G. R. (1996). Manufacture and use of hook-tools by New Caledonian crows. *Nature*, **379**, 249–251.

Hunt, G. R. (2016). Social and spatial reintegration success of New Caledonian crows (*Corvus moneduloides*) released after aviary confinement. *Wilson Journal of Ornithology*, **128**, 168–173.

Kabadayi, C., and Osvath, M. (2017). Ravens parallel great apes in flexible planning for tool-use and bartering. *Science*, **357**, 202–204.

(cont.)

Klump, B. C., Sugasawa, S., St Clair, J. J. H., and Rutz, C. (2015). Hook tool manufacture in New Caledonian crows: behavioural variation and the influence of raw materials. *BMC Biology*, **13**, 97.

Loretto, M.-C., Schuster, R., Itty, C., Marchand, P., Genero, F., and Bugnyar, T. (2017). Fission–fusion dynamics over large distances in raven non-breeders. *Scientific Reports*, **7**, 380.

Massen, J. J. M., Pašukonis, A., Schmidt, J., and Bugnyar, T. (2014). Ravens notice dominance reversals among conspecifics within and outside their social group. *Nature Communications*, **5**, 3679.

Raby, C. R., Alexis, D. M., Dickinson, A., and Clayton, N. S. (2007). Planning for the future by western scrub-jays. *Nature*, **445**, 919–921.

Rutz, C., Bluff, L. A., Weir, A. A. S., and Kacelnik, A. (2007). Video cameras on wild birds. *Science*, **318**, 765.

Rutz, C., Klump, B. C., Komarczyk, L., *et al.* (2016a). Discovery of species-wide tool use in the Hawaiian crow. *Nature*, **537**, 403–407.

Rutz, C., Sugasawa, S., van der Wal, J. E. M., Klump, B. C., and St Clair, J. J. H. (2016b). Tool bending in New Caledonian crows. *Royal Society Open Science*, **3**, 160439.

St Clair, J. J. H., Burns, Z. T., Bettaney, E., *et al.* (2015). Experimental resource pulses influence social-network dynamics and the potential for information flow in tool-using crows. *Nature Communications*, **6**, 7197.

Swift, K. N., and Marzluff, J. M. (2015). Wild American crows gather around their dead to learn about danger. *Animal Behaviour*, **109**, 187–197.

Taylor, A. H., Hunt, G. R., Holzhaider, J. C., and Gray, R. D. (2007). Spontaneous metatool use by New Caledonian crows. *Current Biology*, **17**, 1504–1507.

Wascher, C. A. F., Hillemann, F., Canestrari, D., and Baglione, V. (2015). Carrion crows learn to discriminate between calls of reliable and unreliable conspecifics. *Animal Cognition*, **18**, 1181–1185.

Field Guide

There are only two handfuls of study sites where chimpanzees allow researchers to approach, without altering their behaviour (Wilson *et al.*, 2014). Study sites with wild chimpanzees are lifetime investments, not only because habituation of chimpanzees to human observers can take up to 10 years (Boesch and Boesch-Achermann, 2000), but also because habituated chimpanzees are an easy target for poachers, and scientists have an ethical obligation to ensure the long-term survival of their study population. Research helps to protect chimpanzees, as the presence of researchers has a repelling effect on poaching in protected areas (Campbell *et al.*, 2011). Observing chimpanzees usually means following them on foot, from the morning nest to the evening nest. Before planning a study on chimpanzee cognition, researchers should take time to extensively observe their behaviour, to ensure the correct questions are asked and the right procedures used. For example, chimpanzees might not solve a cooperation task because the possible cooperation partner has social attributes that prevent it, or certain behaviours may be culturally biased and individuals may be inhibited from solving problems in a different way (Gruber *et al.*, 2009). Considering the ecological relevance of a stimulus or the local traditions of particular chimpanzee populations will produce clearer results, and experiments will more likely reflect the true abilities of chimpanzees, if they represent natural problems.

Behavioural Observations

Detailed behavioural observations are paramount for observational and experimental studies and can be informative about underlying cognitive abilities. During the last decade, new statistical methods were developed, enabling analysis of observational data sets while testing and controlling for a number of potentially influencing factors. General Linear Mixed Models, for example, are helpful in controlling for multiple observations of the same subject or dyad, and other possible factors influencing the variance (e.g. age, sex, rank), while focusing on the variables most relevant to the question (Bates *et al.*, 2015). Planning the ideal statistical models, however, requires at least as much thought before starting with the data collection as experiments do (Mundry, 2017). Behavioural observations, in combination with complex statistical methods, revealed that Taï chimpanzees plan their breakfast when choosing the nest site for the night (Janmaat *et al.*, 2014), use spatial cognition to detect food (Ban *et al.*, 2014), take into account object physical properties when choosing tools to crack nuts (Sirianni *et al.*, 2015a), and examine when and with whom to intervene in others' grooming bouts (Mielke *et al.*, 2017). These studies indicate that some aspects of cognition can be studied relying purely on observations.

Another way to collect data on cognitive abilities is to collect behavioural sequences on video, either using HD video cameras or distributing trophy camera systems at interesting spots in the research area (Kühl *et al.*, 2016), for instance at nut-cracking sites or where other tool use happens (Sanz and Morgan, 2007; Estienne *et al.*, 2017). Trophy cameras are automatically triggered by movement and have a night vision option, which sometimes needs to be covered, because chimpanzees are known to react to light sources. Researchers have even created experiments with trophy cameras filming the experiment, so that observers are not present when chimpanzees conduct the experiment (Sirianni *et al.*, 2015b). Rechargeable battery-powered cameras can operate for several weeks, cameras are waterproof (although they need additional protection against tropical rains) and chimpanzees rarely touch the cameras. Detailed observations are impossible without video coding, although this can be extremely time-consuming. Video analysis requires remeasuring techniques with different observers blind to the conditions in the video (Lonsdorf, 2006).

Field Experiments and How to Conduct Them

Experiments are manipulations of the social or physical environment of the target animal by the experimenter, making the target animal believe something simulated is real (Zuberbühler and Wittig, 2011; Fischer *et al.*, 2013). Field experiments enable the experimenter to choose the interaction partners, create the interaction without waiting for its natural occurrence, and choose the most appropriate situation for the test. Conducting a field experiment, however, is not a guarantee for a fast lane to results. Most experiments need careful preconditions that are not frequently met, and many days may pass without a successfully conducted experiment.

Having conducted field experiments on both baboons and chimpanzees, we need to point out that some crucial differences between species need to be considered. Chimpanzees seem exceptionally aware of context and circumstances. Even chimpanzees that are well-habituated to humans may react to subtle changes in human behaviour, making the difference between an experimental design that works and one that does not. For example, in populations where chimpanzees almost always observe humans together with chimpanzees, suddenly seeing a human who is alone ahead of them may be enough to cause them to divert away from their current travel trajectory and miss seeing a placed object.

Acoustic Simulations

Chimpanzees use a range of vocalizations in different contexts. Their repertoire consists of four main vocalization types grading into each other, namely 'barks', 'grunts', 'hoos' and 'screams' (Crockford and Boesch, 2003; Slocombe and Zuberbühler, 2007, 2010; Crockford *et al.*, 2015). Call combinations created from these four vocalization types are associated with different contexts (Crockford and Boesch, 2005). Sequences of grunts ('rough-grunts') can be given in a food context (Slocombe *et al.*, 2010), but a 'pant-grunt' (whereby sequences of grunts are joined together by ingressive pants) indicates the vocalizer's subordination to the receiver of the signal (Wittig and Boesch, 2003a).

In chimpanzees, vocalizations are crucial for deducing social events, given their low-visibility tropical forest habitat. Using chimpanzee vocalizations in playback experiments, therefore, allows the experimenter to simulate either the signaller or the receiver of an interaction, in the absence of that individual. In a playback experiment with the Sonso chimpanzees, for instance, Wittig and colleagues (2014b) used pre-recorded bark vocalizations of known community members to simulate aggressive interactions and test whether chimpanzees reacted differently depending on the relationship of the caller to their previous aggressor.

When conducting a successful play-back experiment (i.e. an acoustic simulation of the social environment, by playing back to an audience a recorded call or noise through a concealed speaker; Table 6.1; Figure 6.3), several steps have to be taken (Cheney and Seyfarth, 2008; Zuberbühler and Wittig, 2011; Fischer *et al.*, 2013).

- High-quality recordings of the desired vocalization have to be obtained from the required number of individuals in the study group, using a high-quality microphone and a digital recording device (Table 6.1). Note that this can take weeks or months. The recorder should have a pre-recording option, so that the last 2 seconds before the pause button is released are already recorded. Otherwise,

Table 6.1. Equipment needed for investigating cognition in wild chimpanzees using field experiments and observational methods.

Equipment	Function
Playback speaker	Playing back of stimuli
Microphone	Recording of vocalizations
Recorder	Recording of vocalizations and playing back stimuli
Radios/GPS units	Communication between experimenters
Objects	Good replicas of natural objects (use e.g. 3D printer)
Video cameras	Video recording of experiments and behaviour
Remote control action camera	Close-up videos of experiments
Trophy cameras	Monitoring and recording of experiments without the presence of the experimenter
Sound meter	Calibrating the playback stimuli
Acoustic software	Producing and cleaning of acoustic stimuli
	PRAAT (Phonetic Sciences Amsterdam: fon.hum.uva.nl/praat/) *FREE*
	Raven interactive sound analysis software (Cornell Lab of Ornithology: birds.cornell.edu/brp/raven/) *FREE*
Video coding software	Coding of video footage
	Boris (Behavioral Observation Research Interactive Software: boris.unito.it) *FREE*
Binoculars (8 × 40, waterproof)	Identifying individuals even when in the trees
Hand-held computer	For data collection of behavioural observations
Computer	Video coding of experiments in the field

you will rarely catch the beginning of the call, until you can predict when calling occurs. Recordings need to be prepared as playback stimuli. Using acoustic editing software, calls need to be cut to length, need to show a similar, but natural, call structure, and need to be of high acoustic quality. Although it is better not to remove the background noise through acoustic software filters (as the filter process alters the recording), sometimes it might be necessary (Table 6.1).

- Stimuli need to be calibrated to the natural volume of the call. The speaker should be placed at the same distance as during experiments, and the call volume should be adjusted to the experimenter's ear, so it sounds natural. This needs to be done far away from any chimpanzees, so they are unable to hear. Finally, to standardize call volume, the call should be played back at 1 m distance from a sound meter (dB measures should be similar, but within the natural variation; Table 6.1).
- On days when playback experiments are planned, two teams with means of communication (handheld radios; Table 6.1) are needed. One follows the individual that will be the subject of the experiment, while the other follows the

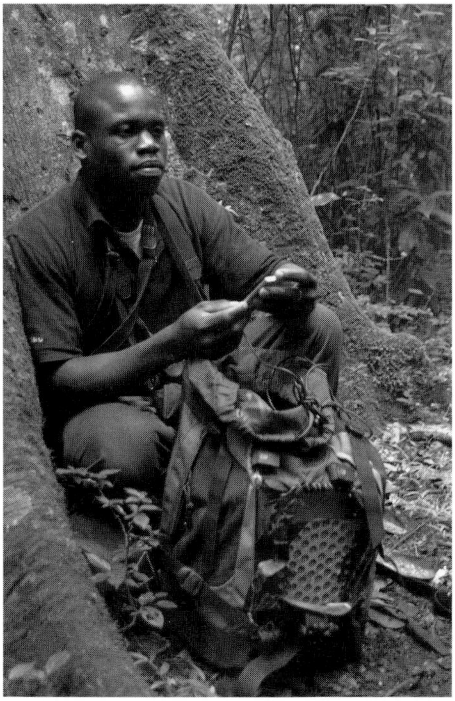

Figure 6.3. BCFS field assistant Jacob Ariyo demonstrates how to operate the playback speaker, which is placed in a backpack for transport. During a playback experiment the speaker and its operator will be concealed in the vegetation.
Photo by Roman Wittig.

individual whose call will be played back, to check that the call provider remains out of the speaker's auditory range.

- When the opportunity arises, the experiment needs to be conducted fast, but with precision. The subject should be resting, without sleeping or interacting. The speaker needs to be placed at the right distance and angle to the subject, and the correct stimuli need to be selected for play back. Before giving the command or pressing the play button for the play back, it must be confirmed that the call provider is far away, and the experimenter needs to start filming the subject. Filming should happen about 10 seconds before and continue as long as subjects respond to the stimulus. Make sure the subject does not see the speaker and its operator, even when moving into the speaker's direction.
- The same evening, the video material should be downloaded and viewed, and all important information documented.

Visual Simulations

Some of the dangers chimpanzees encounter in the forest can only be detected by seeing them. Predators, like leopards or pythons, are chased away after they are detected, triggering aggressive behaviours and bark vocalizations (Crockford and Boesch, 2003). Sedentary

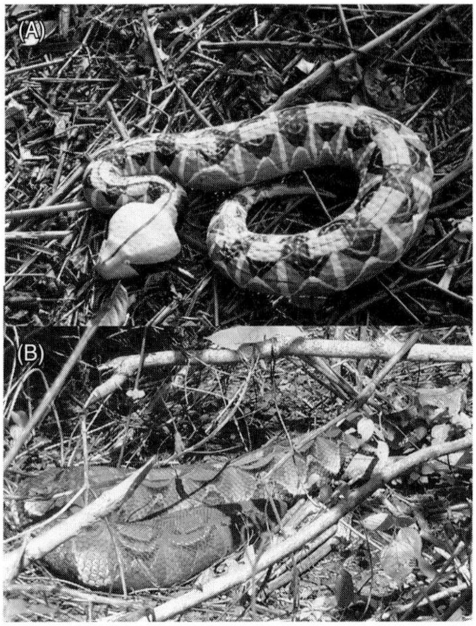

Figure 6.4. (A) The model of a Gaboon viper used in experiments. Photo by Cedric Girard-Buttoz. (B) A real Gaboon viper discovered in Budongo Forest, Uganda.
Photo by Roman Wittig.

snakes like Gaboon vipers (*Bitis gabonica*), on the other hand, are highly camouflaged, but extremely venomous snakes (Figure 6.4A). Although they do not prey on chimpanzees, it is easy to fail to see them and get bitten. Chimpanzees therefore warn each other about these snakes, using alert hoos or alarm barks (Crockford *et al.*, 2012, 2015; Schel *et al.*, 2013b).

Chimpanzees also mark the spot where the snake is sitting, using gaze-alternation between the snake and the receivers (Schel *et al.*, 2013b; Crockford *et al.*, 2017). Observing how chimpanzees react to such external stimuli and to each other, in the presence of such stimuli, can be revealing in terms of both social cognition and communication. One way to increase and control observations to such events, especially those that are rare, is by producing models, such as model Gaboon vipers (Figure 6.4A). Again, this takes some prior experience, as the placement of models needs to be conducted without any chimpanzee seeing the placement and in a place where chimpanzees will pass close enough to see the model (Crockford *et al.*, 2012; Schel *et al.*, 2013b). For experiments like this, the shape and colour of the stimuli should be convincing replicas of the real objects (Figure 6.4A).

The experimenter needs to place an object in the projected line of travel of the subject, so the subject is likely to find it. Although this sounds trivial for animals that use the same paths again and again, it can be nerve-wracking for experimenters trying to set up an object in the path of chimpanzees. One possibility can be to use natural feeding trees or areas that are revisited (Gruber *et al.*, 2009; Sirianni *et al.*, 2015b). Researchers in Bossou have set up an outdoor laboratory where they provide oil palm nuts (*Elaeis guineensis*) and stones to the Bossou chimpanzees to crack nuts (Inoue-Nakamura and

Matsuzawa, 1997). This laboratory is often revisited and it allows study of the nut-cracking techniques and the ontogeny of nut-cracking.

Once the object is placed, the experimenter gets ready to film the reaction of the subject. A remote-controlled camera close to the object (e.g. action camera) can also help to record the subject's reaction. Given that vegetation is always a confound, it is best to conduct experiments in open areas and to have one member of the team following the subject, to film the experiment from another angle, making it less likely that the subject is simultaneously hidden from view from two cameras. Three problems need to be pointed out here: (a) dehabituation trials (i.e. identical trials, but without the snake in place) are needed to avoid subjects learning to expect the object whenever researchers are filming or standing in specific positions; (b) subjects should never see the experimenter handling the object, to avoid associating them and becoming unreceptive to this type of simulation; and (c) subjects should not handle the object, or the objects should be treated to avoid disease transmissions (see Pitfalls).

Combinations of Several Stimuli

In some cases, information about a situation is incomplete, if giving only one stimulus. When simulating the separation of two individuals, for instance, it may be necessary to play the call of both individuals in two distant positions, which requires good coordination between experimenters (Crockford *et al.*, 2007). Also the combination of multi-sensory information (e.g. object presentation and playback experiment; Crockford *et al.*, 2017) is complicated to conduct and requires experience. However, multistimuli experiments can help to remove more confounding effects from the context. Finally, although olfaction may play an important role in chimpanzees (see above), the potential of olfactory simulations has not yet been tested in the wild.

Pitfalls

Although field experiments are very attractive to answer complex questions, they are accompanied by a number of problems that can make a study worthless, if one is not careful to address them. Moreover, if conducted without understanding the natural social dynamics, field experiments could alter the social dynamics in the long term. Below, readers will find a list of the main pitfalls of field experiments (for more information, see Zuberbühler and Wittig, 2011; Fischer *et al.*, 2013).

Authenticity. Experimental stimuli have to be of sufficient quality, so that subjects are taken in by simulation. If the stimuli are of low quality, reactions may be ambiguous or not happen at all.

Habituation. Presenting the same stimuli (e.g. snake models) several times to the same individual can lead to a reduced salience of the stimulus and subjects may stop reacting. Thus, stimuli should not be presented more frequently than they occur naturally. Subjects might also get habituated to specific calls played back multiple times. Thus, the same call should only be used multiple times when the experimenter has to keep certain values of the call (e.g. the aggressiveness) constant (Wittig *et al.*, 2014a). Otherwise, several recordings of the same call type by the same individual may limit habituation effects.

Altering chimpanzee behaviour. Conserving chimpanzees as a species means to also protect the uniqueness of their behavioural traditions. Researchers should thus be careful not to use experiments that may permanently alter their behaviour. For instance, special caution is needed with the experimental manipulation of intergroup contexts, as it can deeply impact between and within-group behaviour (Radford *et al.*, 2016). In birds (Mennill *et al.*, 2002), even a single experiment can have drastic implications for the animals involved, altering paternity choices of female birds exposed to playbacks. In mammals, the implications are not yet well explored, but experiments suggesting changes in outgroup pressure are likely to strongly impact in-group dynamics, 'with lasting effect' (Radford *et al.*, 2016). Any simulated intergroup activity should thus be conducted with extreme caution, and only after a good understanding of the natural dynamics. A playback experiment with captive chimpanzees suggests that even one or two exposures to simulated encounters spaced over weeks may increase territorial activity and hostile behaviour (Cronin *et al.*, 2015).

Teamwork. Often, the opportunity to conduct an experiment when all criteria are met can last only a few minutes before a critical variable changes. Thus, team coordination is critical, and teams need to be ready to spring into action within a moment's notice. All electronic equipment must be kept in perfect working order, batteries and cables checked repeatedly through the day, with backups available just in case. All team members need to thoroughly know and have rehearsed their role ahead of time. The fewer trials that fail due to lack of team cooperation or equipment failure, the more data you will end up with.

Disease transmission. Due to the close genetic relationship between chimpanzees and humans, human pathogens can easily jump the species barrier. Pathogens that cause a cold in humans can be fatal in chimpanzees (e.g. Köndgen *et al.*, 2008). In most study sites, researchers have therefore implemented rules to reduce the possibility of zoonotic disease transmission, keeping a distance from chimpanzees, wearing surgical face masks or going through quarantine procedures before seeing the chimpanzees (Grützmacher *et al.*, 2017). However, experiments can bridge the distance that is usually kept between chimpanzees and observers and create indirect contact between humans and chimpanzees through the stimuli. A notorious problem for indirect contact is the presentation of food as stimuli (Gruber *et al.*, 2009; Sirianni *et al.*, 2015b). One possibility is to treat the food with a kind of quarantine. Sirianni and colleagues (2015b) collected nuts in the forest wearing surgical gloves and face masks and transported them back in a fresh plastic liner. Once arrived at the camp, the nuts were stored on a dry-rack at the forest edge, next to the research camp, exposing the nuts to UV light and eliminating human contact. Before any manipulation of nuts, experimenters disinfected hands and slipped on gloves and face masks. Nuts were then placed in fresh plastic liners and placed on the forest floor, ensuring the same precautions as during storing. Chimpanzees might also touch model objects that have been placed to create a certain situation for them. We recommend disinfecting these models before taking them into the forest, keeping them in a clean plastic liner, disinfecting hands and wearing gloves before handling. However, the best practice is to choose objects that chimpanzees are unlikely to touch.

Wild vs. Lab

Box 6.2 Cognitive Testing: From the Field into the Lab, and Back

Julia Fischer

Studies of primate cognitive abilities are typically following two quite disjunct research traditions. Investigations in captivity are mostly conducted within an experimental psychological framework, where paradigms are often borrowed from developmental research on human children. Because such experiments aim to confront the animal with novel problems, the aim is to rule out or control for learning by trial and error. Such experiments can thus provide insights into the animals' problem-solving and reasoning skills. By systematically varying different parameters, it is also possible to probe the cognitive limits of the animals. Experimental manipulations in the lab are extremely powerful to investigate the mechanisms supporting the animals' choices.

Field researchers, in contrast, are typically following an ethological/ecological approach, and ground their questions in the actual problems the animals face in their natural environments – such as choosing a mating partner, finding food or avoiding predators. Field experiments standing in the ethological tradition thus make use of stimuli that also occur in nature, such as vocalizations of other group members, or indicators of predator presence. Food items may be placed strategically in the animals' way to assess their spatial cognition. While such investigations have much higher ecological validity – especially when based on detailed observations of the animals' unperturbed behaviour – they are hampered by the lack of control the researchers have over current and recent contextual variation. For instance, one might set up an experiment, unbeknownst to the fact that the animals had spotted a lion in the early morning. The animals respond strongly in the experiment, but this is because they are still skittish after the encounter with the predator. Field researchers are thus often trapped between a rock and a hard place: because of the resulting higher noise in the data, they want to increase the number of trials in experiments, but this might cause the animals to habituate to the stimuli. Detailed knowledge of natural rates of occurrence of specific situations and a good intuition are thus needed when field experiments are devised.

Unfortunately, there has been considerable disdain and/or ignorance in the communities concerning the value of either approach. Some field researchers have quipped that work under captive conditions is meaningless, while researchers working in captivity abhor the lack of control associated with field experiments. A big step forward would be to recognize that both approaches have their strengths and weaknesses. To understand both the mechanisms supporting cognitive abilities as well as their function, both sides can learn a great deal from each other, and conversely serve as sources of inspiration. Finally, both camps have to keep in mind what Wolfgang Köhler, one of the pioneers of cognitive tests with chimpanzees, once remarked: 'The successful outcome of intelligence assessments is, as a general rule, far more easily

(*cont.*)

jeopardized by the experimenter than by the animal . . . and, generally, every investigator should recognize that, besides the creature being investigated, every intelligence test necessarily tests the tester' (cited from Fischer, 2017).

References

Fischer, J. (2017). *Monkeytalk: inside the worlds and minds of primates*. Chicago, IL: University of Chicago Press.

Resources

Films/movies:

- *Too close for comfort?* (1992) Film by the BBC Natural History Unit about the Taï Chimpanzees, their hunting behaviour, their nut-cracking culture and their social life: www.wildfilmhistory.org/film/162/Too+Close+For+Comfort%3F.html
- *Chimpanzee* (2012) Film by Disney Nature about the orphan Oscar, who gets adopted by the old male Freddy: https://en.wikipedia.org/wiki/Chimpanzee_(film)
- *Rise of the warrior apes* (2017) Documentary about research on the Ngogo chimpanzees: www.youtube.com/watch?v=dQn1-mLkIHwandapp=desktop

Chimpanzee long-term study sites across Africa (Figure 6.1):

- Bossou – the chimpanzees of Bossou and Mount Nimba: www.greencorridor.info/
- Budongo – Budongo Conservation Field Station: www.budongo.org/
- Fongoli – Fongoli Savannah Chimpanzee Project: http://savannachimp.blogspot.de
- Gashaka – The Gashaka Primate Project: www.ucl.ac.uk/gashaka/
- Gombe – Gombe Chimpanzees: www.gombechimpanzees.org/
- Goualougo – Goualougo Triangle Ape Project: www.congo-apes.org/
- Kanyawara – Kibale Chimpanzee Project: https://kibalechimpanzees.wordpress.com/
- Loango – Loango Ape Project: www.eva.mpg.de/primat/research-groups/chimpanzees/field-sites/loango-chimpanzee-project.html?Fsize=vcxcvwdvavat
- Ngogo – The Ngogo Chimpanzee Project: http://ngogochimpanzeeproject.org/
- Taï – Taï Chimpanzee Project: www.taichimps.org

Profile

Roman is Max Planck Research Group Leader at the EVA-MPI in Leipzig, Germany, and Director of the Taï Chimpanzee Project in Côte d'Ivoire. He studied Biology at the

University of Bielefeld, Germany, receiving his PhD from the University of Leipzig, for research on 'Conflict management in wild chimpanzees'.

Catherine is ERC Research Group Leader for Ape Attachment at the EVA-MPI, and scientific Co-director of the Taï Chimpanzee Project. She trained as a Clinical Speech and Language Therapist (University of Newcastle, UK), before becoming interested in chimpanzee communication. She received her PhD from the University of Leipzig, for research on 'Vocal communication in wild chimpanzees'.

In 2004, Roman and Catherine teamed up, studying sociality and social cognition of chacma baboons in Botswana and Eastern chimpanzees in Uganda, during their post-docs at the University of Pennsylvania, USA, and the University of St Andrews, UK. They returned to Leipzig in 2012 to investigate chimpanzee sociality, competition, cooperation, cognition, communication, culture, conservation and health.

References

Arnold, K., and Whiten, A. (2001). Post-conflict behaviour of wild chimpanzees (*Pan troglodytes schweinfurthii*) in the Budongo forest, Uganda. *Behaviour*, **138**, 649–690.

Ban, S. D., Boesch, C., and Janmaat, K. R. L. (2014). Taï chimpanzees anticipate revisiting high-valued fruit trees from further distances. *Animal Cognition*, **17**, 1353–1364.

Bates, D., Kliegl, R., Vasishth, S., and Baayen, H. (2015). Parsimonious mixed models. *ArXiv:1506.04967 [Stat]*. Retrieved from http://arxiv.org/abs/1506.04967

Boesch, C. (1991). Teaching among wild chimpanzees. *Animal Behaviour*, **41**, 530–532.

Boesch, C. (1996). Hunting strategies of Gombe and Tai chimpanzees. In *Chimpanzee cultures* (pp. 77–91). Cambridge, MA: Harvard University Press.

Boesch, C. (2002). Cooperative hunting roles among Taï chimpanzees. *Human Nature*, **13**, 27–46.

Boesch, C. (2007). What makes us human (*Homo sapiens*): the challenge of cognitive cross-species comparison. *Journal of Comparative Psychology*, **121**, 227–240.

Boesch, C., and Boesch, H. (1982). Optimisation of nut-cracking with natural hammers by wild chimpanzees. *Behaviour*, **83**, 265–286.

Boesch, C., and Boesch, H. (1989). Hunting behavior of wild chimpanzees in the Taï National Park. *American Journal of Physical Anthropology*, **78**, 547–573.

Boesch, C., and Boesch-Achermann, H. (2000). *The chimpanzees of the Taï forest: behavioural ecology and evolution*. Oxford: Oxford University Press.

Boesch, C., Kohou, G., Néné, H., and Vigilant, L. (2006). Male competition and paternity in wild chimpanzees of the Taï forest. *American Journal of Physical Anthropology*, **130**, 103–115.

Boesch, C., Crockford, C., Herbinger, I., Wittig, R., Moebius, Y., and Normand, E. (2008). Intergroup conflicts among chimpanzees in Taï National Park: lethal violence and the female perspective. *American Journal of Primatology*, **70**, 519–532.

Boesch, C., Head, J., and Robbins, M. M. (2009). Complex tool sets for honey extraction among chimpanzees in Loango National Park, Gabon. *Journal of Human Evolution*, **56**, 560–569.

Boesch, C., Bolé, C., Eckhardt, N., and Boesch, H. (2010). Altruism in forest chimpanzees: the case of adoption. *PLoS ONE*, **5**(1), e8901.

Brüne, M., and Brüne-Cohrs, U. (2006). Theory of mind – evolution, ontogeny, brain mechanisms and psychopathology. *Neuroscience and Biobehavioral Reviews*, **30**, 437–455.

Byrne, R., and Whiten, A. (1989). *Machiavellian intelligence: social expertise and the evolution of intellect in monkeys, apes, and humans*. Oxford: Oxford University Press.

Call, J. (2009). Contrasting the social cognition of humans and nonhuman apes: the shared intentionality hypothesis. *Topics in Cognitive Science*, **1**, 368–379.

Campbell, G., Kuehl, H., Diarrassouba, A., N'Goran, P. K., and Boesch, C. (2011). Long-term research sites as refugia for threatened and over-harvested species. *Biology Letters*, **7**, 723–726.

Carter, C. S., Harris, J., and Porges, S. W. (2011). Neural and evolutionary perspectives on empathy. In *The social neuroscience of empathy* (pp. 169–182). Cambridge, MA: MIT Press.

Cheney, D. L., and Seyfarth, R. M. (2008). *Baboon metaphysics: the evolution of a social mind*. Chicago, IL: University of Chicago Press.

Christel, M. (1993). Grasping techniques and hand preferences in Hominoidea. In *Hands of primates* (pp. 91–108). Vienna: Springer.

Coolidge, H. J., and Shea, B. T. (1982). External body dimensions of *Pan paniscus* and *Pan troglodytes* chimpanzees. *Primates*, **23**, 245–251.

Crockford, C., and Boesch, C. (2003). Context-specific calls in wild chimpanzees, *Pan troglodytes verus*: analysis of barks. *Animal Behaviour*, **66**, 115–125.

Crockford, C., and Boesch, C. (2005). Call combinations in wild chimpanzees. *Behaviour*, **142**, 397–421.

Crockford, C., Herbinger, I., Vigilant, L., and Boesch, C. (2004). Wild chimpanzees produce group-specific calls: a case for vocal learning? *Ethology*, **110**, 221–243.

Crockford, C., Wittig, R. M., Seyfarth, R. M., and Cheney, D. L. (2007). Baboons eavesdrop to deduce mating opportunities. *Animal Behaviour*, **73**, 885–890.

Crockford, C., Wittig, R. M., Mundry, R., and Zuberbühler, K. (2012). Wild chimpanzees inform ignorant group members of danger. *Current Biology*, **22**, 142–146.

Crockford, C., Wittig, R. M., Langergraber, K., Ziegler, T. E., Zuberbühler, K., and Deschner, T. (2013). Urinary oxytocin and social bonding in related and unrelated wild chimpanzees. *Proceedings of the Royal Society of London B: Biological Sciences*, **280**, 20122765.

Crockford, C., Wittig, R. M., and Zuberbühler, K. (2015). An intentional vocalization draws others' attention: a playback experiment with wild chimpanzees. *Animal Cognition*, **18**, 581–591.

Crockford, C., Wittig, R. M., and Zuberbuehler, K. (2017). Vocalizing in chimpanzees is influenced by social cognitive processes. *Science Advances*, 3(11), e1701742.

Cronin, K. A., Pieper, B., van Leeuwen, E. J., Crockford, C., and Haun, D. B. (2015). Cooperating to compete: evaluating behavioral coordination in response to simulated territorial intrusion in chimpanzees (*Pan troglodytes*). *American Journal of Primatology*, **77**(S1), 64.

Duffy, K. G., Wrangham, R. W., and Silk, J. B. (2007). Male chimpanzees exchange political support for mating opportunities. *Current Biology*, **17**, 586–587.

Estienne, V., Stephens, C., and Boesch, C. (2017). Extraction of honey from underground bee nests by central African chimpanzees (*Pan troglodytes troglodytes*) in Loango National Park, Gabon: techniques and individual differences. *American Journal of Primatology*, **79**, 101–109.

Fischer, J., Noser, R., and Hammerschmidt, K. (2013). Bioacoustic field research: a primer to acoustic analyses and playback experiments with primates. *American Journal of Primatology*, **75**, 643–663.

Fraser, O. N., Koski, S. E., Wittig, R. M., and Aureli, F. (2009). Why are bystanders friendly to recipients of aggression? *Communicative and Integrative Biology*, **2**, 285–291.

Gilby, I. C. (2006). Meat sharing among the Gombe chimpanzees: harassment and reciprocal exchange. *Animal Behaviour*, **71**, 953–963.

Gilby, I. C., and Connor, R. C. (2010). The role of intelligence in group hunting: are chimpanzees different from other social predators? In *The mind of the chimpanzee: ecological and experimental perspectives* (pp. 220–232). Chicago, IL: University of Chicago Press.

Gilby, I. C., Thompson, M. E., Ruane, J. D., and Wrangham, R. (2010). No evidence of short-term exchange of meat for sex among chimpanzees. *Journal of Human Evolution*, **59**, 44–53.

Gomes, C. M., and Boesch, C. (2009). Wild chimpanzees exchange meat for sex on a long-term basis. *PLoS ONE*, **4**(4), e5116.

Gomes, C. M., Mundry, R., and Boesch, C. (2009). Long-term reciprocation of grooming in wild West African chimpanzees. *Proceedings of the Royal Society of London B: Biological Sciences*, **276**, 699–706.

Goodall, J. (1986). *The chimpanzees of Gombe: patterns of behavior*. Cambridge, MA: Harvard University Press.

Gruber, T., Muller, M. N., Strimling, P., Wrangham, R., and Zuberbühler, K. (2009). Wild chimpanzees rely on cultural knowledge to solve an experimental honey acquisition task. *Current Biology*, **19**, 1806–1810.

Grützmacher, K., Keil, V., Leinert, V., *et al.* (2017). Human quarantine: toward reducing infectious pressure on chimpanzees at the Taï Chimpanzee Project, Côte d'Ivoire. *American Journal of Primatology*, **80**, e22619.

Hare, B., Call, J., and Tomasello, M. (2001). Do chimpanzees know what conspecifics know? *Animal Behaviour*, **61**, 139–151.

Herrmann, E., Call, J., Hernàndez-Lloreda, M. V., Hare, B., and Tomasello, M. (2007). Humans have evolved specialized skills of social cognition: the cultural intelligence hypothesis. *Science*, **317**, 1360–1366.

Herrmann, E., Hernández-Lloreda, M. V., Call, J., Hare, B., and Tomasello, M. (2010). The structure of individual differences in the cognitive abilities of children and chimpanzees. *Psychological Science*, **21**, 102–110.

Heymann, E. W. (2006). The neglected sense – olfaction in primate behavior, ecology, and evolution. *American Journal of Primatology*, **68**, 519–524.

Hobaiter, C., Schel, A. M., Langergraber, K., and Zuberbühler, K. (2014). 'Adoption' by maternal siblings in wild chimpanzees. *PLoS ONE*, **9**(8), e103777.

Hockings, K. J., Humle, T., Anderson, J. R., *et al.* (2007). Chimpanzees share forbidden fruit. *PLoS ONE*, **2**(9), e886.

Horner, V., and Whiten, A. (2005). Causal knowledge and imitation/emulation switching in chimpanzees (*Pan troglodytes*) and children (*Homo sapiens*). *Animal Cognition*, **8**, 164–181.

Humle, T., and Matsuzawa, T. (2002). Ant-dipping among the chimpanzees of Bossou, Guinea, and some comparisons with other sites. *American Journal of Primatology*, **58**, 133–148.

Inoue, S., and Matsuzawa, T. (2007). Working memory of numerals in chimpanzees. *Current Biology*, **17**, 1004–1005.

Inoue-Nakamura, N., and Matsuzawa, T. (1997). Development of stone tool use by wild chimpanzees (*Pan troglodytes*). *Journal of Comparative Psychology*, **111**, 159–173.

Janmaat, K. R. L., Ban, S. D., and Boesch, C. (2013). Taï chimpanzees use botanical skills to discover fruit: what we can learn from their mistakes. *Animal Cognition*, **16**, 851–860.

Janmaat, K. R. L., Polansky, L., Ban, S. D., and Boesch, C. (2014). Wild chimpanzees plan their breakfast time, type, and location. *Proceedings of the National Academy of Sciences*, **111**, 16343–16348.

Kahlenberg, S. M., Thompson, M. E., Muller, M. N., and Wrangham, R. W. (2008a). Immigration costs for female chimpanzees and male protection as an immigrant counterstrategy to intrasexual aggression. *Animal Behaviour*, **76**, 1497–1509.

Kahlenberg, S. M., Thompson, M. E., and Wrangham, R. W. (2008b). Female competition over core areas in *Pan troglodytes schweinfurthii*, Kibale National Park, Uganda. *International Journal of Primatology*, **29**, 931.

Köhler, W. (2013). *Intelligenzprüfungen an Menschenaffen: mit einem Anhang zur Psychologie des Schimpansen* (Vol. 134). Berlin: Springer.

Kojima, S. (1990). Comparison of auditory functions in the chimpanzee and human. *Folia Primatologica*, **55**, 62–72.

Köndgen, S., Kühl, H., N'Goran, P. K., *et al.* (2008). Pandemic human viruses cause decline of endangered great apes. *Current Biology*, **18**, 260–264.

Krupenye, C., Kano, F., Hirata, S., Call, J., and Tomasello, M. (2016). Great apes anticipate that other individuals will act according to false beliefs. *Science*, **354**, 110–114.

Kühl, H. S., Kalan, A. K., Arandjelovic, M., *et al.* (2016). Chimpanzee accumulative stone throwing. *Scientific Reports*, **6**, 22219.

Kutsukake, N., and Castles, D. L. (2004). Reconciliation and post-conflict third-party affiliation among wild chimpanzees in the Mahale Mountains, Tanzania. *Primates*, **45**, 157–165.

Langergraber, K. E., Mitani, J. C., and Vigilant, L. (2007). The limited impact of kinship on cooperation in wild chimpanzees. *Proceedings of the National Academy of Sciences*, **104**, 7786–7790.

Langergraber, K. E., Boesch, C., Inoue, E., *et al.* (2010). Genetic and 'cultural' similarity in wild chimpanzees. *Proceedings of the Royal Society of London B: Biological Sciences*, **278**, 20101112.

Langergraber, K. E., Prüfer, K., Rowney, C., *et al.* (2012). Generation times in wild chimpanzees and gorillas suggest earlier divergence times in great ape and human evolution. *Proceedings of the National Academy of Sciences*, **109**, 15716–15721.

Lonsdorf, E. V. (2006). What is the role of mothers in the acquisition of termite-fishing behaviors in wild chimpanzees (*Pan troglodytes schweinfurthii*)? *Animal Cognition*, **9**, 36–46.

Luncz, L. V., Mundry, R., and Boesch, C. (2012). Evidence for cultural differences between neighboring chimpanzee communities. *Current Biology*, **22**, 922–926.

Luncz, L. V., Wittig, R. M., and Boesch, C. (2015). Primate archaeology reveals cultural transmission in wild chimpanzees (*Pan troglodytes verus*). *Philosophical Transactions of the Royal Society B: Biological Sciences*, **370**, 20140348.

Martin-Ordas, G., Haun, D., Colmenares, F., and Call, J. (2010). Keeping track of time: evidence for episodic-like memory in great apes. *Animal Cognition*, **13**, 331–340.

Matsumoto-Oda, A., Kutsukake, N., Hosaka, K., and Matsusaka, T. (2007). Sniffing behaviors in Mahale chimpanzees. *Primates*, **48**, 81–85.

Matsuno, T., Kawai, N., and Matsuzawa, T. (2004). Color classification by chimpanzees (*Pan troglodytes*) in a matching-to-sample task. *Behavioural Brain Research*, **148**, 157–165.

Matsuzawa, T., Biro, D., Humle, T., Inoue-Nakamura, N., Tonooka, R., and Yamakoshi, G. (2008). Emergence of culture in wild chimpanzees: education by master-apprenticeship. In *Primate origins of human cognition and behavior* (pp. 557–574). Japan: Springer.

Mennill, D. J., Ratcliffe, L. M., and Boag, P. T. (2002). Female eavesdropping on male song contests in songbirds. *Science*, **296**, 873.

Menzel, C. R. (1999). Unprompted recall and reporting of hidden objects by a chimpanzee (*Pan troglodytes*) after extended delays. *Journal of Comparative Psychology*, **113**, 426–434.

Mielke, A., Samuni, L., Preis, A., Gogarten, J. F., Crockford, C., and Wittig, R. M. (2017). Bystanders intervene to impede grooming in Western chimpanzees and sooty mangabeys. *Royal Society Open Science*, **4**(11), 171296.

Mitani, J. C., and Watts, D. P. (2001). Why do chimpanzees hunt and share meat? *Animal Behaviour*, **61**, 915–924.

Mitani, J. C., Merriwether, D. A., and Zhang, C. (2000). Male affiliation, cooperation and kinship in wild chimpanzees. *Animal Behaviour*, **59**, 885–893.

Mitani, J. C., Watts, D. P., and Amsler, S. J. (2010). Lethal intergroup aggression leads to territorial expansion in wild chimpanzees. *Current Biology*, **20**, 507–508.

Mulcahy, N. J., and Call, J. (2006). Apes save tools for future use. *Science*, **312**, 1038–1040.

Mundry, R. (2017). From nonparametric tests to mixed models: a brief overview of statistical tools frequently used in comparative psychology. In *APA Handbook of comparative psychology*, Vol. 1 (pp. 157–177). Philadelphia, PA: American Psychological Association.

Newton-Fisher, N. E., and Lee, P. C. (2011). Grooming reciprocity in wild male chimpanzees. *Animal Behaviour*, **81**, 439–446.

Nishida, T. (1968). The social group of wild chimpanzees in the Mahali Mountains. *Primates*, **9**, 167–224.

Nishida, T., Hasegawa, T., Hayaki, H., Takahata, Y., and Uehara, S. (1992). Meat-sharing as a coalitionary strategy by an alpha male chimpanzee. In *Topics in primatology* (pp. 159–174). Tokyo: University of Tokyo Press.

Normand, E., and Boesch, C. (2009). Sophisticated Euclidean maps in forest chimpanzees. *Animal Behaviour*, **77**, 1195–1201.

Normand, E., Ban, S. D., and Boesch, C. (2009). Forest chimpanzees (*Pan troglodytes verus*) remember the location of numerous fruit trees. *Animal Cognition*, **12**, 797–807.

Povinelli, D. J., and Vonk, J. (2003). Chimpanzee minds: suspiciously human? *Trends in Cognitive Sciences*, **7**, 157–160.

Premack, D., and Woodruff, G. (1978). Does the chimpanzee have a theory of mind? *Behavioral and Brain Sciences*, **1**, 515–526.

Pruetz, J. D., and Bertolani, P. (2007). Savanna chimpanzees, *Pan troglodytes verus*, hunt with tools. *Current Biology*, **17**, 412–417.

Radford, A. N., Majolo, B., and Aureli, F. (2016). Within-group behavioural consequences of between-group conflict: a prospective review. *Proceedings of the Royal Society of London B: Biological Sciences*, **283**, 1843.

Ramsey, G., Bastien, M. L., and van Schaik, C. (2007). Animal innovation defined and operationalized. *Behavioural and Brain Sciences*, **30**, 393–437.

Rilling, J. K., and Young, L. J. (2014). The biology of mammalian parenting and its effect on offspring social development. *Science*, **345**, 771–776.

Samuni, L., Preis, A., Mundry, R., Deschner, T., Crockford, C., and Wittig, R. M. (2017). Oxytocin reactivity during intergroup conflict in wild chimpanzees. *Proceedings of the National Academy of Sciences*, **114**, 268–273.

Sanz, C. M., and Morgan, D. B. (2007). Chimpanzee tool technology in the Goualougo Triangle, Republic of Congo. *Journal of Human Evolution*, **52**, 420–433.

Schel, A. M., Machanda, Z., Townsend, S. W., Zuberbühler, K., and Slocombe, K. E. (2013a). Chimpanzee food calls are directed at specific individuals. *Animal Behaviour*, **86**, 955–965.

Schel, A. M., Townsend, S. W., Machanda, Z., Zuberbuehler, K., and Slocombe, K. E. (2013b). Chimpanzee alarm call production meets key criteria for intentionality. *PLoS ONE*, **8**(10), e76674.

Schino, G., and Aureli, F. (2010). Primate reciprocity and its cognitive requirements. *Evolutionary Anthropology*, **19**, 130–135.

Seyfarth, R. M., and Cheney, D. L. (2012). The evolutionary origins of friendship. *Annual Review of Psychology*, **63**, 153–177.

Seyfarth, R. M., and Cheney, D. L. (2013). Affiliation, empathy, and the origins of theory of mind. *Proceedings of the National Academy of Sciences*, **110**, 10349–10356.

Sirianni, G., Mundry, R., and Boesch, C. (2015a). When to choose which tool: multidimensional and conditional selection of nut-cracking hammers in wild chimpanzees. *Animal Behaviour*, **100**, 152–165.

Sirianni, G., Wittig, R. M., and Boesch, C. (2015b). Do chimpanzees anticipate an object's weight? A field experiment on the kinematics of hammer-lifting movements in the nut-cracking Tai chimpanzees. *Folia Primatologica*, **86**, 360–361.

Slocombe, K. E., and Zuberbühler, K. (2007). Chimpanzees modify recruitment screams as a function of audience composition. *Proceedings of the National Academy of Sciences*, **104**, 17228–17233.

Slocombe, K. E., and Zuberbühler, K. (2010). Vocal communication in chimpanzees. In *The mind of the chimpanzee: ecological and experimental perspectives* (pp. 192–207). Chicago, IL: Chicago University Press.

Slocombe, K. E., Kaller, T., Turman, L., *et al.* (2010). Production of food-associated calls in wild male chimpanzees is dependent on the composition of the audience. *Behavioral Ecology and Sociobiology*, **64**, 1959–1966.

Surbeck, M., Boesch, C., Girard-Buttoz, C., Crockford, C., Hohmann, G., and Wittig, R. M. (2017a). Comparison of male conflict behavior in chimpanzees (*Pan troglodytes*) and bonobos (*Pan paniscus*), with specific regard to coalition and post-conflict behavior. *American Journal of Primatology*, **79**, e22641.

Surbeck, M., Girard-Buttoz, C., Boesch, C., *et al.* (2017b). Sex-specific association patterns in bonobos and chimpanzees reflect species differences in cooperation. *Royal Society Open Science*, **4**, 161081.

Tomasello, M. (2009a). *The cultural origins of human cognition*. Cambridge, MA: Harvard University Press.

Tomasello, M. (2009b). *Why we cooperate*. Cambridge, MA: MIT Press.

Tomasello, M., and Call, J. (1997). *Primate cognition*. Oxford: Oxford University Press.

Uehara, S., and Nishida, T. (1987). Body weights of wild chimpanzees (*Pan troglodytes schweinfurthii*) of the Mahale Mountains National Park, Tanzania. *American Journal of Physical Anthropology*, **72**, 315–321.

van Lawick-Goodall, J. (1968). The behaviour of free-living chimpanzees in the Gombe Stream Reserve. *Animal Behaviour Monographs*, **1**, 161-IN12.

Watts, D. P. (2000). Grooming between male chimpanzees at Ngogo, Kibale National Park. I. Partner number and diversity and grooming reciprocity. *International Journal of Primatology*, **21**, 189–210.

Watts, D. P., and Mitani, J. C. (2001). Boundary patrols and intergroup encounters in wild chimpanzees. *Behaviour*, **138**, 299–327.

Whiten, A., Goodall, J., McGrew, W. C., *et al.* (1999). Cultures in chimpanzees. *Nature*, **399**, 682–685.

Wilson, M. L., and Wrangham, R. W. (2003). Intergroup relations in chimpanzees. *Annual Review of Anthropology*, **32**, 363–392.

Wilson, M. L., Kahlenberg, S. M., Wells, M., and Wrangham, R. W. (2012). Ecological and social factors affect the occurrence and outcomes of intergroup encounters in chimpanzees. *Animal Behaviour*, **83**, 277–291.

Wilson, M. L., Boesch, C., Fruth, B., *et al.* (2014). Lethal aggression in *Pan* is better explained by adaptive strategies than human impacts. *Nature*, **513**, 414–417.

Wittig, R. M., and Boesch, C. (2003a). Food competition and linear dominance hierarchy among female chimpanzees of the Taï National Park. *International Journal of Primatology*, **24**, 847–867.

Wittig, R. M., and Boesch, C. (2003b). The choice of post-conflict interactions in wild chimpanzees (*Pan troglodytes*). *Behaviour*, **140**, 1527–1559.

Wittig, R. M., and Boesch, C. (2010). Receiving post-conflict affiliation from the enemy's friend reconciles former opponents. *PLoS ONE*, **5**(11), e13995.

Wittig, R. M., Crockford, C., Seyfarth, R. M., and Cheney, D. L. (2007a). Vocal alliances in Chacma baboons (*Papio hamadryas ursinus*). *Behavioral Ecology and Sociobiology*, **61**, 899–909.

Wittig, R. M., Crockford, C., Wikberg, E., Seyfarth, R. M., and Cheney, D. L. (2007b). Kin-mediated reconciliation substitutes for direct reconciliation in female baboons. *Proceedings of the Royal Society of London B: Biological Sciences*, **274**, 1109–1115.

Wittig, R. M., Crockford, C., Deschner, T., Langergraber, K. E., Ziegler, T. E., and Zuberbühler, K. (2014a). Food sharing is linked to urinary oxytocin levels and bonding in related and unrelated wild chimpanzees. *Proceedings of the Royal Society of London B: Biological Sciences,* **281**, 20133096.

Wittig, R. M., Crockford, C., Langergraber, K. E., and Zuberbühler, K. (2014b). Triadic social interactions operate across time: a field experiment with wild chimpanzees. *Proceedings of the Royal Society of London B: Biological Sciences*, **281**, 20133155.

Wittig, R. M., Crockford, C., Weltring, A., Langergraber, K. E., Deschner, T., and Zuberbühler, K. (2016). Social support reduces stress hormone levels in wild chimpanzees across stressful events and everyday affiliations. *Nature Communications*, **7**, 13361.

Wroblewski, E. E. (2008). An unusual incident of adoption in a wild chimpanzee (*Pan troglodytes*) population at Gombe National Park. *American Journal of Primatology*, **70**, 995–998.

Wroblewski, E. E., Murray, C. M., Keele, B. F., Schumacher-Stankey, J. C., Hahn, B. H., and Pusey, A. E. (2009). Male dominance rank and reproductive success in chimpanzees, *Pan troglodytes schweinfurthii. Animal Behaviour*, **77**, 873–885.

Zuberbühler, K., and Byrne, R. W. (2006). Social cognition. *Current Biology*, **16**, 786–790.

Zuberbühler, K., and Wittig, R. M. (2011). Field experiments with nonhuman primates: a tutorial. In *Field and laboratory methods in primatology: a practical guide* (pp. 207–224). Cambridge: Cambridge University Press.

7 Dolphins and Whales – Taking Cognitive Research Out of the Tanks and into the Wild

Volker B. Deecke

Species Description

Anatomy

The whales and dolphins (order Cetacea) are a highly diverse group of animals. They have some commonalities (e.g. mammalian body plan and reproductive strategy, complete adaptation to an aquatic lifestyle), but there are several key differences in feeding ecology, social structure and sensory perception that have considerable repercussions on their cognitive abilities.

While the taxonomic position of the cetaceans was disputed for a long time, it now seems reasonably clear that they are located within the superorder Cetartiodactyla, along with the even-toed ungulates (e.g. Price *et al.*, 2005; Agnarsson and May-Collado, 2008). Molecular studies (e.g. Price *et al.*, 2005; Agnarsson and May-Collado, 2008) have confirmed that within the Cetacea, the major taxonomic distinction lies between the toothed whales (suborder Odontoceti) and the baleen whales (suborder Mysticeti), and this distinction is delineated by major behavioural and ecological differences. The taxonomic position of the three species of sperm whales (families Physeteridae and Kogiidae) has been subject to some discussion, but they are now generally included within the suborder Odontoceti (e.g. Heyning, 1997; Nikaido *et al.*, 2001; May-Collado and Agnarsson, 2005; Agnarsson and May-Collado, 2008).

The mysticetes range in adult size from 6 m (the pygmy right whale, *Caperea marginata*) to over 30 m (the blue whale, *Balaenoptera musculus*), and are characterized by their use of baleen plates to filter small prey from the water. Most baleen whales feed in the water column on crustaceans or small schooling fish. However, grey whales (*Eschrichtius robustus*) can also feed on benthic invertebrates by filtering them from the sediment. Ten extant species in four major clades (Balaenidae, Neobalaenidae, Eschrichtiidae and Balaenopteridae) are currently recognized.

With the exception of the sperm whale (*Physeter macrocephalus*), with an adult male size of up to 20 m, the odontocetes tend to be smaller, with adult sizes ranging from 1.4 m (the vaquita or Gulf of California porpoise, *Phocoena sinus*) to 13 m (Baird's beaked whale, *Berardius bairdii*). Diets of odontocetes are varied and range from cephalopods and crustaceans to fish, sea mammals, seabirds or marine turtles. Rather than filter-feeding on schools of prey, odontocetes typically single out individual prey animals, which they pursue and capture. Whereas baleen whales are found exclusively in the marine environment and are relatively shallow divers (to 500 m), some toothed whales, such as the river dolphin, live exclusively in freshwater habitats, and other species such as beaked whales and sperm whales have evolved a deep-diving lifestyle and are capable of descending to depths of almost 3000 m (Schorr *et al.*, 2014). The toothed whales are comprised of 10 major clades (Delphinidae, Phocoenidae, Monodontidae, Iniidae, Pontoporiidae, Lipotidae, Ziphiidae, Platanistidae, Kogiidae and Physeteridae), with a total of 73 species currently recognized (Nikaido *et al.*, 2001).

Along with the sirenids (manatees and dugongs), cetaceans are the only mammals fully adapted to an aquatic existence. Whereas marine mammals, such as seals and sealions, return to land for reproduction and essential body maintenance, cetaceans have evolved the physiological adaptations to complete all life processes in the aquatic environment. They are characterized by a more or less torpedo-shaped body and the absence of hind legs. The forelimbs have evolved into flippers and most species have a dorsal fin that presumably evolved for stability. A broad tail fluke reinforced by collagen-rich connective tissue, rather than bone, is the primary means of propulsion. Through evolutionary elongation of the premaxillary bones, the entrance of the nasal passage has migrated to the top of the head forming the blowhole (Thewissen, 1994).

Perception

The adaptation to a fully aquatic existence has meant a reduced reliance on the traditional mammalian sensory systems of vision and olfaction, and an evolution towards using sound as the primary means of perception and communication. Whereas light is absorbed quickly in the aquatic environment, sound waves transmit freely through water, travelling at greater speed and experiencing less attenuation than in air. Underwater, vision is limited to distances of approximately 100 m in the best conditions, and not useful at depths below 200 m. Sound, on the other hand, allows cetaceans to sense their environment and communicate over distances for tens if not hundreds of kilometres (e.g. Madsen *et al.*, 2002; Janik, 2005).

Many mysticetes and odontocetes use sound extensively for communication. Some baleen whales produce highly structured songs, thought to function in mate attraction and/or male–male competition (e.g. humpback whales, *Megaptera novaeangliae*: Helweg *et al.*, 1992; bowhead whales, *Balaena mysticetus*: Stafford *et al.*, 2008), and various sounds related to feeding and social behaviour have also been described (e.g. Cerchio and Dahlheim, 2001; Dunlop *et al.*, 2008). Toothed whales use a variety of tonal sounds mostly for social communication (e.g. May-Collado *et al.*, 2007). However, in addition to social sounds, all odontocete species studied so far have been shown to produce broadband clicks for echolocation. True echolocation has not been documented in baleen whales (but see Stimpert *et al.*, 2007).

Sound production in mysticetes remains poorly understood, but at least some species appear to use the larynx as their main sound-generating organ (Reidenberg and Laitman, 2007). Odontocetes, on the other hand, have evolved an independent sound production mechanism: sound is generated by nasal plugs located at the junction between the nasal passage and adjacent air sacs (Madsen *et al.*, 2013). This system allows the recycling of air between the different air sacs while diving, rather than expelling it into the water. Except for the sperm whales, these nasal plugs are paired structures, and studies using animal-attached hydrophones or small catheters to measure air pressure in different parts of the nasal passage suggest that echolocation clicks are generated with the right nasal plug, whereas the left one serves to produce tonal sounds (Cranford *et al.*, 2011; Madsen *et al.*, 2013).

In toothed whales, outgoing sound passes though the melon, an organ comprised of fatty tissue overlying the premaxillary bones, thought to function to focus the sound. The shape of the melon is controlled by various muscles, which allows the animal to modify the structure of the sound beams (Harper *et al.*, 2008).

Resonant volumes in the trachea, nasal passage and adjacent air sacs are subject to pressure-related change, as animals ascend and descend in the water column. This means that acoustic features related to resonance, such as formants, important in the communication of many terrestrial mammals, do not provide reliable markers to encode information such as individual identity.

Sound reception in baleen whales remains poorly understood. However, in toothed whales, incoming sounds are thought to be received by the jaws, and conducted directly to the inner ear via special fatty channels (Ketten, 2000). The oral cavity and gular region may also play a role in conducting sound to the inner ear (Cranford *et al.*, 2008). Echolocating species are able to use the returning echoes to identify objects, including prey or underwater features for orientation. The functional range over which echolocation provides useful information remains unclear, but is bound to vary depending on the echolocation task. Prey detection is thought to be possible over a few hundred metres (e.g. Au *et al.*, 2004, 2010). Some species may be able to obtain useful information for navigation (e.g. depth of the water column) over a few kilometres. The echolocation signals of some species are audible to conspecifics over tens of kilometres (thus providing potentially useful information on prey aggregations; Madsen *et al.*, 2002).

Audiogram data are available for many odontocete species, but limited for mysticetes. However, hearing sensitivity at different frequencies has been estimated from the dimensions of the ear bones and the basilar membrane in the inner ear (e.g. Ketten, 1997, 2000; Hemilä *et al.*, 1999). Most toothed whales have sensitive hearing between 10 and 100 kHz (Au, 2000), although for some porpoises and small dolphins, the range of sensitive hearing extends considerably above 100 kHz (e.g. Kastelein *et al.*, 2002). Baleen whales are thought to hear best at frequencies below 10 kHz, with some species adapted to hearing at very low frequencies of a few tens of Hz (Ketten, 2000).

Cetaceans are not thought to have sensitive chemosensory abilities (Kremers *et al.*, 2016), although taste buds and chemoreceptor cells have been found in some species, and bottlenose dolphins have been shown to be able to perceive sour, bitter and sweet tastes (Kremers *et al.*, 2016)

Most cetaceans have well-developed eyes, which are generally located on the side of the head, rather than facing forward. Whales and dolphins were originally thought to be colour-blind, but at least some species of delphinids appear to have basic colour vision (Mobley and Helweg, 1990; Kremers *et al.*, 2016). Visual acuity is high among marine delphinids, whereas some river dolphins appear to have limited capability or are even functionally blind (e.g. Mass and Supin, 1990, 1999).

The skin of cetaceans has rich innervation and may be capable of sensing fine differences in water pressure (Ridgway and Carder, 1990). This may aid in maintaining laminar flow around the body, but also help sense approaching conspecifics, predators or prey at close range. While the body of adult cetaceans largely lacks hair, many species have hairs as embryos and neonates, and some species retain functional sensory hairs into adulthood, which appear to play a role in prey sensing and capture (e.g. Pyenson *et al.*, 2012; Drake *et al.*, 2015).

Life Cycle

All cetaceans are slow reproducing, with females giving birth to single calves. In most species, birthing appears to occur at specific times of year. While the females of some small odontocetes are able to reproduce annually, most whales and dolphins have interbirth intervals of multiple years, with females of some species only reproducing every 5 years (Whitehead and Mann, 2000). Lactation ranges from 6 months in some baleen whales to several years in sperm whales (Best *et al.*, 1984; Whitehead and Mann, 2000), and the young of several toothed whale species appear to remain dependent on their mother beyond the age of weaning (e.g. Bigg *et al.*, 1990; Olesiuk *et al.*, 1990).

Reproduction is costly in terms of energetic resources: female cetaceans mobilize a large amount of their body fat to produce a foetus and nurse a young calf. Females of migratory baleen whale species do not feed during this time, and rely entirely on stored fat reserves to sustain themselves and their offspring. However, reproduction also has cognitive costs, because breathing in cetaceans is a voluntary response and the animals need to be conscious to breathe, so that both mothers and newborn calves of some species appear not to sleep during the first month after birth (Lyamin *et al.*, 2005).

Some toothed whale species have been shown to undergo menopause, with the females of some delphinids living almost half of their lives in a post-reproductive state. For example, female resident killer whales (*Orcinus orca*) typically stop reproducing around age 45, but may live well into their 90s (Olesiuk *et al.*, 1990). The presence of post-reproductive females has a significant effect on the survival probability of their sons (Foster *et al.*, 2012), either because they act as repositories for ecological knowledge (Brent *et al.*, 2015), or through active provisioning of food (Wright *et al.*, 2016).

Cetaceans are generally long-lived, with large overlaps between generations. With a maximum longevity of 22–23 years (Koschinski, 2001), the harbour porpoise (*Phocoena phocoena*) is probably on the lower end of cetacean life expectancies. Killer whales are thought to live for a maximum of 80–90 years for females and a maximum of 50–60 years for males (Olesiuk *et al.*, 1990). Maximum longevity for Atlantic bottlenose dolphins has been estimated at 50 and 30 years for females and males, respectively (Stolen and Barlow, 2003). Female narwhals (*Monodon monoceros*) are thought to reach at least 115 years of age (Garde *et al.*, 2007). Life expectancy data for baleen whales are scarce, but photographic and morphological data suggest maximum longevity of 60–90 years for most baleen whale species (e.g. Hamilton *et al.*, 1998; Arrigoni *et al.*, 2011). However, novel molecular ageing methods suggest longevity exceeding 200 years for bowhead whales, *Balaena mysticetus* (George *et al.*, 1999).

Individual Identification

Photographic identification of cetaceans using natural marking was first pioneered in the late 1970s (Hammond *et al.*, 1982) and has been used effectively in studies of population structure, social behaviour and cognition. While in some species every individual can be reliably identified from high-quality photographs (e.g. killer whales: Bigg, 1982; Bain, 1990; humpback whales: Stevick *et al.*, 2001), populations of other species, especially the smaller odontocetes, typically contain a proportion of poorly marked individuals (e.g. Wilson *et al.*, 1999), so that conclusions are often drawn from a sample of well-marked individuals that may not be representative of the population as a whole.

A number of long-term studies using photographic identification have now been running for several decades, yielding a wealth of social information. These studies have largely focused on bottlenose dolphins (*Tursiops* spp.; e.g. Wells, 1991; Wilson *et al.*, 1997; Connor *et al.*, 2001) and killer whales (e.g. Bigg *et al.*, 1990; Similä *et al.*, 1996), providing valuable baseline information, on which to base research into the social cognition of these species (e.g. Sayigh *et al.*, 1999; Deecke *et al.*, 2010).

Other marking techniques, such as roto- or spaghetti-tags, tags bolted through the dorsal fin or freeze brands, were explored in the 1970s and 1980s (e.g. Irvine *et al.*, 1982), but largely abandoned once photo-ID became established. Small satellite tags, deployed using a crossbow or air rifle and embedded into the animals' blubber or dorsal fin with barbs, are also used to track movement patterns of some of the larger cetaceans (e.g. Mate *et al.*, 2007).

A fundamental problem when studying cetacean behaviour and cognition is that direct observation is only possible when the animals are at the surface to breathe, but most behavioural responses to social or environmental stimuli happen underwater out of our sight. In the last 20 years, miniaturization of technology has permitted the development of on-animal data loggers (e.g. Johnson and Tyack, 2003; see Figure 7.1), which have provided fascinating insights into the underwater lives of whales and dolphins. Such tags are typically attached with suction cups and remain on the animal for hours or days. Most tags contain accelerometers, magnetometers and pressure sensors, which allow researchers to reconstruct the detailed underwater movement of the tagged individuals in three dimensions. In addition, some tags also contain hydrophones and sufficient storage capacity to record high-quality underwater sound, which allows the study of echolocation behaviour, and the responses to anthropogenic noise and communicative events (e.g. Johnson *et al.*, 2009). Digital archival tags have so far mostly been used to investigate foraging behaviour and responses to anthropogenic sounds. However, they present valuable tools to investigate other aspects of cognition (particularly social ones) as well.

Ecological Characteristics

Baleen and toothed whales differ fundamentally in the way they obtain food, and this distinction has shaped their cognitive evolution. Mysticetes typically feed on small schooling prey, engulfing a large number of prey items in a single gulp. Their sensory

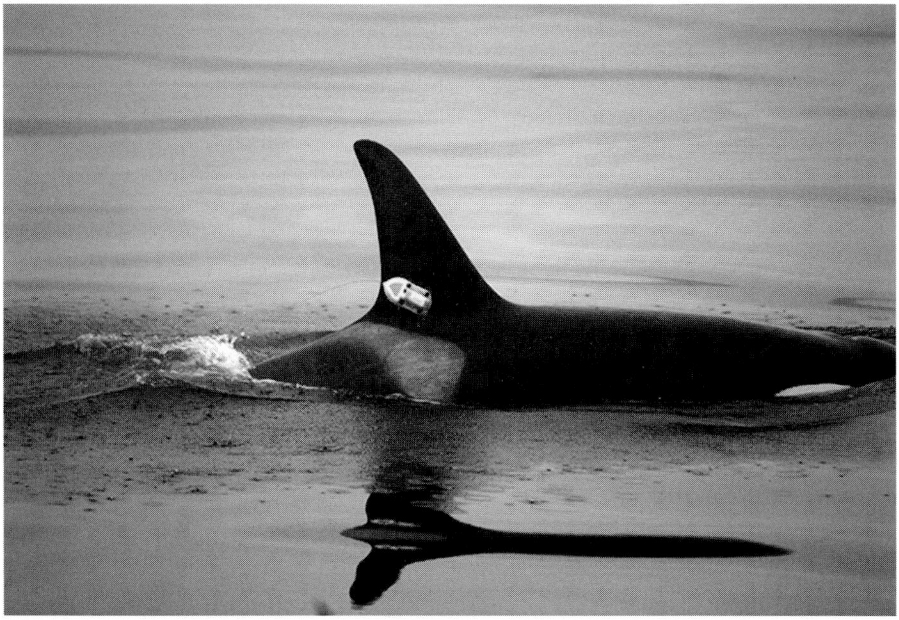

Figure 7.1. Photograph of a juvenile killer whale (*Orcinus orca*) carrying an archival digital recording tag (Dtag; Johnson and Tyack, 2003). The tag is attached by four suction cups, and records the animal's underwater movements, as well as any sounds it hears or emits. It was used to study the echolocation behaviour and hunting strategies of killer whales, while feeding on Pacific salmon (*Oncorhynchus* spp.; Wright *et al.*, 2017).
Photograph by Volker Deecke.

systems are therefore adapted to effectively detect such large aggregations and to sense their density and profitability. Odontocetes, on the other hand, typically feed on individual prey items, which they must detect, pursue and capture. They have therefore evolved sensory capability to detect and track fast-moving and manoeuvrable prey, presumably using their echolocation (e.g. Au *et al.*, 2004).

Aside from some river dolphins, which appear to have few predators other than humans, most cetaceans are subject to predation by sharks and killer whales. Anti-predator strategies include morphological adaptations (e.g. countershading: Caro *et al.*, 2011; false gill slits in dwarf and pygmy sperm whales, *Kogia simus* and *K. breviceps*: Bloodworth and Odell, 2008), as well as behavioural strategies such as vertical and horizontal avoidance, aggression and mobbing (Ford and Reeves, 2008). Playbacks of killer whale sounds to various cetacean species have provided valuable insights into such behavioural anti-predator strategies (e.g. Tyack *et al.*, 2011; Curé *et al.*, 2012, 2013).

The movement ecology of baleen and toothed whales shows fundamental differences, and these are likely to affect spatial cognition and memory. Many odontocetes remain in the same habitats year-round or follow movements that are not seasonally defined, whereas most mysticetes follow a clear seasonal migration. Baleen whales typically give birth on low-latitude breeding grounds, which they visit in the winter months, but then migrate to high-latitude feeding grounds, where they spend the summer. In some species, feeding activity appears to be entirely limited to the summer months. This migratory behaviour may be due to the lower thermoregulatory capacity and higher predation risk of calves (Corkeron and Connor, 1999; Clapham, 2001).

Social Characteristics

Photographic identification has played a critical role in identifying the social structure of many species. Like other mammals, cetaceans have strong bonds between mothers and dependent young. In many species, however, such bonds can persist beyond independence. Odontocetes exhibit a variety of social structures (Connor *et al.*, 1998), ranging from closed groups in killer whales (Bigg *et al.*, 1990) and sperm whales (Whitehead *et al.*, 1991), to fission–fusion societies (e.g. bottlenose dolphins, *Tursiops aduncus*: Smolker *et al.,* 1992; Möller *et al.*, 2006) or stratified societies (e.g. Risso's dolphins, *Grampus griseus*: Hartman *et al.*, 2008). Social behaviour varies between age and sex groups, but can also exhibit pronounced differences between populations of the same species (e.g. killer whales: Bigg, 1990; Baird and Whitehead, 2000; Tavares *et al.*, 2017).

Several species of toothed whales have been shown to have a distinct matrilineal social organization, with closed groups consisting of individuals from three or four generations, related through matrilineal descent. Matrilineal social structure has so far been documented in sperm whales (Richard *et al.*, 1996; Lyrholm and Gyllensten, 1998), killer whales and long-finned pilot whales (*Globicephala melas*: Amos *et al.*, 1993), but is probably also found in other species, particularly in the subfamily Globicephalinae.

The social structure of both Atlantic and Indo-Pacific bottlenose dolphins is characterized by weak and/or temporary associations between females, but remarkably strong and lasting associations between adult males (Wells, 1991; Smolker *et al.*, 1992; Möller *et al.*, 2006). Such male alliances have been documented in all bottlenose dolphin populations studied to date. Alliance members are sometimes, but not always, close relatives (e.g. Möller *et al.*, 2001; Parsons *et al.*, 2003) and maintain very high levels of association, sometimes for the majority of their lives. These male alliances are thought to increase access to females in reproductive condition. In Shark Bay, higher-order alliances of several groups of males, joining forces against rivals in contests for females, have also been documented (Krützen *et al.*, 2003; Connor *et al.*, 2010).

The social structure of baleen whales remains poorly understood, but is thought to be more fluid than that of odontocetes. The period of dependency is generally much shorter in baleen whales. Calves of many baleen whale species are weaned and independent after 6–7 months (Whitehead and Mann, 2000). Little is currently known about adult association behaviour in baleen whales, although long-term association between individuals does exist in at least some species (e.g. Weinrich, 1991; Ramp *et al.*, 2010).

State of the Art

In captivity, most species of odontocetes appear to respond readily to training, if using positive reinforcement and acoustic or visual bridges, so that fundamental aspects of cognition, such as perception and memory, can be readily assessed. The challenges of a comprehensive assessment of cetacean cognitive abilities lie principally in the fact that many species are difficult or impossible to maintain in captivity, and that captive animals are unlikely to express the full cognitive repertoire of their wild counterparts. This is particularly problematic in studies of social cognition and communication. Most of our knowledge on cetacean cognition comes from toothed whales, and much of this research has been done in a captive setting. Bottlenose dolphins (*Tursiops* spp.) have received the vast majority of research attention, with only a handful of cognitive studies on a few other species (belugas, *Delphinapterus leucas*, killer whales, harbour porpoise and Pacific white-sided dolphins, *Lagenorhynchus obliquidens*).

Because sound is the principal means by which most cetacean species receive and transmit information, playback experiments are the primary research tool by which cetacean cognition has been assessed in the field (Deecke, 2006). Playbacks offer an effective way to present controlled stimuli to wild whales and dolphins in order to assess their response. So far, playback has been used primarily to understand social cognition in toothed whales, including individual and group recognition. With the exception of research on the production, perception and learning of song in humpback whales, very little cognitive research has been done on baleen whales – these species are almost impossible to maintain in captivity and present substantial challenges for research in the wild.

The aim of this section is to review the research on cetacean cognition with a focus on studies conducted in the wild. This will help identify future approaches using the novel technologies now available and can also inform strategies to study cognition in the more challenging species, such as the deep-diving odontocetes and the baleen whales.

Perception and Attention

Studies on perception have investigated hearing abilities in toothed whales, and behavioural or neurophysiological audiogram information is available for several species (e.g. Thomas *et al.*, 1988; Sauerland and Denhardt, 1998; Szymanski *et al.*, 1999; Kastelein *et al.*, 2002; Houser *et al.*, 2008; Branstetter *et al.*, 2017). Studies on baleen whale perception are currently limited to a few preliminary studies on grey whales (*Eschrichtius robustus*; Dahlheim and Ljungblad, 1990; Ridgway and Carder, 2001).

The echolocation abilities of toothed whales have been largely studied in captivity, and have shown to provide very detailed resolution of size, shape and texture (e.g. Herman *et al.*, 1998; DeLong *et al.*, 2006) as well as cross-modal transfer between echoic and visual recognition (e.g. Harley *et al.*, 2003). Whereas in visual cognition tasks, gaze direction can provide information on where an animal focuses its attention, the rate and direction of echolocation can provide this information in echoic cognition of toothed whales (e.g. Wisniewska *et al.*, 2012). Few studies have looked at echoic perception in the wild. Studies on free-ranging bottlenose dolphins show that the animals adjust both interclick intervals and source levels to ensure good signal-to-noise ratios and effective signal processing with varying range to the echolocation target (Jensen *et al.*, 2009). Wild bottlenose dolphins appear to be able to echolocate through sandy sediments to detect visually hidden fish (Herzing, 2004). The fact that individual echolocation rates decrease with increasing group size in many species may mean that toothed whales are able to extract information from echoes returning from clicks of other group members (Götz *et al.*, 2006). Madsen and colleagues (2005) present exciting insights into the echoic perception of Blainville's beaked whale (*Mesoplodon densirostris*). They show that strategically placed acoustic tags can not only be used to record outgoing echolocation clicks but also their returning echoes. Using echograms, they were able to visualize the echoic information obtained by the tagged whale as it homed in on individual targets or schools of prey.

In addition to active use of echolocation to obtain information about objects in their environments, some toothed whales have been shown to use passive listening, for example, for sounds produced by prey animals (e.g. Gannon *et al.*, 2005). Because baleen whales are not known to echolocate, passive listening may be their primary way of orientation and prey detection.

Physical Cognition: Spatial Relationships, Numerical Competence and Tool Use

While there has been a fair amount of research into echolocation (the primary method by which most toothed whales obtain information about their environments), we know very little about how cetaceans integrate spatial information and use it for orientation and navigation, or to remember and localize food sources. Studies from the wild are largely limited to mapping movement patterns and migratory routes. Bottlenose dolphins appear to be able to use their echolocation to detect fish hidden from view and buried in sediments (Herzing, 2004). When it comes to tracking objects that are hidden both visually and acoustically, studies in captivity suggest that, like many terrestrial mammals, bottlenose dolphins (*Tursiops truncatus*) are able to identify the location of objects that they are able to track visually, but perform poorly when tracking hidden objects (i.e. the object is placed in a secondary container before being moved to a hiding place: Jaakkola *et al.*, 2010).

Only a few studies have so far investigated numerical competence in cetaceans, and none of these were conducted in the wild. Captive bottlenose dolphins, which were trained to choose sets of fewer items physically presented in their tank, were able to generalize this response to novel numbers and items, thus suggesting that the animals had a sense of the numerical concept 'less' (Kilian *et al.*, 2003). Dolphins exhibit similar performance when presented with visual representations, rather than physical items, suggesting that their numerical competence does not require echolocation, but is expressed equally well in the visual domain (Kilian *et al.*, 2003; Jaakkola *et al.*, 2005).

Similarly, captive bottlenose dolphins are also able to generalize the concept of 'same' and 'different' (Mercado *et al.*, 2000).

Tool use may be defined as the use of a freely manipulable object to modify the physical properties of a target object, through some form of complex mechanical interaction (e.g. Seed and Byrne, 2010). Bottlenose dolphins (*Tursiops* sp.) in Shark Bay are known to pick marine sponges off the sea floor and carry them on their rostrum, while probing in the substrate for fish (Smolker *et al.*, 1997). The precise function of sponging remains unclear, but it may serve to protect the rostrum from physical injury or harmful fish, such as stingrays. The behaviour is more common in females and appears to be transmitted through social learning along maternal lines (Krützen *et al.*, 2005). Many species of baleen and toothed whales emit bubbles as part of the foraging process, and this can be interpreted as tool use in the widest sense. The most complex use of bubbles comes from humpback whales: some northeast Pacific populations exhibit a feeding behaviour, where up to 20 individuals feed cooperatively on schooling herring (*Clupea pallasii*; e.g. D'Vincent *et al.*, 1985). One group member swims in a circle below the school, exhaling air and thus creating a curtain of bubbles that encircle the fish. All group members then swim upwards through the bubble net, engulfing the fish. These feeding groups are stable over the years, and show a remarkable level of coordination (D'Vincent *et al.*, 1985). During the herding phase, one or two individuals emit a series of low-frequency calls that may serve to manipulate the schooling behaviour of the fish (Cerchio and Dahlheim, 2001). Similar feeding vocalizations have also been documented in killer whales in the Northeast Atlantic (Simon *et al.,* 2006; Deecke *et al.*, 2011). Because a physical structure, a sound, is apparently being used to modify the behaviour of the prey, such herding calls can also be seen as tool use in the widest sense.

Learning and Memory

In captivity, odontocetes can readily be trained to learn associations between different visual, acoustic or echoic stimuli in their environment, or to respond with conditioned behaviours (see Schusterman *et al.*, 1986; Jaakkola, 2012). In captivity, novel associations or behavioural responses can also be socially transmitted through observational learning (e.g. Yeater *et al.*, 2010). There is limited, mostly anecdotal, evidence for associative and social learning in the wild (e.g. Guinet, 1991; Guinet and Bouvier, 1995; Yeater *et al.*, 2010). Some of the best field evidence for complex associative learning in odontocetes comes from the social transmission of sponging (Krützen *et al.*, 2005), as well as associations of killer whales and bottlenose dolphins with artisanal fisheries, where certain individuals have learned to cooperate with fishermen in often complex behavioural interactions in order to increase their own foraging success (e.g. Wellings, 1944; Pryor and Lindbergh, 1990; Neil, 2002). At least some species of mysticetes are similarly capable of complex social learning: in humpback whales, novel feeding behaviours are far more likely to spread between frequent social associates (Allen *et al.*, 2013).

Cetaceans are one of only a few mammalian taxa capable of complex vocal learning. Captive odontocetes can be trained to copy sounds in their environment and to associate existing vocal patterns and sound stimuli with novel contexts (Janik and Slater, 1997). Captive animals will furthermore spontaneously copy each other's vocalizations (e.g. Crance *et al.*, 2014). There is also good evidence for complex vocal production learning from both toothed and baleen whales in the field: modifications to stereotyped call types of killer whales are transferred between groups that do not interbreed (Deecke *et al.*, 2000). In Sarasota, Florida, pairs of male bottlenose dolphins in an alliance converge on a common signature whistle pattern (Watwood *et al.*, 2004). Wild bottlenose dolphins are able to copy the signature whistles of close social associates (King *et al.*, 2013), and killer whales occasionally appear to copy call types of other social groups (Weiß *et al.*, 2011). All male humpback whales on a common breeding ground typically share the same song type, which changes within and between seasons (e.g. Cerchio *et al.*, 2001), and song changes can propagate very rapidly throughout a population (Noad *et al.*, 2000) and even across ocean basins (Garland *et al.*, 2011).

Field playbacks to wild bottlenose dolphins have shown that the animals are able to recognize the signature whistles of relatives, including offspring that have been independent for several years (Sayigh *et al.*, 1999). Playback experiments have furthermore shown that wild bottlenose dolphins recognize the structural properties of their own signature whistle and typically respond by matching it (King and Janik, 2013). Humpback whales show different behavioural responses to playbacks of song and social sounds (Tyack, 1983; Mobley *et al.*, 1988), suggesting different functions of the sounds. While recognition of individual or group identity or behavioural context from vocalizations is well established, both in captivity and the wild, the evidence for categorical matching is limited and controversial. Vergara and Barrett-Lennard (2017) trained a captive beluga to match two sound categories (screams and pulse trains): while the individual eventually achieved a high degree of accuracy on the training set, it failed to generalize the discrimination to novel exemplars. Reverting to an achievable training task showed that the poor performance was not due to lack of motivation, but may suggest a fundamental difference in the way humans and cetaceans perceive tonal and pulsed sounds.

In captivity, cetaceans have shown good capacity for both short- and long-term memory. Bottlenose dolphins can be successfully trained to respond to a specific command by repeating the last behaviour exhibited (Mercado *et al.*, 1998) and to repeat actions performed with specific objects (Mercado *et al.*, 1999), which shows that they maintain a working memory of their behaviour. Captive bottlenose dolphins, furthermore, recognized playbacks of signature whistles of former social associates, even after decades of separation (Bruck, 2013). The results of field playbacks, showing that wild dolphins recognize the signature whistles of their offspring that have been independent for several years (Sayigh *et al.*, 1999), are also suggestive of long-term social memory.

Social Cognition and Communication

Cetaceans live in complex social environments, and the evidence suggests that they have evolved complex social cognitive faculties to guide social decisions. Long and stable associations between individuals have been shown among both mysticetes and odontocetes. There is solid evidence for recognition of individuals from signature whistles in bottlenose dolphins (e.g. Sayigh *et al.*, 1999), but such individual recognition is probably more widespread, especially among the toothed whales. Playback experiments in the field (King and Janik, 2013; King *et al.*, 2013) and captivity (King *et al.*, 2014) further suggest that bottlenose dolphins copy the signature whistles of other individuals and may effectively use them as labels to address specific individuals. Quick and Janik (2012) showed that the usage of signature whistles increased in situations when individuals rejoined after some period of separation.

In contrast to the individual signatures of bottlenose dolphins, many killer whale populations exhibit group-specific variation in their vocalizations that identifies social groups rather than individuals. Resident killer whales in the northeast Pacific live in stable matrilineal social groups that typically consist of three or four generations of animals, related through matrilineal descent. All members of such a matriline share the same vocal repertoire of 8–15 highly stereotyped call types (Ford, 1991). Some of the call types may be shared with other, presumably related, matrilines; however, the population also contains matrilines that frequently associate yet have no call types in common. All groups that share at least one call type are grouped together into a common acoustic clan. The Northern Resident population of killer whales contains three such clans (Ford, 1991). Examples of repertoires from matrilines belonging to different clans are given in Figure 7.2. Call types that are shared among matrilines often show subtle structural differences between groups. Weiß and colleagues (2006) showed that the usage of matriline-specific call types increased after the birth of a new calf.

Comparisons with microsatellite DNA data suggest that structural variation of at least some call types reflects genetic relatedness, as well as social affiliations (Deecke *et al.*, 2010). The vocal dialects, therefore, may allow resident killer whales to identify maternal relatives with a high degree of precision. Like bottlenose dolphins, killer whales occasionally mimic call types of another acoustic clan (Weiß *et al.*, 2011). Whether such copied calls also function in labelling has yet to be established.

While the social cognition and communication systems of a few odontocete species are relatively well understood, we are a long way from a comprehensive understanding of the acquisition, processing and transmission of social information for the taxon as a whole. Many oceanic dolphin species habitually live in groups of hundreds and in some cases, thousands of individuals. Living in groups of such size likely requires constant processing of social information and behavioural decision-making, yet studying individual behaviour in such large groups is extremely challenging. Some beaked whale species appear to have very unusual social structures and mating systems (e.g. Connor *et al.*, 1998), yet due to their pelagic habitat and deep-diving lifestyles, their social cognition is very difficult to study. Finally, we know very little about the social lives of mysticetes, even though some species clearly show long-term social association between individuals and a high degree of behavioural cooperation. New technologies (such as animal-attached recording tags that can record behavioural and acoustic responses to social stimuli) promise to be extremely helpful in providing novel insights into the complex social lives of a large number of cetacean species.

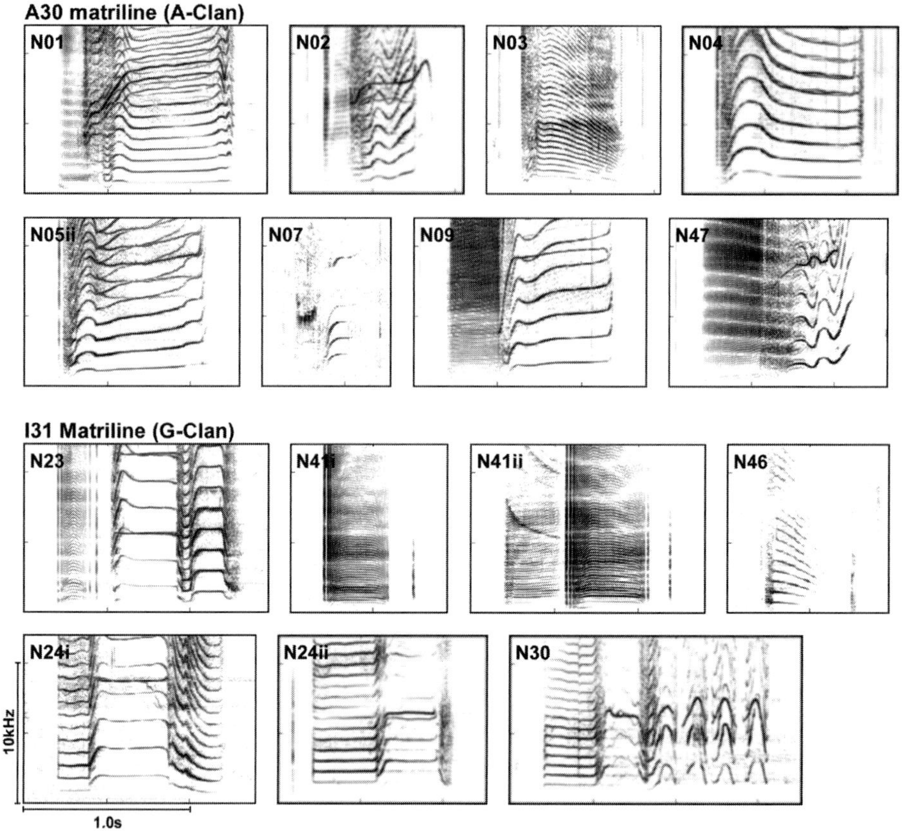

Figure 7.2. Spectrograms of the most common call types from recordings of two matrilines of Northern Resident killer whales (*Orcinus orca*) belonging to different acoustic clans. In spite of the fact that these groups frequently associate, they do not share any stereotyped call types.

Future Directions

Cetaceans are long-lived species, and it can therefore take decades to build up informative social histories of individuals. Long-term studies, such as those conducted on bottlenose dolphins in Sarasota Bay, USA (e.g. Wells, 1991) and Shark Bay, Australia (e.g. Connor *et al.*, 2001), or on killer whales in British Columbia, Canada, and Washington State, USA (e.g. Bigg *et al.*, 1990), are therefore invaluable to provide the background of social information against which complex questions of social cognition can be framed. In addition to information on maternal (and in some cases also paternal) genealogies, these studies have provided records of social associations for large numbers of individuals, often for the entirety of their lives. Because of such wealth of social information, we are now in a position to address fine-scale questions on the manifestation and evolution of social cognition in these species.

Captive research has provided valuable insights into the cognitive abilities of toothed whales. Some aspects of perception, physical cognition and learning do not lend themselves to be studied in the field. On the other hand, research into many aspects of social cognition can only be valid if conducted on functional social groups in the wild. Aside from a few juvenile grey whales, baleen whales have not been held in captivity, and captive research is therefore not an option for this clade. Ultimately, we will need to arrive at an integrative approach, where an understanding of cognitive mechanisms elucidated from captive studies can be complemented by rigorously designed experiments on wild animals, providing ecological validity. The ability to obtain long-term acoustic data sets using autonomous recorders and to reconstruct underwater movements from animal-borne tags, and thus analyse the fine-scale behavioural responses to playbacks or to natural social and communicative events, finally gives us the ability to complement captive studies with data of similar quality and detail from the field.

All for One and One for All

Box 7.1 Fission–Fusion Dynamics and Cognition

Filippo Aureli and Colleen M. Schaffner

Kummer (1971) used the term 'fission–fusion' to explain the social system of some group-living primates, in which the size of their groups changes by means of the fission and fusion of subgroups. Since then, different fission–fusion types have been described. For example, the 'multilevel societies' of geladas, hamadryas baboons and snub-nosed monkeys are characterized by different grouping levels, from large night aggregations to small foraging one-male units with a fixed composition (Grueter *et al.*, 2012). In contrast, chimpanzees, bonobos and spider monkeys live in groups in which individuals belonging to the same group are rarely all together, but rather spend most of their time in temporary subgroups that frequently merge and split again with different composition. Fission–fusion patterns are also typical of modern humans (Rodseth *et al.*, 1991) and other animals, such as dolphins, elephants, spotted hyenas, bats and parrots. A careful examination leads to the conclusion that there is pronounced variation in the fission–fusion patterns across and within species, which cannot be captured with modal fission–fusion types. Thus, Aureli and colleagues (2008) proposed the term 'fission–fusion dynamics' to refer to the extent of variation in spatial cohesion and individual membership in a (sub)group over time. As a consequence, any animal social system can be characterized by its degree of fission–fusion dynamics, varying from highly cohesive with fixed membership to highly fluid with flexible membership.

The degree of fission–fusion dynamics influences the possibility for group members to interact with one another. In groups with a higher degree of fission–fusion dynamics, individuals spend longer periods apart from at least some group members, and subgroup composition is highly variable, introducing uncertainty about interacting with group members (Ramos-Fernandez and Aureli, 2018). This situation creates specific challenges and opportunities, which may require the enhancement of certain cognitive abilities. For example, when individuals meet at fusions after

(*cont.*)

a period of separation, they need to confirm the status of their own relationships. This requires memory to retain knowledge about partners, as well as the ability to pick up subtle social cues for relationship assessment via emotional mediation (Aureli and Schaffner, 2002), and use behaviours designed to probe others and extract relevant information from them (Zahavi, 1977). More challenging, individuals need to reassess the relationships between other members that were in another subgroup, as they may have changed during the separation (Aureli *et al.*, 2008). In addition, soon after fusion, members of different subgroups may need to inhibit prepotent behavioural responses and better assess the situation before acting, given that the appropriate response may vary depending on subgroup composition (Amici *et al.*, 2008). Moreover, there is evidence that individuals preferentially fission into subgroups with group members with whom they have more valuable and secure relationships (Busia *et al.*, 2017). Therefore, enhanced planning skills can be advantageous to 'engineer' subgroup composition by associating with the most profitable partners and avoiding unreliable or dangerous individuals (Aureli *et al.*, 2008).

References

Amici, F., Aureli, F., and Call, J. (2008). Fission–fusion dynamics, behavioral flexibility and inhibitory control in primates. *Current Biology*, **18**, 1415–1419.

Aureli, F., and Schaffner, C. M. (2002). Relationship assessment through emotional mediation. *Behaviour*, **139**, 393–420.

Aureli, F., Schaffner, C. M., Boesch, C., *et al.* (2008). Fission–fusion dynamics: new research frameworks. *Current Anthropology*, **48**, 627–654.

Busia, L., Schaffner, C. M., and Aureli, F. (2017). Relationship quality affects fission decisions in wild spider monkeys (*Ateles geoffroyi*). *Ethology*, **123**, 405–411.

Grueter, C. C., Chapais, B., and Zinner, D. (2012). Evolution of multilevel social systems in nonhuman primates and humans. *International Journal of Primatology*, **33**, 1002–1037.

Kummer, H. (1971). *Primate societies: group techniques of ecological adaptation*. Chicago, IL: Aldine.

Ramos-Fernandez, G., and Aureli, F. (2018). Fission–fusion. In *Encyclopedia of animal cognition and behavior*. Berlin: Springer.

Rodseth, L., Wrangham, R. W., Harrigan, A. M., and Smuts, B. B. (1991). The human community as a primate society. *Current Anthropology*, **32**, 221–254.

Zahavi, A. (1977). The testing of a bond. *Animal Behaviour*, **25**, 246–247.

Field Guide

It is an overcast and calm day in late August in Goletas Channel, off the north-eastern coast of Vancouver Island, Canada. After initial light fog in the morning, the air is now clear and the sea only slightly rippled – ideal fieldwork conditions. We are following a group of 10 killer whales, as they are travelling northwest in the channel, in a loose formation. The group is led by its matriarch, A30, thought to be around 60 years old. With her are her adult sons A38 (aged 38 years) and A39 (aged 34). A30 also has two adult daughters accompanying her: A50 (aged 25) and A54 (aged 20). Both now have offspring of their own: A50 is the mother of the 10-year-old female A72 (characterized by a very distinctive nick in the leading edge of her dorsal fin) and A84, a 4-year-old juvenile, whose sex is yet to be determined. A54 gave birth to female A75 7 years ago and to A86 (sex unknown) 3 years ago. She also has a new calf, A93, who is only a few months old and typically swims in echelon formation, close to her mother. All individuals in the group can be readily identified from photographs or by trained eye, based on the shape and size of their dorsal fin and nicks in the fin, as well as pigmentation patterns and scars in the saddle, the grey patch behind the fin.

A30 and her matriline are members of the Northern Resident population of killer whales, and typically range from central Vancouver Island north to the border with southeast Alaska. Like other members of their population, the A30s frequent the waters off northern Vancouver Island in late summer and autumn to intercept Pacific salmon (*Oncorhynchus* spp.), passing through the straits and fjords on their way to the spawning rivers. Northern resident killer whales have been the subjects of a systematic study into killer whale life history and social behaviour since 1972, for which group composition is documented on a regular basis. Because the A30 matriline is one of the most commonly encountered groups, we have a plethora of information on association patterns, social interactions and life-history data for this group (e.g. Bigg *et al.*, 1990; Olesiuk *et al.*, 1990).

A72, the 10-year-old female, is wearing a digital recording tag (Dtag; Johnson and Tyack, 2003; Johnson *et al.*, 2009; see Figure 7.1), attached below her dorsal fin with four suction cups. The tag has a magnetometer, accelerometers and a depth sensor to record A72's underwater movements with very high resolution. In addition, the tag also contains two hydrophones to record high-quality underwater sound, including the echolocation clicks and communicative calls and whistles of A72 and the other members of her group, but also the noise generated by passing vessels. All data are stored on the tag. To aid in tracking the whale and recovering the tag, the tag sends out VHF radio signals that we can pick up, using our antenna array every time A72 surfaces and the antenna clears the surface. We have programmed the tag to detach from the animal at 7 p.m. At this point, the tag will shunt its remaining battery power to two loops of galvanic wire, causing them to corrode in the seawater over the next 20 minutes or so. This will open up four small rubber tubes, each leading to one of the suction cups, and break the vacuum, causing the tag to float free.

The whales are heading north-west in the channel, in a loose formation. A72 is with A30, A50 and A84, travelling within 50 m of the shoreline. A54 and her offspring A75, A86 and A93 are swimming in a tight subgroup behind them, while the two adult males, A38 and A39, are paralleling them mid-channel. We encountered the whales earlier this morning, some 12 km to the south-east. It took us just over an hour to deploy the Dtag. This was done by slowly paralleling the group with one team member on the bow of the vessel, holding a 5-m carbon fibre pole with the tag attached to its end. Eventually, A72 surfaced close to the boat and the tag was deployed. The animal gave a short flinch as the tag attached, but quickly resumed her previous behaviour. The vessel we are using for this research is a 10-m aluminium-hulled vessel, specially designed to minimize disturbance to the animals: the vessel is powered by a surface-drive propulsion system, which is extremely quiet. In addition, the engines are mounted on rubber shock-absorbers, to limit sound propagation through the hull, and the exhaust is expelled through two water-filled mufflers. In addition, we are using a 21-m steel-hulled sailboat for cooking and accommodation.

We are following the whales at a distance of 50–100 m, looking for signs of feeding activity. The aim of our study is to use the tag data to gain a better understanding of the behavioural strategies deployed by resident killer whales to detect, pursue and capture their primary prey, Pacific salmon. Northern resident killer whales preferentially feed on Chinook salmon (*Oncorhynchus tshawytscha*), but will also take chum (*O. keta*) and other salmon species (Ford and Ellis, 2006). The health of the population appears intricately linked to Chinook salmon returns to the major river systems within the animals' range (Ford *et al.*, 2010), and by better understanding their foraging process we hope to be able to ultimately minimize anthropogenic influences on their feeding success. If we find evidence that A72 may have caught a salmon, we will take the boat closer and look for fish scales near the surface where the animal surfaced. These will not only help us confirm a salmon capture, but also provide information on the species and age of the fish taken, and allow us to determine later how the whale used its echolocation to detect and track the fish. The results of this study have since been published by Wright and colleagues (2017).

However, today we have a second objective to our research: having a tag on a killer whale and being able to track its underwater movements in response to sound stimuli gives us the opportunity to test whether playback experiments can be used to address questions about social cognition in this species. Specifically, we want to see whether killer whales extract social information from the call types of other clans in their population, call types that they are presumably familiar with, but which they do not usually produce themselves. The A30 matriline is a member of the A-clan, an assemblage of several dozen matrilines that all share at least one call type. The Northern Resident population contains two other clans, G-clan and R-clan, and members of different clans do not share any call types (Ford, 1991). We have therefore prepared a short playback sequence containing eight calls produced by members of the I31 matriline. This matriline forms part of the G-clan, occasionally associated with the A30 matriline, but does not share any of its call types (see Figure 7.2 for an illustration of the vocal repertoires of both groups). Playing back calls of a different acoustic clan can rule out call-type matching as the primary reason for a vocal response. As a control, we can then use recordings from another killer whale population (e.g. Icelandic or Norwegian killer whales) containing call types that the A30s will also not produce themselves, but will also be unfamiliar with.

The whales have reached the western end of Nigei Island, where Bate Passage meets Goletas Channel from the north. After some milling and foraging activity at the

Table 7.1. Essential experimental equipment required to study cetaceans in the field.

Tool	Function
Digital SLR camera	A high-quality camera with telephoto lens is essential for identifying individuals from natural markings. A 300–400-mm image-stabilized lens works best on small boats. Choose a fixed lens for larger species, but an adjustable zoom lens (e.g. 80–300 mm) is preferable for smaller species that have a tendency to approach the boat for bow-riding
Boats	A good research boat must be stable, fast and manoeuverable enough to keep up with the animals and capable of handling the sea conditions where the animals live. Power supply and space for research equipment that is protected from the elements are additional considerations. Any boat used for cetacean research should be designed with the reduction of underwater noise output in mind to minimize disturbance to the animals
Hydrophone	Hydrophones are required to monitor and record underwater vocalizations and should be sensitive in the full frequency range produced by the study species. Simple hydrophones deployed over the side of the boat are useful while the boat is stationary, but need to be retrieved before the boat moves. Towable or hull-mounted systems allow monitoring and recording while underway as well (but may receive interference from engine noise)
Digital recorder	A sound recorder should be capable of capturing the full range of sound frequencies produced by the species studied. Standard systems sampling at 48 kHz are adequate for baleen whales, but most toothed whales require sampling rates of 96 kHz or higher. Two-channel recorders are adequate for general recording, but projects where identifying the direction of localization of sounds is important require multichannel recorders
Acoustic analysis software	Several programs are available. Adobe Audition (Adobe Systems, San Jose, USA) or Audacity (Audacity Development Team) work well for rapidly scanning large sound files. Sound analysis programs such as Raven (Cornell Lab of Ornithology, Ithaca, USA), Avisoft (Avisoft Bioacoustics, Glienicke, Germany) allow more detailed measuring of sounds and also some simple manipulations. MATLAB (The Math Works, Natick, USA) is useful for more complex signal-processing tasks
Theodolite	A theodolite can be useful in situations where animal movements need to be tracked from shore (e.g. to document movements towards or away from a sound source)
Underwater loudspeaker	Realistic playback experiments require a high-quality sound source. Underwater loudspeakers developed for synchronous swimming (e.g. Lubell Labs LL916, Columbus, USA) are adequate in some circumstances. However, for playback of ultrasonic vocalizations, systems with better high-frequency response are required
Digital recording tags	Accelerometry tags are invaluable to record the underwater movement of animals, and some tags are able to also record underwater sound (e.g. Dtag: Johnson and Tyack, 2003) and GPS location. Tags attached with suction cups are minimally invasive, and if applied correctly they can remain attached for hours or days. Various propulsion systems (crossbows, pneumatic devices) have been used for deployment, but a long, lightweight carbon fibre pole works best for species that are reasonably habituated to boats
Autonomous recorders	In situations where long-term records of communication signals are required, autonomous recorders can be helpful. These are deployed on the ocean floor, and can be set to record continuously or on a duty cycle (e.g. 5 min every hour). Deployments of several weeks of continuous recording are possible, whereas duty-cycling can extend recording time to over a year

junction, they start heading north in Bate Passage, and we decide that this is a good time for the playback experiment, as this is a location where other groups could be approaching from the west. The whales have gone into resting behaviour: the group members are lined up beside each other in a line, almost touching. They are diving for 3–4 minutes and moving very slowly. We ask the sailboat to assume a position approximately 1.5 km behind the whales, and lower the playback speaker into the water, while we continue to follow the group in the smaller boat and monitor their underwater vocalizations using a hydrophone array towed behind the boat. Currently, the whales are largely silent, except for the occasional N03 call (Figure 7.2).

We start the playback at 5:11 p.m. The playback system had been calibrated to transmit the calls with a source level of 152 dB, the typical source level of stereotyped call for this population (Miller, 2006). After the first few playback calls, the members of A30 matriline that had been silent for the last 20 minutes start vocalizing prolifically. Interestingly, they are producing N47 calls, the signature call type of this particular matriline (Weiß *et al.*, 2006). A spectrogram showing the vocal response recorded on A72's Dtag is given in Figure 7.3. Later, analysis of the tag data also shows rapid acceleration and a 180° turn towards the playback source. The whales remain agitated for the next 30 min, frequently changing direction, although little further vocal behaviour is recorded on the tag. Eventually, they resume their resting behaviour and slowly continue northwards in Bate Passage. We continue to follow them through the Passage and into Gordon Channel. The tag detaches on time at 7:30 p.m., and we manage to recover it within minutes. We head for anchorage to get some food and rest, and to begin the long process of downloading the tag data.

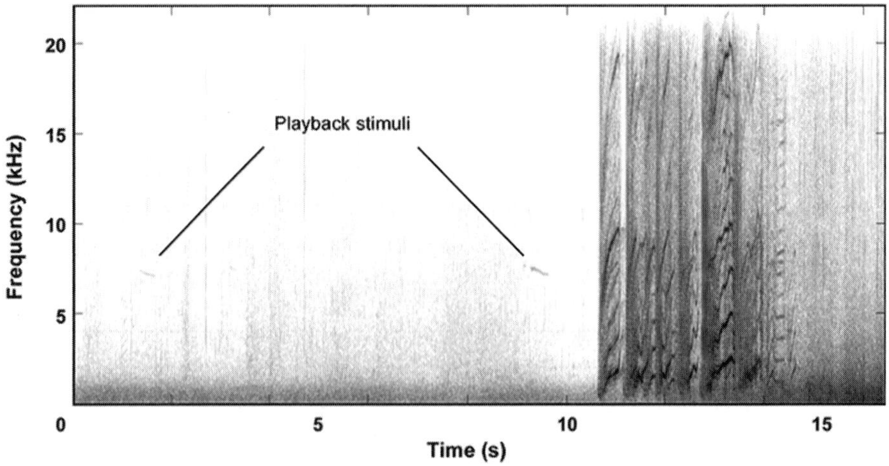

Figure 7.3. Spectrogram of the vocal response of the A30 matriline of the Northern Resident population of killer whales to the playback of G-clan calls. The recording was made on an archival digital recording tag (Dtag; Johnson and Tyack, 2003), deployed on one of the group members. The playback was conducted from a distance of approximately 1.5 km. The playback stimuli are faintly visible.

This experiment illustrates not only the value of conducting cognitive research on cetaceans in the field, but also some of its challenges. Many replicates will be necessary to draw firm conclusions about call recognition in killer whales, and opportunities to conduct playback trials under similarly ideal conditions and appropriate contexts can be hard to come by. However, the preliminary data suggest that the members of the A30 matriline responded to the playback, by orientating towards the source, communicating their presence and signalling their identity by producing the one call type most useful for identifying this group. The experiment was only made possible by the long-term data available for Northern Resident killer whales. Without an understanding of the animals' association patterns and repertoire variation within the population, choosing appropriate playback stimuli and interpreting responses would have been impossible. With several long-term studies on free-ranging cetaceans now having reached maturity, and with new technologies that allow us to obtain detailed behavioural data from free-ranging unrestrained animals, we now have the ability to tackle fine-scale questions and to finally take cognitive research on whales and dolphins out of the tanks and into the field.

The Devil Is in the Details

Box 7.2 Cognition of Deep-Diving Toothed Whales

Frants Havmand Jensen

A subset of toothed whales has adapted to exploit deep-water food resources in the open ocean. Several delphinid species including pilot whales (*Globicephala* spp.) and Risso's dolphins (*Grampus griseus*) exploit prey at depths of up to 1000 m. Sperm whales (*Physeter macrocephalus*) and the few studied species of beaked whales (*Ziphiidae* spp.) routinely dive beyond 1000 m, but have been recorded going as far as 2–3 km. Adapting to these foraging niches has entailed extensive improvements to diving physiology and further shifted sensory focus from vision to sound and echolocation, because light does not penetrate to typical foraging depths.

A few deep-diving species are particularly interesting: sperm whales are long-lived animals that live in matrilineal social groups structured within sympatric clans. Each clan is recognized easily by distinct, clan-specific stereotyped click series known as codas (Rendell and Whitehead, 2003), which have been suggestive of vocal culture in these animals. This relatively simple and well-understood communication system lends itself well to manipulation experiments, through playback experiments in populations with long-term photo-ID studies, including the Pacific (Whitehead *et al.*, 1998) and the Caribbean (Gero *et al.*, 2016) populations.

Pilot whales are highly social and curious animals structured in matrilineal social groups, with short-finned (but not long-finned) pilot whales exhibiting a pronounced period of menopause (Kasuya and Marsh, 1984). Pilot whales have a more complex vocal repertoire than sperm whales, and they share a propensity for vocal imitation and

(cont.)

copying with other delphinids, with functions that are as yet not well understood. While pilot whales have a higher degree of unmarked (and not easily identified) individuals compared to bottlenose dolphins and killer whales, several field sites have ongoing long-term studies documenting identity and social associations. For short-finned pilot whales, these sites include Hawaii (Mahaffy *et al.*, 2015) and Madeira (Alves *et al.*, 2013). For long-finned pilot whales, extensive work has been done off Nova Scotia (Augusto *et al.*, 2017), but the small population resident to the Strait of Gibraltar (de Stephanis *et al.*, 2008; Verborgh *et al.*, 2009) may be more ideal in situations where resighting the same individuals over short time periods is a priority.

Deep-divers rely on open ocean habitats and typically range widely. As described for other cetaceans, suction cup acoustic tags have become an increasingly effective tool to track the movement and acoustics of individual animals and are used to track social interactions and social coordination between simultaneously tagged individuals in both pilot and sperm whales. Additionally, developments in multicopter battery life are making drones an increasingly viable method for tracking surface-oriented movement, or monitoring responses to relatively short-duration playback experiments.

These new tools are opening up possibilities for testing a wide range of cognitive questions. From a sensory perspective, tags allow studying foraging decisions (Fais *et al.*, 2015), integration of echoic information (Johnson *et al.*, 2004; Madsen *et al.*, 2013) and potentially the role of memory in informing individual movement decisions. Because tags record outgoing echolocation sounds, along with foraging events, it is increasingly feasible to probe the ways animals explore the environment and integrate their own accumulated experience about prey location with information about activity and location of group members to improve foraging success. As for other delphinids, tags and drones may facilitate data collection from playback experiments that can investigate social communication in a natural context and test how different species, such as sperm whales or pilot whales, recognize familiar individuals or social groups. Finally, simultaneous tagging of multiple individuals or combinations of overhead video and acoustic array recordings may allow us to investigate how specific group members in heterogeneous social groups, such as older individuals in matrilineal groups, affect decision-making of conspecifics.

References

Alves, F., Quérouil, S. Dinis, A., *et al.* (2013). Population structure of short-finned pilot whales in the oceanic archipelago of Madeira based on photo-identification and genetic analyses: implications for conservation. *Aquatic Conservation: Marine and Freshwater Ecosystems*, **23**, 758–776.

Augusto, J. F., Frasier, T. R., and Whitehead, H. (2017). Social structure of long-finned pilot whales (*Globicephala melas*) off northern Cape Breton Island, Nova Scotia. *Behaviour*, **154**, 509–540.

(*cont.*)

De Stephanis, R., Verborgh, P., Perez, S., Esteban, R., Minvielle-Sebastia, L., and Guinet, C. (2008). Long-term social structure of long-finned pilot whales (*Globicephala melas*) in the Strait of Gibraltar. *Acta Ethologica*, **11**, 81–94.

Fais, A., Soto, N. A., Johnson, M., Perez-Gonzalez, C., Miller, P. J. O., and Madsen, P. T. (2015). Sperm whale echolocation behaviour reveals a directed, prior-based search strategy informed by prey distribution. *Behavioral Ecology and Sociobiology*, **69**, 663–674.

Gero, S., Bøttcher, A., Whitehead, H., and Madsen, P. T. (2016). Socially segregated, sympatric sperm whale clans in the Atlantic Ocean. *Royal Society Open Science*, **3**, 160061.

Johnson, M., Madsen, P. T., Zimmer, W. M. X., De Soto, N. A., and Tyack, P. L. (2004). Beaked whales echolocate on prey. *Proceedings of the Royal Society of London B: Biological Sciences*, **271**, 383–386.

Kasuya, T., and Marsh, H. (1984). Life history and reproductive biology of the short-finned pilot whale, *Globicephala macrorhynchus*, off the Pacific coast of Japan. *IWC Special Issue*, **6**, 259–310.

Madsen, P. T., De Soto, N. A., Arranz, P., and Johnson, M. (2013). Echolocation in Blainville's beaked whales (*Mesoplodon densirostris*). *Journal of Comparative Physiology A*, **199**, 451–469.

Mahaffy, S. D., Baird, R. W., Mcsweeney, D. J., Webster, D. L., and Schorr, G. S. (2015). High site fidelity, strong associations, and long-term bonds: short-finned pilot whales off the island of Hawai'i. *Marine Mammal Science*, **31**, 1427–1451.

Rendell, L. E., and Whitehead, H. (2003). Vocal clans in sperm whales (*Physeter macrocephalus*). *Proceedings of the Royal Society of London B: Biological Sciences*, **270**, 225–231.

Verborgh, P., De Stephanis, R., Pérez, S., Jaget, Y., Barbraud, C., and Guinet, C. (2009). Survival rate, abundance, and residency of long-finned pilot whales in the Strait of Gibraltar. *Marine Mammal Science*, **25**, 523–536.

Whitehead, H., Dillon, M., Dufault, S., Weilgart, L., and Wright, J. (1998). Non-geographically based population structure of South Pacific sperm whales: dialects, fluke-markings and genetics. *Journal of Animal Ecology*, **67**, 253–262.

Resources

- Au, W. W. L., Popper, A. N., and Fay, R. R. (2000). *Hearing by whales and dolphins*. New York, NY: Springer.
- Jaakkola, K. (2012). Cetacean cognitive specializations. In *The Oxford handbook of comparative evolutionary psychology* (pp. 144–165). Oxford: Oxford University Press.
- Kastelein, R. A., Supin, A. Ya., and Thomas, J. A. (eds) (1992). *Marine mammal sensory systems*. New York, NY: Springer.
- Kremers, D., Célérier, A., Schaal, B., *et al.* (2016). Sensory perception in cetaceans: part I – current knowledge about dolphin senses as a representative species. *Frontiers in Ecology and Evolution*, **4**, 49.

- Mann, J., Connor, R. C., Tyack, P. L., and Whitehead, H. (2000). *Cetacean societies: field studies of dolphins and whales*. Chicago, IL: University of Chicago Press.
- Perrin, W. F., Würsig, B., and Thewissen, J. G. M. (2009). *Encyclopedia of marine mammals*. Burlington, MA: Academic Press.
- Thomas, J. A., and Kastelein, R. A. (1990). *Sensory abilities of cetaceans: laboratory and field evidence*. New York, NY: Springer.
- Society for Marine Mammalogy: www.marinemammalscience.org
- European Cetacean Society: www.europeancetaceansociety.eu
- European Association for Aquatic Mammals: https://eaam.org

Profile

Born far from the sea in southern Germany, Volker grew up in land-locked Austria. An interest for wildlife and human languages led him to study animal communication, first in Berlin, Germany, and then in Vancouver, Canada, where he acquired the necessary boating skills and a masters degree from the University of British Columbia. He received his doctorate from the University of St Andrews, UK, on vocal behaviour of mammal-eating killer whales in British Columbia and Alaska. After post-doctoral research at the University of British Columbia's Marine Mammal Research Unit, Volker returned to the UK, where he is currently Associate Professor in Wildlife Conservation at the University of Cumbria. Volker has studied acoustic communication and population structure of killer whales in Canada, Alaska, Shetland and Iceland, and has also been involved in behavioural and cognitive research on grey whales, humpbacks, brown bears and snow leopards.

References

Agnarsson, I., and May-Collado, L. J. (2008). The phylogeny of Cetartiodactyla: the importance of dense taxon sampling, missing data, and the remarkable promise of cytochrome b to provide reliable species-level phylogenies. *Molecular Phylogenetics and Evolution*, **48**, 964–985.

Allen, J., Weinrich, M., Hoppitt, W., and Rendell, L. (2013). Network-based diffusion analysis reveals cultural transmission of lobtail feeding in humpback whales. *Science*, **340**, 485–488.

Amos, B., Schlötterer, C., and Tautz, D. (1993). Social-structure of pilot whales revealed by analytical DNA profiling. *Science*, **260**, 670–672.

Arrigoni, M., Manfredi, P., Panigada, S., Bramanti, L., and Santangelo, G. (2011). Life-history tables of the Mediterranean fin whale from stranding data. *Marine Ecology*, **32**, 1–9.

Au, W. W. L. (2000). Hearing in whales and dolphins: an overview. In *Hearing by whales and dolphins* (pp. 1–42). New York, NY: Springer.

Au, W. W. L., Ford, J. K. B., Horne, J. K., and Allman, K. A. N. (2004). Echolocation signals of free-ranging killer whales (*Orcinus orca*) and modeling of foraging for Chinook salmon (*Oncorhynchus tshawytscha*). *Journal of the Acoustical Society of America*, **115**, 901–909.

Au, W. W. L., Horne, J. K., and Jones, C. (2010). Basis of acoustic discrimination of chinook salmon from other salmons by echolocating *Orcinus orca*. *Journal of the Acoustical Society of America*, **28**, 2225–2232.

Bain, D. (1990). Examining the validity of inferences drawn from photo-identification data, with special reference to studies of the killer whale (*Orcinus orca*) in British Columbia. *Report of the International Whaling Commission*, **12**, 93–100.

Baird, R. W., and Whitehead, H. (2000). Social organization of mammal-eating killer whales: group stability and dispersal patterns. *Canadian Journal of Zoology*, **78**(12), 2096–2105.

Best, P. B., Canham, P. A. S., and Macleod, N. (1984). Patterns of reproduction in sperm whales, *Physeter macrocephalus*. *Report of the International Whaling Commission*, **6**, 51–79.

Bigg, M. A. (1982). An assessment of killer whale (*Orcinus orca*) stocks off Vancouver Island, British Columbia. *Report of the International Whaling Commission*, **32**, 655–666.

Bigg, M. A., Olesiuk, P. F., Ellis, G. M., Ford, J. K. B., and Balcomb, K. C. (1990). Social organization and genealogy of resident killer whales (*Orcinus orca*) in the coastal waters of British Columbia and Washington State. *Report of the International Whaling Commission*, **12**, 383–405.

Bloodworth, B. E., and Odell, D. K. (2008). *Kogia breviceps* (Cetacea: Kogiidae). *Mammalian Species*, 1–12.

Branstetter, B. K., Leger, J. S., Acton, D., *et al.* (2017). Killer whale (*Orcinus orca*) behavioral audiograms. *Journal of the Acoustical Society of America*, **141**, 2387–2398.

Brent, L. J., Franks, D. W., Foster, E. A., Balcomb, K. C., Cant, M. A., and Croft, D. P. (2015). Ecological knowledge, leadership, and the evolution of menopause in killer whales. *Current Biology*, **25**, 746–750.

Bruck, J. N. (2013). Decades-long social memory in bottlenose dolphins. *Proceedings of the Royal Society of London B: Biological Sciences*, **280**, 20131726.

Caro, T., Beeman, K., Stankowich, T., and Whitehead, H. (2011). The functional significance of colouration in cetaceans. *Evolutionary Ecology*, **25**, 1231.

Cerchio, S., and Dahlheim, M. E. (2001). Variation in feeding vocalizations of humpback whales (*Megaptera novaeangliae*) from Southeast Alaska. *Bioacoustics*, **11**, 277–295.

Cerchio, S., Jacobsen, J. K., and Norris, T. N. (2001). Temporal and geographical variation in songs of humpback whales, *Megaptera novaeangliae*: synchronous change in Hawaiian and Mexican breeding assemblages. *Animal Behaviour*, **62**, 313–329.

Clapham, P. J. (2001). Why do baleen whales migrate? A response to Corkeron and Connor. *Marine Mammal Science*, **17**, 432–436.

Connor, R. C., Mann, J., Tyack, P. L., and Whitehead, H. (1998). Social evolution in toothed whales. *Trends in Ecology and Evolution*, **13**, 228–232.

Connor, R. C., Heithaus, M. R., and Barre, L. M. (2001). Complex social structure, alliance stability and mating access in a bottlenose dolphin 'super-alliance'. *Proceedings of the Royal Society of London B: Biological Sciences*, **268**, 263–267.

Connor, R. C., Watson-Capps, J. J., Sherwin, W. B., and Krützen, M. (2010). A new level of complexity in the male alliance networks of Indian Ocean bottlenose dolphins (*Tursiops* sp.). *Biology Letters*, 20100852.

Corkeron, P. J., and Connor, R. C. (1999). Why do baleen whale migrate? *Marine Mammal Science*, **15**, 1228–1245.

Crance, J. L., Bowles, A. E., and Garver, A. (2014). Evidence for vocal learning in juvenile male killer whales, *Orcinus orca*, from an adventitious cross-socializing experiment. *Journal of Experimental Biology*, **217**, 1229–1237.

Cranford, T. W., Krysl, P., and Hildebrand, J. A. (2008). Acoustic pathways revealed: simulated sound transmission and reception in Cuvier's beaked whale (*Ziphius cavirostris*). *Bioinspiration and Biomimetics*, **3**, 016001.

Cranford, T. W., Elsberry, W. R., Van Bonn, W. G., *et al.* (2011). Observation and analysis of sonar signal generation in the bottlenose dolphin (*Tursiops truncatus*): evidence for two sonar sources. *Journal of Experimental Marine Biology and Ecology*, **407**, 81–96.

Curé, C., Antunes, R. N., Samarra, F. I. P., *et al.* (2012). Pilot whales attracted to killer whale sounds: acoustically-mediated interspecific interactions in cetaceans. *PLoS ONE*, **7**(12), e52201.

Curé, C., Antunes, R. N., Alves, A. C., Visser, F., Kvadsheim, P. H., and Miller, P. J. O. (2013). Responses of male sperm whales (*Physeter macrocephalus*) to killer whale sounds: implications for anti-predator strategies. *Scientific Reports*, **3**, 1579.

D'Vincent, C. G., Nilson, R. M., and Hanna, R. E. (1985). Vocalization and coordinated feeding behaviour of the humpback whale in southeastern Alaska. *Scientific Reports of the Whales Research Institute*, **36**, 41–47.

Dahlheim, M. E., and Ljungblad, D. K. (1990). Preliminary hearing study on gray whales *Eschrichtius robustus* in the field. In *Sensory abilities of cetaceans* (pp. 335–346). New York, NY: Plenum Press.

Deecke, V. B. (2006). Studying marine mammal cognition in the wild – a review of four decades of playback experiments. *Aquatic Mammals*, **32**, 461–482.

Deecke, V. B., Ford, J. K. B., and Spong, P. (2000). Dialect change in resident killer whales (*Orcinus orca*): implications for vocal learning and cultural transmission. *Animal Behaviour*, **60**, 629–638.

Deecke, V. B., Barrett-Lennard, L. G., Spong, P., and Ford, J. K. B. (2010). The structure of stereotyped calls reflects kinship and social affiliation in resident killer whales (*Orcinus orca*). *Naturwissenschaften*, **97**, 513–518.

Deecke, V. B., Nykänen, M., Foote, A. D., and Janik, V. M. (2011). Vocal behaviour and feeding ecology of killer whales (*Orcinus orca*) around Shetland, UK. *Aquatic Biology*, **13**, 79–88.

DeLong, C. M., Au, W. W., Lemonds, D. W., Harley, H. E., and Roitblat, H. L. (2006). Acoustic features of objects matched by an echolocating bottlenose dolphin. *Journal of the Acoustical Society of America*, **119**, 1867–1879.

Drake, S. E., Crish, S. D., George, J. C., Stimmelmayr, R., and Thewissen, J. (2015). Sensory hairs in the bowhead whale, *Balaena mysticetus* (Cetacea, Mammalia). *Anatomical Record*, **298**, 1327–1335.

Dunlop, R. A., Cato, D. H., and Noad, M. J. (2008). Non-song acoustic communication in migrating humpback whales (*Megaptera novaeangliae*). *Marine Mammal Science*, **24**, 613–629.

Ford, J. K. B. (1991). Vocal traditions among resident killer whales (*Orcinus orca*) in coastal waters of British Columbia, Canada. *Canadian Journal of Zoology*, **69**, 1454–1483.

Ford, J. K. B., and Ellis, G. M. (2006). Selective foraging by fish-eating killer whales *Orcinus orca* in British Columbia. *Marine Ecology Progress Series*, **316**, 185–199.

Ford, J. K. B., and Reeves, R. R. (2008). Fight or flight: antipredator strategies of baleen whales. *Mammal Review*, **38**, 50–86.

Ford, J. K. B., Ellis, G. M., Olesiuk, P. F., and Balcomb, K. C. (2010). Linking killer whale survival and prey abundance: food limitation in the oceans' apex predator? *Biology Letters*, **6**, 139–142.

Foster, E. A., Franks, D. W., Mazzi, S., *et al.* (2012). Adaptive prolonged postreproductive life span in killer whales. *Science*, **337**, 1313.

Gannon, D. P., Barros, N. B., Nowacek, D. P., Read, A. J., Waples, D. M., and Wells, R. S. (2005). Prey detection by bottlenose dolphins, *Tursiops truncatus*: an experimental test of the passive listening hypothesis. *Animal Behaviour*, **69**, 709–720.

Garde, E., Heide-Jørgensen, M. P., Hansen, S. H., Nachman, G., and Forchhammer, M. C. (2007). Age-specific growth and remarkable longevity in narwhals (*Monodon monoceros*) from West Greenland as estimated by aspartic acid racemization. *Journal of Mammalogy*, **88**, 49–58.

Garland, E. C., Goldizen, A. W., Rekdahl, M. L., *et al.* (2011). Dynamic horizontal cultural transmission of humpback whale song at the ocean basin scale. *Current Biology*, **21**, 687–691.

George, J. C., Bada, J., Zeh, J., *et al.* (1999). Age and growth estimates of bowhead whales (*Balaena mysticetus*) via aspartic acid racemization. *Canadian Journal of Zoology*, **77**, 571–580.

Götz, T., Verfuss, U. K., and Schnitzler, H.-U. (2006). 'Eavesdropping' in wild rough-toothed dolphins (*Steno bredanensis*)? *Biology Letters*, **2**, 5–7.

Guinet, C. (1991). Intentional stranding apprenticeship and social play in killer whales (*Orcinus orca*). *Canadian Journal of Zoology*, **69**, 2712–2716.

Guinet, C., and Bouvier, J. (1995). Development of intentional stranding hunting techniques in killer whale (*Orcinus orca*) calves at Crozet Archipelago. *Canadian Journal of Zoology*, **73**, 27–33.

Hamilton, P. K., Knowlton, A. R., Marx, M. K., and Kraus, S. D. (1998). Age structure and longevity in North Atlantic right whales *Eubalaena glacialis* and their relation to reproduction. *Marine Ecology Progress Series*, **171**, 285–292.

Hammond, P. S., Mizroch, S. A., and Donovan, G. P. (1982). *Individual recognition of cetaceans: use of photo-identification and other techniques to estimate population parameters*. International Whaling Commission.

Harley, H. E., Putman, E. A., and Roitblat, H. L. (2003). Bottlenose dolphins perceive object features through echolocation. *Nature*, **424**, 667–669.

Harper, C., Mclellan, W. A., Rommel, S., Gay, D. M., Dillaman, R., and Pabst, D. A. (2008). Morphology of the melon and its tendinous connections to the facial muscles in bottlenose dolphins (*Tursiops truncatus*). *Journal of Morphology*, **269**, 820–839.

Hartman, K. L., Visser, F., and Hendriks, A. J. E. (2008). Social structure of Risso's dolphins (*Grampus griseus*) at the Azores: a stratified community based on highly associated social units. *Canadian Journal of Zoology*, **86**, 294–306.

Helweg, D. A., Frankel, A. S., Mobley Jr, J. R., and Herman, L. M. (1992). Humpback whale song: our current understanding. In *Marine mammal sensory systems* (pp. 459–483). New York, NY: Springer.

Hemilä, S., Nummela, S., and Reuter, T. (1999). A model of the odontocete middle ear. *Hearing Research*, **133**, 82–97.

Herman, L. M., Pack, A. A., and Hoffmann-Kuhnt, M. (1998). Seeing through sound: dolphins (*Tursiops truncatus*) perceive the spatial structure of objects through echolocation. *Journal of Comparative Psychology*, **11**, 292.

Herzing, D. L. (2004). Social and nonsocial uses of echolocation in free-ranging *Stenella frontalis* and *Tursiops truncatus*. In *Echolocation in bats and dolphins* (pp. 404–409). Chicago, IL: University of Chicago Press.

Heyning, J. E. (1997). Sperm whale phylogeny revisited: analysis of the morphological evidence. *Marine Mammal Science*, **13**, 596–613.

Houser, D. S., Gomez-Rubio, A., and Finneran, J. J. (2008). Evoked potential audiometry of 13 Pacific bottlenose dolphins (*Tursiops truncatus gilli*). *Marine Mammal Science*, **24**, 28–41.

Irvine, A. B., Wells, R. S., and Scott, M. D. (1982). An evaluation of techniques for tagging small odontocete cetaceans. *Fishery Bulletin*, **80**, 135–143.

Jaakkola, K. (2012). Cetacean cognitive specializations. In *The Oxford handbook of comparative evolutionary psychology* (pp. 144–165). Oxford: Oxford University Press.

Jaakkola, K., Fellner, W., Erb, L., Rodriguez, M., and Guarino, E. (2005). Understanding of the concept of numerically "less" by bottlenose dolphins (*Tursiops truncatus*). *Journal of Comparative Psychology*, **119**, 296.

Jaakkola, K., Guarino, E., Rodriguez, M., Erb, L., and Trone, M. (2010). What do dolphins (*Tursiops truncatus*) understand about hidden objects? *Animal Cognition*, **13**, 103.

Janik, V. M. (2005). Underwater acoustic communication networks in marine mammals. In *Animal communication networks* (pp. 390–415). Cambridge: Cambridge University Press.

Janik, V. M., and Slater, P. J. B. (1997). Vocal learning in mammals. *Advances in the Study of Behavior*, **26**, 59–99.

Jensen, F. H., Bejder, L., Wahlberg, M., and Madsen, P. T. (2009). Biosonar adjustments to target range of echolocating bottlenose dolphins (*Tursiops* sp.) in the wild. *Journal of Experimental Biology*, **212**, 1078–1086.

Johnson, M., Aguilar de Soto, N., and Madsen, P. T. (2009). Studying the behaviour and sensory ecology of marine mammals using acoustic recording tags: a review. *Marine Ecology Progress Series*, **395**, 55–73.

Johnson, M. P., and Tyack, P. L. (2003). A digital acoustic recording tag for measuring the response of wild marine mammals to sound. *IEEE Journal of Oceanic Engineering*, **28**, 3–12.

Kastelein, R. A., Bunskoek, P., Hagedoorn, M., Au, W. W. L., and de Haan, D. (2002). Audiogram of a harbor porpoise (*Phocoena phocoena*) measured with narrow-band frequency-modulated signals. *Journal of the Acoustical Society of America*, **112**, 334–344.

Ketten, D. R. (1997). Structure and function in whale ears. *Bioacoustics*, **8**, 103–135.

Ketten, D. R. (2000). Cetacean ears. In *Hearing by whales and dolphins* (pp. 43–108). New York, NY: Springer.

Kilian, A., Yaman, S., von Fersen, L., and Güntürkün, O. (2003). A bottlenose dolphin discriminates visual stimuli differing in numerosity. *Animal Learning and Behavior*, **31**, 133–142.

King, S. L., and Janik, V. M. (2013). Bottlenose dolphins can use learned vocal labels to address each other. *Proceedings of the National Academy of Sciences*, **110**, 13216–13221.

King, S. L., Sayigh, L. S., Wells, R. S., Fellner, W., and Janik, V. M. (2013). Vocal copying of individually distinctive signature whistles in bottlenose dolphins. *Proceedings of the Royal Society of London B: Biological Sciences*, **280**, 20130053.

King, S. L., Harley, H. E., and Janik, V. M. (2014). The role of signature whistle matching in bottlenose dolphins, *Tursiops truncatus*. *Animal Behaviour*, **96**, 79–86.

Koschinski, S. (2001). Current knowledge on harbour porpoises (*Phocoena phocoena*) in the Baltic Sea. *Ophelia*, **55**, 167–197.

Kremers, D., Célérier, A., Schaal, B., *et al.* (2016). Sensory perception in cetaceans: part I – current knowledge about dolphin senses as a representative species. *Frontiers in Ecology and Evolution*, **4**, 49.

Krützen, M., Sherwin, W. B., Connor, R. C., *et al.* (2003). Contrasting relatedness patterns in bottlenose dolphins (*Tursiops* sp.) with different alliance strategies. *Proceedings of the Royal Society of London B: Biological Sciences*, **270**, 497–502.

Krützen, M., Mann, J., Heithaus, M. R., Connor, R. C., Bejder, L., and Sherwin, W. B. (2005). Cultural transmission of tool use in bottlenose dolphins. *Proceedings of the National Academy of Sciences*, **102**, 8939–8943.

Lyamin, O., Pryaslova, J., Lance, V., and Siegel, J. (2005). Continuous activity in cetaceans after birth. *Nature*, **435**, 1177.

Lyrholm, T., and Gyllensten, U. (1998). Global matrilineal population structure in sperm whales as indicated by mitochondrial DNA sequences. *Proceedings of the Royal Society of London B: Biological Sciences*, **265**, 1679–1684.

Madsen, P., Wahlberg, M., and Møhl, B. (2002). Male sperm whale (*Physeter macrocephalus*) acoustics in a high-latitude habitat: implications for echolocation and communication. *Behavioral Ecology and Sociobiology*, **53**, 31–41.

Madsen, P. T., Johnson, M., Aguilar de Soto, N., Zimmer, W. M. X., and Tyack, P. L. (2005). Biosonar performance of foraging beaked whales (*Mesoplodon densirostris*). *Journal of Experimental Biology*, **208**, 181–194.

Madsen, P. T., Lammers, M., Wisniewska, D., and Beedholm, K. (2013). Nasal sound production in echolocating delphinids (*Tursiops truncatus* and *Pseudorca crassidens*) is dynamic, but unilateral: clicking on the right side and whistling on the left side. *Journal of Experimental Biology*, **216**, 4091–4102.

Mass, A., and Supin, A. (1990). Best vision zones in the retinae of some cetaceans. In *Sensory abilities of cetaceans* (pp. 505–517). New York, NY: Springer.

Mass, A. M., and Supin, A. Y. (1999). Retinal topography and visual acuity in the riverine tucuxi (*Sotalia fluviatilis*). *Marine Mammal Science*, **15**, 351–365.

Mate, B., Mesecar, R., and Lagerquist, B. (2007). The evolution of satellite-monitored radio tags for large whales: one laboratory's experience. *Deep Sea Research Part II: Topical Studies in Oceanography*, **54**, 224–247.

May-Collado, L. J., and Agnarsson, I. (2005). Cytochrome *b* and Bayesian inference of whale phylogeny. *Molecular Phylogenetics and Evolution*, **38**, 344–354.

May-Collado, L. J., Agnarsson, I., and Wartzok, D. (2007). Phylogenetic review of tonal sound production in whales in relation to sociality. *BMC Evolutionary Biology*, **7**, 136.

Mercado, E. I., Murray, S. O., Uyeyama, R. K., Pack, A. A., and Herman, L. M. (1998). Memory for recent actions in the bottlenosed dolphin (*Tursiops truncatus*): repetition of arbitrary behaviors using an abstract rule. *Learning and Behavior*, **26**, 210–218.

Mercado, E. I., Uyeyama, R. K., Pack, A. A., and Herman, L. M. (1999). Memory for action events in the bottlenosed dolphin. *Animal Cognition*, **2**, 17–25.

Mercado, E., Killebrew, D. A., Pack, A. A., Mácha, I. V., and Herman, L. M. (2000). Generalization of 'same–different'classification abilities in bottlenosed dolphins. *Behavioural Processes*, **50**, 79–94.

Miller, P. J. O. (2006). Diversity in sound pressure levels and estimated active space of resident killer whale vocalizations. *Journal of Comparative Physiology A*, **192**, 449–459.

Mobley Jr., J. R., and Helweg, D. A. (1990). Visual ecology and cognition in cetaceans. In *Sensory abilities of cetaceans* (pp. 519–536). New York, NY: Springer.

Mobley, J. R., Herman, L. M., and Frankel, A. S. (1988). Responses of wintering humpback whales (*Megaptera novaeangliae*) to playback of recordings of winter and summer vocalizations and of synthetic sound. *Behavioral Ecology and Sociobiology*, **23**, 211–223.

Möller, L. M., Beheregaray, L. B., Harcourt, R. G., and Krützen, M. (2001). Alliance membership and kinship in wild male bottlenose dolphins (*Tursiops aduncus*) of southeastern Australia. *Proceedings of the Royal Society of London B: Biological Sciences*, **268**, 1941–1947.

Möller, L. M., Beheregaray, L. B., Allen, S. J., and Harcourt, R. G. (2006). Association patterns and kinship in female Indo-Pacific bottlenose dolphins (*Tursiops aduncus*) of southeastern Australia. *Behavioral Ecology and Sociobiology*, **61**, 109–117.

Neil, D. T. (2002). Cooperative fishing interactions between Aboriginal Australians and dolphins in eastern Australia. *Anthrozoos*, **15**, 3–18.

Nikaido, M., Matsuno, F., Hamilton, H., *et al.* (2001). Retroposon analysis of major cetacean lineages: the monophyly of toothed whales and the paraphyly of river dolphins. *Proceedings of the National Academy of Sciences*, **98**, 7384–7389.

Noad, M. J., Cato, D. H., Bryden, M. M., Jenner, M. N., and Jenner, K. C. S. (2000). Cultural revolution in whale songs. *Nature*, **408**, 537.

Olesiuk, P. F., Bigg, M. A., and Ellis, G. M. (1990). Life history and population dynamics of resident killer whales (*Orcinus orca*) in the coastal waters of British Columbia and Washington State. *Reports of the International Whaling Commission*, **12**, 209–243.

Parsons, K. M., Durban, J. W., Claridge, D. E., Balcomb, K. C., Noble, L. R., and Thompson, P. M. (2003). Kinship as a basis for alliance formation between male bottlenose dolphins, *Tursiops truncatus*, in the Bahamas. *Animal Behaviour*, **66**, 185–194.

Price, S. A., Bininda-Emonds, O. R. P., and Gittleman, J. L. (2005). A complete phylogeny of the whales, dolphins and even-toed hoofed mammals (Cetartiodactyla). *Biological Reviews*, **80**, 445–473.

Pryor, K., and Lindbergh, J. (1990). A dolphin–human fishing cooperative in Brazil. *Marine Mammal Science*, **6**, 77–82.

Pyenson, N. D., Goldbogen, J. A., Vogl, A. W., Szathmary, G., Drake, R. L., and Shadwick, R. E. (2012). Discovery of a sensory organ that coordinates lunge feeding in rorqual whales. *Nature*, **485**, 498–501.

Quick, N. J., and Janik, V. M. (2012). Bottlenose dolphins exchange signature whistles when meeting at sea. *Proceedings of the Royal Society of London B: Biological Sciences*, **279**, 2539–2545.

Ramp, C., Hagen, W., Palsbøll, P., Bérubé, M., and Sears, R. (2010). Age-related multi-year associations in female humpback whales (*Megaptera novaeangliae*). *Behavioral Ecology and Sociobiology*, **64**, 1563–1576.

Reidenberg, J. S., and Laitman, J. T. (2007). Discovery of a low frequency sound source in Mysticeti (baleen whales): anatomical establishment of a vocal fold homolog. *Anatomical Record*, **290**, 745–759.

Richard, K. R., Dillon, M. C., Whitehead, H., and Wright, J. M. (1996). Patterns of kinship in groups of free-living sperm whales (*Physeter macrocephalus*) revealed by multiple molecular genetic analyses. *Proceedings of the National Academy of Sciences*, **93**, 8792–8795.

Ridgway, S. H., and Carder, D. A. (1990). Tactile sensitivity, somatosensory responses, skin vibrations, and the skin surface ridges of the bottle-nose dolphin, *Tursiops truncatus*. In *Sensory abilities of cetaceans* (pp. 163–179). New York, NY: Springer.

Ridgway, S. H., and Carder, D. A. (2001). Assessing hearing and sound production in cetaceans not available for behavioral audiograms: experiences with sperm, pygmy sperm, and gray whales. *Aquatic Mammals*, **27**, 267–276.

Sauerland, M., and Dehnhardt, G. (1998). Underwater audiogram of a tucuxi (*Sotalia fluviatilis guianensis*). *The Journal of the Acoustical Society of America*, **103**, 1199–1204.

Sayigh, L. S., Tyack, P. L., Wells, R. S., Solow, A. R., Scott, M. D., and Irvine, A. B. (1999). Individual recognition in wild bottlenose dolphins: a field test using playback experiments. *Animal Behaviour*, **57**, 41–50.

Schorr, G. S., Falcone, E. A., Moretti, D. J., and Andrews, R. D. (2014). First long-term behavioral records from Cuvier's beaked whales (*Ziphius cavirostris*) reveal record-breaking dives. *PLoS ONE*, **9**(3), e92633.

Schusterman, R., Thomas, J. A., and Wood, F. G. (1986). *Dolphin cognition and behavior: a comparative approach*. Hillsdale, NJ: Lawrence Erlbaum Associates.

Seed, A., and Byrne, R. W. (2010). Animal tool-use. *Current Biology*, **20**, 1032–1039.

Similä, T., Holst, J. C., and Christensen, I. (1996). Occurrence and diet of killer whales in northern Norway: seasonal patterns relative to the distribution and abundance of Norwegian spring-spawning herring. *Canadian Journal of Fisheries and Aquatic Sciences*, **53**, 769–779.

Simon, M., Ugarte, F., Wahlberg, M., and Miller, L. A. (2006). Icelandic killer whales *Orcinus orca* use a pulsed call suitable for manipulating the schooling behaviour of herring *Clupea harengus*. *Bioacoustics*, **26**, 57–74.

Smolker, R. A., Richards, A. F., Connor, R. C., and Pepper, J. W. (1992). Sex-differences in patterns of association among Indian Ocean bottle-nosed dolphins. *Behaviour*, **123**, 38–69.

Smolker, R., Richards, A., Connor, R., Mann, J., and Berggren, P. (1997). Sponge carrying by dolphins (Delphinidae, *Tursiops* sp.): a foraging specialization involving tool use? *Ethology*, **103**, 454–465.

Stafford, K. M., Moore, S. E., Laidre, K. L., and Heide-Jørgensen, M. (2008). Bowhead whale springtime song off West Greenland. *Journal of the Acoustical Society of America*, **124**, 3315–3323.

Stevick, P. T., Palsbøll, P. J., Smith, T. D., Bravington, M. V., and Hammond, P. S. (2001). Errors in identification using natural markings: rates, sources and effects on capture–recapture estimates of abundance. *Canadian Journal of Fisheries and Aquatic Sciences*, **58**, 1861–1870.

Stimpert, A. K., Wiley, D. N., Au, W. W. L., Johnson, M. P., and Arsenault, R. (2007). 'Megapclicks': acoustic click trains and buzzes produced during night-time foraging of humpback whales (*Megaptera novaeangliae*). *Biology Letters*, **3**, 467–470.

Stolen, M. K., and Barlow, J. (2003). A model life table for bottlenose dolphins (*Tursiops truncatus*) from the Indian River Lagoon system, Florida, USA. *Marine Mammal Science*, **19**, 630–649.

Szymanski, M. D., Bain, D. E., Kiehl, K., Pennington, S., Wong, S., and Henry, K. R. (1999). Killer whale (*Orcinus orca*) hearing: auditory brainstem response and behavioral audiograms. *Journal of the Acoustical Society of America*, **106**, 1134–1141.

Tavares, S. B., Samarra, F. I. P., and Miller, P. J. O. (2017). A multilevel society of herring-eating killer whales indicates adaptation to prey characteristics. *Behavioral Ecology*, **28**, 500–514.

Thewissen, J. G. M. (1994). Phylogenetic aspects of cetacean origins: a morphological perspective. *Journal of Mammalian Evolution*, **2**, 157–184.

Thomas, J., Chun, N., Au, W., and Pugh, K. (1988). Underwater audiogram of a false killer whale (*Pseudorca crassidens*). *Journal of the Acoustical Society of America*, **84**, 936–940.

Tyack, P. L. (1983). Differential response of humpback whales, *Megaptera novaeangliae*, to playback of song or social sounds. *Behavioral Ecology and Sociobiology*, **13**, 49–55.

Tyack, P. L., Zimmer, W. M., Moretti, D., *et al.* (2011). Beaked whales respond to simulated and actual navy sonar. *PLoS ONE*, **6**(3), e17009.

Vergara, V., and Barrett-Lennard, L. (2017). Call usage learning by a beluga (*Delphinapterus leucas*) in a categorical matching task. *International Journal of Comparative Psychology*, **30**.

Watwood, S. L., Tyack, P. L., and Wells, R. S. (2004). Whistle sharing in paired male bottlenose dolphins, *Tursiops truncatus*. *Behavioral Ecology and Sociobiology*, **55**, 531–543.

Weinrich, M. T. (1991). Stable social associations among humpback whales (*Megaptera novaeangliae*) in the southern Gulf of Maine. *Canadian Journal of Zoology*, **69**, 3012–3019.

Weiß, B. M., Ladich, F., Spong, P., and Symonds, H. K. (2006). Vocal behavior of resident killer whale matrilines with newborn calves: the role of family signatures. *Journal of the Acoustical Society of America*, **119**, 627–635.

Weiß, B. M., Symonds, H. K., Spong, P., and Ladich, F. (2011). Call sharing across vocal clans of killer whales: evidence for vocal imitation? *Marine Mammal Science*, **27**, 1–13.

Wellings, C. E. (1944). The killer whales of Twofold Bay, N.S.W., Australia, *Grampus orca*. *Australian Journal of Zoology*, **10**, 291–293.

Wells, R. S. (1991). The role of long-term study in understanding the social structure of a bottlenose dolphin community. In *Dolphin societies: discoveries and puzzles* (pp. 199–225). Berkeley, CA: University of California Press.

Whitehead, H., and Mann, J. (2000). Female reproductive strategies of cetaceans. In *Cetacean societies: field studies of dolphins and whales* (pp. 219–246). Chicago, IL: University of Chicago Press.

Whitehead, H., Waters, S., and Lyrholm, T. (1991). Social organization of female sperm whales and their offspring: constant companions and casual acquaintances. *Behavioral Ecology and Sociobiology*, **29**, 385–389.

Wilson, B., Thompson, P. M., and Hammond, P. S. (1997). Habitat use by bottlenose dolphins: seasonal distribution and stratified movement patterns in the Moray Firth, Scotland. *Journal of Applied Ecology*, **34**, 1365–1374.

Wilson, B., Hammond, P. S., and Thompson, P. M. (1999). Estimating size and assessing trends in a coastal bottlenose dolphin population. *Ecological Applications*, **9**, 288–300.

Wisniewska, D. M., Johnson, M., Beedholm, K., Wahlberg, M., and Madsen, P. T. (2012). Acoustic gaze adjustments during active target selection in echolocating porpoises. *Journal of Experimental Biology*, **215**, 4358–4373.

Wright, B. M., Stredulinsky, E. H., Ellis, G. M., and Ford, J. K. B. (2016). Kin-directed food sharing promotes lifetime natal philopatry of both sexes in a population of fish-eating killer whales, *Orcinus orca*. *Animal Behaviour*, **115**, 81–95.

Wright, B. M., Ford, J. K. B., Ellis, G. M., *et al.* (2017). Fine-scale foraging movements by fish-eating killer whales (*Orcinus orca*) relate to the vertical distributions and escape responses of salmonid prey (*Oncorhynchus* spp.). *Movement Ecology*, **5**, 3.

Yeater, D., Kuczaj, I., and Stan, A. (2010). Observational learning in wild and captive dolphins. *International Journal of Comparative Psychology*, **23**, 379–385.

8 Elephants – Studying Cognition in the African Savannah

Lucy A. Bates

Species Description

Elephants are not funny-nosed, one-handed primates. This mantra should be repeated *ad nauseam* by students of elephant cognition. Yes, they are large-brained, long-lived and highly social – like some of the more charismatic primate species – and people often claim that elephants share many of humankind's most positive traits. For example, they are considered empathic, playful, fiercely protective of their kin and mournful at the death of another. However, despite these apparent similarities, elephants remain elephants. Not primates. In this chapter, I will attempt to demonstrate that elephants deserve to be studied in their own right, because they have much to teach us about the possibilities (and limits) of cognition – of what a brain can do, and why. But more fundamentally, I hope to show why it is imperative to remember that elephants must be studied *as elephants*, if we are to learn anything interesting about their specific cognitive skills, as well as the wider evolution of cognition.

Extant elephants are divided into two genera, the African *Loxodonta* and the Asian *Elephus*. Asian elephants (*Elephus maximus*) are divided into three or sometimes four subspecies, the Indian, Sri Lankan, Sumatran and Bornean elephants (Sukumar, 2006; Choudhury *et al.*, 2008). African elephants remain officially listed by the IUCN as one species divided into two subspecies (savannah elephants: *Loxodonta africana africana*, and forest elephants *L. africana cyclotis*; Blanc, 2008), but recent data on the status of forest elephants may soon lead to officially changing this classification (Roca *et al.*, 2001). Indeed, many biologists already record savannah and forest elephants as two separate species, *L. africana* and *L. cyclotis* (Grubb *et al.*, 2000; Meyer *et al.*, 2017).

My primary experience is in studying free-ranging African savannah elephants. Relatively little is known about the behaviour and cognition of forest elephants, and the cognition of *Elephus maximus* has largely been studied in various captive settings, of which I have little experience but quite strong opinions. For behavioural scientists, there are some obvious reasons why studies of captive elephants of either genus might be preferable, but I shall highlight the difficulties that these captive situations present.

Anatomy

Elephants look unlike any other animal. Even their closest extant phylogenetic relatives, the Hyracoidea (hyraxes) and Sirenia (dugongs and manatees), bare little resemblance.

The most striking physical characteristics of elephants, beyond their sheer size, are their perilously valuable tusks (evolved from incisor teeth) and their long trunks – a fusion of the nose and upper lip (Spinage, 1994). Interestingly, Asian elephants have one 'finger' on the top tip of their trunks, whereas African elephants have one on the lower half as well, which they can oppose to pick up objects (Figure 8.1).

Adult elephants are very sexually dimorphic. Adult female savannah elephants weigh up to 3 tonnes, with a maximum height of around 2.5 m, while mature males can become 3.5 or even 4 m tall, and weigh up to 6 tonnes. Asian elephants are slightly smaller, with adult males typically weighing around 5 tonnes and standing 3 m tall. Even infants are large, at around 75 cm high and 100 kg at birth. Any studies of elephants must therefore take very particular care to both protect personnel and use equipment that can withstand unrelenting interactions with the strongest and heaviest terrestrial animal on the planet.

Perception

Contrary to popular belief, elephant eyesight is not terrible, although it can be limited in bright light (Yokoyama *et al.*, 2005). Indeed, a lot of communication between elephants is visual, based on gesture and body language (Kahl and Armstrong, 2000; Poole and Granli, 2011). However, while it is difficult to decide which perceptual system is most important to elephants, their well-developed olfactory bulb and disproportionately large temporal lobe suggest that smell and hearing are particularly significant (Hakeem *et al.*, 2005; Shoshani *et al.*, 2006).

Elephants derive so much information from scent and sounds (Langbauer, 2000), probably more than we can readily conceive, and tests must take this into account (see below). Consideration of olfactory and auditory cues is crucial when designing and evaluating studies of elephant cognition. Unlike studies with some birds or primates, manipulation of visual cues alone will probably teach us only a very limited amount about elephant cognition.

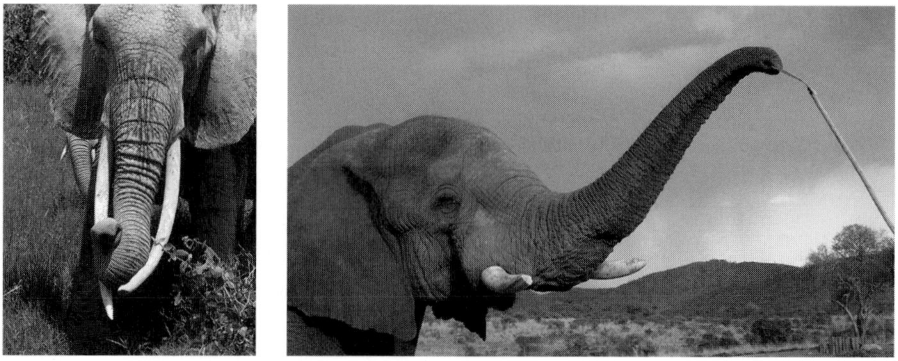

Figure 8.1. (Left) African elephants have two 'fingers' on the top and bottom of their trunk-tip, which (right) can be opposed to pick up and hold objects.

Life Cycle

Elephants are very long-lived. Female savannah elephants have been known to live over 70 years, and males can survive and reproduce into their 60s (Moss, 2001; Lee *et al.*, 2016). Females typically become sexually receptive between the ages of 10 and 15 years, with an average age at first birth of 14 in Amboseli, Kenya (Moss and Lee, 2011a). Pregnancy is famously long, with a 22-month gestation. Although not strictly seasonal breeders, savannah elephants tend to optimize timing of reproductive events to coincide with periods of maximum food availability (Lee *et al.*, 2011a). This obviously means there are peak birth periods as well (Moss, 2001). These reproductive and birthing peaks may offer spectacular observational opportunities, but they are not optimal periods for experimental testing.

Infants are precocial, standing and walking within an hour or two of birth, but it takes years to learn all the necessary life skills, for example to use the trunk properly for drinking and eating (Lee, 1987). Although calves start trying solid food from around 3 months old, they tend to suckle throughout the typical 4-year interbirth interval, with weaning often only occurring because a new infant has been born (Lee, 1987). Studies of female elephants must not entail any risks to – or come between – mothers and their calves. Even after weaning, juveniles remain dependent on their natal family groups, with females maintaining close proximity for life, and males becoming independent around age 10–15.

Despite being sexually mature by their early 20s, males are not considered socially mature until much later. Males typically in their 30s and older enter annual 'musth' phases – periods of greatly heightened testosterone that can last several months, which signal social and sexual maturity (Poole and Moss, 1981; Poole, 1987, 1989a). During musth, males become considerably more aggressive, wandering far and searching for sexually receptive females. Musth males seek to maintain exclusive access to any sexually receptive females, chasing non-musth males away and even fighting with other males in musth. These fights can last several hours, and may result in severe injury or even death to the losing male (Poole, 1987, 1989b). Unless individuals are very well known, and highly experienced researchers are present, musth males are best avoided (both in the wild and in captivity), as they can be unpredictable and dangerous.

Individual Identification

Individual identification of elephants does not require any specific devices other than a camera, notebook and good memory. Sexing adult elephants is relatively easy given their dimorphism, which becomes apparent from about age 10 onwards (Lee and Moss, 1995). Adult females tend to reach the same height as a male of around age 20 (~2.5 m). Mature males are much bigger than females in all ways, including having thicker tusks. The belly line slopes down in mature males, and they have more rounded heads, with an hourglass shape. Adult females have narrower and often more angular heads, a more horizontal belly line, and often visible breasts between their front legs (Figure 8.2).

Sexing immature elephants is harder, tending to require a specific view of the genital area, but ageing them is easier. For example, calves under 1 year can walk under their mother's stomach. Calves who are still drinking with their mouth (rather than their trunk) are likely under 2 years old. Tusks tend to start erupting from 3 years old, and males moving away from their family group are likely 10 or more.

For individual identification, ears are the best source of information, as they vary in shape, size, and patterns of tears, holes and wrinkles. Tusks can also give cues to identity, but this method is not always reliable, as tusks do break. Body height and shape, injuries, scars, warts, head shape and wrinkle patterns also provide valuable clues to aid identification. All this information must be noted down with photos and/or drawings.

Alternatively, it is possible to use GPS collars to identify and track individual elephants. These collars are expensive and dangerous to fit, requiring sedation by a qualified veterinary team (after permits have been acquired from the relevant authorities). However, they give brilliantly accurate information about the location of specific individuals and all that that reveals, such as movement routes, land-use information, travel speed, and timing and location of resting behaviour.

Social Characteristics

Savannah elephants live in hierarchical societies, where the mother–calf unit is fundamental. Families are led by a matriarch, typically the oldest female in the family, and are composed of her close female kin (sisters, daughters, granddaughters, nieces) and their dependent offspring, typically numbering around 20 animals (varying from 3 to over 40; Moss and Poole, 1983; Moss and Lee, 2011b). Elephants form a fission–fusion society, with families breaking into smaller units at times. Fusion with family

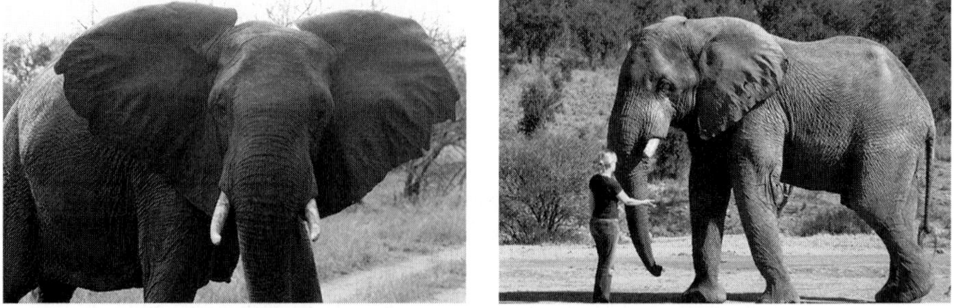

Figure 8.2. Elephants can be readily identified by their ear patterns, and sexed by their body shapes. Females (left) have sloping stomachs, often visible breasts, and narrower and more angular heads than males (right), who are much larger with much wider and more rounded heads.

members is often associated with intense and dramatic 'greeting ceremonies' (Poole and Granli, 2011). Two or more families may form bond-groups, and bond-groups can form clans or subpopulations within the population (Wittemyer *et al.*, 2005, 2009; Archie *et al.*, 2006; see de Silva and Wittemyer, 2012, for a synopsis of Asian elephant society).

Dominance hierarchies are not strong in female savannah elephants, and we tend to consider females as egalitarian and cooperative (Moss and Lee, 2011a). This egalitarian society involves a lot of play (Lee and Moss, 2014), allomothering of calves by females, and a lot of touching and/or caressing (Lee, 1987). Male society exhibits clearer dominance hierarchies based on musth status and physical size and strength. Young males seek out the company of other (preferably older) males, and spend a lot of time sparring with peers, at least in part to ascertain their relative strength (Chiyo *et al.*, 2011; Lee *et al.*, 2011b).

This means you cannot rely on testing single elephants in the wild. Female or immature elephants are almost never alone, and even independent males are often in the company of other males and/or family groups. Moreover, when one elephant interacts with something (including experimental equipment), the others present are also likely to become interested, so often there will be multiple elephants reacting to or interacting with the apparatus (Figure 8.3); therefore, independence of reactions cannot be assumed.

Ecological Characteristics

Elephants drink between 100 and 200 litres of water per day, ideally every day. Water sources are often the site of congregation of many elephants, so a lot of social interactions may be observed once the elephants have drunk. Bathing and mud wallowing are also important for elephants as a mechanism for keeping cool. Studies should not interrupt these activities. After mud bathing, elephants often rub their bodies against large objects

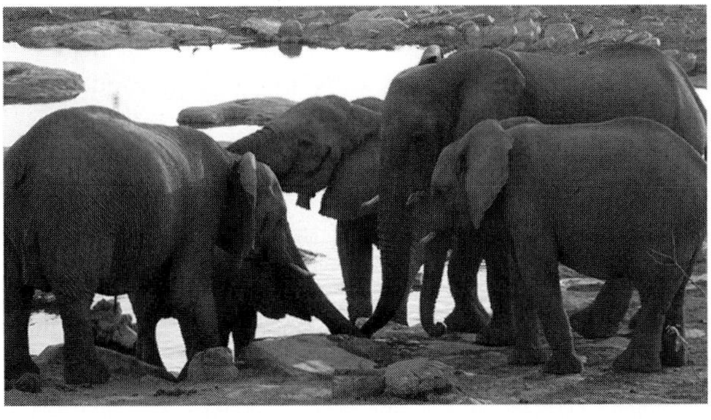

Figure 8.3. When one elephant shows interest by sniffing something, others often tend to smell the same area, which can make analysing responses difficult.

(such as trees or rocks) to remove parasites. They may use any large object that is available, which can sometimes include research vehicles and/or study equipment.

The preferred food in wild savannah elephants is fresh grass, but they also browse on leaves, twigs, bark and roots. They can tolerate quite a poor-quality diet, and this generality allows them to live in many habitats, although they will spend longer foraging in arid areas or during dry seasons, when no grass is available. Elephants are considered habitat architects (Owen-Smith *et al.*, 2006; van Aarde *et al.*, 2006; Guldemond *et al.*, 2017), with adult female savannah elephants consuming about 250 kg of food per day and males about 300–400 kg. Competition for food sources is rare, however.

Elephants often travel on well-worn and visible paths (Fishlock *et al.*, 2016), and it is possible to use these paths to increase the chances of wild elephants noticing and interacting with any experimental apparatus (e.g. Bates *et al.*, 2008a). However, during dry periods, elephants may be less inclined to interact with or investigate an apparatus, as they are primarily motivated by searching for food and water, although they do tend to move in smaller groups during these periods. In wet seasons or in areas with plentiful grass, elephants tend to be more playful and investigative, but they often move in larger groups, which can make data recording and analysis very troublesome.

Despite their size, elephants are not immune to predation. Very young calves are vulnerable to hyenas, and lions can also take down juvenile elephants. Humans also pose a significant and increasing risk to elephants, including the effects of human–elephant conflict (such as retaliatory killings by people after elephants raid crops or attack livestock), poaching for ivory or bushmeat, and even ill-regulated tourism or infrastructure-related accidents (for example, being hit by cars or trains, electrocuted by fences and power lines, or drowning in wells and drainage systems). Elephants are thus wary of, and may be aggressive towards, hyenas, lions *and* people.

In general, elephants who have been highly disturbed by humans in the past will be much more wary of people (especially people they do not know, such as new researchers). This could result in them being shy and attempting to evade observation, or even becoming aggressive and threatening. Due consideration of a population's history (predation and poaching levels, human–elephant conflict rates, frequency and type of management intervention) is thus necessary before commencing a research project with wild elephants, to ensure the aims are not confounded by ecology and human interference.

State of the Art

Elephants are large-brained (Cozzi *et al.*, 2001; Shoshani *et al.*, 2006) and highly social (Moss and Poole, 1983; Moss and Lee, 2011b), so we might expect them to possess advanced cognitive skills (Byrne and Bates, 2007, 2010). Yet, a great deal remains unknown about the extent of elephant cognition (Byrne and Bates, 2011). Here I outline what is known about cognition among African and Asian elephants, focusing particularly on the strengths and weaknesses of study designs. As will become apparent, the importance of *ecological validity* – basing the studies on elephants' natural behaviour and on the abilities they require – is paramount.

Experimental studies have demonstrated that wild savannah elephants possess sophisticated categorization skills. They are able to categorize a single species (humans) into subclasses, based on olfactory (Bates *et al.*, 2007) and, separately, auditory cues (McComb *et al.*, 2014). Thuppil and Coss (2013) showed that wild Asian elephants discriminate between the growls of tigers and leopards. These naturalistic, wild-based studies demonstrate that learning and classifying ecologically relevant information appears to be a highly refined skill in elephants.

We tested working memory in savannah elephants with an 'expectancy-violation' paradigm, which involved moving urine deposits from known individuals to positions where they would be discovered by target individuals from the same family (Bates *et al.*, 2008a). After varying the placement of deposits between feasible and impossible ('unexpected') locations, we concluded that elephants continually track the locations of family members in relation to themselves. It is important to note that the initial measure of 'expectancy violation' – that of 'smelling time' – did not reveal differences across conditions. Instead, 'trunk reaching' was the appropriate measure, an illustration of the importance of considering natural behaviour, to ensure measures are appropriate and relevant.

These discrimination and working memory skills are counterparts to the most famed elephant cognitive characteristic: long-term memory. McComb and colleagues (2000) employed experimental playback of long-distance contact calls to show that adult female savannah elephants are familiar with the vocalizations of multiple individuals in other families in the population, including some whose calls they had not heard for many years. They also showed that this knowledge is more pronounced in families with older matriarchs, indicating social knowledge accrues with age (McComb *et al.*, 2001), and older females make better leaders, as also shown in tests of reactions to lions (McComb *et al.*, 2011). Impressive feats of long-term memory have also been demonstrated by observations of elephants' spatial knowledge, including their ability to access remote sources of water during times of drought (e.g. see Blake *et al.*, 2003; Leggett, 2006; Foley *et al.*, 2008; Polansky *et al.*, 2015).

Tests of learning and memory have been conducted in captive Asian elephants. Rensch (1957) tested one zoo elephant in a visual discrimination, object-choice task. The female was slow at learning the task (as might be expected in such an arbitrary and abstract task), but once she understood the object-choice paradigm, she learned each discrimination increasingly rapidly. She could remember the 'correct' pattern in 20 pairs at the same time, and retained this knowledge long-term, still performing well a year later. Arvidsson and colleagues (2012) and Plotnik and colleagues (2014) showed captive Asian elephants also use olfactory cues to solve object-choice tasks, again with long retention. Savannah elephants are able to detect the smell of TNT and are being trained as landmine 'biosensors' (Miller *et al.*, 2015).

Problem-solving remains an intriguing question in elephants. Hart and colleagues (2008) report an unpublished study with captive Asian elephants that failed to show 'insight'. The elephants did not use sticks placed in their enclosure to obtain out-of-reach food rewards, despite the authors' belief that this should have been an easy task (because elephants frequently reach their trunks toward high food and separately pick up and hold sticks). Foerder and colleagues (2011) subsequently modified this task, providing blocks for the elephants to stand on, as well as sticks. Again, none of the test elephants used the sticks, but one male did spontaneously stand on a block to reach the food. Foerder and colleagues argued that expecting elephants to use a stick to reach food ignores the most important function of the trunk: it is primarily a sensory organ and not a hand to reach for things. Elephants rarely use trunk-held tools to acquire food, as this would preclude the trunk's principal task of sniffing out the food. Therefore, it seems that disregarding natural behaviour led to a false negative in the study by Hart and colleagues.

Elephants in a Burmese logging camp were trained to remove food from a bucket only after they had touched the bucket lid, which was always placed on top of the bucket during training (Nissani, 2006). In the test phase, the lid was placed next to the bucket, eliminating the need to touch it before accessing the food. Elephants almost always continued to touch the lid, which, according to Nissani, showed a lack of causal understanding. However, working elephants are trained to follow precise sequences of behaviour and may be punished for deviating from these routines. The subjects may have understood that the lid was irrelevant in the test phase, but persisted in touching it because that is what they had previously learned and experience had shown them not to deviate from learned patterns. It is therefore unwise to draw conclusions about problem-solving and causal understanding from elephants that are not free to make their own choices.

Mizuno and colleagues (2016) reported another example of spontaneous behaviour to solve a problem, with captive Asian elephants accessing food by blowing it towards themselves. The study draws parallels between using the trunk in this novel way and tool use. Both Asian and African elephants have been seen to use different tool types (Chevalier-Skolnikoff and Liska, 1993), and Asian elephants have been shown to modify sticks before using them as fly switches (Hart and Hart, 1994; Hart *et al.*, 2001). Elephants may thus be added to the small number of animals that *modify* tools. However, this tool modification does not compare in complexity to the manufacture of tools by chimpanzees (Goodall, 1986; Boesch and Boesch, 1990; Sanz *et al.*, 2009) or New Caledonian crows (Hunt, 1996, 2000).

Based on decades of field observations of savannah elephants, my colleagues and I found clear evidence of coalitions and alliances, cooperative problem-solving and helping, and understanding of others' emotions and intended goals (Bates *et al.*, 2008b). Observations of captive Asian elephants also demonstrate compassionate empathy, with more physical contact and communication occurring between elephants after a distressing event (Plotnik and de Waal, 2014). Plotnik and colleagues (2011) also found that captive Asian elephants can learn to coordinate with a partner to simultaneously pull the two ends of a rope and bring food within reach – a classic paradigm used to explore cooperation in primates.

Data on theory of mind among elephants are sketchy but tantalizing. Smet and Byrne (2013, 2014b) presented initial evidence that captive African elephants follow and understand human pointing gestures to locate hidden food in an object-choice task. Moreover, these elephants could discriminate the human experimenter's visual attention (Smet and Byrne, 2014a). However, Plotnik and colleagues (2013) found little evidence for comprehension of pointing in captive Asian elephants. Therefore, it is not yet clear if this difference represents a genuine cognitive disparity between African and Asian elephants.

To date, there are few experimental data on social learning or behavioural traditions in elephants (Greco *et al.*, 2013). However, information exchange between savannah elephants is well documented (Lee and Moss, 1999), and it seems feasible that such a long-lived and highly social species would learn from observing others. The possibility of behavioural traditions in path use (Fishlock *et al.*, 2016) suggests the transmission of spatial knowledge from older relatives to young individuals. Familiar social network positions are also likely learned and traditional (Goldenberg *et al.*, 2016). Elephants may possess social learning abilities absent in non-human primates. For instance, there is evidence of vocal imitation in both a savannah elephant (Poole *et al.*, 2005) and a captive Asian elephant (Stoeger *et al.*, 2012). Observational data further suggest that older female African elephants *might* teach young, naïve, nulliparous females how to behave when they come into oestrous for the first time (Bates *et al.*, 2010).

A particularly enticing area of study concerns elephants' awareness of self. Two tests of self-awareness in Asian elephants have been published, with contradictory results. Both relied on Gallup's 'mark test' paradigm, developed for apes (Gallup, 1970). Povinelli (1989) observed no signs of self-recognition in two elephants he tested, but these elephants were only given a few days' prior exposure to the mirror before being tested. In contrast, apes that passed the test have typically had weeks or months of prior experience. In the second experiment, Plotnik and colleagues report that one of three adult females they tested did show mirror self-recognition, suggesting that elephants can recognize themselves in a mirror, and thus have some concept of the self as an entity (also see Dale and Plotnik, 2017).

Observations of savannah elephants' reactions to dying or dead family members further support the notion that they have a concept of self and act empathically (Douglas-Hamilton *et al.*, 2006), and experimental data show they distinguish elephant bones from those of other animals (McComb *et al.*, 2006). However, there is currently no evidence for elephants' capacity to understand others' knowledge or beliefs. Explicit tests of their understanding of others' mental states are required, but these tests *must* be carefully designed and reflect elephants' natural behaviour.

All for One and One for All

Box 8.1 Social Cognition and Social Strategies in Wild Elephants and Other Taxa

Phyllis Lee

Bates describes elephants' ability to monitor their world using different modalities – scent, sound, touch – and apply this knowledge to responses to challenges. Further

(*cont.*)

details on responses to environmental and social challenges are useful. An elephant's brain, like macaques, chimpanzees, humans and dolphins, has Von Economo neurons for processing complex cognitive and social stimuli. How do elephants respond to social stimuli, e.g. their social decision-making?

Elephants have distinct individual responses to their world (Lee and Moss, 2012). These behavioural syndromes or personalities reliably predict the way different elephants cope with social or physical stresses. Personality differences are found across a vast range of species (from octopus to dolphins, and humans); holding a playful personality in elephants is associated with traits like a long lifespan (Lee and Moss, 2014). Enabling quick and efficient responses to threats, being confident and exploratory, or getting others to follow signals and directions (traits of leadership) produces elephants who can cope with their risky environments.

Sociable and likeable elephants attract others; central social females are anchors for expanded social networks (de Silva and Wittemyer, 2012), and in humans and baboons the size of a network and the embeddedness of individuals in networks predicts longevity. Sociability is more than a measure of time spent with others; it reflects tolerance of others' nearness, positive responses to approaches and contacts with others (including via vocalizations), and friendly concern and care for other's infants (called allomothering).

Elephant groups form and dissolve on a minute-to-minute or day-to-day basis. How they manage this feat of social coordination, with individuals they know and like, as well as with less-preferred associates, requires decisions about when, where and with whom to group. These decisions are based on knowledge and memory of others described by Bates, and represent ongoing challenges to elephants. Forest elephants, typically found in pairs or trios, aggregate in 100 s in clearings using knowledge based on scent, sounds and holding memories of their past interactions; elephants can follow scent trails of individuals. Although simple joint movement rules can coordinate large groups in the absence of any cognitive representations, the underlying choices of specific 'others' over space and many years suggests that for elephants, knowledge, memory and active choice are all involved. In these aspects, elephants are more like people than like fish, birds or even baboons (Hill *et al.*, 2008).

The likes, dislikes and personalities of elephants are reflected in their emotions, which can be positive and intense (Safina, 2015) and differ from ours (imagine if your experience of life was constantly like being in a crowd at a football game); these may be more similar to highly excitable species, such as chimpanzees or some breeds of domestic dogs. Elephants appear phlegmatic (because of their large size, deliberate movements and low affect in captivity – where what we see is boredom), but field observers recognize the emotionality inherent in their communication, interactions with the environment and other elephants. Imagine being bombarded with the smell of nearby and distant friends and relatives, plus vocalizations from several kilometres away, signalling the location and activities of up to 100 friends,

(cont.)

all part of the dynamic, fluctuating emotional environment. We have sufficient information on arousal, rate and nature of responses to stimuli, and changes to affect or emotion to compare between varieties of cognitively complex, highly social species like elephants in their emotional excitability.

References

de Silva, S., and Wittemyer, G. (2012). A comparison of social organization in Asian elephants and African savannah elephants. *International Journal of Primatology*, **33**, 1125–1141.

Hill, R. A., Bentley, R. A., and Dunbar, R. I. (2008). Network scaling reveals consistent fractal pattern in hierarchical mammalian societies. *Biology Letters*, **4**, 748–751.

Lee, P. C., and Moss, C. J. (2012). Wild female African elephants (*Loxodonta africana*) exhibit personality traits of leadership and social integration. *Journal of Comparative Psychology*, **126**, 224.

Lee, P. C., and Moss, C. J. (2014). African elephant play, competence and social complexity. *Animal Behavior and Cognition*, **1**, 144–156.

Safina, C. (2015). *Beyond words: what animals think and feel.* New York, NY: Macmillan Press.

Field Guide

What to Study

In my experience, there are two ways to approach questions of elephant cognition. The first is to look at cognitive research being conducted with other species, typically preverbal human infants and other great apes, and try to apply those questions and designs to elephants. This can result in captivating studies of key questions (self-awareness, theory of mind, insight), but it runs the risk of foregoing ecological validity, if designs are simply lifted from studies of two-handed primates, with highly developed vision and a relatively poor sense of smell. If taking this approach, it is important to be very careful, to make sure that both (a) the questions are relevant to elephants and (b) the design is valid. For example, it took years to realize that in a species like chimpanzees, competitive interactions were a better way to experimentally study theory-of-mind processes (Hare and Tomasello, 2004), but this is unlikely to yield much in elephants as they are so rarely competitive (except between males, over access to oestrus females). Cooperative or affiliative interactions will probably be a more productive avenue from which to explore elephants' knowledge of others' minds.

The second approach is to base studies on interesting things that have been observed and noted in the field, reading about field studies, or talking to field researchers who often have a wealth of 'anecdotal' observations and ideas that are crying out to be tested empirically (Bates and Byrne, 2007; de Waal, 2016). This approach guarantees ecological validity, exploring underlying and complex cognitive processes by testing existing behaviour – the things that elephants actually do. However, it does mean that studies and results may not be easily comparable to what we know about behaviour and cognition in other species, and it may not show us how flexible elephants are in the application of their cognitive skills – two pervasive problems in comparative psychology research (Shettleworth, 1993; Stevens, 2010; Burkart *et al.*, 2017).

Where to Conduct your Research

Of course, the first step in conducting animal cognition research is to decide upon the research topic and question that are of most interest, and then to determine which animal is most appropriate for studying that question. If these decisions have led you to research with elephants, you must then further decide which species of elephant to study, and whether your research questions and logistics are best suited to a study of wild (field-based) or captive elephants.

As shown above, field studies may be difficult to manage and can – although not necessarily – yield small sample sizes. However, they have the huge advantage of offering tests of real behaviour, as actually used by real elephants. Captive studies are likely easier to arrange and manage, and offer opportunities to study questions that are virtually intractable with wild populations. However, captive studies often do not provide any larger sample sizes (as elephant groups in zoos are generally very small), and captivity often entails serious confounds. Crucially, there is much evidence that captivity can be genuinely damaging to the psychological well-being of elephants (Clubb and Mason, 2002; Clubb *et al.*, 2008; Mason and Veasey, 2010), so we are forced to question whether results from captive individuals really represent 'normal' elephants.

Wherever your research questions lead you – be it to the wilds of Africa or Asia, or a captive facility – it is then necessary to locate a specific, viable research site where the study can be conducted. This is likely to be an established field research station or a zoo with an interest in accommodating animal research and enrichment.

Field Research Considerations

If you have decided field research is most appropriate for your specific aims, you must find an appropriate site that can accommodate you and support the research. Think about your research question and the particular set-up at potential research sites. For example, some research sites mostly concentrate on male elephants, or some may have a lot of GPS-collared elephants for tracking data, whereas others have many fewer. Bear in mind that some research sites are very small, with very little or no capacity to host students (for example, the Amboseli Trust for Elephants research camp has very little space to accommodate visiting researchers).

After you have established collaboration with a suitable research site, it is then necessary to obtain the appropriate permissions before any fieldwork can be conducted (see Table 8.1). Such permissions include ethical clearance from your home institution and research partners, and research permits from the host country, if working abroad (as well as an appropriate visa, where necessary). Research personnel at the site you will be visiting can usually provide information about what is required to obtain such permits. Furthermore, it is essential to ensure you have enough funding to cover all research costs, including research fees and national park fees where applicable, as well as travel, accommodation fees and subsistence, any equipment and apparatus costs, and fuel costs for using a vehicle in the field. Preparing an expansive budget while still in the early planning phase is a very good idea.

One other significant thing to note about field research is that it takes time. Therefore, fieldwork is probably not appropriate when you only have a few weeks available to conduct your research. The planning and preparation can be laborious, and even once in the field both observational and experimental studies can progress slowly. You have to wait for the right opportunities and set-up to occur naturally, which involves you being in the right place at the right time. This often comes down in no small way to pure luck. Also, it is likely that at least some of your days in the field will actually be spent dealing

Table 8.1. Aspects to consider when planning fieldwork with wild elephants.

Planning	Items to consider
Research administration	Where to study elephants? Ethical approval from home research institution. Where and how to acquire research permits? Research fees. How to travel to research site? Expenses at research site (food, accommodation, etc.).
Data collection	What assistance do you require to collect data? What equipment do you need? How long will it likely take to collect sufficient data?
Standard research equipment	Binoculars; camera and video cameras; notebooks or tablet containing data sheets; laptop computer; mobile phone (with local SIM); GPS; spare batteries and/or chargers for all devices; humidity and shock-proof cases for all equipment.
Specific research equipment	Depending on the nature of your research, additional equipment (e.g. loudspeakers and/or microphones) or specific apparatus (e.g. 'puzzle boxes') may be necessary. Make sure this is wellprotected and as robust as possible. Is it adequately protected from dust, wind and rain? Will it withstand being swung repeatedly around the head of an elephant and then thrown several metres up in the air? If not, how will you make sure the elephants do not come into physical contact with the apparatus?
Personal well-being	Sunglasses; sun hat; sun block; mosquito repellent and bite cream; anti-malaria prophylaxis and/or treatment; clothes for keeping cool and covering up from sun; warmer clothes for evenings and early mornings; sturdy shoes; waterproof clothing and shoes depending on season.
Personality	Patience; ability to live in close proximity with other researchers, field assistants, camp staff; flexibility to cope with changing situations and plans; toughness to get through some difficult scenes (the chances of observing the tragedies of HEC are high); sense of humour!

with fall-out from HEC (human–elephant conflict) – be it damaged infrastructure, such as broken fences or lost crops, or injured or killed elephants, livestock or people. These are serious issues that are unfortunately widespread across elephants' range and must be dealt with extremely sensitively by the researchers. You must accept that dealing with these issues will take precedence over conducting your research.

Of course, it is possible to conduct fieldwork without partnering with an established elephant research project. However, this is not recommended for most finite research studies. The logistics could be immense and require a very significant investment of time and money. Where will you stay; what will you eat; how will you power your computer; what vehicle will you use in the field; how will you find any elephants; how will you identify the elephants; how will you habituate the elephants, so they are not aggressive or fearful of your presence; who will help you set up experiments and/or record data; will your research suffer if you are not permitted to drive 'off-road' in reserves (a privilege that is usually only afforded to established and well-respected research projects); how will you fund the costs of the research project; what will happen to the elephants once your research project ends? These are just a few of the problems that will require solutions before any research can begin. Arranging the logistics and preparing the science (the elephants would have to be habituated to your presence, and you would have to be able to identify them before any cognitive research gets underway, which could take several years), as well as the difficulties in even finding a suitable research population and obtaining agreement and permission to start a research project from all the relevant national and local authorities, means that, for most research aims, collaborating with an established research project site is likely to be the best solution.

Captive Elephant Research Considerations

As an alternative to field research on wild elephants, which necessarily requires months (at least) living in reasonably remote parts of Africa or Asia, it is also possible to conduct research projects on captive elephants living in zoos. As stated above, this may entail very small sample sizes – unless collaboration with a number of institutions is achieved, and can add confounds to your study in terms of the psychological well-being of the animals. However, it is likely that not all zoo animals are affected in this way, and the fact remains that some research questions probably cannot be answered experimentally with wild elephants.

If a captive setting is logistically and/or scientifically the most appropriate option for your study, it is important to first do some research on the life histories of the elephants at the potential facility. This is a sensitive issue, and zoos may be reticent with detailed information about their elephant collections, as they may be wary of any potentially negative information becoming widely available. But wherever possible, it would be useful to determine the sex and approximate ages of the potential elephant participants, as well as their relatedness and basic life histories (were they born in captivity or the wild; how long have they been at this institution; how many times have they moved institution; have they been moved with their family members/social group or separated from them; what is their social set-up now; are they housed in large groups or alone; do they appear to have strong social ties to the other elephants?). The answers to these types of questions will help you judge the potential stress levels of the animals and the extent of possible confounds on their psychological performance and well-being.

If possible, also find out what training and husbandry methods are used on the elephants. Hands-off, 'protected contact', for instance, implies that people usually remain behind a fence to prevent accidents, while 'free-contact' implies that handlers and elephants freely interact and touch each other, which often requires strict handling of the elephant by a person carrying an ankus or other means of physical control. The latter method may allow more freedom in test design, but in some settings may also render elephants more stressed and fearful, and so even more removed from 'normal' wild counterparts. The answers to at least some of these questions can usually be gleaned from simply visiting the zoo, spending some time observing the elephants and reading the information provided as part of the exhibit.

Once an appropriate captive facility has been identified, and you have sought and obtained permission to conduct your research there, the specific design of your study should be developed in consultation with zoo personnel and elephant handlers. For example, they may have specific rules about test rewards, or the time and duration of testing, among other things. Obesity can be a problem in captive elephants, so food rewards in particular will likely have to be carefully controlled. However, many zoos encourage enrichment and want to provide the elephants with new challenges to stimulate them, so such institutions may well be happy to collaborate.

Captive elephants can be encouraged to interact with equipment by handlers or induced by food rewards. However, there are individual differences in how quickly or easily they will become distracted, and it must be expected that females will be much less cooperative if they have been separated from their calves for the purposes of testing (although they are prone to being distracted if their calves are present).

Elephants can readily learn to identify people. There are lots of anecdotal reports of elephants remembering individual humans (both those that were kindly, and those that were not) and treating the people accordingly, years or decades later. So it is important to bear in mind that if testing or observations disrupt or stress the elephants and they associate this disruption with you, they may avoid you or act aggressively towards you for a long time afterwards. Captive research may be dependent on the handlers being present, but this could introduce confounds to the study if the elephants and handlers have a negative relationship. Assessing the relationship between elephants and handlers could thus be important.

A Day in the Life

As Table 8.1 suggests, there is much to plan and consider when conducting research with animals that are not housed in a laboratory situation. Both field and captive research requires careful consideration of all aspects of the process, from what research equipment is required and which data collection methods are most appropriate, to consideration of how you will maintain your own safety and well-being, in what can sometimes be very difficult, lonely or uncomfortable conditions. That being said, studying elephants is hugely enjoyable, and the rewards have always far outweighed the difficulties for me. I will describe a typical day in the field as I have experienced them, to help you decide if it sounds worth it to you.

Wake up before dawn, quickly freshen up and drink a cup of coffee, check you have all necessary equipment for field, apply sunscreen, drink more coffee, then head to the research vehicle. Fight with research vehicle to get it started (including but not limited to several bouts of mindless hammering on the bonnet), eventually prevail and head out into the field with fingers crossed.

Search for an elephant group to approach. Without the aid of radio-collars, elephants are usually encountered by luck, some judgement and seeking from higher ground (which usually means scanning the horizon with powerful binoculars, from the roof of a four-wheel drive vehicle, concentrating on the direction you saw most elephants moving yesterday). When elephants are spotted, drive closer to identify them, and then decide if that is a suitable group on which to begin data collection. If not, return to search mode. If yes, count and/or identify the animals present, and then begin data collection.

If observational study, ensure vehicle is parked in a suitable position to view the focal animals or behaviours, and make sure all required equipment is to hand (e.g. binoculars, cameras, notebooks or tablets, microphones and recording equipment, range-finders, etc.). If urine or dung samples are required, ensure the samples can be easily reached to bag/tube them once the elephants have moved away, without having to travel large distances by foot. If conducting experimental trials, attempt to predict the movements and activities of the elephants, prepare and wait for an opportune moment, and then attempt to set-up the experimental protocol in record-breaking time before the elephants move, change activity or otherwise stymie a potentially excellent trial. Take a deep breath and have a cup of coffee when elephants either suddenly change paths for no fathomable reason, and so miss experimental apparatus by a hundred metres, or start doing some particularly amazing and compelling behaviour just as they are entering a swamp where you cannot possibly get close enough to adequately record what is happening.

When the observations or trials are complete for that particular group, move away from the elephants, have a ‘comfort break’ behind the vehicle, while reprimanding self for drinking so much coffee; reapply sunscreen; have a snack and a drink (probably coffee); then resume search efforts to find another suitable elephant group. Depending on the habitat and season, this pattern may continue for much of the day, in which case make sure you carry a bucket of sunscreen, a hamper full of snacks and packed lunch, plenty of water, and – of course – several flasks of coffee.

Upon returning to the research camp in the afternoon or early evening, unload equipment from the vehicle; clean it (as necessary); recharge equipment batteries; download and back-up photo or data files; and write up any notes (remind self to not leave this to ‘later’, as you will forget the important little details and fail to make sense of your hasty scribbles from the field). Once this is complete, contemplate and then reject doing some kind of exercise to make up for having spent most of the day sat in a vehicle; attempt shower to wash off at least the surface layer of dusty sun cream; drown self in mosquito repellent; eat supper (which will taste eerily like mosquito repellent); check on all equipment; and prepare for the subsequent day in the field. Set pre-dawn alarm clock; make solemn promise to drink less coffee and do more squat-jumps tomorrow; collapse into bed, exhausted, sore and very happy.

Resources

The ElephantVoices website (www.elephantvoices.org), set up by Dr Joyce Poole and Petter Granli, contains a wealth of information about elephant life history, behaviour, communication and identification, as well as information about the anthropogenic threats that elephants currently face and the ethics of keeping them in captivity.

There are many brilliant documentaries about elephant behaviour and conservation. The recent 'Mind of a Giant' by Vulcan Productions for National Geographic explores and illustrates some of the cognition studies discussed here. However, the all-time best documentaries have to be the series of films produced for the BBC, beginning with 'Echo of the elephants', and the subsequent 'Echo of the elephants: the next generation'; 'Echo of the elephants: the final chapter?' and 'Echo – an unforgettable elephant', all filmed in Amboseli, Kenya, in collaboration with the Amboseli Trust for Elephants (www.elephanttrust.org).

The Elephant Specialist Advisory Group of South Africa (ESAG) recently published a field guide, *Understanding elephants: guidelines for safe and enjoyable elephant viewing* (2017), with information on behaviour and ecology, as well as chapters on how to safely observe wild savannah elephants and recognize their warning and threat signals. It is available from Amazon and other retailers.

There are several ongoing research projects studying various topics related to savannah elephants across Africa, with conservation being the common theme between them. Here are the very interesting websites of a few of them: Elephants Alive (www.elephantsalive.org); Elephants for Africa (www.elephantsforafrica.org); Elephants and Bees (www.elephantsandbees.com); Elephants without Borders (www.elephantswithoutborders.org); and Save the Elephants (www.savetheelephants.org).

Much of the information we have about African forest elephants comes from the work of the Elephant Listening Project, established by Dr Katy Payne and Andrea Turkalo (www.birds.cornell.edu/brp/elephant/index.html) and from a Wildlife Conservation Society research project at Mbeli Bai, in Congo (www.mbelibaistudy.org). Dr Vicki Fishlock and Dr Thomas Breuer edited a volume, *Studying forest elephants* (2015) which gives excellent practical advice and background information on forest elephants, available via the Wildlife Conservation Society press release pages. The best resource for studies of cognition in Asian elephants can be found at Think Elephants International (www.thinkelephants.org).

Profile

After an undergraduate research project on social learning in guppies, Lucy conducted her Masters and PhD research on wild chimpanzees in Budongo, Uganda.

She then decided she needed an even bigger challenge and started studying cognition in African elephants in 2005, with Professor Byrne at the University of St Andrews, UK, and in partnership with the Amboseli Trust for Elephants. From this privileged position, she began exploring elephant cognition with field-based experiments and analysis of observational data recorded by the Trust. Lucy then got sucked into the conservation world for several years, before returning to academic research in 2016, to continue her studies on elephant social cognition. Clearly, there is something very special about elephants, and while we know quite a bit about their social interactions and ecology, we still know almost nothing about their cognition. Those enormous brains are doing some remarkable things; she longs to find out what.

References

Archie, E. A., Morrison, T. A., Foley, C. A. H., Moss, C. J., and Alberts, S. C. (2006). Dominance rank relationships among wild female African elephants, *Loxodonta africana*. *Animal Behaviour*, **71**, 117–127.

Arvidsson, J., Amundin, M., and Laska, M. (2012). Successful acquisition of an olfactory discrimination test by Asian elephants, *Elephas maximus*. *Physiology and Behavior*, **105**, 809–814.

Bates, L. A., and Byrne, R. W. (2007). Creative or created: using anecdotes to investigate animal cognition. *Methods*, **42**, 12–21.

Bates, L. A., Sayialel, K. N., Njiraini, N. W., Moss, C. J., Poole, J. H., and Byrne, R. W. (2007). Elephants classify human ethnic groups by odor and garment color. *Current Biology*, **17**, 1–5.

Bates, L. A., Sayialel, K. N., Njiraini, N. W., Poole, J. H., Moss, C. J., and Byrne, R. W. (2008a). African elephants have expectations about the locations of out-of-sight family members. *Biology Letters*, **4**, 34–36.

Bates, L. A., Lee, P. C., Njiraini, N., *et al.* (2008b). Do elephants show empathy? *Journal of Consciousness Studies*, **15**, 204–225.

Bates, L. A., Handford, R., Lee, P. C., *et al.* (2010). Why do African elephants (*Loxodonta africana*) simulate oestrus? An analysis of longitudinal data. *PLoS ONE*, **5**(4), e10052.

Blake, S., Bouché, P., Rasmussen, H., Orlando, A., and Douglas-Hamilton, I. (2003). *The last Sahelian elephants: ranging behavior, population status and recent history of the desert elephants of Mali*. Report by Save the Elephants. Available at http://savetheelephants.org/wp-content/uploads/2016/11/2003Sahelianelephants.pdf

Blanc, J. (2008). *Loxondonta africana* IUCN status report. Retrieved from http://www.iucnredlist.org/details/12392/0

Boesch, C., and Boesch, H. (1990). Tool use and tool making in wild chimpanzees. *Folia Primatologica*, **54**, 86–99.

Burkart, J. M., Schubiger, M. N., and van Schaik, C. P. (2017). The evolution of general intelligence. *Behavioural and Brain Sciences*, **40**, e195.

Byrne, R. W., and Bates, L. A. (2007). Sociality, evolution and cognition. *Current Biology*, **17**, 714–723.

Byrne, R. W., and Bates, L. A. (2010). Review: primate social cognition: uniquely primate, uniquely social, or just unique? *Neuron*, **65**, 815–830.

Byrne, R. W., and Bates, L. A. (2011). Elephant cognition: what we know about what elephants know. In *The Amboseli elephants* (pp. 174–182). Chicago, IL: Chicago University Press.
Chevalier-Skolnikoff, S., and Liska, J. (1993). Tool use by wild and captive elephants. *Animal Behaviour*, **46**, 209–219.
Chiyo, P. I., Archie, E. A., Hollister-Smith, J. A., *et al.* (2011). Association patterns of African elephants in all-male groups: the role of age and genetic relatedness. *Animal Behaviour*, **81**, 1093–1099.
Choudhury, A., Lahiri Choudhury, D. K., Desai, A., *et al.* (2008). *Elephas maximus* status report. Retrieved from www.iucnredlist.org/details/7140/0.
Clubb, R., and Mason, G. (2002). A review of the welfare of zoo elephants in Europe. Report commissioned by the RSPCA. Available from https://science.rspca.org.uk/sciencegroup/wildlife/reportsandresources/captivity
Clubb, R., Rowcliffe, M., Lee, P., Mar, K. U., Moss, C., and Mason, G. J. (2008). Compromised survivorship in zoo elephants. *Science*, **322**, 1649.
Cozzi, B., Spagnoli, S., and Bruno, L. (2001). An overview of the central nervous system of the elephant through a critical appraisal of the literature published in the XIX and XX centuries. *Brain Research Bulletin*, **54**, 219–227.
Dale, R., and Plotnik, J. M. (2017). Elephants know when their bodies are obstacles to success in a novel transfer task. *Scientific Reports*, **7**, 46309.
De Silva, S., and Wittemyer, G. (2012). A comparison of social organization in Asian elephants and African savannah elephants. *International Journal of Primatology*, **33**, 1125–1141.
de Waal, F. B. M. (2016). *Are we smart enough to know how smart animals are?* New York, NY: W.W. Norton and Company.
Douglas-Hamilton, I., Bhalla, S., Wittemyer, G., and Vollrath, F. (2006). Behavioural reactions of elephants towards a dying and deceased matriarch. *Applied Animal Behaviour Science*, **100**, 87–102.
Fishlock, V., and Breuer, T. (2015). *Studying forest elephants*. Kerpen: Rettet die Elefanten Afrikas e.V.
Fishlock, V., Caldwell, C., and Lee, P. C. (2016). Elephant resource-use traditions. *Animal Cognition*, **19**, 429–433.
Foerder, P., Galloway, M., Barthel, T., Moore, D. E., and Reiss, D. (2011). Insightful problem solving in an Asian elephant. *PLoS ONE*, **6**(8), e23251.
Foley, C., PettorelliI, N., and Foley, L. (2008). Severe drought and calf survival in elephants. *Biology Letters*, **4**, 541–544.
Gallup, G. G. (1970). Chimpanzees: self-recognition. *Science*, **167**, 86–87.
Goldenberg, S. Z., Douglas-Hamilton, I., and Wittemyer, G. (2016). Vertical transmission of social roles drives resilience to poaching in elephant networks. *Current Biology*, **26**, 75–79.
Goodall, J. (1986). *The chimpanzees of Gombe*. Cambridge: Cambridge University Press.
Greco, B. J., Brown, T. K., Andrews, J. R. M., Swaisgood, R. R., and Caine, N. G. (2013). Social learning in captive African elephants (*Loxodonta africana africana*). *Animal Cognition*, **16**, 459–469.
Grubb, P., Groves, C., Dudley, J., and Shoshani, J. (2000). Living African elephants belong to two species: *Loxodonta africana* (Blumenbach, 1797) and *Loxodonta cyclotis* (Matschie, 1900). *Elephant*, **2**, 1–4.
Guldemond, R. A. R., Purdon, A., and Van Aarde, R. J. (2017). A systematic review of elephant impact across Africa. *PLoS ONE*, **12**(6), e0178935.
Hakeem, A. Y., Hof, P. R., Sherwood, C. C., Switzer, III, R. C., Rasmussen, L. E. L., and Allman, J. M. (2005). Brain of the African elephant (*Loxodonta africana*): neuroanatomy from magnetic

resonance images. *The Anatomical Record Part A: Discoveries in Molecular, Cellular, and Evolutionary Biology*, **287**, 1117–1127.

Hare, B., and Tomasello, M. (2004). Chimpanzees are more skilful in competitive than in cooperative cognitive tasks. *Animal Behaviour*, **68**, 571–581.

Hart, B., Hart, L. A., McCoy, M., and Sarath, C. (2001). Cognitive behaviour in Asian elephants: use and modification of branches for fly switching. *Animal Behaviour*, **62**, 839–847.

Hart, B. L., and Hart, L. A. (1994). Fly switching by Asian elephants: tool use to control parasites. *Animal Behaviour*, **48**, 35–45.

Hart, B. L., Hart, L. A., and Pinter-Wollman, N. (2008). Large brains and cognition: Where do elephants fit in? *Neuroscience and Biobehavioral Reviews*, **32**, 86–98.

Hunt, G. (1996). Manufacture and use of hook-tools by New Caledonian crows. *Nature*, **379**, 249–251.

Hunt, G. (2000). Human-like, population-level specialization in the manufacture of Pandanus tools by New Caledonian crows *Corvus moneduloids*. *Proceedings of the Royal Society of London B: Biological Sciences*, **267**, 403–413.

Kahl, M. P., and Armstrong, B. D. (2000). Visual and tactile displays in African elephants, *Loxodonta africana*: a progress report (1991–1997). *Elephant*, **2**, 19–21.

Langbauer, W. R. (2000). Elephant communication. *Zoo Biology*, **19**, 425–445.

Lee, P. (1987). Allomothering among African elephants. *Animal Behaviour*, **35**, 278–291.

Lee, P. C., and Moss, C. J. (1995). Statural growth in known-age African elephants (*Loxodonta africana*). *Journal of Zoology*, **236**, 29–41.

Lee, P. C., and Moss, C. J. (1999). The social context for learning and behavioural development amond wild African elephants. In *Mammalian social learning* (pp. 102–125). Cambridge: Cambridge University Press.

Lee, P. C., and Moss, C. J. (2014). African elephant play, competence and social complexity. *Animal Behavior and Cognition*, **2**, 144.

Lee, P. C., Lindsay, W. K., and Moss, C. J. (2011a). Ecological patterns of variability in demographic rates. In *The Amboseli elephants* (pp. 74–88). Chicago, IL: Chicago University Press.

Lee, P. C., Poole, J. H., Njiraini, N., Sayialel, K. N., and Moss, C. J. (2011b). Male social dynamics: independence and beyond. In *The Amboseli elephants* (pp. 260–271). Chicago, IL: Chicago University Press.

Lee, P. C., Fishlock, V., Webber, C. E., and Moss, C. J. (2016). The reproductive advantages of a long life: longevity and senescence in wild female African elephants. *Behavioral Ecology and Sociobiology*, **70**, 337–345.

Leggett, K. E. A. (2006). Home range and seasonal movement of elephants in the Kunene Region, northwestern Namibia. *African Zoology*, **41**, 17–36.

Mason, G. J., and Veasey, J. S. (2010). What do population-level welfare indices suggest about the well-being of zoo elephants? *Zoo Biology*, **29**, 256–273.

McComb, K., Moss, C., Sayialel, S., and Baker, L. (2000). Unusually extensive networks of vocal recognition in African elephants. *Animal Behaviour*, **59**, 1103–1109.

McComb, K., Moss, C., Durant, S. M., Baker, L., and Sayialel, S. (2001). Matriarchs act as repositories of social knowledge in African elephants. *Science*, **292**, 491–494.

McComb, K., Baker, L., and Moss, C. (2006). African elephants show high levels of interest in the skulls and ivory of their own species. *Biology Letters*, **2**, 26–28.

McComb, K., Shannon, G., Durant, S. M., Sayialel, K., Slotow, R., *et al.* (2011). Leadership in elephants: the adaptive value of age. *Proceedings of the Royal Society of London B: Biological Sciences*, **278**, 3270–3276.

McComb, K., Shannon, G., Sayialel, K. N., and Moss, C. (2014). Elephants can determine ethnicity, gender, and age from acoustic cues in human voices. *Proceedings of the National Academy of Sciences*, **111**, 5433–5438.

Meyer, M., Palkopoulou, E., Baleka, S., *et al.* (2017). Palaeogenomes of Eurasian straight-tusked elephants challenge the current view of elephant evolution. *eLife*, **6**, e25413.

Miller, A. K., Hensman, M. C., Hensman, S., *et al.* (2015). African elephants (*Loxodonta africana*) can detect TNT using olfaction: implications for biosensor application. *Applied Animal Behaviour Science*, **171**, 177–183.

Mizuno, K., Irie, N., Hiraiwa-Hasegawa, M., and Kutsukake, N. (2016). Asian elephants acquire inaccessible food by blowing. *Animal Cognition*, **19**, 215–222.

Moss, C. J. (2001). The demography of an African elephant (*Loxodonta africana*) population in Amboseli, Kenya. *Journal of Zoology*, **255**, 145–156.

Moss, C. J., and Lee, P. C. (2011a). Female reproductive strategies: individual life histories. In *The Amboseli elephants* (pp. 187–204). Chicago, IL: Chicago University Press.

Moss, C. J., and Lee, P. C. (2011b). Female social dynamics: fidelity and flexibility. In *The Amboseli elephants* (pp. 205–223). Chicago, IL: Chicago University Press.

Moss, C. J., and Poole, J. H. (1983). Relationships and social structure of African elephants. In *Primate social relationships: an integrated approach* (pp. 314–325). Oxford: Blackwells.

Nissani, M. (2006). Do Asian elephants (*Elephas maximus*) apply causal reasoning to tool-use tasks? *Journal of Experimental Psychology. Animal Behavior Processes*, **32**, 91–96.

Owen-Smith, N., Kerley, G. I. H., Page, B., Slotow, R., and Van Aarde, R. J. (2006). A scientific perspective on the management of elephants in the Kruger National Park and elsewhere. *South African Journal of Science*, **102**, 389–394.

Plotnik, J. M., and de Waal, F. B. M. (2014). Asian elephants (*Elephas maximus*) reassure others in distress. *PeerJ*, **2**, e278.

Plotnik, J. M., Lair, R., Suphachoksahakun, W., and de Waal, F. B. M. (2011). Elephants know when they need a helping trunk in a cooperative task. *Proceedings of the National Academy of Sciences*, **108**, 5116–5121.

Plotnik, J. M., Pokorny, J. J., Keratimanochaya, T., *et al.* (2013). Visual cues given by humans are not sufficient for Asian elephants (*Elephas maximus*) to find hidden food. *PLoS ONE*, **8**(4), e61174.

Plotnik, J. M., Shaw, R. C., Brubaker, D. L., Tiller, L. N., and Clayton, N. S. (2014). Thinking with their trunks: elephants use smell but not sound to locate food and exclude nonrewarding alternatives. *Animal Behaviour*, **88**, 91–98.

Polansky, L., Kilian, W., and Wittemyer, G. (2015). Elucidating the significance of spatial memory on movement decisions by African savannah elephants using state-space models. *Proceedings of the Royal Society of London B: Biological Sciences*, **282**, 20143042.

Poole, J. H. (1987). Rutting behaviour in African elephants: the phenomenon of musth. *Behaviour*, **102**, 283–316.

Poole, J. H. (1989a). Announcing intent: the aggressive state of musth in African elephants. *Animal Behaviour*, **37**, 140–152.

Poole, J. H. (1989b). Mate guarding, reproductive success and female choice in African elephants. *Animal Behaviour*, **37**, 842–849.

Poole, J. H., and Granli, P. (2011). Signals, gestures, and behavior of African elephants. In *The Amboseli elephants* (pp. 125–161). Chicago, IL: Chicago University Press.

Poole, J. H., and Moss, C. J. (1981). Musth in the African elephant *Loxodonta africana*. *Nature*, **292**, 830–831.

Poole, J. H., Tyack, P. L., Stoeger-Horwath, A. S., and Watwood, S. (2005). Elephants are capable of vocal learning. *Nature*, **434**, 455–456.

Povinelli, D. J. (1989). Failure to find self-recognition in Asian elephants (*Elephus maximus*) in contrast to their use of mirror cues to discover hidden food. *Journal of Comparative Psychology*, **103**, 122–131.

Rensch, B. (1957). The intelligence of elephants. *Scientific American*, **196**, 44–49.

Roca, A. L., Georgiadis, N., Pecon-Slattery, J., and Brien, S. J. O. (2001). Genetic evidence for two species of elephant in Africa. *Science*, **293**, 1473–1478.

Sanz, C., Call, J., and Morgan, D. (2009). Design complexity in termite-fishing tools of chimpanzees (*Pan troglodytes*). *Biology Letters*, **5**, 293–296.

Shettleworth, S. J. (1993). Where is the comparison in comparative cognition? Alternative research programs. *Psychological Science*, **4**, 179–184.

Shoshani, J., Kupsky, W. J., and Marchant, G. H. (2006). Elephant brain. Part I: gross morphology, functions, comparative anatomy, and evolution. *Brain Research Bulletin*, **70**, 124–157.

Smet, A. F., and Byrne, R. W. (2013). African elephants can use human pointing cues to find hidden food. *Current Biology*, **23**, 2033–2037.

Smet, A. F., and Byrne, R. W. (2014a). African elephants (*Loxodonta africana*) recognize visual attention from face and body orientation. *Biology Letters*, **10**, 20140428.

Smet, A. F., and Byrne, R. W. (2014b). Interpretation of human pointing by African elephants: generalisation and rationality. *Animal Cognition*, **17**, 1365–1374.

Spinage, C. (1994). *Elephants*. London: T and AD Poyser Ltd.

Stevens, J. R. (2010). The challenges of understanding animal minds. *Frontiers in Psychology*, **1**, 203.

Stoeger, A. S., Mietchen, D., Oh, S., *et al.* (2012). An Asian elephant imitates human speech. *Current Biology*, **22**, 2144–2148.

Sukumar, R. (2006). A brief review of the status, distribution and biology of wild Asian elephants. *International Zoo Yearbook*, **40**, 1–8.

Thuppil, V., and Coss, R. G. (2013). Wild Asian elephants distinguish aggressive tiger and leopard growls according to perceived danger. *Biology Letters*, **9**, 20130518.

van Aarde, R. J., Jackson, T. P., and Ferreira, S. M. (2006). Conservation science and elephant management in southern Africa. *South African Journal of Science*, **102**, 385–388.

Wittemyer, G., Douglas-Hamilton, I., and Getz, W. M. (2005). The socioecology of elephants: analysis of the processes creating multitiered social structures. *Animal Behaviour*, **69**, 1357–1371.

Wittemyer, G., Okello, J. B. A., Rasmussen, H. B., *et al.* (2009). Where sociality and relatedness diverge: the genetic basis for hierarchical social organization in African elephants. *Proceedings of the Royal Society of London B: Biological Sciences*, **276**, 3513–3521.

Yokoyama, S., Takenaka, N., Agnew, D. W., and Shoshani, J. (2005). Elephants and human color-blind deuteranopes have identical sets of visual pigments. *Genetics*, **170**, 335–344.

9 Fish – How to Ask Them the Right Questions

Catarina Vila Pouca and Culum Brown

Species Description

Brain

Arguably, the anatomical trait most relevant to fish cognition is the brain. Many fish brain regions are involved in specific cognitive tasks (see Broglio *et al.*, 2011). For example, the lateral telencephalic pallium is involved in encoding spatial information and in spatial learning, while the medial pallium is involved in emotional behaviour and emotional learning (Broglio *et al.*, 2005; Vargas *et al.*, 2009). Despite the morphological and architectural differences, most fish brain areas are homologous or analogous to tetrapod brain areas. Among other examples, there is strong evidence for the homology between the lateral telencephalic pallium of teleost fishes and the hippocampal pallium of land vertebrates, or between the teleost medial pallium and the tetrapod amygdala (Broglio *et al.*, 2011). This parallel in neural systems for learning and memory suggests a common evolutionary ancestry of cognitive functions, deeming fish an excellent group for comparative and evolutionary cognition studies.

Despite a common 'vertebrate brain plan', fish have far more neural plasticity than other vertebrates. The physical structure and functional organization of their brain is constantly moulded by environmental and behavioural inputs, and is continually gaining and losing neural connections throughout life (Ebbesson and Braithwaite, 2012). Furthermore, neurogenesis in fish during adulthood occurs in dozens of brain regions, while in mammals it is restricted to two (Zupanc *et al.*, 2005). Moreover, fish, like all vertebrates, have cerebral lateralization (i.e. a preference to use one side of the brain over the other one, to analyse specific stimuli or cues which often manifest as a side bias during experiments; Bisazza and Brown, 2011). Cognitive performance can be influenced by the complexity of the rearing environment, its habitat, and the direction and strength of lateralization of each fish (Brown *et al.*, 2003; Brown and Braithwaite, 2005; Bisazza and Brown, 2011).

Another anatomical characteristic of fish that has implications for comparative cognition studies is the absence of limbs and hand-like appendages. Nonetheless, fish can use their mouth to touch targets and even manipulate objects. For example, Bisazza and colleagues (2014a) successfully trained guppies to dislodge small plastic disks to retrieve food rewards.

Perception

Acquiring information from the environment is essential to cognition. Water differs from air in many ways, and fish have evolved special adaptations and senses for the aquatic environment.

The process of hearing in fish is quite diverse, with big anatomical variation in the ears across species. Some fish, such as sticklebacks, can only detect the particle motion component of sounds, while others like zebrafish or goldfish possess accessory hearing structures and can detect the pressure component (Fay and Popper, 2012). Fish also possess a lateral line system, additional to the conventional vertebrate inner ear, which allows them to detect vibration and water displacement information over the body surface (Higgs and Radford, 2013). Even though lots of fish rely on sound for many aspects of their life, there are surprisingly few cognition studies involving sound.

Most fish species have very good visual acuity, and tetrachromatic vision is the ancestral state. Goldfish, sticklebacks and guppies can all see ultraviolet (UV) light, which is important for communication and mate choice (Smith *et al.*, 2002). Many fish (e.g. goldfish) can even see polarized light, which is beneficial in enhancing contrast and object recognition, communication and navigation (Hawryshyn and McFarland, 1987; Cronin *et al.*, 2003). Because most fish have such good vision, researchers often use visual learning and memory tasks, including the use of mirrors, video playbacks and computer animations (Gori *et al.*, 2014; Qin *et al.*, 2014). These are generally useful, but we should be aware that the subjects might not be seeing the world as we do. As humans, fish are fooled by optical illusions (Agrillo *et al.*, 2013; Gori *et al.*, 2014), but in other situations there might be perceptual differences at the physiological and molecular level that we cannot identify from observing their behaviour. Mirrors are often used to study male aggression in sticklebacks, Siamese fighting fish and cichlids, and for a long time it was thought that fish do not show self-recognition and treat the mirror image as an opponent (Tinbergen, 1951; Thompson and Sturm, 1965; Franck and Ribowski, 1987). However, recent studies have found different brain activation, gene expression and hormonal levels between males fighting a mirror image and a real fish, which suggests some level of cognitive distinction between real life and mirror images (Desjardins and Fernald, 2010; Oliveira *et al.*, 2016). Adapting mirror tasks to a more natural setting, such as preventing the focal fish from getting too close to the mirror, reduces behavioural differences between tasks with mirror and live conspecifics (Cattelan *et al.*, 2017).

The senses of smell and taste of most fishes are also highly developed, and their taste buds are present in many body regions (mouth, barbels, gills and pharynx to fins or whole body surface; Hara, 2012). Fish use chemosensory abilities for foraging, navigation, predator recognition, mate choice or individual and self-recognition (Milinski, 2003; Mehlis *et al.*, 2008; Thünken *et al.*, 2009; Brown *et al.*, 2011b; Hara, 2012). For this reason, the way reinforcement is provided during learning experiments, as well as the potential interference of alarm or social cues, needs to be carefully assessed.

In addition to conventional senses, some species of fish have electrogenic, electroreceptive or magnetoreceptive abilities, meaning they can produce electricity and/or detect and respond to electric or magnetic fields (including the Earth's), respectively (Nelson, 2011; Putman *et al.*, 2014). These senses are especially important for foraging, navigation and communication.

Life Cycle

In general, fish have a faster life cycle than most vertebrates and reach sexual maturity at an early age, but there are major variations between species. For example, guppies and zebrafish can be sexually mature at approximately 3 months and have a lifespan of 1–2 years in the wild. Sticklebacks can take up to 2 years to reach sexual maturity and may live about 4 years in the wild. Goldfish, on the other hand, are sexually mature at the age of one, and typically live for 5–10 years, but in large outdoor ponds they can live for up to 30 years. Lungfish and coelacanth live for more than 100 years.

As fish have substantial neural plasticity and neurogenesis throughout their life, the most significant transition in their cognitive development is reaching sexual maturity. This activates hormonal and behavioural differences between sexes, as well as sensory and behavioural biases that we need to consider when designing cognitive tasks, especially in species with strong sexual dimorphism and mate choice. Breeding male sticklebacks and guppies, for example, have conspicuous red and orange carotenoid coloration, respectively, and both sexes show a strong bias for red/orange objects in non-mating contexts (Rodd *et al.*, 2002; Smith *et al.*, 2004). Even species that do not show strong sexual dimorphism, or red coloration, such as zebrafish, may display a bias towards red, which may mirror a foraging preference (Spence and Smith, 2008). This preference can be disruptive when training fish against the colour red (Laland and Williams, 1997), and it may be better to use other stimuli colours (e.g. green, yellow or white; Reader *et al.*, 2003; Brown and Braithwaite, 2005).

During the breeding season, many fish species show strong male aggression and competition. Researchers have taken advantage of these behaviours to investigate personality and laterality traits, mate choice, individual recognition and transitive inference (Sovrano *et al.*, 1999; Grosenick *et al.*, 2007; Archard and Braithwaite, 2011). In particular, fish deduced overall social hierarchy relationships between all males, after observing pairwise fights between them (Grosenick *et al.*, 2007). Numerous species school and live in social groups for most of their lives, so we can use conspecifics as rewards in learning tasks, or even as choice stimuli in numerical discrimination experiments (Al-Imari and Gerlai, 2008; Agrillo *et al.*, 2014a). As fish tend to prefer bigger schools, one can present them with schools of differing sizes, and infer from their choices if they can distinguish between them (Agrillo *et al.*, 2014a). In this context, we often use female subjects because they show stronger schooling behaviour, while males in mixed-sex schools tend to disrupt behaviour with their mating attempts (Swaney *et al.*, 2001).

Besides considering biological and social differences between species and sexes, we often must consider variability in learning ability at the population level, which is due to both evolutionary and developmental factors. Environmental complexity and predation risk, for instance, are related to variability in individual behaviour, personality and cognition (Brown and Braithwaite, 2005; Brown *et al.*, 2011a). Moreover, captivity may remove, modify or intensify some selective pressures, and in just a few generations we can see differences in behaviour, learning and memory between wild fish and domestic strains (Brown and Braithwaite, 2005; Spence *et al.*, 2011; White and Brown, 2014).

Individual Identification

Identification of individuals is a must in some behavioural experiments, but artificial marking might be stressful and affect aspects of behaviour (Frommen *et al.*, 2015; Fürtbauer *et al.*, 2015). Strong sexual dimorphism is helpful with some species (e.g. Brown and Laland, 2002b). In sticklebacks, disc-shaped tags that carry specific markings identifiable by the researcher or by video software can be mounted on their dorsal spines, removing the need for invasive markings (e.g. Kleinhappel *et al.*, 2014). In the absence of distinctive colour markings (i.e. zebrafish and goldfish), it is common to mark the fish with injected visible implant fluorescent elastomers (VIE) or subcutaneous dyes (e.g. Croft *et al.*, 2004).

Fish can be quite engaging and show rapid learning in many cognitive tasks, but they are also prone to stress or motivation loss during experimentation. Most fish release alarm substances when stressed, and this can impact all other fish in the group, as well as fish tested in the apparatus in the future. Frequent water changes prevent this from being an issue. To reduce the initial stress of being moved to the experimental tank, we can catch the fish in containers so they remain submerged, or even set up testing arenas within their housing tanks, to avoid moving them at all (Brown and Laland, 2002a; Agrillo *et al.*, 2012). If animals must be moved, sufficient recovery time is required. As with other animals, fish can also be distracted by noise when performing tasks that require concentration (Purser and Radford, 2011).

Fish have low metabolic rates and thus will soon loose motivation to feed. This can be overcome by using alternative rewards such as a shelter (e.g. White and Brown, 2014), or by studying escape responses (e.g. Brown and Warburton, 1999). In social species, it is common to have mirrors or conspecifics in sight behind a transparent partition, to avoid social isolation stress (e.g. Bisazza *et al.*, 2014b). In other cases, dominance hierarchies can prevent fish from performing when the alpha is within sight (Brown *et al.*, 2003). Shoaling preference can be used as a reinforcer (e.g. Al-Imari and Gerlai, 2008), yet fish may become familiar with the procedure, and the shoal might lose reward value after repeated testing (Agrillo *et al.*, 2012). Loss of motivation is generally counterbalanced with quick tasks, small delays between start of the trial and stimulus presentation, small intertrial intervals, and few trials per session (e.g. Brown, 2001). In some contexts, fish are better at learning with stimuli in motion, as compared to static stimuli (Agrillo *et al.*, 2014b).

State of the Art

Sticklebacks

Sticklebacks have been used as model species for investigating cognition for well over a century. Notably, all three joint 1973 Nobel prize winners, Tinbergen, Lorenz and von

Frisch, used sticklebacks as model organisms. Their popularity is largely due to their whole Arctic distribution, and the ease with which they adjust to life in aquaria.

Sticklebacks rely on learning for nearly all aspects of their behaviour. In the context of social behaviour, they have preferred partners when inspecting predators and can use tit-for-tat rules during cooperation (Milinski, 1987; Milinski *et al.*, 1990). They prefer shoaling with familiar individuals (Barber and Ruxton, 2000) and in familiar groups with reduced aggression (Utne-Palm and Hart, 2000). Their ability to distinguish between individuals is driven by their keen sense of smell, but they can also distinguish between conspecifics using visual cues alone (Waas and Colgan, 1994). Sticklebacks can distinguish kin from non-kin based on MHC alleles (Mehlis *et al.*, 2008), and they optimize mate choice accordingly (Milinski, 2003). Despite the very stereotyped mating behaviour, they can modify their courtship preferences through learning (Sevenster and Van Roosmalen, 1985; Jenkins and Rowland, 1997). They also differentiate individuals and preferentially associate with them, based on diet and habitat occupancy (Ward *et al.*, 2005). This high selectivity for schooling partners facilitates social learning. Sticklebacks weigh up their own private knowledge against public knowledge (i.e. social learning) when making decisions (van Bergen *et al.*, 2004), and the social network is a good predictor of the discovery of novel information (Atton *et al.*, 2012). Sticklebacks adopt a 'follow the majority' rule (Pike and Laland, 2010) and prefer to follow large, presumably experienced demonstrators (Duffy *et al.*, 2009). The demonstrator they choose to follow also varies depending on their perception of how successful the demonstrator is (Pike *et al.*, 2010). Reliance on social learning varies between species; three-spined sticklebacks are less inclined than nine-spined sticklebacks to use public information, possibly because they are less prone to predation (Coolen *et al.*, 2003).

Population differences in stickleback learning abilities are driven by a mixture of genes and environment. Freshwater sticklebacks in environments with higher prey stability, for instance, have better memory retention than marine sticklebacks from unstable habitats (Mackney and Hughes, 1995). Sticklebacks from different environments vary in learning rates and the cues they use to navigate (Girvan and Braithwaite, 1998; Odling-Smee *et al.*, 2008). Sticklebacks from high-predation populations, for example, learn a conditioned avoidance task significantly faster than those from low-predation areas (Huntingford and Wright, 1992). The maternal environment may also influence cognitive development. Young sticklebacks whose mothers were chased by a model predator learned to associate food rewards with coloured chambers more slowly than fish whose mother had not been harassed (Roche *et al.*, 2012). Many of these differences in learning between populations are underpinned by variation in brain morphology (Gonda *et al.*, 2009).

Goldfish

Like sticklebacks, goldfish have a long history of being used in the lab, largely because they have been domesticated for over 1000 years and are relatively easy to maintain. However, there has been less emphasis on ecological approaches to cognition and a primary focus on comparative psychology. Goldfish rank alongside pigeons and rats as the model species of choice for comparative studies.

Their learning and memory consolidation in shock avoidance paradigms is well documented (e.g. Bitterman, 1964). For example, goldfish swim spontaneously against a flow to access calm water, but show avoidance behaviour after a single shock (Riege and Cherkin, 1971). Goldfish are also willing to trade-off shock avoidance to access conspecifics (Dunlop *et al.*, 2006), indicating that their avoidance behaviour is not reflexive, and that they can make complex decisions when balancing out conflicts between various motivators.

Goldfish have also been commonly tested with positive reinforcement paradigms. Among the early experiments on learning in goldfish, Perkins and Wheeler (1930) used a food conditioning paradigm to show that goldfish could discriminate different levels of light intensity. Goldfish trained with large rewards took longer to extinguish their learned behaviour than those trained with small rewards (Mackintosh, 1971), and reinforcement was stronger with shorter delays between stimulus and reward (Breuning *et al.*, 1981).

Early studies on spatial learning showed that goldfish can learn to swim a maze of 'moderate difficulty' and retain their learning for 13 days (Churchill, 1916). Fish trained in a four-arm maze rapidly solve the task using egocentric, allocentric and a combination of both cue types. Interestingly, fish trained in the allocentric set-up move directly towards the goal, even from novel starting points, which indicates the formation of a mental map (Rodríguez *et al.*, 1994). Moreover, goldfish can rely on both direct landmarks (e.g. a beacon on the food patch) and indirect landmarks (e.g. a beacon on the opposite side of the tank) to locate hidden food patches (Warburton, 1990), relying on different cognitive strategies (i.e. guidance strategy versus spatial mapping system, respectively; López *et al.*, 1999).

Goldfish indirectly learn about predators by recognizing the smell of dead conspecifics in the predator's diet and then pairing it with the predator's smell. Their response to the chemical cues is risk-sensitive, varying depending on the perceived level of risk (Zhao *et al.*, 2006). Goldfish are willing to pay a cost for access to conspecifics, suggesting that being in large groups has benefits other than deterring predators (Pitcher and Magurran, 1983), including increased foraging efficiency through social learning (Pitcher *et al.*, 1982). Goldfish can recognize other goldfish using chemical cues alone (Sisler and Sorensen, 2008), and isolation stress can interfere with memory formation (Laudien *et al.*, 1986).

Early research on object discrimination showed that goldfish have no problem discriminating between geometric shapes (Herter, 1929). Moreover, fish trained to discriminate between squares and triangles transfer that training to Kanizsa squares and triangles, suggesting their visual perception is similar to humans (Wyzisk and Neumeyer, 2007).

Finally, there has been a huge amount of work on various parts of the goldfish brain responsible for learning. Their brain is very similar to other vertebrates in terms of its functional capabilities (see Broglio *et al.*, 2011).

Guppies

Guppies have been long used as model species to investigate the impacts of environmental variation (especially in predation pressure) in a range of life-history and behaviour traits, including cognition (Reznick *et al.*, 2001). Guppies have featured heavily in work focusing on social learning, social cognition, predator–prey interactions, numerical cognition and laterality (see Evans *et al.*, 2011). Here, we briefly describe some of the research on numerical skills and social learning.

Overall, fish numerical skills compare favourably with terrestrial vertebrates, and the underlying cognitive mechanisms seem to be much the same (Agrillo and Bisazza, 2014). Fish can accurately track around four objects and use an approximation system for comparing larger numbers following Weber's law. Although untrained guppies only discriminate three versus four social companions (Bisazza *et al.*, 2010), increased training improves their discrimination capabilities to five versus six (Bisazza *et al.*, 2014a). Numerical skills are also greater in fish that have stronger cerebral lateralization (Bisazza and Brown, 2011), which is consistent with work in other animals showing that laterality is linked to cognition (e.g. parrots: Magat and Brown, 2009).

Social learning has been a topic of immense interest, and guppies often serve as ideal models (see Brown and Laland, 2011). Social learning offers a more rapid mode of learning than individual learning (Brown and Laland, 2002b) and can be used by guppies to gain a variety of information, including on predators and prey (Reader *et al.*, 2003). However, social learning can also lead to the adoption of maladaptive information (Laland and Williams, 1998) in the absence of 'proof checking' through individual assessment. Close examination of social interactions (e.g. through social network analysis) can reveal how information passes through populations (Reader and Laland, 2000). Interestingly, social learning is facilitated by both shoaling (Laland and Williams, 1997) and familiarity among individuals (Swaney *et al.*, 2001).

Although larger brains are costly, they can lead to better cognitive performance, including in numerical associative learning tasks (Kotrschal *et al.*, 2013). Brain size and learning rate are similar for guppies from high- and low-predation regimes, although the former take longer to make decisions (Burns and Rodd, 2008).

Zebrafish

Zebrafish are a model organism for neurobiological and genetic studies and can thus help identify the mechanisms of cognition (Sison *et al.*, 2006). They are a reasonably social species, and their attraction to conspecifics can provide a useful reward in associative learning trials (Al-Imari and Gerlai, 2008). Shoal interactions are non-random structured social networks, with key individuals playing important leadership roles (Vital and Martins, 2011). Like many fish, zebrafish show a preference for familiar conspecific phenotypes from the juvenile phases (Engeszer *et al.*, 2007) and for larger and more active shoals (Pritchard *et al.*, 2001). Social recognition, including kin recognition, can occur through chemosensory as well as visual cues, and seems to rely on phenotype matching (Gerlach and Lysiak, 2006). Close social ties facilitate social learning of predator cues (Hall and Suboski, 1995). Zebrafish can also learn novel escape routes by following demonstrators, maintaining arbitrary preferences for one escape route, after demonstrators have been removed (Lindeyer and Reader, 2010). Zebrafish also eavesdrop on social signals between conspecifics to obtain information (Lopes *et al.*, 2016). Abril-de-Abreu and colleagues (2015) showed that the attention of zebrafish is more likely to be directed towards interacting conspecifics, and that they pay attention to different details during different fight phases.

A series of experiments examining the learning and memory mechanisms in zebrafish has shown them to be very similar to those observed in terrestrial vertebrates (a consistent emerging theme in all fish cognition research), reinforcing the notion that these mechanisms are highly conserved (Xu *et al.*, 2007). For example, zebrafish learn to feed on alternating sides of a fish tank following the onset of a light cue in just 14 trials and retain the information for 10 days in the absence of reinforcement (Williams *et al.*, 2002). Spence and colleagues (2011) showed that spatial learning ability in two strains of zebrafish was improved by increasing the complexity of the rearing environment, with implications for lab housing conditions when testing cognitive performance. Likewise, zebrafish showed rapid learning to avoid a moving net and could also be trained to move to the left or right, as part of the avoidance response (Arthur and Levin, 2001).

All for One and One for All

Box 9.1 Investigating Memory in Novel Animal Models

Jonathon D. Crystal

Zebrafish (*Danio rerio*) is increasingly being used as an animal model of cognition, given its widespread use in developmental biology and genetics. One area of cognition focuses on episodic memory, which stores personal past experiences. The central hypothesis of an animal model of episodic memory is that, at the moment of a memory assessment, the animal retrieves a memory of the specific earlier event (Crystal, in press). In addition to episodic memory, an animal may rely on familiarity with a stimulus; notably, according to this alternative, the strength of a memory trace may provide a useful cue, because memory traces passively decline after presentation of a stimulus.

A prominent approach to evaluating episodic memory in animals (e.g. Eacott and Norman, 2004; Dere *et al.*, 2005; Kart-Teke *et al.*, 2006; Belblidia *et al.*, 2015; de Souza Silva *et al.*, 2015; Hamilton *et al.*, 2016) capitalizes on animals' natural tendency to explore novel situations. Novelty-seeking may be based on the widespread phenomenon of habituation. Habituation is typically defined as learning about a stimulus (Thompson and Spencer, 1966). For example, when a loud noise is presented, many animals display a startle response. When the same noise is presented repeatedly, the magnitude of the startle response tends to decline.

How can novelty approaches be used to explore episodic memory in animals? A recent demonstration of episodic memory in zebrafish serves as an example. Hamilton and colleagues (2016) exposed zebrafish to a tank of water with multiple

(cont.)

features, including two objects placed on left or right sides of the tank, with the tank surrounded by one of two distinctive colours. In the first presentation of features, one object appeared on the left, and the other object appeared on the right, both in a yellow tank. In the second presentation of features, the left–right locations of the objects were reversed, and the tank was blue. In the memory assessment, one object was presented in both left and right locations of a blue tank. If the fish remembers the object, location and colour, it will spend more time inspecting the object that appears at the location that was not previously presented in that colour context. Although the scenario described above gives an example sequence of features, the features were counterbalanced across different fish. Overall, individual fish spent more time inspecting the novel object–location–colour item.

Why does the fish explore the novel object–location–colour combination? According to the episodic-memory proposal, the fish retrieves an episodic memory of the initial presentation of item, location and context; the item–location–context is compared to the current options, namely two object–location–contexts (only the location feature varies in the memory assessment), and chooses to spend more time in the location that does not match the retrieved object–location–context. Notice that familiarity is inherently embedded in the proposed episodic-memory explanation outlined above: one object–location–context is more familiar than the other, and the novelty preference is expressed by spending more time in the less-familiar option.

The increasing use of zebrafish in cognitive studies provides opportunities to take approaches commonly used with other animals and import for use with fish. Some examples include: episodic memory, source memory, what-where-when memory and retrieval practice (Babb and Crystal, 2005, 2006; Zhou *et al.*, 2012; Crystal *et al.*, 2013a, b; Panoz-Brown *et al.*, 2016) – all approaches that have been successfully used with rats and could be adapted to study fish cognition.

References

Babb, S. J., and Crystal, J. D. (2005). Discrimination of what, when, and where: Implications for episodic-like memory in rats. *Learning & Motivation*, **36**, 177–189.

Babb, S. J., and Crystal, J. D. (2006). Episodic-like memory in the rat. *Current Biology*, **16**, 1317–1321.

Belblidia, H., Abdelouadoud, A., Jozet-Alves, C., *et al.* (2015). Time decay of object, place and temporal order memory in a paradigm assessing simultaneously episodic-like memory components in mice. *Behavioural Brain Research*, **286**, 80–84.

Crystal, J. D. (in press). Animal models of episodic memory. *Comparative Cognition & Behavior Reviews*.

Crystal, J. D., Alford, W.T., Zhou, W., and Hohmann, A. G. (2013a). Source memory in the rat. *Current Biology*, **23**, 387–391.

Crystal, J. D., Ketzenberger, J. A., and Alford, W. T. (2013b). Practicing memory retrieval improves long-term retention in rats. *Current Biology*, **23**, 708–709.

(cont.)

de Souza Silva, M. A., Huston, J. P., Wang, A. L., Petri, D., and Chao, O.Y. H. (2015). Evidence for a specific integrative mechanism for episodic memory mediated by AMPA/kainate receptors in a circuit involving medial prefrontal cortex and hippocampal CA3 region. *Cerebral Cortex*, **26**, 3000–3009.

Dere, E., Huston, J. P., and de Souza Silva, M. A. (2005). Episodic-like memory in mice: simultaneous assessment of object, place and temporal order memory. *Brain Research Protocols*, **16**, 10–19.

Eacott, M. J., and Norman, G. (2004). Integrated memory for object, place, and context in rats: a possible model of episodic-like memory? *The Journal of Neuroscience*, **24**, 1948–1953.

Hamilton, T. J., Myggland, A., Duperreault, E., *et al.* (2016). Episodic-like memory in zebrafish. *Animal Cognition*, **19**, 1071–1079.

Kart-Teke, E., de Souza Silva, M. A., Huston, J. P., and Dere, E. (2006). Wistar rats show episodic-like memory for unique experiences. *Neurobiology of Learning and Memory*, **85**, 173–182.

Panoz-Brown, D. E., Corbin, H. E., Dalecki, S. J., *et al.* (2016). Rats remember items in context using episodic memory. *Current Biology*, **26**, 2821–2826.

Thompson, R. F., and Spencer, W. A. (1966). Habituation: a model phenomenon for the study of neuronal substrates of behavior. *Psychological Review*, **73**, 16–43.

Zhou, W., Hohmann, A. G., and Crystal, J. D. (2012). Rats answer an unexpected question after incidental encoding. *Current Biology*, **22**, 1149–1153.

Field Guide

Husbandry

Starting a fish lab is reasonably straightforward. The models discussed here are all freshwater fish, thus maintaining them is very easy. There are two basic set-ups. The first one is a flow-through system that is very popular with zebrafish researchers. A single large sump and filtration system supplies a number of small aquariums on a racking system. Water quality is monitored regularly, paying attention to pH and the ammonia cycle. Low water quality is best prevented by water changes. In most countries, aged tapwater is sufficient. It is vital to ensure that the chlorine in town water has had time to breakdown, as it is toxic to most aquatic animals. Water temperature is typically maintained by adjusting room temperature.

The second system is better suited to situations where fish will be sourced from multiple, wild populations. Here, isolated aquaria are a better option for quarantine reasons, so each aquarium has its own filtration system, nets and cleaning accessories. Water temperature can be adjusted using heaters in each aquarium or maintained by room temperature. This set-up will prevent diseases and parasites moving between aquaria.

When sourcing fish from the wild, most countries will insist on the researcher obtaining permits first. Sourcing captive fish, on the other hand (e.g. guppies or zebrafish), is simply a matter of identifying a reputable supplier. Running fish through multiple cognition tasks is often not a problem, as long as sufficient time has passed between experiments. Often, however, it may be simpler to rehome fish.

Spatial Learning

One of the most common methods for studying fish cognition is to use spatial learning tasks. Spatial learning is often studied using a T-maze or a plus maze, which has its roots in the rodent literature. In our lab, a modified plus maze (so that one of the arms can be partitioned off to form a T) is commonly used (Figure 9.1). The subjects learn one of two possible routes to access a reward (food, shelter, mirror, etc.). Once subjects have made a choice, they can be returned to the start position, or their current position can become the new start position. By rotating the start position, one can eliminate reliance on extra-maze cues and reduce handling stress. Thus, multiple tests can be run in rapid succession.

In spatial learning tests, it is important that the fish are first given a chance to become familiar with the testing environment (Brown, 2001) by allowing them free access to the apparatus for 24 hours before testing begins. This can occur in small groups to improve efficiency. Feeding can take place in the apparatus in random locations during the orientation period. We often employ two identical mazes, so we can alternate between them: one batch of fish can be familiarized in one maze, while the other group of fish is run in the other maze.

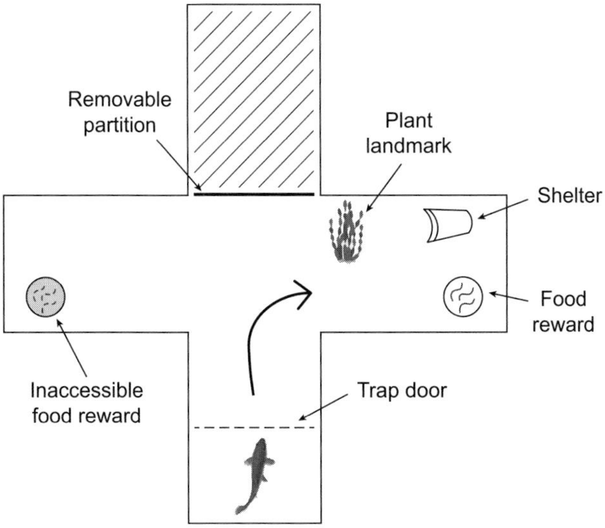

Figure 9.1. Diagram of a plus maze (top view), modified to work as a T-maze. The arrow indicates the correct route a fish trained to the right arm had to take in order to obtain food and shelter. In this example, the fish can use either direct cues (plant landmark) or a body-centred algorithm ('turn right') to learn the task.

Table 9.1. Essential experimental tools required to study fish.

Mask, snorkel and fins
Wetsuit and boots (freshwater tends to be cold), or waders if you are electrofishing
Sunscreen, hat and polarized sunglasses
Fish nets, traps and containers to catch your fish (you can never have too many buckets!)
GPS
Tagging kit (we nearly always use polymer elastomer injection)
Tape measure and fish scale
Stopwatch
Waterproof paper to take notes
Action cameras and all that fancy equipment to record your trials
A lot of patience and an optimistic attitude
Tolerance to a range of weather conditions
Willing to get wet, muddy and potentially scratched
Not afraid of a few leeches and ticks, and the occasional snake or freshwater crocodile
Capable of spending several weeks in the field, without internet access or other commodities
Other useful items include: thermal bottle (and water purification tablets, depending on your sampling location), waterproof torch, dry bag, waterproof phone case, laptop Pelican case (if you can afford it!)

The number of trials to reach learning criteria can vary greatly between species, but up to 50 exposures are generally required. A common success criterion is completing 7/8 or 8/10 trials correctly. One can also record the number of arms entered, the number of mistakes made and the latency to enter the correct arm: all are good indicators of learning. In a typical day, a single fish might only be tested about four times due to motivation constraints.

T-mazes can also be used to examine the types of cues fish use to navigate, or whether they learn body-centred algorithms, such as 'always turn right' (e.g. White and Brown, 2014). One can also run probe trials where cues are placed into conflict. For example, a fish may have been trained to turn right and follow a landmark (Figure 9.1), but in the probe trial the landmark can be switched to the left, and the fish must decide whether to follow an egocentric or cue-based strategy. In this manner, one can determine the hierarchical organization of orientation strategies.

Memory retention is typically investigated by withdrawing individuals from training and testing them at pre-determined intervals (e.g. 1 day, 2 days, 3 days, 1 week, 1 month). Fish will often remember training for several weeks or months in the absence of any reinforcement. Reversal learning is also possible using this paradigm, where the fish are trained to an alternative location or using different cues.

Social Learning

To study social learning in fish (see Brown and Laland, 2011), the key is to illustrate that the subject learns the task significantly faster in a group than alone (i.e. via trial and error). The simplest test is to teach fish to swim through a doorway to access food. The food might be delivered manually with tweezers in a specific place, such as a floating ring (Figure 9.2A), or attached with petroleum jelly to a Petri dish or some other part of the tank. In all cases, we first need to train *demonstrator* fish that will later be used to demonstrate the behaviour to the naïve *observers*. We can use these data as control data to illustrate how long naïve individuals take to learn the task in isolation. However, further controls also account for the number of fish present, by testing naïve fish in pairs (which sometimes perform worse than solitary individuals; Brown and Laland, 2002b). Also, keep in mind that your demonstrators can be so quick that the observer has no chance to copy it! Thus, mediocre demonstrators may be better (Swaney *et al.*, 2001).

In general, there are two approaches to expose the observer fish to the demonstrators' performance. Observers may watch the demonstrator perform the task while constrained behind a partition or can interact with the demonstrator directly (i.e. they get to do the

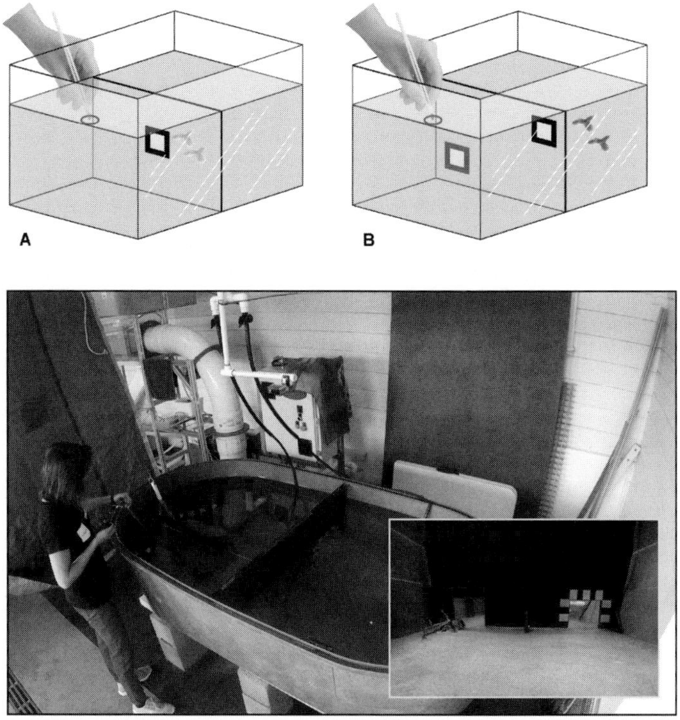

Figure 9.2. Top: diagram of a common experimental apparatus to study social learning in fish, illustrating (A) one- or (B) two-route options, to access a food reward manually provided in a floating feeder ring. Bottom: photo of Catarina giving a food reward to a juvenile Port Jackson shark, which swam through the correct door. Inset: in-water view of the shark as it swims through the door. Note that with two-route options, fish must make a choice as to which foraging route they will use.

task alongside the demonstrator). To some degree, the approach will depend on the species being tested. Highly anti-social, aggressive species are best tested with the partition method (e.g. Brown *et al.*, 2003; but see Trompf and Brown, 2014), while social species do well using the latter approach (e.g. guppies: Brown and Laland, 2002b).

We can also ask fish to swim through one of two holes, making a choice as to which foraging route they will use (e.g. Laland and Williams, 1997; Brown and Laland, 2002b; Figure 9.2B). In this instance, demonstrators are trained to swim through one of two routes to access a food reward, so we can test whether observers (1) pass through any door more quickly than control fish, and (2) show fidelity to the door used by the demonstrator. This arbitrary use of one route or the other is how even maladaptive cultural traditions start and are maintained (Laland and Williams, 1998).

Finally, one can determine how long information is retained by the observers, in the absence of the demonstrators. The simplest version of this is a memory retention test, whereby the observers are tested at various time points post-demonstrator experience. A more complicated version is to run a transmission chain test, where demonstrators are gradually removed from the population and replaced by naïve observers (Figure 9.3; e.g. Laland and Williams, 1997). This process more closely mimics the situation in wild animal populations, where old knowledgeable leaders die, and new recruits take their place.

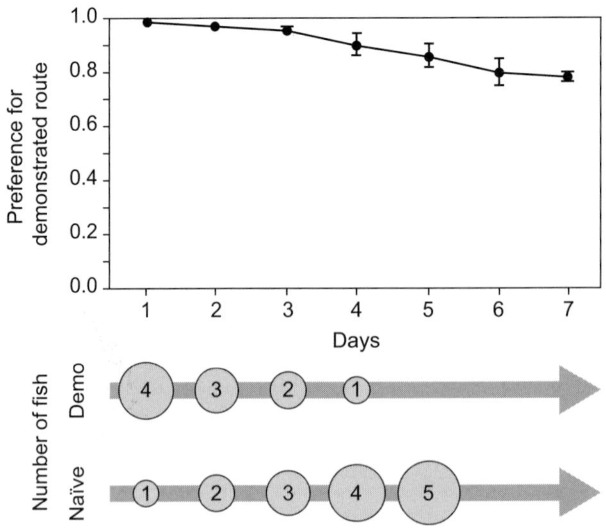

Figure 9.3. The proportion of trials per day, in which naïve observer fish took the demonstrated route to a food source, in a transmission chain design. Each day, one of the demonstrator fish is replaced by a new observer.

Adapted from: Laland, K.N., and Williams, K. (1997). Shoaling generates social learning of foraging information in guppies, *Animal Behaviour*, **53**, 1161–1169. Copyright (1997), with permission from Elsevier.

The Devil Is in the Details

Box 9.2 Cichlid Social Cognition

Michael Taborsky and Barbara Taborsky

Cichlids are different. Among fishes, they strike through their great behavioural repertoire, advanced sociality, adaptive radiation and associated evolvability of behaviour (Barlow, 2000; Taborsky, 2016; Taborsky and Wong, 2017). This renders them ideal candidates for studies of cognitive mechanisms involved in social interactions.

Visual communication in cichlids is conspicuous, variable with context and between species, and often complex (Baerends and Baerends van Roon, 1950; Keenleyside, 1991; Barlow, 2000). This involves graded signals between individuals competing for resources in the form of an escalation cascade or the mutual exchange of signals between partners in courtship. The great responsiveness of cichlids to visual cues and signals has led to the widespread application of a simple technique to release measurable and predictable aggressive responses: the use of mirrors. However, this method is by no means appropriate for all cichlid species. Its suitability depends primarily on the preferred orientation of rivals in aggressive encounters, which can be frontal or sideways (Balzarini *et al.*, 2014).

The exchange of signals is not confined to the visual domain. Chemical and acoustic signals may be similarly important, and the transfer of information may be greatly enhanced by multimodal signalling. In the cooperatively breeding cichlid *Neolamprologus pulcher*, for example, chemical signals can change both the visual display patterns of territory owners and their response to the presence and behaviour of competitors (Bayani *et al.*, 2017). It is hence important to consider all modalities of potential importance when studying information exchange between social partners and the underlying cognitive processes.

The social environment is the most complex and fluctuating component of an animal's ecology, as it involves interactions with other unpredictable behavioural agents. In highly social animals, such as *N. pulcher*, virtually all daily activities involve social interactions. Therefore, these fish would benefit from cognitive mechanisms allowing them to assess, integrate and process cues of the internal state of conspecifics and social context, to fine-tune their behaviour according to the situation. The ability of individuals to flexibly regulate the expression of their social behaviour in order to optimize their social relationships is referred to as 'social competence' (Taborsky and Oliveira, 2012).

In the social cichlid *N. pulcher*, the acquisition of social competence is influenced by early social experience, and it involves 'learning-by-doing' of appropriate social behaviour, when interacting with same-aged peers (Arnold and Taborsky, 2010). Comparing *N. pulcher* reared in impoverished versus enriched social environments in a battery of social tests suggests that social competence is a *general* ability pertaining to different social contexts and social roles, which remains a life-long ability of individuals (Arnold and Taborsky, 2010; Taborsky *et al.*, 2012). Individual

(cont.)

variation of social competence is reflected by differences in the programming of the stress axis, as revealed by the stable, differential expression of stress genes in the brain (Taborsky *et al.*, 2013; Nyman *et al.*, 2017).

Nevertheless, there is no evidence that early-life social experience in cichlids affects cognitive abilities outside the social domain. When testing the ability to associate food rewards with spatial location or visual patterns, performance depended on early experience of predation risk (Bannier *et al.*, 2017) or on the predictability of food availability during early life (Kotrschal and Taborsky, 2010), but not on social competence. Combined, these findings highlight the importance of incorporating early social and ecological experiences when studying cognition in fish.

References

Arnold, C., and Taborsky, B. (2010). Social experience in early ontogeny has lasting effects on social skills in cooperatively breeding cichlids. *Animal Behaviour*, **79**, 621–630.

Baerends, G. P., and Baerends van Roon, J. M. (1950). An introduction to the study of the ethology of cichlid fishes. *Behaviour*, **S1**, 1–242.

Balzarini, V., Taborsky, M., Wanner, S., Koch, F., and Frommen, J. G. (2014). Mirror, mirror on the wall: the predictive value of mirror tests for measuring aggression in fish. *Behavioral Ecology and Sociobiology*, **68**, 871–878.

Bannier, F., Tebbich, S., and Taborsky, B. (2017). Early experience affects learning performance and neophobia in a cooperatively breeding cichlid. *Ethology*, **123**, 712–723.

Barlow, G. W. (2000). *The cichlid fishes: nature's grand experiment in evolution*. New York, NY: Perseus Publishing.

Bayani, D. M., Taborsky, M., and Frommen, J. G. (2017). To pee or not to pee: urine signals mediate aggressive interactions in the cooperatively breeding cichlid *Neolamprologus pulcher*. *Behavioral Ecology and Sociobiology*, **71**, 37.

Keenleyside, M. H. A. (1991). *Cichlid fishes*. London: Chapman and Hall.

Kotrschal, A., and Taborsky, B. (2010). Environmental change enhances cognitive abilities in fish. *PLoS Biology*, **8**, e1000351.

Nyman, C., Fischer, S., Aubin-Horth, N., and Taborsky, B. (2017). Effect of the early social environment on behavioural and genomic responses to a social challenge in a cooperatively breeding vertebrate. *Molecular Ecology*, **26**, 3186–3203.

Taborsky, M. (2016). Cichlid fishes: a model for the integrative study of social behavior. In *Cooperative breeding* (pp. 272–293). Cambridge: Cambidge University Press.

Taborsky, B., and Oliveira, R. F. (2012). Social competence: an evolutionary approach. *Trends in Ecology and Evolution*, **27**, 679–688.

Taborsky, M., and Wong, M. (2017). Sociality in fishes. In *Comparative social evolution* (pp. 354–389). Cambridge: Cambridge University Press.

Taborsky, B., Arnold, C., Junker, J., and Tschopp, A. (2012). The early social environment affects social competence in a cooperative breeder. *Animal Behaviour*, **83**, 1067–1074.

Taborsky, B., Tschirren, L., Meunier, C., and Aubin-Horth, N. (2013). Stable reprogramming of brain transcription profiles by the early social environment in a cooperatively breeding fish. *Proceedings of the Royal Society of London B: Biological Sciences*, **280**, 20122605.

Resources

Fish cognition and behaviour (Brown *et al.*, 2011a) includes comprehensive reviews on just about all aspects of fish cognition. There are several key research labs around the world working in this field. Cosme Salas and his lab at the University of Sevilla, Spain, use goldfish to study aspects of neural mechanisms of learning. Kevin Laland at the University of St Andrews, UK, is an expert on social learning and cultural evolution. Theresa Burt de Perera at the University of Oxford, UK, has special interests in spatial learning in three dimensions. Angelo Bisazza's lab at the University of Padova, Italy, studies laterality and numerical competence. Lastly, Culum Brown's lab at Macquarie University, Australia, studies fish cognition from a behavioural ecology perspective.

Profile

Culum has studied fish cognition for over 20 years (ouch). His fascination with fish started when he was very young, snorkelling on coral reefs throughout south-east Asia. He had a fish tank and a pond by the age of 6, and was scuba diving by 16. His childhood dream was to become a marine biologist. Now, Culum spends his time convincing people that fishes are smarter than usually believed and worthy of welfare attention.

Catarina has always had a passion for sharks and decided early on she would become a marine biologist, even if it meant working with birds for a while. She thinks fish and sharks are fascinating creatures, and that the fear they instigate comes from knowing very little about their behaviour and intelligence. Studying fish cognition allowed her to spend a lot of time in the water with sharks and help changing public perception of these amazing animals.

References

Abril-de-Abreu, R., Cruz, J., and Oliveira, R. F. (2015). Social eavesdropping in zebrafish: tuning of attention to social interactions. *Scientific Reports*, **5**, 12687.

Agrillo, C., and Bisazza, A. (2014). Spontaneous versus trained numerical abilities. A comparison between the two main tools to study numerical competence in non-human animals. *Journal of Neuroscience Methods*, **234**, 82–91.

Agrillo, C., Petrazzini, M. E. M., Piffer, L., Dadda, M., and Bisazza. A. (2012). A new training procedure for studying discrimination learning in fish. *Behavioural Brain Research*, **230**, 343–348.

Agrillo, C., Miletto Petrazzini, M. E., and Dadda, M. (2013). Illusory patterns are fishy for fish, too. *Frontiers in Neural Circuits*, **7**, 137.

Agrillo, C., Petrazzini, M. E. M., and Bisazza, A. (2014a). At the root of math: numerical abilities in fish. In *Evolutionary origins and early development of number processing*, vol. 1 (pp. 3–34). New York, NY: Academic Press.

Agrillo, C., Petrazzini, M. E. M., and Bisazza, A. (2014b). Numerical acuity of fish is improved in the presence of moving targets, but only in the subitizing range. *Animal Cognition*, **17**, 307–316.

Al-Imari, L., and Gerlai, R. (2008). Sight of conspecifics as reward in associative learning in zebrafish (*Danio rerio*). *Behavioural Brain Research*, **189**, 216–219.

Archard, G. A., and Braithwaite, V. A. (2011). Variation in aggressive behaviour in the poeciliid fish *Brachyrhaphis episcopi*: population and sex differences. *Behavioural Processes*, **86**, 52–57.

Arthur, D., and Levin, E. D. (2001) Spatial and non-spatial visual discrimination learning in zebrafish. *Animal Cognition*, **4**, 125–131.

Atton, N., Hoppitt, W., Webster, M. M., Galef, B. G., and Laland, K. N. (2012). Information flow through threespine stickleback networks without social transmission. *Proceedings of the Royal Society of London B: Biological Sciences*, **279**, 4272–4278.

Barber, I., and Ruxton, G. D. (2000). The importance of stable schooling: do familiar sticklebacks stick together? *Proceedings of the Royal Society of London B: Biological Sciences*, **267**, 151–155.

Bisazza, A., and Brown, C. (2011). Lateralization of cognitive functions in fish. In *Fish cognition and behaviour* (pp. 298–324). Oxford: Wiley-Blackwell.

Bisazza, A., Piffer, L., Serena, G., and Agrillo, C. (2010). Ontogeny of numerical abilities in fish. *PLoS ONE*, **5**, e15516.

Bisazza, A., Agrillo, C., and Lucon-Xiccato, T. (2014a). Extensive training extends numerical abilities of guppies. *Animal Cognition*, **17**, 1413–1419.

Bisazza, A., Butterworth, B., Piffer, L., Bahrami, B., Petrazzini, M. E. M., and Agrillo, C. (2014b). Collective enhancement of numerical acuity by meritocratic leadership in fish. *Scientific Reports*, **4**, 4560.

Bitterman, M. E. (1964) Classical conditioning in the goldfish as a function of the CS–US interval. *Journal of Comparative and Physiological Psychology*, **58**, 356–366.

Breuning, S. E., Ferguson, D. G., and Poling, A. D. (1981). Second-order schedule effects with goldfish: a comparison of brief-stimulus, chained, and tandem schedules. *Pyschological Record*, **31**, 437–445.

Broglio, C., Gómez, A., Durán, E., *et al.* (2005). Hallmarks of a common forebrain vertebrate plan: specialized pallial areas for spatial, temporal and emotional memory in actinopterygian fish. *Brain Research Bulletin*, **66**, 277–281.

Broglio, C., Gómez, A., Durán, E., Salas, C., and Rodríguez, F. (2011). Brain and cognition in teleost fish. In *Fish cognition and behaviour* (pp. 325–358). Oxford: Wiley-Blackwell.

Brown, C. (2001). Familiarity with the test environment improves escape responses in the crimson spotted rainbowfish, *Melanotaenia duboulayi*. *Animal Cognition*, **4**, 109–113.

Brown, C., and Braithwaite, V. A. (2005). Effects of predation pressure on the cognitive ability of the poeciliid *Brachyraphis episcopi*. *Behavioural Ecology*, **16**, 482–487.

Brown, C., and Laland, K. N. (2002a). Social enhancement and social inhibition of foraging behaviour in hatchery-reared Atlantic salmon. *Journal of Fish Biology*, **61**, 987–998.

Brown, C., and Laland, K. N. (2002b). Social learning of a novel avoidance task in the guppy: conformity and social release. *Animal Behaviour*, **64**, 41–47.

Brown, C., and Laland, K. N. (2011). Social learning in fishes. In *Fish cognition and behaviour* (pp. 186–202). Oxford: Wiley-Blackwell.

Brown, C., and Warburton, K. (1999). Social mechanisms enhance escape responses in shoals of rainbowfish, *Melanotaenia duboulayi*. *Environmental Biology of Fishes*, **56**, 455–459.

Brown, C., Markula, A., and Laland, K. (2003). Social learning of prey location in hatchery-reared Atlantic salmon. *Journal of Fish Biology*, **63**, 738–745.

Brown, C., Laland, K., and Krause, J. (2011a). *Fish cognition and behaviour*. Oxford: Wiley-Blackwell.

Brown, G. E., Ferrari, M. C., and Chivers, D. P. (2011b). Learning about danger: chemical alarm cues and threat-sensitive assessment of predation risk by fishes. In *Fish cognition and behaviour* (pp. 59–80). Oxford: Wiley-Blackwell.

Burns, J. G., and Rodd, F. H. (2008). Hastiness, brain size and predation regime affect the performance of wild guppies in a spatial memory task. *Animal Behaviour*, **76**, 911–922.

Cattelan, S., Lucon-Xiccato, T., Pilastro, A., and Griggio, M. (2017). Is the mirror test a valid measure of fish sociability? *Animal Behaviour*, **127**, 109–116.

Churchill, E. P. (1916). The learning of a maze by goldfish. *Journal of Animal Behaviour*, **6**, 247–255.

Coolen, I., van Bergen, Y., Day, R. L., and Laland, K. N. (2003). Species difference in adaptive use of public information in sticklebacks. *Proceedings of the Royal Society of London B: Biological Sciences*, **270**, 2413–2419.

Croft, D. P., Krause, J., and James, R. (2004). Social networks in the guppy (*Poecilia reticulata*). *Proceedings of the Royal Society of London B: Biological Sciences*, **271**, 516–519.

Cronin, T. W., Shashar, N., Caldwell, R. L., Marshall, J., Cheroske, A. G., and Chiou, T. H. (2003). Polarization vision and its role in biological signaling. *Integrative and Comparative Biology*, **43**, 549–558.

Desjardins, J. K., and Fernald, R. D. (2010). What do fish make of mirror images? *Biology Letters*, **6**, 744–747.

Duffy, G. A., Pike, T. W., and Laland, K. N. (2009). Size-dependent directed social learning in nine-spined sticklebacks. *Animal Behaviour*, **78**, 371–375.

Dunlop, R., Millsopp, S., and Laming, P. (2006). Avoidance learning in goldfish (*Carassius auratus*) and trout (*Oncorhynchus mykiss*) and implications for pain perception. *Applied Animal Behaviour Science*, **97**, 255–271.

Ebbesson, L., and Braithwaite, V. (2012). Environmental effects on fish neural plasticity and cognition. *Journal of Fish Biology*, **81**, 2151–2174.

Engeszer, R. E., da Barbiano, L. A., Ryan, M. J., and Parichy, D. M. (2007). Timing and plasticity of shoaling behaviour in the zebrafish, *Danio rerio*. *Animal Behaviour*, **74**, 1269–1275.

Evans, J. P., Pilastro, A., and Schlupp, I. (2011). *Ecology and evolution of poeciliid fishes*. Chicago, IL: University of Chicago Press.

Fay, R. R., and Popper, A. N. (2012). Fish hearing: new perspectives from two 'senior' bioacousticians. *Brain, Behaviour and Evolution*, **79**, 215–217.

Franck, D., and Ribowski, A. (1987). Influences of prior agonistic experiences on aggression measures in the male swordtail (*Xiphophorus helleri*). *Behaviour*, **103**, 217–240.

Frommen, J. G., Hanak, S., Schmidl, C. A., and Thünken, T. (2015). Visible implant elastomer tagging influences social preferences of zebrafish (*Danio rerio*). *Behaviour*, **152**, 1765–1777.

Fürtbauer, I., King, A., and Heistermann, M. (2015). Visible implant elastomer (VIE) tagging and simulated predation risk elicit similar physiological stress responses in three-spined stickleback *Gasterosteus aculeatus*. *Journal of Fish Biology*, **86**, 1644–1649.

Gerlach, G., and Lysiak, N. (2006). Kin recognition and inbreeding avoidance in zebrafish, *Danio rerio*, is based on phenotype matching. *Animal Behaviour*, **71**, 1371–1377.

Girvan, J. R., and Braithwaite, V. A. (1998). Population differences in spatial learning in three-spined sticklebacks. *Proceedings of the Royal Society of London B: Biological Sciences*, **265**, 913–918.

Gonda, A., Herczeg, G., and Merilä, J. (2009). Adaptive brain size divergence in nine-spined sticklebacks (*Pungitius pungitius*)? *Journal of Evolutionary Biology*, **22**, 1721–1726.

Gori, S., Agrillo, C., Dadda, M., and Bisazza, A. (2014). Do fish perceive illusory motion? *Scientific Reports*, **4**, 6443.

Grosenick, L., Clement, T. S., and Fernald, R. D. (2007). Fish can infer social rank by observation alone. *Nature*, **445**, 429–432.

Hall, D., and Suboski, M. (1995). Visual and olfactory stimuli in learned release of alarm reactions by zebra danio fish (*Brachydanio rerio*). *Neurobiology of Learning and Memory*, **63**, 229–240.

Hara, T. J. (2012). Fish chemoreception. In *Fish and fisheries series*, vol. 6. Dordrecht: Springer.

Hawryshyn, C. W., and McFarland, W. N. (1987). Cone photoreceptor mechanisms and the detection of polarized light in fish. *Journal of Comparative Physiology A*, **160**, 459–465.

Herter, K. (1929). Dressurversuche an Fischen. *Zeitschrift für Vergleichende Physiologie*, **10**, 688–711.

Higgs, D. M., and Radford, C. A. (2013). The contribution of the lateral line to 'hearing' in fish. *The Journal of Experimental Biology*, **216**, 1484–1490.

Huntingford, F. A., and Wright, P. J. (1992). Inherited population differences in avoidance-conditioning in 3-spined sticklebacks, *Gasterosteus aculeatus*. *Behaviour*, **122**, 264–273.

Jenkins, J. R., and Rowland, W. J. (1997). Learning influences courtship preferences of male threespine sticklebacks (*Gasterosteus aculeatus*). *Ethology*, **103**, 954–965.

Kleinhappel, T., Al-Zoubi, A., Al-Diri, B., *et al.* (2014). A method for the automated long-term monitoring of three-spined stickleback *Gasterosteus aculeatus* shoal dynamics. *Journal of Fish Biology*, **84**, 1228–1233.

Kotrschal, A., Rogell, B., Bundsen, A., *et al.* (2013). The benefit of evolving a larger brain: big-brained guppies perform better in a cognitive task. *Animal Behaviour*, **86**, 4–6.

Laland, K., and Williams, K. (1997). Shoaling generates social learning of foraging information in guppies. *Animal Behaviour*, **53**, 1161–1169.

Laland, K., and Williams, K. (1998). Social transmission of maladaptive information in the guppy. *Behavioural Ecology*, **9**, 493–499.

Laudien, H., Freyer, J., Erb, R., and Denzer, D. (1986). Influence of isolation stress and inhibited protein biosynthesis on learning and memory in goldfish. *Physiology and Behaviour*, **38**, 621–628.

Lindeyer, C. M., and Reader, S. M. (2010). Social learning of escape routes in zebrafish and the stability of behavioural traditions. *Animal Behaviour*, **79**, 827–834.

Lopes, J. S., Abril-de-Abreu, R., and Oliveira, R. F. (2016). Brain transcriptomic response to social eavesdropping in zebrafish (*Danio rerio*). *PLoS ONE*, **10**, e0145801.

López J. C., Broglio, C., Rodríguez, F., Thinus-Blanc, C., and Salas, C. (1999). Multiple spatial learning strategies in goldfish (*Carassius auratus*). *Animal Cognition*, **2**, 109–120.

Mackintosh, N. J. (1971). Reward and aftereffects of reward in the learning of goldfish. *Journal of Comparative and Physiological Psychology*, **76**, 225–232.

Mackney, P. A., and Hughes, R. N. (1995). Foraging behaviour and memory window in sticklebacks. *Behaviour*, **132**, 1241–1253.

Magat, M., and Brown, C. (2009). Laterality enhances cognition in Australian parrots. *Proceedings of the Royal Society of London B: Biological Sciences*, **276**, 4155–4162.

Mehlis, M., Bakker, T. C. M., and Frommen, J. G. (2008). Smells like sib spirit: kin recognition in three-spined sticklebacks (*Gasterosteus aculeatus*) is mediated by olfactory cues. *Animal Cognition*, **11**, 643–650.

Milinski, M. (1987). Tit for tat in sticklebacks and the evolution of cooperation. *Nature*, **325**, 433–435.

Milinski, M. (2003). The function of mate choice in sticklebacks: optimizing MHC genetics. *Journal of Fish Biology*, **63**, 1–16.

Milinski, M., Kulling, D., and Kettler, R. (1990). Tit for tat: sticklebacks trusting a cooperating partner. *Behavioural Ecology*, **1**, 7–10.

Nelson, M. E. (2011). Electric fish. *Current Biology*, **21**, 528–529.

Odling-Smee, L., Boughman, J., and Braithwaite, V. (2008). Sympatric species of threespine stickleback differ in their performance in a spatial learning task. *Behavioural Ecology and Sociobiology*, **62**, 1935–1945.

Oliveira, R. F., Simões, J. M., Teles, M. C., Oliveira, C. R., Becker, J. D., and Lopes, J. S. (2016). Assessment of fight outcome is needed to activate socially driven transcriptional changes in the zebrafish brain. *Proceedings of the National Academy of Sciences*, **113**, 654–661.

Perkins, F. T., and Wheeler, R. H. (1930). Configurational learning in the goldfish. *Comparative Psychology Monographs*, **7**, 50.

Pike, T. W., and Laland, K. N. (2010). Conformist learning in nine-spined sticklebacks' foraging decisions. *Biology Letters*, **6**, 466–468.

Pike, T. W., Kendal, J. R., Rendell, L. E., and Laland, K. N. (2010). Learning by proportional observation in a species of fish. *Behavioural Ecology*, **21**, 570–575.

Pitcher T. J., and Magurran A. E. (1983). Shoal size, patch profitability and information exchange in foraging goldfish. *Animal Behaviour*, **31**, 546–555.

Pitcher, T. J., Magurran, A. E., and Winfield, I. (1982). Fish in larger shoals find food faster. *Behavioural Ecolology and Sociobiology*, **10**, 149–151.

Pritchard, V. L., Lawrence, J., Butlin, R. K., and Krause, J. (2001). Shoal choice in zebrafish, *Danio rerio*: the influence of shoal size and activity. *Animal Behaviour*, **62**, 1085–1088.

Purser, J., and Radford, A. N. (2011). Acoustic noise induces attention shifts and reduces foraging performance in three-spined sticklebacks (*Gasterosteus aculeatus*). *PLoS ONE*, **6**, e17478.

Putman, N. F., Scanlan, M. M., Billman, E. J., *et al.* (2014). An inherited magnetic map guides ocean navigation in juvenile Pacific salmon. *Current Biology*, **24**, 446–450.

Qin, M., Wong, A., Seguin, D., and Gerlai, R. (2014). Induction of social behaviour in zebrafish: live versus computer animated fish as stimuli. *Zebrafish*, **11**, 185–197.

Reader, S., and Laland, K. (2000). Diffusion of foraging innovation in the guppy. *Animal Behaviour*, **60**, 175–180.

Reader, S. M., Kendal, J. R., and Laland, K. N. (2003). Social learning of foraging sites and escape routes in wild Trinidadian guppies. *Animal Behaviour*, **66**, 729–739.

Reznick, D., Butler, M. J., IV, and Rodd, H. (2001). Life-history evolution in guppies. VII. The comparative ecology of high- and low-predation environments. *The American Naturalist*, **157**, 126–140.

Riege, W. H., and Cherkin, A. (1971). One-trial learning and biphasic time course of performance in the goldfish. *Science*, **172**, 966–968.

Roche, D. P., McGhee, K. E., and Bell, A. M. (2012). Maternal predator-exposure has lifelong consequences for offspring learning in three-spined sticklebacks. *Biology Letters*, **8**, 932–935.

Rodd, F. H., Hughes, K. A., Grether, G. F., and Baril, C. T. (2002). A possible non-sexual origin of mate preference: are male guppies mimicking fruit? *Proceedings of the Royal Society of London B: Biological Sciences*, **269**, 475–481.

Rodríguez, F., Duran, E., Vargas, J. P., Torres, B., and Salas, C. (1994). Performance of goldfish trained in allocentric and egocentric maze procedures suggests the presence of a cognitive mapping system in fishes. *Learning and Behaviour*, **22**, 409–420.

Sevenster, P., and Van Roosmalen, M. E. (1985). Cognition in sticklebacks: some experiments on operant conditioning. *Behaviour*, **93**, 170–183.

Sisler, S. P., and Sorensen, P. W. (2008). Common carp and goldfish discern conspecific identity using chemical cues. *Behaviour*, **145**, 1409–1425.

Sison, M., Cawker, J., Buske, C., and Gerlai, B. (2006). Fishing for genes influencing vertebrate behaviour: zebrafish making headway. *Lab Animal*, **35**, 33.

Smith, C., Barber, I., Wootton, R. J., and Chittka, L. (2004). A receiver bias in the origin of three-spined stickleback mate choice. *Proceedings of the Royal Society of London B: Biological Sciences*, **271**, 949–955.

Smith, E. J., Partridge, J. C., Parsons, K. N., *et al.* (2002). Ultraviolet vision and mate choice in the guppy (*Poecilia reticulata*). *Behavioural Ecology*, **13**, 11–19.

Sovrano, V., Rainoldi, C., Bisazza, A., and Vallortigara, G. (1999). Roots of brain specializations: preferential left-eye use during mirror-image inspection in six species of teleost fish. *Behavioural Brain Research*, **106**, 175–180.

Spence, R., and Smith, C. (2008). Innate and learned colour preference in the zebrafish, *Danio rerio*. *Ethology*, **114**, 582–588.

Spence, R., Magurran, A. E., and Smith, C. (2011). Spatial cognition in zebrafish: the role of strain and rearing environment. *Animal Cognition*, **14**, 607–612.

Swaney, W., Kendal, J., Capon, H., Brown, C., and Laland, K. N. (2001). Familiarity facilitates social learning of foraging behaviour in the guppy. *Animal Behaviour*, **62**, 591–598.

Thompson, T., and Sturm, T. (1965). Classical conditioning of aggressive display in Siamese fighting fish. *Journal of the Experimental Analysis of Behaviour*, **8**, 397–403.

Thünken, T., Waltschyk, N., Bakker, T. C. M., and Kullmann, H. (2009). Olfactory self-recognition in a cichlid fish. *Animal Cognition*, **12**, 717–724.

Tinbergen, N. (1951). *The study of instinct*. New York, NY: Oxford University Press.

Trompf, L., and Brown, C. (2014). Personality affects learning and trade-offs between private and social information in guppies, *Poecilia reticulata*. *Animal Behaviour*, **88**, 99–106.

Utne-Palm, A. C., and Hart, P. J. (2000). The effects of familiarity on competitive interactions between three-spined sticklebacks. *Oikos*, **91**, 225–232.

van Bergen, Y., Coolen, I., and Laland, K. N. (2004). Nine-spined sticklebacks exploit the most reliable source when public and private information conflict. *Proceedings of the Royal Society of London B: Biological Sciences*, **271**, 957–962.

Vargas, J. P., Lopez, J. C., and Portavella, M. (2009). What are the functions of fish brain pallium? *Brain Research Bulletin*, **79**, 436–440.

Vital, C., and Martins, E. P. (2011). Strain differences in zebrafish (*Danio rerio*) social roles and their impact on group task performance. *Journal of Comparative Psychology*, **125**, 278–285.

Waas, J. R., and Colgan, P. W. (1994). Male sticklebacks can distinguish between familiar rivals on the basis of visual cues alone. *Animal Behaviour*, **47**, 7–13.

Warburton, K. (1990). The use of local landmarks by foraging goldfish. *Animal Behaviour*, **40**, 500–505.

Ward, A. J. W., Holbrook, R. I., Krause, J., and Hart, P. J. B. (2005). Social recognition in sticklebacks: the role of direct experience and habitat cues. *Behavioural Ecology and Sociobiology*, **57**, 575–583.

White, G. E., and Brown, C. (2014). Cue choice and spatial learning ability are affected by habitat complexity in intertidal gobies. *Behavioural Ecology*, **26**, 178–184.

Williams, F. E., White, D., and Messer, W. S. (2002). A simple spatial alternation task for assessing memory function in zebrafish. *Behavioural Processes*, **58**, 125–132.

Wyzisk, K., and Neumeyer, C. (2007). Perception of illusory surfaces and contours in goldfish. *Visual Neuroscience*, **24**, 291–298.

Xu, X., Scott-Scheiern, T., Kempker, L., and Simons, K. (2007). Active avoidance conditioning in zebrafish (*Danio rerio*). *Neurobiology of Learning and Memory*, **87**, 72–77.

Zhao, X., Ferrar, M. C., and Chivers, D. P. (2006). Threat-sensitive learning of predator odours by a prey fish. *Behaviour*, **143**, 1103–1121.

Zupanc, G. K. H., Hinsch, K., and Gage, F. H. (2005). Proliferation, migration, neuronal differentiation, and long-term survival of new cells in the adult zebrafish brain. *The Journal of Comparative Neurology*, **488**, 290–319.

10 Hermit Crabs – Information Gathering by the Hermit Crab, *Pagurus bernhardus*

Robert W. Elwood

Species Description

Anatomy

Hermit crabs are crustaceans, classified as part of the infraorder Anomura within the order Decapoda (Bracken-Grissom *et al.*, 2013). There are two main groups of hermits: the Paguridae, which includes *Pagurus bernhardus*, and the Diogenidae. Both are marine and found in the littoral zone as well as the sublittoral. There is a smaller but nevertheless well-known group, the Coenobitidae, comprising terrestrial species commonly kept as pets, and the coconut crab, *Birgus latro*, which is the largest terrestrial arthropod. These three groups typically inhabit gastropod shells for at least part of their life cycle; *B. latro* stops using shells after the juvenile stage. By contrast, the Pylochelidae inhabit various sponges, holes in rocks or bamboo, and the Parapaguridae cover themselves with anemones, but have received relatively little study (Elwood and Neil, 1992; Bracken-Grissom *et al.*, 2013).

The common European hermit crab, *Pagurus bernhardus*, has a complement of head and thoracic appendages typical for decapod crustaceans (Figure 10.1). As befits a decapod, the first three pairs of thoracic appendages, the maxillipeds, are closely associated with the mouth and not easily observed. The following five are known as pereiopods. The first are the large chelipeds that have claws, but the right cheliped is larger than the left, as is the case in most pagurids. The next two pairs of pereiopods are much larger than the last two pairs. The former two are used for walking, whereas the latter two usually remain within the shell and likely play a role in maintaining posture. There is a large coiled abdomen that lacks a hard exoskeleton, and some of the abdominal appendages have been lost. Decapods typically have five pairs of pleopods and a final pair of uropods on each side of a symmetrical abdomen, but in *P. bernhardus* the pleopods on the right side are absent and those on the left are sexually dimorphic. Females have four pleopods that are clearly biramous, with the ramii approximately equal in size. The male has only three pleopods that are also biramous, but the ramii are very different in size and the overall size of the pleopods is smaller than in the female. These provide the most obvious way of determining the sex of these animals. However, another way is to note that males have gonopores on the fifth pereiopods, whereas females have them on the third. The uropods are the final pair of abdominal appendages, but these are asymmetrically developed (Elwood and Neil, 1992). The unusual anatomy

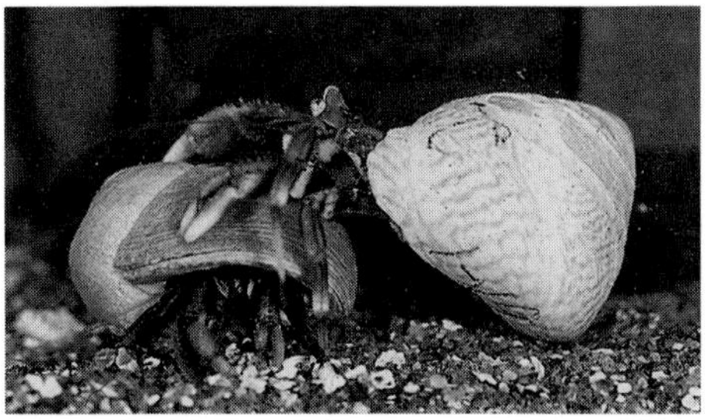

Figure 10.1. *Pagurus bernhardus* compete for shells, with the crab on the right assuming the role of attacker and causing the other crab to withdraw and assume the role of defender. The crab on the right is in a *Gibbula cineraria* shell that is less preferred than the *Littorina obtusata* shell on the left.
Photo by R. W. Elwood.

enables these crabs to inhabit empty gastropod shells, with the right side of the abdomen devoid of pleopods where they wrap around the columella of the shell, and the uropods provide an anchor that prevents the animal from being easily extracted. The crab can partially emerge from the shell when walking and feeding, but the delicate abdomen is rarely exposed and remains within the shell, which provides protection from predators and conspecifics (Laidre, 2007). If disturbed, the hermit can withdraw entirely into its shell and use the broad side of the large right cheliped to occlude the shell aperture.

Although shells are important for these animals, they are not cost-free. The shells are heavy relative to the mass of the crab: for example, a crab that weighs 0.3 g will inhabit a shell of approximately 1.3 g, i.e. more than four times the crab's weight (Elwood and Neil, 1992). When the crabs live in water, the problem of carrying the weight is not as great as for terrestrial hermit crabs (Herreid and Full, 1986). However, when the crabs move, the friction between the shell and the water imposes an energetic cost, especially for large, heavy shells (Elwood and Neil, 1992). Thin-walled shells have lower energetic costs, but might be more easily broken by a predator. There may be no such thing as a perfect shell on the shore for any crab, and a series of compromises are required (Bertness, 1981). However, what is clear is that there is huge competition for shells, and some crabs may be found in shells that are obviously too small or occasionally too large, that are broken and offer limited protection, or of non-preferred species (Elwood *et al.*, 1979). Thus, most crabs on a shore will readily examine any empty shell they encounter to assess if it offers an improvement to the one they have. Empty shells, however, are typically rare where hermits are common, and probably the most common method of obtaining a new shell, at least in *P. bernhardus*, is to fight another crab to evict it from its shell (Dowds and Elwood, 1983).

Perception

Hermit crabs have compound eyes on flexible stalks and appear to have good vision (Kinosita and Okajima, 1968; Ping *et al.*, 2015). They orient to shells and the distance at which that is achieved depends on the contrast between the shell and background (Reese, 1963). They are easily startled by a moving shadow (Jackson and Elwood, 1990). Hermits also use chemical cues to locate shells at predation sites (Ritschoff, 1980). The chemical composition of shells affects shell choice, and hermit crabs prefer artificial shells that have some calcium rather than those without calcium (Mesce, 1982). Finally, crabs are sensitive to vibration (Elwood *et al.*, 1998; Roberts *et al.*, 2016).

Reproduction

Pagurus bernhardus mate at least once a year and the female attaches the eggs to the filamentous pleopods, so that the eggs are protected within the shell. Small specimens of less than 0.2 g may have less than 100 eggs per brood and just one brood in the first year (Elwood and Stewart, 1987; Lancaster, 1990). However, somewhat larger specimens of approximately 0.8 g on the shore produce two broods per year, each with up to 2000 eggs. The largest *P. bernhardus* of 10 g or more are found offshore and carry up to 48,000 eggs. Eggs are brooded for about 3 months (Pike and Williamson, 1959), and the young hatch as free-swimming larvae that remain in the plankton for 2 months before settling to the substrate as glaucothoe. The survival of these young hermits and their subsequent life depend largely on the availability of small shells. These crabs may live for 10 or more years, and as they grow, they become too large for their existing shells and seek larger shells. On UK shores, small crabs primarily use either *Littorina obtusata* shells or those of *Gibbula cineraria* and *G. umbilicalis*, but these shells vary in size, and the crabs will first inhabit the smallest available ones and then move up in size. They subsequently use either *Nucella lapilus* or *Littorina littorea* shells, and the largest crabs inhabit *Neptuna antiqua* or *Buccinum undatum* shells (Elwood *et al.*, 1979). Thus, these crabs attempt to find a long succession of shells during their life, and they are totally dependent upon shells for their survival. Further, the largest species of shell are sublittoral, and crabs in these shells are very rarely found on the shore (Elwood and Neil, 1992).

Social Organization

Pagurus bernhardus shows little to no social organization. It often occurs in aggregations, but this is probably because of specific environmental conditions rather than social activity. Interactions between crabs are primarily agonistic, and they compete for space and food with various cheliped displays. The fights for shells are more elaborate (Dowds and Elwood, 1983; Figure 10.1). These involve one crab, the attacker, holding the opponent's shell and causing the defender to withdraw, and then repeatedly pulling the two shells together so that they impact, creating a sound, called rapping, that can be clearly heard in the laboratory and field (Briffa et al., 1998). The defender might then give up and allow itself to be pulled out of the shell by the winner. It may be thrown to one side, while the winner decides which shell to occupy. The loser will stay in the locality and wait until one shell is finally discarded by the winner, and the loser gets into that shell.

The raps are grouped into bouts of 2–16 raps with short pauses between bouts, during which the attacker readjusts its hold on the shell, probes the aperture (Briffa *et al.*, 1998) and may rock the defender's shell, which is less vigorous than rapping (Dowds and Elwood, 1983). The power of the rapping has a marked effect on the defender, which is more likely to get out of the shell when the raps are of high power (Briffa and Elwood, 2000a). When the power of the raps is dampened by placing silicon on the shells at the point of impact, attackers are less able to evict the defender (Briffa and Elwood, 2000a), but there is an increase in shell rocking (Edmonds and Briffa, 2017). Therefore, attackers appear to monitor their own performance and adjust their fight tactics accordingly.

Attackers that maintain a high temporal rate of rapping are also more likely to evict the opponent (Briffa *et al.*, 1998; Briffa and Elwood, 2002). This is most noted towards the end of contests, and attackers that rap with particularly short gaps between individual raps, and have more raps per bout of rapping, are more likely to win (Briffa *et al.*, 1998). That is, losers show signs of tiring before they give up. This is not surprising, because rapping is costly in energetic terms and haemolymph lactic acid shows a marked increase, even after just a few bouts of rapping (Briffa and Elwood, 2005). Attackers' lactate at the end of contests is positively related to the number of bouts and total raps, indicating the high cost of persisting in the contest; moreover, high lactate is also associated with longer pauses between bouts, suggesting that longer rest periods are required when lactate is high (Briffa and Elwood, 2001). Unsurprisingly, winners also have higher concentrations of the respiratory pigment haemocyanin than losers (Mowles *et al.*, 2009), as concentration is positively related to size. When residuals of this relation were examined, however, attackers with particularly high concentrations for their size were more likely to win. Thus, winning is influenced by the physiological state of the attacker. Further, if the attackers were maintained in low oxygen water prior to the contest, their chance of winning was reduced (Briffa and Elwood, 2000b). Curiously, defenders maintained in low oxygen did not differ from normal defenders in their chance of resisting eviction, possibly because defending does not entail vigorous activity (Briffa and Elwood, 2000b).

The most prolonged social interactions occur at mating, and a male may hold the female's shell for several days prior to sperm transfer (Contreras-Garduño and Córdoba-Aguilar, 2006). Males may also engage in fights for females. These contests do not involve the shell rapping noted above, but rather the two males engage in cheliped displays and grappling (Yasuda *et al.*, 2012). Another curious social behaviour occurs in some species when crabs appear to queue in decreasing order of size behind a large crab that is about to take a new shell and leave its original shell to be taken by the next crab. Each crab then takes its turn to move to a slightly larger shell, a process called vacancy chains (Chase *et al.*, 1988).

State of the Art

Exploration of Unoccupied Shells

Shells vary in size, weight, internal volume, shape, damage, manoeuvrability and presence of a range of colonizing organisms. These factors, and more, will affect the benefit to the crab in occupying a shell and, hence, the motivation to keep using that shell. These variables will also affect the net benefit of changing from the current shell to an alternative shell. How crabs gather information about shells and make decisions about which shell to occupy has been the subject of various studies that provide crucial information on their cognitive skills.

When a hermit crab encounters an empty shell, it typically approaches and makes contact, first with the antennae or possibly a walking leg or cheliped (Elwood and Neil, 1992). It then grasps the shell, the chelipeds are moved over the exterior, and the shell is then turned so that the aperture is facing upwards. The chelipeds, and possibly some walking legs, are then inserted into the aperture and are moved around within the shell (Kinosita and Okajima, 1968). Often the crab reverts to exterior examination and then again to interior examination. The shell may be rejected at any stage during this process. Alternatively, the crab may grasp the shell and then release its abdominal hold on its existing shell and swiftly move its abdomen out of one shell and into the other. A sequence of events typically starts with the crab turning to grasp its original shell and then investigating the original shell in a manner just described above. It may also let go of the old shell and repeatedly withdraw into the new shell, it may feel the exterior of the new shell with its walking legs, and it may hold the new shell aloft while supporting itself on its chelipeds and walking legs. Sometimes, the crab will move back to its original shell and either move away in that shell or start the whole process again by investigating the new shell. Eventually, the crab makes a final decision and moves away, either in the new shell or in its old shell (Elwood and Stewart, 1985).

These activities have been called 'shell investigation', because they appear to be a process of gathering information about the new shell and possibly a means of comparing that information with existing information about the old shell (or with newly gained information, if the old shell is reinvestigated). A key aspect of our early studies, and studies in other laboratories on different species, was to determine what information was gathered, when it was gathered and which sensory modalities were used to gather the information (e.g. Reese, 1963; Kinosita and Okajima, 1968; Rittschof, 1980; Elwood and Stewart, 1985; Jackson and Elwood, 1989a, 1990). We have used three main experimental approaches to test how the motivational state might have been influenced by the information acquired.

First, to assess if information is gathered about the shell on offer, and if the current shell also affects the motivation to change, Elwood and Stewart (1985) set up an experiment in which crabs that were naked were in a shell of only 50 per cent of the preferred weight (and hence was too small) for each crab, in a shell of 100 per cent of the preferred weight or 150 per cent of the preferred weight (and hence too heavy and large). Thirty crabs in each of these situations were then offered empty shells that were 50 per cent, 100 per cent or 150 per cent of the preferred weight for each crab. All the shells were *L. obtusata*. The quality of the occupied shell influenced the number of crabs approaching the new shell and contacting it, suggesting that crabs maintain information about their current shell, which is presumably gained from the fit and/or weight of that shell. Further, information about the new shell was gathered from a distance, presumably by visual input, because good-quality shells were more likely to be approached and contacted. Crabs in optimal shells were the least likely to investigate the new shell, indicating that progress in the sequence was influenced by information about the current shell. However, the quality of the new shell did not affect whether investigation took place. That is, there is no further information gain between making contact and initiating investigation. However, information about the new shell was gathered during the active investigation, because those investigating optimal shells were the most likely to enter those shells (Elwood and Stewart, 1985). Moreover, crabs with a high motivation should move from one stage (i.e. approaching, investigating, entering) to another more quickly than those with low motivation. Therefore, the proportion of crabs that approach, investigate and enter the new shell should reflect the average motivation of crabs in each experimental group to obtain the new shell (Elwood and Stewart, 1985). Results showed that the speed with which each stage was conducted was related to the motivation to gain a new shell. In particular, there was a negative relationship between the proportion of crabs that approached the shell and the time taken to approach, the proportion that actively investigated and the time being in contact prior to investigation, and the proportion that entered the new shell and the duration of aperture investigation.

A second method of determining if information has been gathered and has altered motivation is to prevent the change from one stage of investigation (i.e. approaching, investigating, entering) to the next stage (Neil and Elwood, 1986). Male crabs were induced to occupy *L. obtusata* shells that were 25 per cent, 50 per cent, 75 per cent or 100 per cent of their optimum weight, and were then offered shells that were either 25 per cent or 100 per cent of their optimum weight, but with the apertures blocked with a quick-setting resin (various types are sold as wood or stone fillers at hardware stores). Crabs with particularly poor shells moved towards the new shell more quickly and remained in contact with the new shell for a shorter duration prior to active investigation. However, those in poor shells persisted with active investigation for longer than did those in good shells (Figure 10.2), confirming that the quality of the current shell influences motivation in terms of persistence. Further, crabs investigating optimal shells (100 per cent) persisted for longer than crabs that were offered much too small shells (25 per cent; Figure 10.2). That is, information must have been gathered in the early stages and altered the motivation of the crabs to access the aperture (Neil and Elwood 1986). A similar result was found if the shell of preferred or less-preferred species were stuck, aperture down, to a piece of slate, so that they could not be moved: crabs persisted with attempting to turn the preferred species longer than the less-preferred species (Elwood and Briffa, 2001).

This technique of recording persistence was extended to investigate how crabs discriminate between the preferred *L. obtusata* shells and those of the much less preferred *G. cineraria* (Jackson and Elwood, 1989a). All subjects were induced to occupy *L. obtusata* shells that were too small (50 per cent of optimum weight), and each was then offered either a preferred species of *L. obtusata* or the less-preferred species of *G. cineraria* shell of optimal weight. These offered shells, however, could be (1) normal, (2) have their apertures blocked or (3) have been externally modified by the application of dental cement and paint (so that the exteriors were the same shape and the

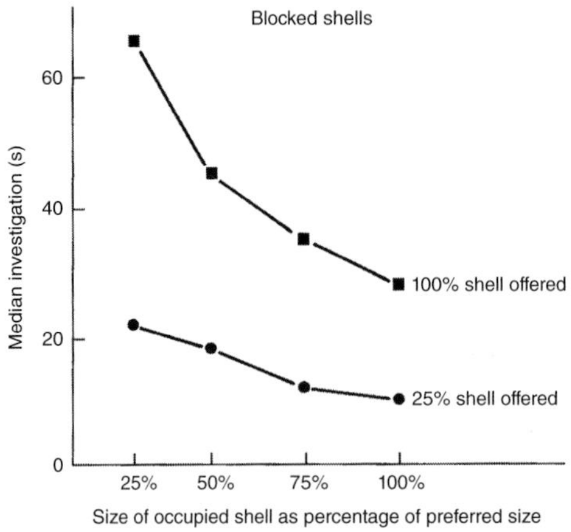

Figure 10.2. Crabs investigate shells with the aperture blocked for longer, if those shells are of optimum size/weight rather than much too small. They also investigate for longer when their own shell is much too small. That is, information about both shells influences persistence times. Photo reprinted with kind permission of John Wiley and Sons, originally published in Neil and Elwood (1986).

same colour, but the interiors were still characteristic for each species). Again, we found that crabs investigating shells with the aperture blocked persisted for longer with the preferred species. Moreover, when the shells had normal exteriors, crabs investigated the exteriors of *L. obtusta* shells for a shorter time than *G. cineraria* shells, indicating a higher motivation to take the preferred species. However, when the exteriors were modified to be similar, crabs investigated each species for similar times. Thus, crabs encountering the modified exteriors could not discriminate the species at this stage and presumably started the stage of internal investigation with the same motivation (Elwood, 1995). Any subsequent difference in investigation was due to information being gathered from the different interiors of the shells: modified *L. obtusta* shells were internally investigated more quickly than *G. cineraria* shells, suggesting higher motivation to obtain the preferred species (Jackson and Elwood, 1989a; Elwood, 1995).

The third method to assess information crabs have gathered is to induce a startle response that interrupts the ongoing behaviour. The more quickly animals resume their behaviour, the greater is the motivation to achieve the goal associated with that behaviour (Culshaw and Broom, 1980; Jackson and Elwood, 1990; Elwood *et al.*, 1998). For example, crabs housed in 75 per cent *L. obtusata* shells were offered the same species of shells that were either 50 per cent (poor quality) or 100 per cent (good quality; Jackson and Elwood, 1990). They were startled by a moving shadow created by a black card, which was moved overhead between the crab and the light source. Crabs investigating 50 per cent shells showed longer startle responses when the stimulus was applied at the holding stage and when they had just initiated external investigation. Thus, the motivation of the crabs differed according to the size of the new shell, even before they had initiated active investigation. A second experiment involved crabs in either 50 per cent or 75 per cent *L. obtusata* shells that were offered either *L. obtusta* or the less-preferred

G. cineraria shells, all of which were 100 per cent of the preferred size. In this experiment, the crabs were startled as they were approaching and had reached about 1 cm distance from the new shell (Figure 10.3). Those in the poorer shells (50 per cent) had shorter startle responses than those in intermediate shells (75 per cent), and those approaching the preferred species had shorter startles than those approaching the less-preferred species. Thus, the crabs had gained information about the species and the shell quality before making contact (Figure 10.3). Further information, however, is clearly gathered during subsequent stages of investigation. A final validation of these techniques was achieved by examining the relationship between the startle durations with the subsequent aperture investigation durations. This relationship was positive and significant, indicating that crabs judged as having low motivation by one technique also had a low motivation towards the end of investigation as judged by a separate technique (Jackson and Elwood, 1990).

Unoccupied shells on the shore often have various debris within the aperture, which must be removed before the shell can be occupied (Elwood and Adams, 1990). In marked contrast to empty shells, those containing loose sand are almost always rotated in the direction that causes the sand to fall out (Imafuku, 1994). Further, although empty shells are typically investigated by inserting the chelipeds, this behaviour is markedly increased when sand is present and a scraping motion may extract some of the sand. Should the shell contain gravel within the aperture, about half of the crabs rotate the shell to tip the obstruction out of the shell, and the remaining crabs pick the gravel out

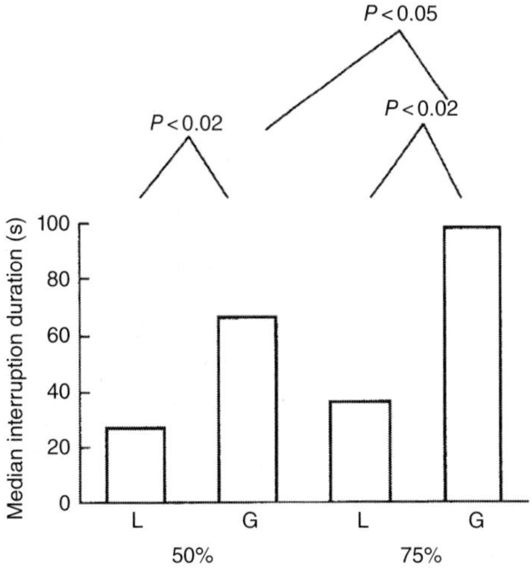

Figure 10.3. Crabs housed in *Littorina* shells of either 50 per cent or 75 per cent of their preferred weight/size approaching either *Littorina* (L) or *Gibbula* (G) shells show shorter startle responses when they approach the preferred species (L), and also show shorter startle responses if they are in very small shells (50 per cent) rather than ones that are only slightly too small (75 per cent). Thus, information about both shells influences motivation as measured by startle responses.

Photo reprinted from *Animal Behaviour*, 39(6), Nicholas W. Jackson and Robert W. Elwood, Interrupting an assessment process to probe changes in the motivational state, 1068–1077, Copyright (1990), with permission from Elsevier (Jackson and Elwood, 1990).

using their chelipeds. Clearly, crabs obtain information about the nature of obstructions and select activities appropriate for their removal (Elwood and Adams, 1990).

Algae and animals may settle and grow on a shell exterior and, in some cases, anemones are placed on the shells by the hermit crab, because anemones provide protection from predators (Williams and McDermott, 2004). These additions, however, alter the 'balance' of the shell and crabs need to adapt to walk normally. Indeed, when plastic plates were attached to shells occupied by the terrestrial hermit, *Coenobita rugosus*, the crabs first appeared unsteady and showed deficits in walking ability. This quickly changed, however, and not only did crabs adjust their walking, but they also quickly came to adjust turning of their body, shell and plate to manoeuvre through space (Sonoda *et al.*, 2012). That is, they seemed to have gained information about the external changes and use the shell as an extension of their body, similarly to other animals adjusting to using tools as by-extensions (i.e. embodiment).

Crabs that investigate a shell and reject it are likely to see that shell again and could waste time if they investigated it again. We therefore tested if they avoid this problem, by allowing crabs to investigate and reject a shell of poor quality and then offer the same shell or a novel shell either in the same or a different location. When a crab encountered the previously rejected shell, whether in the same location or a different location, the second investigation was of a shorter duration than the first one (Jackson and Elwood, 1989b). There was no reduction in the second investigation if a novel shell was encountered in either location. Further, the longer the time between the first investigation and the re-encounter with that same shell, the less was the reduction. The data are thus consistent with the idea of a short-term memory of information gathered about the shell, although it cannot be excluded that there was a chemical marking of the shell that faded rapidly.

Shell Fights

As noted above, hermit crabs fight over ownership of shells, and these fights may be largely viewed as a process of gathering information that alters the motivation of each crab to persist with the contest. Recall that the attacker grasps the shell of the defender, and the defender typically withdraws into the shell. The attacker may then rap the two shells together in a highly vigorous and energetically demanding activity (Briffa and Elwood, 2005). Because of the high energetic costs of shell rapping, attackers should adjust costs according to the potential gain or loss from shell exchange. While the energetic costs to defenders seem not to be as great as for attackers, there are time costs and possible injury costs, and defenders should also adjust these costs depending on the gain or loss that might result from shell exchange. Therefore, both attacker and defender must gather information about their own shell and that of the opponent. However, the ability to gather information about the opponent's shell might be different in attackers and defenders. The attacker feels over the exterior of the defender's shell and partially accesses the aperture during the contest, gathering information, in a similar manner to that achieved with an empty shell. By contrast, the defender withdraws into the shell and might be less able to gather information, although some information should be available just prior to withdrawing.

To examine assessment of shells in shell fights, Dowds and Elwood (1983) placed pairs of crabs that differed in size in *L. obtusata* or *G. cineraria* shells (Figure 10.1), with both shells being the correct size for the larger crab. Some attackers and some defenders were in *L. obtusata* shells and others in *G. cineraria* shells, in a 2 × 2 design. The larger crab of each pair was considerably more likely to assume the role of attacker. The larger crab was also more likely to attack if it was in the less-preferred species, but the defender's shell did not influence whether the larger crab initiated the contest, suggesting that attackers do not discriminate between species prior to starting the contest. This is in marked contrast to previous studies showing that some information about empty shells could be gathered during the approach (Jackson and Elwood, 1990). Further, there was no evidence that the defender could gather information about the attacker's shell at any stage of the contest, even though the defender could see the approaching attacker and its shell (Elwood and Glass, 1981; Dowds and Elwood, 1983). It appears that the presence of the potential opponent makes it more difficult to attend to features of the shell, presumably because the crabs attend to each other, reducing their ability to gather other information. When the attacker grasps the defender's shell, however, it feels over the exterior, and the quality of both shells influences whether the attacker escalates to shell rapping. Further, both shells influence the probability of the defender being evicted (Dowds and Elwood, 1983). While there is no indication that the defender is more willing to be evicted when it can gain in shell quality, defenders have information about their current shells. They employ a tactic called cheliped flicking (i.e. the major cheliped is repeatedly moved against the intruding cheliped of an attacker) more when being in the preferred species. However, attackers put more effort into fights when they are in particularly small shells, and those that are successful rap more than those that give up (Briffa *et al.*, 1998; Figure 10.4).

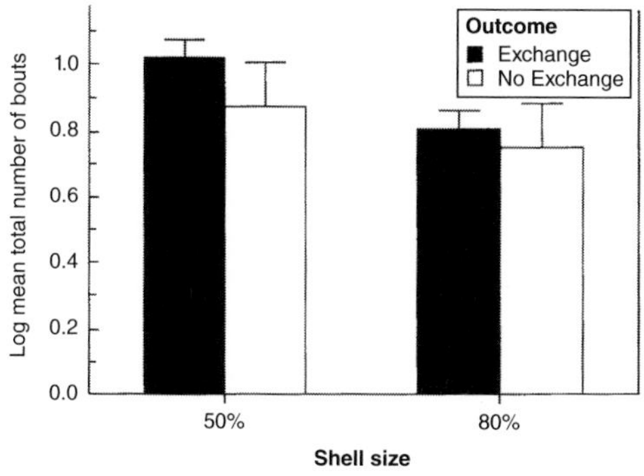

Figure 10.4. Crabs housed in poor shells (50 per cent) persist for longer than those in moderate quality shells (80 per cent), by using more bouts of rapping, and winners (exchange) use more bouts than losers (no exchange).
Photo reprinted with kind permission of The Royal Society, originally published in Briffa *et al.*, 1998.

That attackers gain information about the opponent's shell was also demonstrated using an interruption technique. Curiously, a stronger stimulus was required to interrupt a fight than to interrupt an investigation of an empty shell (Elwood *et al.*, 1998), confirming that the attacker is attending to the other crab and less so to external events. When the novel stimulus was employed at the start of physical contact, interruptions were shorter when the defender was in a good-quality shell for the attacker, indicating that the attacker had assessed the defender's shell.

To test if crabs alter their behaviour depending on private information about shells, the suitability of the shell can be modified in a way that may only be detected by the crab occupying that shell. This was achieved by gluing sand to the shell interior, which makes it much less desirable (Arnott and Elwood, 2007). When contests were set up between one crab forced to occupy a shell with a sandy interior and a crab in a shell without sand, there were marked effects on the behaviour of the occupant of the sandy shell. If the crab with the sandy shell assumed the attacker role, it fought more vigorously and for longer than if in a non-sandy shell. However, if it assumed the role of defender, it gave up far more quickly than crabs in normal shells. Thus, crabs altered their fight tactics according to privately held information. There was no indication that the other crab had any information about the sand, so the information was private to one of the contestants.

Importantly, age and/or experience may be a key factor in refining the information-gathering abilities of hermit crabs. Hazlett (1978), for instance, reported that with very large and old crabs, defenders could gain information about the attacker's shell, and suggested that 'shell negotiation' was a better description for these encounters than 'shell fights' (Hazlett, 1978). Contests involving larger crabs, indeed, resulted in defenders giving up more quickly if the opponent had a good shell for the defender. This ability had not been found in our experiments with small, young crabs (Elwood and Glass, 1981; Dowds and Elwood, 1983). In one later experiment, we needed to use older and larger crabs, but not as large as in Hazlett (1978), because we wished to take haemolymph for physiological measures after the contest (Doake and Elwood, 2011). To our surprise, these crabs showed the same abilities noted by Hazlett (1978). We concluded that age and experience improve the ability to gather information, but how this is achieved has yet to be determined.

All for One and One for All

Box 10.1 Sizing Up the Prize: Information Gathering in Fish Resource Contests

Erin S. McCallum and Sigal Balshine

The round goby (*Neogobius melanostomus*) is a small, territorial fish that uses sheltered rocky spaces in the near-shore regions of lakes and rivers to reproduce, care for offspring and escape from predators (Belanger and Corkum, 2003; Balshine *et al.*, 2005; Kornis *et al.*, 2012). Like the hermit crabs described in this chapter,

(*cont.*)

round goby vigorously compete for access to shelters in both the field and the laboratory. But how do these fish assess and decide which shelters are worth fighting for?

To answer this question, we conducted a series of experiments aimed at uncovering how round goby gather information about shelter value and whether they use this information in resource contests (McCallum *et al.*, 2017). First, we manipulated shelter value by providing the fish with a choice between a high-quality, enclosed, defendable shelter and a low-quality, open shelter that was difficult to defend (Figure B10.1.1A). Round goby strongly prefer the high-quality shelter. We then staged aggressive contests over a high- or low-quality shelter to determine whether fish would fight harder for a highly valuable shelter. Surprisingly, we found that fish fought equally hard for both shelter types. Why might that be, if the fish clearly prefer the high-quality resource?

We wondered whether round goby might need prior experience with the resource to assess its value. To test how resource experience influenced a contest, we housed fish for 24 hours with either a high- or low-quality shelter, and then allowed fish to contest over a single shelter. When fish were given experience with a shelter, they

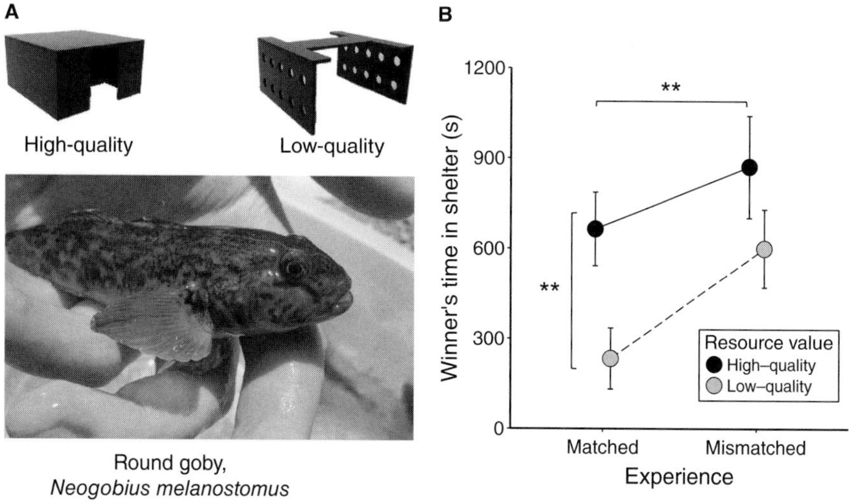

Figure B10.1.1. (A) The high- and low-quality shelter resources used in resource assessment experiments and a photo of a round goby. Photo by E. S. McCallum. (B) Results from our resource assessment experiment, showing that fish spent more time inspecting shelters (both high- and low-quality) when their prior resource experience was 'mismatched' with the resource present during the contest. Photo reprinted from *Animal Behaviour*, **123**, E. S. McCallum, S. T. Gulas and S. Balshine, Accurate resource assessment requires experience in a territorial fish, 249–257, Copyright (2017), with permission from Elsevier (McCallum *et al.*, 2017).

(*cont.*)

fought more intensely over high-quality shelters: these contests began faster and had more aggressive acts. So, round goby are indeed capable of assessing resource value and modulate their aggression in a contest accordingly, but they need time to evaluate the quality of the resource that they are fighting over. Next, we examined whether round goby could 'update' their appraisal of resource value in real-time. We did this by switching the value of the resource encountered during the contest from that of their prior experience. Fish that were housed with a high-quality shelter fought over a low-quality shelter, and vice versa. The fish now had to simultaneously assess both a competitor and the new resource. Here, we found that contest intensity was not purely driven by the previous experienced resource value *or* entirely by the current resource value in the contest. Round goby may therefore have a limited ability to update information of resource value while engaged in a contest. In all experiments, the fish engaged in aggressive behaviour quickly and rarely prioritized shelter inspection before resolving the conflict. Intriguingly, after the contests were resolved and a winner had emerged, winners spent more time investigating the shelter they won, especially in the 'mismatched' treatment (Figure B10.1.1B).

Our research shows that round goby require experience to make accurate assessments of resource value. There is still much to be learned about what physical cues round goby use to judge shelter quality and the limitations of their cognitive abilities for simultaneously assessing both competitors and resources.

References

Balshine, S., Verma, A., Chant, V., and Theysmeyer, T. (2005). Competitive interactions between round gobies and logperch. *Journal of Great Lakes Research*, **31**, 68–77.

Belanger, R. M., and Corkum, L. D. (2003). Susceptibility of tethered round gobies (*Neogobius melanostomus*) to predation in habitats with and without shelters. *Journal of Great Lakes Research*, **29**, 588–593.

Kornis, M. S., Mercado-Silva, N., and Vander Zanden, M. J. (2012). Twenty years of invasion: a review of round goby *Neogobius melanostomus* biology, spread and ecological implications. *Journal of Fish Biology*, **80**, 235–285.

McCallum, E. S., Gulas, S. T., and Balshine, S. (2017). Accurate resource assessment requires experience in a territorial fish. *Animal Behaviour*, **123**, 249–257.

Field Guide

All hermit crab species that use shells have similar problems about locating, evaluating and using shells, and most of these shells are suitable for similar experiments, if found in sufficient numbers. *Pagurus bernhardus* was selected for our experiments simply because it is by far the most common species around the UK and easily found at low tide in the littoral zone. Low tides vary in the time of day and intensity, with very low tides during good light providing the best opportunity to gather crabs. Good tides may not be frequent, and rain makes it difficult to see into the pools of water, again limiting collection chances. *Pagurus bernhardus* is widely distributed and found on virtually any shore that offers pools and some seaweed cover. However, the numbers that may be found vary widely. Local advice will be of great help to find productive beaches. The shores used in our studies in Northern Ireland could provide a hundred crabs on one visit, but on others only a few crabs could be collected. However, on some occasions very few crabs could be collected from previously productive locations. There is also variation between shores in the size of crabs, with those that have plenty of *Nucella lapillus* and *Littorina littorea* shells more likely to have larger crabs than those that just have *L. obtusata* and *Gibbula* spp. shells.

Pagurus bernhardus in the UK and Europe is typically the only hermit species on the shore, and the number of shell species is limited. This offers advantages in tackling a simple system, as opposed to a tropical shore that might have several species of hermits and numerous species of shell. This complexity will add to the preliminary work required to evaluate shell preferences by crabs of different sizes, and it is likely to reduce the ability to use a standard experimental approach with one crab species.

No permits are required to collect crabs in the UK. Wellington boots or waders will protect feet and ankles from sharp rocks and cold water, and thin rubber gloves will provide protection for the hands against the cold in winter. It is surprising how cold bare hands become when collecting in the UK in February, and holding the steering wheel for the drive to the laboratory may be difficult.

We typically collect crabs by searching the various littoral pools until one is located with specimens. They often occur in large numbers, under overhanging seaweed, and then they are easily collected by hand. Crabs will withdraw into their shells and often fall over if climbing on small rocks, and this movement often makes them more easily seen. They are protected by the shell and not damaged when collecting, and may be placed in large buckets or other suitable containers. However, if crabs are crowded, they may fight and some may be evicted from their shell and may not be able to locate a vacant shell. Naked crabs may not survive long in captivity.

Very large hermit crabs may be part of the by-catch of commercial fisheries and it might be possible to have them retained for study. If this is intended, the fishermen should be given instruction on how to keep the crabs in water-filled containers and with a limited number of specimens per container.

Crabs can be transported by car (approximately 1 hour) in buckets with lids and sufficient water to cover the animals, but without any form of cooling. In the laboratory, they are maintained in a temperature-controlled room at 11°C, with lights on a 12:12 cycle, and kept in mixed-sex groups of about 50 crabs in white plastic containers (60 × 30 × 15 cm). Seaweed from the beach provides some complexity and reduces the probability of fights occurring because it allows some avoidance of other crabs. Well-aerated natural seawater of 5 cm depth is sufficient to cover the crabs and is changed every 2–3 days. Crabs are fed on chopped fish or pieces of gastropod about twice a week.

Table 10.1. List of key materials and their use for these studies.

Tools	Function
Tide tables	To determine if collection is possible
Bucket with lid	Collecting crabs and transport without spills
Rubber gloves	To protect from cold in winter
Boots or waders	Foot and ankle protection
Containers	Holding crabs in laboratory
Temperature-controlled room	To maintain crabs in cool conditions
Aeration system	To keep crabs in aerated water
Bench vice	To crack shells so crabs can be removed
Crystallizing dishes	Small observation chambers for experiments
One-way mirror chamber	Enables crabs to be observed without being disturbed
Event recorder package on PC	Enables immediate analysis
Video camera	Allows subsequent detailed analysis
Microphone	Allows recoding and detailed analysis of shell rapping

Empty shells were required for the experiments described above. Sometimes we used live molluscs, killed them and then prepared the shells for the experiments, but only when that was deemed necessary (Doake *et al.*, 2010). For most experiments, we located areas in small bays where shells were washed high on the shore, away from the littoral zone in which the crabs occur. Shells were gathered in large numbers and then washed and dried, ensuring that no material was inside. They were then weighed, marked with the weight and sorted in drawers, like those typically sold in hardware shops to store screws and such like.

We established the relationship between the crab weight and the weight of shells of each species used in preference tests, and we tested preference for each shell species (Elwood *et al.*, 1979). We also determined if there was a sex preference for different species (Elwood and Kennedy, 1988). These data were required so that shells given to crabs (to occupy or evaluate) could be varied in terms of their suitability for the specific size of crabs used in each replicate. In our studies, we extracted crabs from their original shell, sexed them by examining the abdominal appendages under a binocular microscope, weighed them and offered a new shell as determined by the protocol of the experiment. Small crabs in *L. obtusata* shells were the most commonly available on the shore, and these were used in most of the experiments. Females carrying eggs might have different shell requirements, so we typically used males, unless we specifically required females. Each crab was then placed in a crystallizing dish and maintained in the cold room (about 11°C) overnight, to recover from shell extraction and to get used to the new shell provided for the experiment, and then used in the observation the following day.

For our experiments, crabs were brought to an adjacent laboratory at approximately 20°C. The temperature difference was not a problem during the short period required for each replicate. Hermit crabs are easily disturbed by visual stimuli or vibration. To reduce such problems during observations, a one-way mirrored screen was employed, which to be effective required the crab being in bright light and the observer in lower light. All efforts were made not to cause vibration in the laboratory. The behaviour was categorized as required for each experiment, and recorded on a desk-top computer using the Observer events package from Noldus.

It is useful to consider how to effectively extract crabs from their shells. Some workers have used heat on the apex of the shell, but this is not recommended, as the crab may be damaged and subsequent behaviour may be affected (Appel and Elwood, 2009; Elwood and Appel, 2009). We typically used a bench vice to crack the shell, and then touched the exposed abdomen with a fine brush: the crab released its hold of the remaining shell if held in water. This provides a quick and effective method, but it destroys the shell. Do not, however, try to crush the shell with a tool such as a hammer or pliers, because the force will travel through the shell and crush the crab. Should the original shell be required, it may be secured by a large clip, so the animal can no longer move the shell, and might abandon it. These and other techniques have been evaluated for *P. longicarpus* (Pechenik *et al.*, 2015).

We typically do not use crabs that have been in the laboratory for more than 10 days because they could become sluggish. After the experiments, we take the unused females and the males back to the shore, and release them a short distance from where we were collecting that day. This means that the population is not damaged by our regular collections, although it is possible that a crab is collected again on a subsequent visit. However, the crab would have a minimum of 10 days back on the shore to recover from any effects of transport and experimentation. It is also highly likely that it would change shell during the time back on the shore. During the years of work on these shores, it was very rare to find a shell that we had already marked in the laboratory.

Wild vs. Lab

Box 10.2 Social Cognition in the Wild: From Lab to Field in Hermit Crabs

Mark E. Laidre

A rich diversity of over 1000 species of hermit crab exists worldwide, distributed from the tropics to the Arctic, and inhabiting environments ranging from deep sea to intertidal to terrestrial and mountainous habitats kilometres inland (Bracken-Grissom *et al.*, 2013). Many if not most of these species are highly amenable to experimentation. Despite small brains, these species are highly cognitive, utilizing multiple sensory modalities (including visual, chemical, vibrational and tactile senses) to acquire information, learn, make decisions and respond adaptively to their environments.

Elwood provides a fascinating in-depth review of what he and his students have learned over several decades of study on a single European intertidal species in the laboratory. Cognition, however, evolved in the wild, and while studies in the lab offer exquisite opportunities for artificial control, such studies overlook the complex socio-ecological context in which cognition evolved (Shettleworth, 2010). This

(cont.)

context is an essential ingredient in designing experiments, particularly for hermit crabs, which must navigate a 'biological market' (Noë *et al.*, 2001), represented by the local housing market of available shells (Laidre and Vermeij, 2012). An immensely powerful approach for such studies involves field experiments that compare and contrast myriad different species in the wild, as Darwin pioneered.

Species of hermit crab vary dramatically, but perhaps none are more cognitively different from their marine ancestors than terrestrial hermit crabs (Coenobitidae). *Birgus latro*, for instance, has ceased using shells altogether (Laidre, 2018) and evolved into a gigantic predator that hunts large vertebrate prey (Laidre, 2017). Others, in the genus *Coenobita*, have become intensely social (Laidre, 2014) due to a unique behaviour (not performed by any other hermit crab species), in which individuals architecturally remodel shells (Laidre, 2012a; Laidre *et al.*, 2012). This costly construction behaviour has ultimately created extreme social dependence among unrelated conspecifics (Laidre, 2012b), which vie for the passed-down remodelled shells inherited socially across generations (Laidre and Trinh, 2014). Consequently, terrestrial hermit crabs offer unique prospects for studying the evolution of social cognition in the wild (Figure B10.2.1).

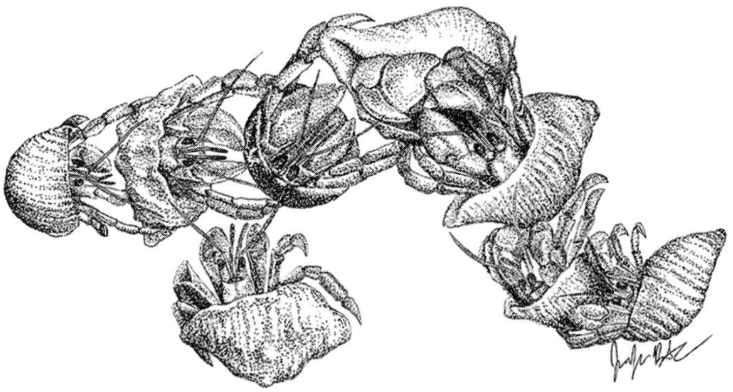

Figure B10.2.1. Social cognition and complexity in wild *Coenobita compressus*. Two individuals form an opportunistic coalition, jointly seeking to pull a third individual out of its shell, while others line up in anticipation of inheriting a shell. A free wandering individual, meanwhile, must decide which of two chains to join to have the greater likelihood of shell inheritance down the line. Drawing by Jennifer Bates.

Within their complex social world, terrestrial hermit crabs must make constant strategic decisions about where to distribute themselves in space and time (Laidre, 2013a) and which social groupings to join or leave, to maximize their chances of shell inheritance (Laidre, 2014). Field experiments with *C. compressus* have revealed that individuals are highly attracted to social groupings, including groupings simulated experimentally in the field using tethered conspecifics (Laidre, 2010). Individuals will

(cont.)

eavesdrop on social groupings, being mostly attracted to those with higher levels of commotion indicative of imminent evictions (Laidre, 2013b). Social structures that form in these groupings can also be experimentally simulated with variable arrays of sham shells (Bates and Laidre, 2018). Intriguingly, unrelated individuals can also team up in opportunistic coalitions, jointly evicting third parties from their shells and generating secondary opportunities for others, which wait in social chains while clinging to one another. With countless opportunities for experimentally manipulating social stimuli and sensory information in the field, as well as applying a Darwinian comparative approach across dozens of species, terrestrial hermit crabs can serve as model systems for studying social cognition in the wild for years to come.

References

Bates, K. M., and Laidre, M. E. (2018). When to socialize: perception of time-sensitive social structures among social hermit crabs. *Animal Behaviour*, **138**, 19–27.

Bracken-Grissom, H. D., Cannon, M. E., Cabezas, P., *et al.* (2013). A comprehensive and integrative reconstruction of evolutionary history for Anomura (Crustacea: Decapoda). *BMC Evolutionary Biology*, **13**, 128.

Laidre, M. E. (2010). How rugged individualists enable one another to find food and shelter: field experiments with tropical hermit crabs. *Proceedings of the Royal Society of London B: Biological Sciences*, **277**, 1361–1369.

Laidre, M. E. (2012a). Homes for hermits: temporal, spatial and structural dynamics as transportable homes are incorporated into a population. *Journal of Zoology*, **288**, 33–40.

Laidre, M. E. (2012b). Niche construction drives social dependence in hermit crabs. *Current Biology*, **22**, 861–863.

Laidre, M. E. (2013a). Foraging across ecosystems: diet diversity and social foraging spanning aquatic and terrestrial ecosystems by an invertebrate. *Marine Ecology*, **34**, 80–89.

Laidre, M. E. (2013b). Eavesdropping foragers use level of collective commotion as public information to target high quality patches. *Oikos*, **122**, 1505–1511.

Laidre, M. E. (2014). The social lives of hermits. *Natural History*, **122**, 24–29.

Laidre, M. E. (2017). Ruler of the atoll. *Frontiers in Ecology and the Environment*, **15**, 527–528.

Laidre, M. E. (2018). Coconut crabs. *Current Biology*, **28**, R58–R60.

Laidre, M. E., and Trinh, R. (2014). Unlike terrestrial hermit crabs, marine hermit crabs do not prefer shells previously used by conspecifics. *Crustaceana*, **87**, 856–865.

Laidre, M. E., and Vermeij, G. J. (2012). A biodiverse housing market in hermit crabs: proposal for a new biodiversity index. *Cuadernos de Investigación UNED*, **4**, 175–179.

Laidre, M. E., Patten, E., and Pruitt, L. (2012). Costs of a more spacious home after remodelling by hermit crabs. *Journal of the Royal Society Interface*, **9**, 3574–3577.

Noë, R., von Hooff, J. A. R. A. M., and Hammerstein, P. (2001). *Economics in nature: social dilemmas, mate choice and biological markets*. Cambridge: Cambridge University Press.

Shettleworth, S. J. (2010). *Cognition, evolution, and behavior*. Oxford: Oxford University Press.

Resources

There are numerous websites that have information about hermit crabs, but many of these refer to those species kept as pets. One website with useful information about *Pagurus bernhardus* is: http://animaldiversity.org/accounts/Pagurus_bernhardus/

Some films of hermit crabs are available on the web. Good ones are:

- *P. bernhardus* walking with good view of walking legs: www.youtube.com/watch?v=c85MrG5XTB8
- Good shell fight between *P. bernhardus*, arranged by Mark Briffa: www.youtube.com/watch?v=Tffgq7eW6uY
- Hermit crab (unknown species) changing shell and then moving anemones: www.youtube.com/watch?v=dYFALyP2e7U
- A delightful film of a vacancy chain for a terrestrial species: www.youtube.com/watch?v=f1dnocPQXDQ

Profile

Robert first saw hermit crabs as a student on a Reading University field course in Coverack, Cornwall, UK. He was immediately fascinated by their behaviour and use of shells. He selected these animals to conduct a brief project and was immediately hooked. However, Robert did his PhD at Reading University, which was well away from the sea, studying social influences on behavioural development in Mongolian gerbils. On obtaining a lectureship at The Queen's University of Belfast, he worked on rodents, amphipods (Dick and Elwood, 1989) and spiders (Prenter *et al.*, 1994), but also sought hermit crabs on nearby shores to supervise studies on them. His latest results show the possibility of pain in crustaceans (Appel and Elwood, 2009; Elwood and Appel, 2009; Magee and Elwood, 2016) and that cognitive limitations often preclude optimal strategies in fights (Elwood and Arnott, 2012).

References

Appel, M., and Elwood R. W. (2009). Gender differences, responsiveness and memory of a potentially painful event in hermit crabs. *Animal Behaviour*, **78**, 1373–1379.

Arnott, G., and Elwood, R. W. (2007). Fighting for shells: how private information about resource value changes hermit crab pre-fight displays and escalated fight behaviour. *Proceedings of the Royal Society of London B: Biological Sciences*, **274**, 3011–3017.

Bertness, M. D. (1981). Conflicting advantages in resource utilization: the hermit crab housing dilemma. *The American Naturalist*, **118**(3), 432–437.

Bracken-Grissom, H. D., Cannon, M. E., Cabezas, P., *et al.* (2013). A comprehensive and integrative reconstruction of evolutionary history for Anomura (Crustacea: Decapoda). *BMC Evolutionary Biology*, **13**, 128.

Bridge, A., Elwood, R. W., and Dick, J. T. A. (2000). Imperfect assessment and limited information preclude optimal strategies in male:male fights in the orb-web spider, *Metellina mengei. Proceedings of the Royal Society of London B: Biological Sciences*, **267**, 273–280.

Briffa, M., and Elwood, R. W. (2000a). The power of rapping influences eviction during hermit crab shell fights. *Behavioural Ecology*, **11**, 288–293.

Briffa, M., and Elwood, R. W. (2000b). Cumulative or sequential assessment during hermit crab shell fights: effects of oxygen on decision rules. *Proceedings of the Royal Society of London B: Biological Sciences*, **267**, 2445–2452.

Briffa, M., and Elwood, R. W. (2001). Decision rules, energy metabolism and vigour in hermit crab fights. *Proceedings of the Royal Society of London B: Biological Sciences*, **268**, 1841–1847.

Briffa, M., and Elwood R. W. (2002). Power of signals influences physiological costs and subsequent decisions during hermit crab fights. *Proceedings of the Royal Society of London B: Biological Sciences*, **269**, 2331–2336.

Briffa, M., and Elwood, R. W. (2005). Rapid change in energetic status in fighting animals: causes and effects of strategic decisions. *Animal Behaviour*, **70**, 119–124.

Briffa, M., Elwood, R. W., and Dick, J. T. A. (1998). Analyses of repeated signals during hermit crab shell fights. *Proceedings of the Royal Society B*, **265**, 1467–1474.

Chase, I. D., Weissburg, M., and Dewitt, T. H. (1988). The vacancy chain process: a new mechanism of resource distribution in animals with application to hermit crabs. *Animal Behaviour*, **36**, 1265–1274.

Contreras-Garduño J., and Córdoba-Aguilar A. (2006). Sexual selection in hermit crabs: a review and outlines of future research. *Journal of Zoology*, **270**, 595–605.

Culshaw, A. D., and Broom, D. M. (1980). The imminence of behavioural change and the startle response. *Behaviour*, **73**, 64–76.

Dick, J. T. A., and Elwood, R. W. (1989). Assessments and decisions during mate choice in *Gammarus pulex* (Amphipoda). *Behaviour*, **109**, 235–246.

Doake, S., and Elwood, R. W. (2011). How resource quality differentially affects motivation and ability to fight in hermit crabs. *Proceedings of the Royal Society of London B: Biological Sciences*, **278**, 567–573.

Doake, S., Scantlebury, M., and Elwood, R. W. (2010). The cost of bearing arms and armour in the hermit crab, Pagurus bernhardus. *Animal Behaviour*, **80**, 637–642.

Dowds, B. M., and Elwood, R. W. (1983). Shell wars: assessment strategies and the timing of decisions in hermit crab fights. *Behaviour*, **85**, 1–24.

Edmonds, E., and Briffa, M. (2017). Weak rappers rock more: hermit crabs assess their own agonistic behaviour. *Biology Letters*, **12**, 20150884.

Elwood, R. W. (1995). Motivational change during resource assessment in hermit crabs. *Journal of Experimental Marine Biology and Ecology*, **193**, 41–55.

Elwood, R. W., and Adams, P. M. (1990). How hermit crabs (*Pagurus bernhardus*) deal with obstructions in the apertures of shells. *Irish Naturalists' Journal*, **23**, 180–185.

Elwood, R. W., and Appel, M. (2009). Pain in hermit crabs? *Animal Behaviour*, **77**, 1243–1246.

Elwood, R. W., and Arnott, G. (2012). Understanding how animals fight with Lloyd Morgan's canon. *Animal Behaviour*, **84**, 1095–1102.

Elwood, R. W., and Briffa, M. (2001). Information gathering during agonistic and non-agonistic shell aquistion by hermit crabs. *Advances in the Study of Behaviour*, **30**, 53–97.

Elwood, R. W., and Glass, C. W. (1981). Negotiation or aggression during shell fights of the hermit crab, *Pagurus bernhardus. Animal Behaviour*, **29**, 1239–1244.

Elwood, R. W., and Kennedy, H. F. (1988). Sex differences in shell preferences in the hermit crab, *Pagurus bernhardus* L. *Irish Naturalists' Journal*, **22**, 436–440.

Elwood, R. W., and Neil, S. J. (1992). *Assessments and decisions: a study of information gathering by hermit crabs*. London: Chapman and Hall.

Elwood, R. W., and Stewart, A. (1985). The timing of decisions during shell investigation by the hermit crab, *Pagurus bernhardus*. *Animal Behaviour*, **33**, 620–627.

Elwood, R. W., and Stewart, A. (1987). Reproduction in the littoral hermit crab, *Pagurus bernhardus*. *Irish Naturalists' Journal*, **22**, 252–255.

Elwood, R. W., McClean, A., and Webb, L. (1979). The development of shell preferences by the hermit crab, *Pagurus bernhardus*. *Animal Behaviour*, **27**, 940–946.

Elwood, R.W., Wood, K., Gallagher, M., and Dick, J. T. A. (1998). Probing motivational state during agonistic encounters in animals. *Nature*, **393**, 66–68.

Hazlett, B. A. (1978). Shell exchanges in hermit crabs: aggression, negotiation, or both? *Animal Behaviour*, **26**, 1278–1279.

Herreid, C. F., and Full, R. J. (1986). Energetics of hermit crabs during locomotion: the cost of carrying a shell. *Journal of Experimental Biology*, **120**, 297–308.

Imafuku, M. (1994). Response of hermit crabs to sinistral shells. *Journal of Ethology*, **12**, 107–114.

Jackson, N. W., and Elwood, R. W. (1989a). How animals make assessments: information gathering by the hermit crab, *Pagurus bernhardus*. *Animal Behaviour*, **38**, 951–957.

Jackson, N. W., and Elwood, R. W. (1989b). Memory of shells in the hermit crab, *Pagurus bernhardus*. *Animal Behaviour*, **37**, 529–534.

Jackson, N. W., and Elwood, R. W. (1990). Interrupting an assessment process to probe changes in the motivational state. *Animal Behaviour*, **39**, 1068–1077.

Kinosita, H., and Okajima, A. (1968). Analysis of shell-searching behaviour of the land hermit crab, *Coenobita rugosus* H. Milne Edwards. *Journal of the Faculty of Science, University of Tokyo, Section IV*, **11**, 293–358.

Laidre, M. E. (2007). Vulnerability and reliable signaling in conflicts between hermit crabs. *Behavioural Ecology*, **18**, 736–741.

Lancaster, I. (1990). Reproduction and life history strategy of the hermit crab *Pagurus bernhardus*. *Journal of the Marine Biological Association UK*, **70**, 129–142.

Magee, B., and Elwood, R. W. (2016). Trade-offs between predator avoidance and electric shock avoidance in hermit crabs demonstrate a non-reflexive response to noxious stimuli consistent with prediction of pain. *Behavioural Processes*, **130**, 31–35.

Mesce, K. A. (1982). Calcium-bearing objects elicit shell selection behaviour in a hermit crab. *Science*, **215**, 993–995.

Mowles, S. L., Cotton, P. A., and Briffa, M. (2009). Aerobic capacity influences giving-up decisions in fighting hermit crabs: does stamina constrain contests? *Animal Behaviour*, 78, 735–740.

Neil, S. J., and Elwood, R. W. (1986). Factors influencing shell selection in the hermit crab, *Pagurus bernhardus*. *Ethology*, **73**, 225–234.

Pechenik, J. A., Diederich, C. M., Burns, R., Pancheri, F. Q., and Dorfmann, L. (2015). Influence of the commensal gastropod *Crepidula plana* on shell choice by the marine hermit crab *Pagurus longicarpus*, with an assessment of the degree of stress caused by different eviction techniques. *Journal of Experimental Marine Biology and Ecology*, **469**, 18–26.

Pike, R. B., and Williamson, D. I. (1959). Observations on the distribution and breeding of British hermit crabs and the stone crab (Crustacea: Diogenidae, Paguridae and Lithodiddae). *Proceedings of the Zoological Society of London*, **132**, 551–567.

Ping, X., Lee, J. S., Garlick, D., Jiang, Z., and Blaisdell, A. P. (2015). Behavioral evidence illuminating the visual abilities of the terrestrial Caribbean hermit crab *Coenobita clypeatus*. *Behavioural Processes*, **118**, 47–58.

Prenter, J., Elwood, R. W., and Montgomery, W. I. (1994). Assessments and decisions in mate guarding in *Metellina segmentata* (Areneae: Metidae). *Behavioural Ecology and Sociobiology*, **35**, 39–43.

Reese, E. S. (1963). The behavioural mechanisms underlying shell selection by hermit crabs. *Behaviour*, **21**, 78–126.

Ritschoff, D. (1980). Chemical attraction of hermit crabs and other attendants to simulated gastropod predation sites. *Journal of Chemical Ecology*, **6**, 103–118.

Roberts, L., Cheesman, S., Elliott, M., and Breithaupt, T. (2016). Sensitivity of *Pagurus bernhardus* (L.) to substrate-borne vibration and anthropogenic noise. *Journal of Experimental Marine Biology and Ecology*, **474**, 185–194.

Sonoda, K., Asakura, A., Minoura, M., Elwood, R. W., and Gunji, P. (2012). Hermit crabs perceive the extent of their virtual bodies. *Biology Letters*, **8**, 495–497.

Williams, J. D., and McDermott, J. J. (2004). Hermit crab biocoenoses: a worldwide review of the diversity and natural history of hermit crab associates. *Journal of Experimental Marine Biology and Ecology*, **305**, 1–128.

Yasuda, C., Takeshita, F., and Wada, S. (2012). Assessment strategy in male-male contests of the hermit crab *Pagurus middendorffi*. *Animal Behaviour*, **84**, 385–390.

11 Hyenas – Testing Cognition in the Umwelt of the Spotted Hyena

Lily Johnson-Ulrich, Kenna D. S. Lehman, Julie W. Turner and Kay E. Holekamp

Species Description

Anatomy

Spotted hyenas (*Crocuta crocuta*) are roughly 1 m tall, 130 cm long and weigh up to 95 kg. In the Serengeti, males weigh on average 41–55 kg, whereas females weigh 45–64 kg (Kruuk, 1972). Although their post-cranial anatomy is adapted for cursorial hunting, spotted hyenas exhibit many morphological specializations for scavenging. They have massive skulls and powerful forequarters, necks and jaws, which permit them to lift or drag entire ungulate carcasses and exert bite forces of at least 14,700 Newtons (unpublished data from an Instron force testing device). The highly specialized skulls of bone-cracking hyenas (Figure 11.1) may constrain brain evolution in these animals (Holekamp *et al.*, 2013). Their tremendous bite forces allow them to destroy most test apparatuses.

Perception and Communication

Hyenas employ various forms of chemical communication, which can be manipulated to test their cognitive abilities. They mark their living spaces with faecal middens, called latrines, and deposit viscous secretions, called 'paste', from their anal scent glands onto grass stalks or other substrates (Kruuk, 1972). Their eyes are dichromatic and exophthalmic (Calderone *et al.*, 2003), allowing for both excellent night vision and human-like visual acuity in daylight (Jacobs, 1993). Their behaviour indicates that hyenas recognize one another based on visual cues. When in close proximity to one another, spotted hyenas communicate by erecting their manes and tails, and using a rich repertoire of facial expressions and body postures.

Spotted hyenas are well known for their complex vocal repertoire. They are often referred to as 'laughing hyenas' because their 'giggle' vocalization sounds like hysterical human laughter. They also emit deep groans to call their cubs out of dens, high-pitched whines to beg for food or milk, and cattle-like lowing sounds to bring group-mates to a common state of arousal (Kruuk, 1972). The hyena's 'whoop' can be heard from distances of at least 5 km.

Life History

Relative to many other carnivores, spotted hyenas have slow life histories, with a protracted ontogenetic development, presumably because their robust skulls and facial musculature take years to develop fully (Watts *et al.*, 2009; Tanner *et al.*, 2010). The hyena's life history can be divided into stages marked by clear milestones (Figure 11.2). After a 110-day gestation period, spotted hyenas give birth in a secluded natal den to one or two cubs (Kruuk, 1972). After 3–4 weeks at the natal den, cubs are moved to the clan's communal den, which they share for 7–12 months with cubs of other females. The communal den is the clan's social hub; virtually all clan members visit it frequently.

Cubs become independent of dens at 8–12 months of age and enter the third life-history stage, during which they continue to nurse but also feed at carcasses. Cubs are weaned at around 13 months of age. When cubs leave the safety of the communal den, a significant spike occurs in their mortality, and fewer than half of all cubs born survive to sexual maturity at 2 years of age (Watts *et al.*, 2009). Females spend their lives in their natal clans, although they occasionally form new clans, by moving *en masse* with other

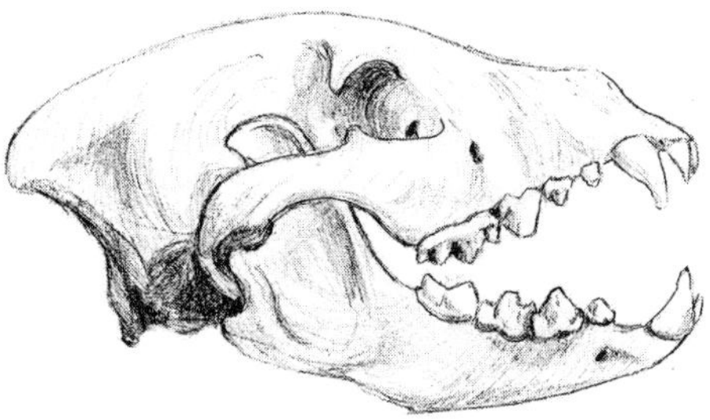

Figure 11.1. The skull of the spotted hyena. Drawing by L. Johnson-Ulrich.

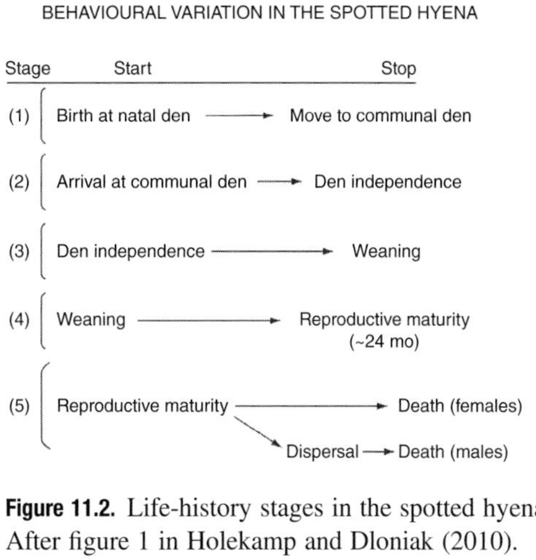

Figure 11.2. Life-history stages in the spotted hyena. After figure 1 in Holekamp and Dloniak (2010).

females to vacant habitat (Mills, 1990; Holekamp *et al.*, 1993); females also sometimes commute outside their natal territories on foraging excursions (Hofer and East, 1993a). In contrast, most males disperse after puberty, forcing them to locate, evaluate and navigate a new physical and, in particular, social environment. In this respect, the cognitive challenges faced by male spotted hyenas exceed those confronting females and may be related to the larger frontal cortex found in male than female hyenas (Arsznov *et al.*, 2010).

Individual Identification

Among adults, females are brawnier than males and have a different body profile, particularly in its ventral aspect. However, the sexes of cubs and subadult hyenas are virtually impossible to distinguish based on body shape. The external genitalia of the female spotted hyena are unique among mammals. The female's clitoris is enlarged to form a fully erectile pseudo-penis, through which she urinates, copulates and gives birth. Additionally, the vaginal labia are fused and filled with connective tissue to form a structure that resembles the male's scrotum. However, the erect pseudo-penis of a female hyena is distinguishable from that of a male from a very young age; it is blunt with little to no constriction near the glans (Figure 11.3A). By contrast, the male's erect penis has a pointed glans with a marked constriction above the glans (Figure 11.3B; Frank *et al.*, 1990).

Hyenas are easy to identify individually by their unique spot patterns, which can be memorized with the help of photographs. In addition, coat colour, ear damage, scarring and other marks help to identify individuals. Young spotted hyenas can be aged to within a few days, based on their appearance. Cubs are born with a solid black natal coat that lightens at the first moult. The spot pattern revealed during this moult is unique and stable throughout the lifespan, although spots tend to fade as hyenas age.

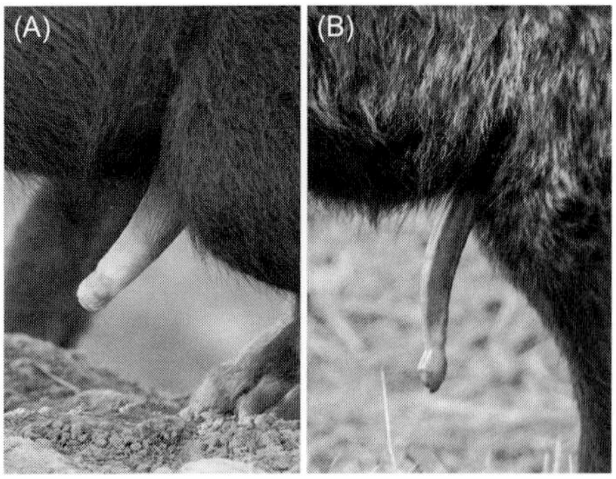

Figure 11.3. The sex of a spotted hyena can be distinguished from a young age, because the pseudo-penis of the female (A) differs in shape from the male's penis (B). In female and male hyenas of the same age, length is not appreciably different between the sexes.
Photos by L. Johnson-Ulrich.

The bone-cracking premolar teeth can be used to determine (± 6 months) ages of hyenas not observed since birth (Van Horn *et al.*, 2003), but this requires immobilization and tooth measurements.

Ecological Characteristics

Spotted hyenas occupy a diverse array of habitats throughout sub-Saharan Africa (Holekamp and Dloniak, 2010), ranging from montane forests to deserts. Seasonal variation in home range use, reproductive behaviour and foraging are related to differential movements of their prey during wet and dry seasons (Trinkel *et al.*, 2006; Holekamp and Dloniak, 2010).

Spotted hyenas have flexible foraging habits, consuming everything from termites to elephants (Holekamp and Dloniak, 2010). They readily exploit novel sources of food, and in Ethiopia, many populations have become adapted to life in cities, where they consume garbage or prey on livestock (Abay *et al.*, 2011). Elsewhere, spotted hyenas kill up to 95 per cent of their own food (Holekamp *et al.*, 1997; Holekamp and Dloniak, 2010), although juveniles do not reach adult hunting proficiency until 5 years of age (Holekamp *et al.*, 1997). Hyenas typically prey on whichever medium- to large-size ungulates are locally most abundant. They are also fond of butchered meat, full-cream powdered milk and eggs, so we often use these as rewards in our test apparatuses. Because spotted hyenas are opportunistic foragers, attracting them to test apparatuses is not difficult, once they catch scent of the bait.

Social Characteristics

Spotted hyenas are highly gregarious, living in stable groups, called clans (Kruuk, 1972), which may contain up to 130 individuals (Holekamp *et al.*, 2015) or as few as 10 individuals (Mills, 1990), but typically contain 25–60 adults in East African savannas (Holekamp and Dloniak, 2010). Clan members defend group territories ranging in size from 20–30 km^2 in prey-rich areas to over 1000 km^2 in deserts (Holekamp and Dloniak, 2010). In prey-rich areas, territorial borders are marked and defended, whereas in areas of low prey abundance, borders may be permeable or separated by unoccupied space. Hyenas in prey-rich areas may forage over 10–12 km/day, whereas hyenas in prey-poor regions may forage over 23–27 km/day (Holekamp and Dloniak, 2010).

Although their clan size, territory size and space use all vary among habitats, the societies of spotted hyenas are remarkably consistent. Spotted hyena clans contain multiple matrilines of females and their young, as well as unrelated immigrant males (Drea and Frank, 2003; Holekamp *et al.*, 2007; Figure 11.4). Relatedness is high within matrilines, but low on average among natal clan-mates due to extensive gene flow via dispersing males (Van Horn *et al.*, 2004a). Hyena clans are structured by linear dominance hierarchies, with the alpha female hyena at the top, followed by her offspring and other members of the alpha matriline, then other matrilines, with immigrant males at the bottom (for aggressive behaviours, see Figure 11.5). Although social

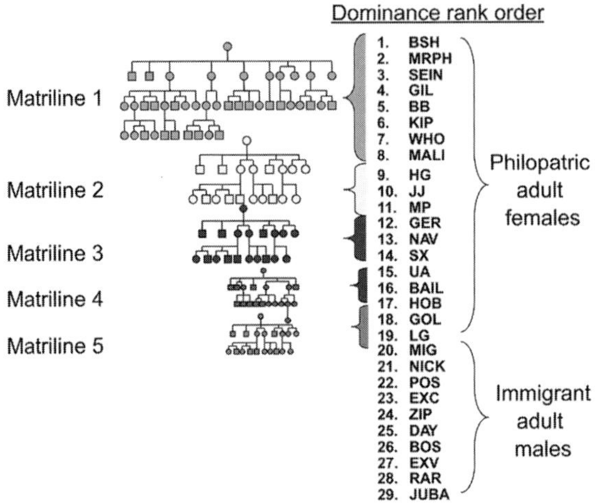

Figure 11.4. Dominance rank order of matrilines, within one cohort of adults present in a single large clan. The dominance hierarchy of natal animals contains multiple matrilineal kin groups, shown on the left; each matriline is represented by a different shade. Squares in genealogies represent males and circles represent females. Although only adult females are shown among the natal animals in the vertical listing on the right, offspring are included in the genealogies shown on the left; offspring slot into the hierarchy immediately below their mothers. Thus all adult females and their young outrank all immigrant males.
After figure 1 in Holekamp *et al.* (2012).

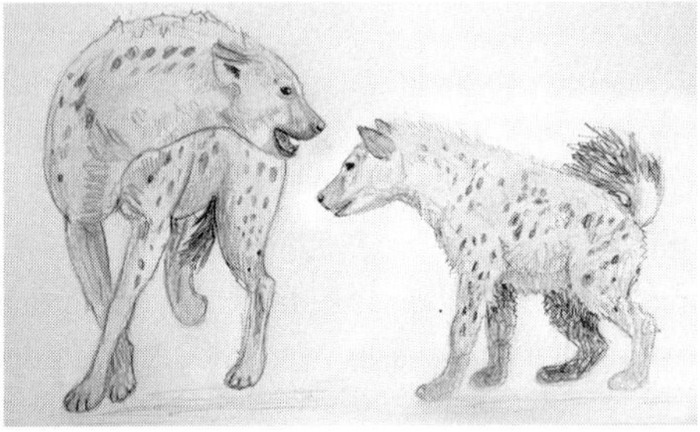

Figure 11.5. A subadult hyena directs aggression towards an adult of lower rank. The subadult has a bristled bristletail and forward-pointing ears to indicate aggressive intent, whereas the adult has its ears back, tail down and mouth open to show appeasement.
Drawing by L. Johnson-Ulrich.

female dominance allows females to defend their offspring with aggression and displace males from kills, so their young juveniles can feed, rates of intrasexual aggression are similar between males and females (Curren *et al.*, 2015).

Spotted hyena clans are fission–fusion societies (Kruuk, 1972; Mills, 1990). Hyenas gather in large groups during clan wars, territory border patrols, lion–hyena conflicts and at large carcasses (Smith *et al.*, 2008). However, they are often found alone, and mean subgroup size is only 2.2 individuals (Smith *et al.*, 2008). The fission–fusion dynamics of spotted hyena clans have both benefits and costs for studies of their cognition. Researchers can easily find individual hyenas alone for testing, but tests may be interrupted by the arrival of clan-mates, and testing at the communal den almost invariably involves multiple hyenas (see below). Moreover, social rank determines priority of access to food, and can thus affect motivation to remove food from test apparatuses. Furthermore, in novel object trials, den-dwelling cubs are bolder when they have a littermate present than when the sibling is absent (Greenberg and Holekamp, 2017). Philopatric members of hyena matrilines form tight lifelong bonds; siblings and female relatives are often found together even as adults (Smith *et al.*, 2010).

Spotted hyenas breed throughout the year. Both sexes mate promiscuously, and twin littermates may have different sires (Engh *et al.*, 2002; East *et al.*, 2003). Reproductive skew is greater among females than males (Engh *et al.*, 2002; Holekamp and Engh, 2009), with alpha females enjoying the greatest reproductive success (Holekamp *et al.*, 1996).

State of the Art

Social Recognition

Spotted hyenas recognize individual group-mates using cues from multiple sensory modalities (Drea, 2002a, b), including whoop vocalizations (Holekamp *et al.*, 1999; Benson-Amram *et al.*, 2011; Gersick *et al.*, 2015) and olfactory cues to discriminate sex, reproductive state, clan membership, social rank and individual identity (Theis, 2008; Burgener *et al.*, 2009; Theis *et al.*, 2012). Although male hyenas do not participate in parental care, sires can recognize their offspring and vice versa (Van Horn *et al.*, 2004b). Hyena littermates can also distinguish full- from half-siblings (Wahaj *et al.*, 2004). Social bonds are stronger among kin than non-kin (Smith *et al.*, 2007), and individuals direct affiliative and cooperative behaviour most frequently towards kin (East *et al.*, 1993; Wahaj *et al.*, 2004; Smith *et al.*, 2007).

Based on both social rank and kinship, spotted hyenas can recognize third-party relationships among their clan-mates (Engh *et al.*, 2005). Hyenas are more likely to attack the relatives of their opponents after a fight than during a matched control period, and after a fight, they are more likely to attack relatives of their opponents than clan-mates unrelated to their opponents (Engh *et al.*, 2005). Spotted hyenas also recognize that their social partners vary in relative value to them and use this knowledge to make adaptive choices regarding which clan-mates to associate with (Smith *et al.*, 2007). Spotted hyenas prefer to spend time with and direct most affiliative behaviour towards high-ranking non-kin (East *et al.*, 1993; Smith *et al.*, 2011), and use unsolicited appeasement and greeting behaviours to reconcile after fights (East *et al.*, 1993; Wahaj *et al.*, 2001).

Rank Learning

The acquisition of social rank by young spotted hyenas involves a protracted process of associative learning (Holekamp and Smale, 1991; Engh *et al.*, 2000). Cubs initially form a rank hierarchy within their den cohort, based on individual differences in aggressiveness (Holekamp and Smale, 1993), but they gradually learn their ranks relative to those of peers and all other clan-mates, a process not complete until cubs are around 18 months of age (Smale *et al.*, 1993). To experimentally test rank acquisition, we mimic the competitive feeding environment experienced by adult hyenas at ungulate carcasses by administering brief tests in which a food item is presented to young hyenas at the communal den when adults are absent. Spotted hyenas clearly remember outcomes of earlier encounters with particular group-mates.

Social Facilitation

Experimental evidence suggests a prominent role for social facilitation in the lives of spotted hyenas (Glickman *et al.*, 1997). Captive hyenas frequently engage in the same behaviours as those exhibited by nearby conspecifics, overcoming a conditioned food aversion when housed with conspecifics that fed on the aversive food (Glickman *et al.*, 1997). Social facilitation promotes synchronous behaviour, which is necessary for coordinated action against rivals, and reduces hyenas' latency to approach a puzzle box, with latency to approach being a significant predictor of success in opening the box (Benson-Amram and Holekamp, 2012).

Cooperation

Despite strong feeding competition, hyenas often hunt cooperatively, and their hunting success increases by 20 per cent with each additional hunter (Holekamp *et al.*, 1997). Male hyenas often form coalitions to cooperatively mob lone females (Szykman *et al.*, 2003; Curren, 2012). The most dramatic cooperation between hyenas takes place during interclan and interspecific competition (Henschel and Skinner, 1991; Boydston *et al.*, 2001). During conflicts with lions, spotted hyenas vocalize and coordinate their movements to approach and mob lions *en masse* (Kruuk, 1972), usurping food and thus enhancing their fitness (Lehmann *et al.*, 2017). Drea and Carter (2009) experimentally tested captive hyenas on a food acquisition task and found that they spontaneously solved cooperation problems requiring both coordination and synchrony and were able to modify their behaviour based on group composition and partner experience.

Social Learning

As generalist carnivores, spotted hyenas may use social learning to exploit novel food sources. In captivity, spotted hyenas show limited social learning, with no effect of observing a demonstrator on successful problem-solving, although there is some evidence for localized stimulus enhancement, focusing more efforts on the same door side of the puzzle box (Benson-Amram *et al.*, 2014).

Deception

Spotted hyenas may conceal their knowledge of hidden food based on social circumstances. Yoerg (in Drea and Frank, 2003) found that high-ranking hyenas approached the location of hidden food regardless of the presence of naïve hyenas, whereas low-ranking hyenas led naïve higher-ranking group-mates astray before returning to consume the food themselves.

Personality

Spotted hyenas exhibit distinct personality traits, including boldness and neophobia (Gosling, 1998; Greenberg and Holekamp, 2017) and these traits affect performance in cognitive tests (e.g. Benson-Amram and Holekamp, 2012). We tested boldness in wild spotted hyenas by presenting them with a mock intruder in the form of a life-size hard foam model of a spotted hyena and measuring their latency to approach it (Turner, 2018). We also assessed boldness in cubs, using experimental presentation of a metal mesh box that a subject must enter to access powdered milk. Using both types of tests, we found that the local level of anthropogenic disturbance affects boldness, suggesting that hyenas' boldness develops at least partially in response to their Umwelt during early ontogeny (Greenberg and Holekamp, 2017; Turner, 2018).

Innovative Problem-Solving

Spotted hyenas are generalist carnivores (Holekamp and Dloniak, 2010), which seems to be broadly associated with the ability to innovate, i.e. to invent a novel solution or solve a novel problem (Reader and Laland, 2003). We tested innovation in wild hyenas using a puzzle box with a hinged door, which could be opened by sliding a bolt with mouth or paws (Benson-Amram and Holekamp, 2012). Only 14.5 per cent of wild hyenas learned to open the box, whereas 73.7 per cent of captive subjects were able to solve this problem. Apparently, wild hyenas were less successful than captives due to greater neophobia and more time constraints (Benson-Amram *et al.*, 2013).

Memory

No systematic study of memory has been conducted in spotted hyenas, but they can live up to 26 years in the wild and are capable of remembering several dozen individual clan-mates, which suggests they have long memories. Interestingly, after an 18-month hiatus, we presented the same puzzle box used by Benson-Amram and Holekamp (2012) to one individual who had learned to open the box in her previous trials, and she immediately opened the box, indicating that she remembered how to solve that problem for at least 18 months without rehearsal.

Numerical Understanding

Although lethal aggression is rare within a clan, interclan fights can cause injury or death. To test numerosity in hyenas, we used playbacks of the whoops of varying numbers of hyenas, whose voices had never been heard by our subjects. In these experiments, hyenas only approached the speaker when they outnumbered their opponents (Benson-Amram *et al.*, 2011).

Spatial Learning

Virtually nothing is known about spatial intelligence in spotted hyenas, although they may regularly commute from their dens as far as 75.2 km, in search of food (Hofer and East, 1993a, b). In the Serengeti, spotted hyenas frequently go on foraging trips that may last a week, to prey upon migrating herds of wildebeest (Hofer and East, 1995). Dispersing male hyenas make exploratory excursions outside their natal territory, and subsequently follow a straight path on return (Booms *et al.*, 2017). These observations suggest that spotted hyenas possess sophisticated cognitive maps and use navigational skills, including path integration, that allow them to find their way home again.

All for One and One for All

Box 11.1 Cognition in Dogs and Wolves

Friederike Range

The current chapter nicely introduced the social ecology and cognitive abilities of hyenas. Another carnivore that, while phylogenetically distant, relies to a high degree on cooperative hunting is the wolf. In contrast to hyenas, however, wolves are also cooperative breeders that live predominantly in family groups composed of a breeding pair (which form a long-term bond) and their adult and subadult offspring, as well as pups from the most recent litter (Packard, 2003). Overall, to successfully hunt, defend their territory and raise pups, wolves highly depend on a cohesive and functional pack structure (Mech and Boitani, 2003). Interestingly, the domesticated form of wolves, dogs, have a very different social ecology when free-ranging: dogs are predominantly scavengers (although they are known to hunt in groups as well), mainly relying on human waste; they forage alone or form multimale multifemale groups of 2–8 individuals; and pups are raised mostly by their mothers (see Marshall-Pescini *et al.*, 2017a, for a review on socio-ecological differences between wolves and dogs).

Using similar tasks as have been used with hyenas, we compared the problem-solving skills of wolves and dogs raised in a similar manner at the Wolf Science Center to study the effects of domestication on dogs and wolves' cognitive and emotional profile. For example, we have found that wolves and dogs, as hyenas, are faster to approach novel objects when in the presence of conspecifics (Moretti *et al.*, 2015), and there is some suggestion that in wolves, conspecifics' aversion to a specific food influences their motivation to relocate the hidden food item afterwards (Range and Virányi, 2013). However, whether wolves and dogs would also overcome aversion to a certain food item by social facilitation, as suggested in hyenas, would have to be confirmed by conducting further experiments along the same lines suggested in the chapter.

Moreover, in contrast to hyenas and dogs, wolves benefit from the demonstration of a conspecific opening a puzzle box. Not only do they manipulate the same side of

(*cont.*)

the apparatus manipulated by the demonstrator, but they also imitate the specific action the demonstrator used to open the box (Range and Virányi, 2014). This difference might be explained by the high dependence of wolves on cooperation with conspecifics, requiring close social attention to each other's actions and high social tolerance – two requisites for social learning. In line with this, we found that while wolves, like hyenas, also spontaneously cooperate in a food acquisition task, dogs fail, most likely due to tolerance issues (Marshall-Pescini *et al.*, 2017b).

Interestingly, wolves and dogs show different conflict management strategies around food resources (tolerant vs. avoidant; Range *et al.*, 2015; Dale *et al.*, 2017), which are in line with their peculiar feeding ecologies (cooperative hunters need to share the prey after hunting, while dogs need to defend scraps from other dogs) and likely explain several of the differences in performance in the various tasks presented. It would be exciting to test and/or observe hyenas using similar methods as we have, to understand how tolerant they are with each other in a feeding context, and compare them to both wolves and dogs. Based on the fact that hyenas rely on both cooperative hunting and scavenging, they might show some behavioural adaptations that are present in wolves but not in dogs, and vice versa.

Finally, we are currently using similar puzzle boxes as those used for hyenas to study wolves and dogs' persistence and innovativeness in independent problem-solving tasks. Overall, from a comparative perspective, using similar methods allows for a more accurate comparison and will ultimately help us to better understand how different species solve different tasks, and how the respective problem-solving strategies are linked to the species-specific socio-ecologies.

References

Dale, R., Range, F., Stott, L., Kotrschal, K., and Marshall-Pescini, S. (2017). The influence of social relationship on food tolerance in wolves and dogs. *Behavioral Ecology and Sociobiology*, **71**, 107–131.

Marshall-Pescini, S., Cafazzo, S., Virányi, Z., and Range, F. (2017a). Integrating social ecology in explanations of wolf-dog behavioral differences. *Current Opinion in Behavioral Sciences*, **16**, 80–86.

Marshall-Pescini, S., Schwarz, J. F. L., Kostelnik, I., Virányi, Z., and Range, F. (2017b). Importance of a species' socioecology: wolves outperform dogs in a conspecific cooperation task. *Proceedings of the National Academy of Sciences*, **114**, 11793–11798.

Mech, L. D., and Boitani, L. (2003). Wolf social ecology. In *Wolves: behavior, ecology and conservation* (pp. 1–35). Chicago, IL: University of Chicago Press.

Moretti, L., Hentrup, M., Kotrschal, K., and Range, F. (2015). The influence of relationships on neophobia and exploration in wolves and dogs. *Animal Behavior*, **107**, 159–173.

Packard, J. M. (2003). Wolf behavior: reproductive, social and intelligent. In *Wolves: behavior, ecology and conservation* (pp. 36–65). Chicago, IL: University of Chicago Press.

(*cont.*)

Range, F., and Virányi, Z. (2013). Social learning from humans or conspecifics: differences and similarities between wolves and dogs. *Frontiers in Psychology*, **4**, 868.

Range, F., and Virányi, Z. (2014). Wolves are better imitators of conspecifics than dogs. *PLoS ONE*, **9**, e86559.

Range, F., Ritter, C., and Virányi, Z. (2015). Testing the myth: tolerant dogs and aggressive wolves. *Proceedings of the Royal Society of London B: Biological Sciences*, **282**, 1807.

Field Guide

Typical Research Day

We study wild hyenas from the safety of our research vehicles. Vehicles must handle rough terrain and contain enough space to accommodate cognitive apparatuses. We observe hyenas and conduct experiements with them around dawn and again around dusk, as equatorial hyenas generally avoid mid-day heat and sleep between 9 AM and 5 PM. We often focus our efforts on the communal den, which is ideal for observing social interactions, assessing demography and conducting cognitive tests in group trials, such as novel object tests or feeding trials. In these experiments, variables such as test group size and littermate presence or absence must be controlled statistically. To conduct cognitive tests on cubs while their mothers and other adults are absent, the best time is often mid to late afternoon, when the sun remains high, as adults usually rest away from the den until closer to dusk. The communal den is also a good place during the morning to reliably find adult female hyenas, which can be followed as they leave the den to be tested alone.

Hyenas can easily be found away from the den, but it is difficult to reliably find specific individuals repeatedly, when they have neither GPS collars nor den-dwelling cubs. Because of this, we opportunistically exploit good situations as soon as they arise, especially when conducting experiments. Although one may be able to find the same individual several days in a row, because it is obliged to visit a den or because it repeatedly uses a particular resting spot, one might never find that individual alone. Thus, experiments involving tests of lone individuals require much time and patience. The best way to locate hyenas away from the den is to find an elevated vantage point and use binoculars to scan the surrounding habitat.

Site Selection

When selecting a study site, researchers should consider both ease of accessibility and the seasonal or environmental factors that might affect test outcomes, which may need to be controlled statistically. We study six spotted hyena clans, chosen for ease of observation and proximity to our research camps, in the Maasai Mara National Reserve, Kenya. The

Mara is covered mainly by open grassland, but grass height, bushes and hidden rocks affect our ability to observe hyenas. Highly nocturnal clans, such as those in areas with much anthropogenic activity, are more difficult to study, even with night vision gear. It is also difficult to monitor clans that den in thickets. The rainy season generates deep mud, which limits our ability to observe hyenas. The annual influx of migratory herbivores from Tanzania makes hyenas more gregarious, relaxed and easier to find, but it does not appear to reduce their motivation to participate in baited cognitive trials.

Collection and Use of Vocalization Data

Before playback experiments can be conducted, one must either obtain call recordings from existing sound libraries, where caller identity is unknown to subjects, or record hyena vocalizations on site. Obtaining recordings from spotted hyenas requires a directional microphone with an effective windscreen, a digital recorder, persistence and luck. Certain types of calls, such as whoops, can be elicited by playbacks of other sounds, such as those of lion–hyena interactions (Gersick *et al.*, 2015), but many vocalizations occur unpredictably, so to capture these, the digital recorder must constantly be switched on. Kills, carcasses and dens are good locations to capture recordings, but hyenas often vocalize over one another when excited, as they often are in these situations.

Many hyena vocalizations are very loud and can transmit over long distances, so speakers must be able to produce undistorted sound at high volume. Speaker sound levels must also be standardized to typical hyena source levels for each vocalization type. Spotted hyenas can quickly become habituated to playback broadcasts if these experiments are not done carefully. The animals readily associate humans with sounds emanating from the vehicle, and if this occurs, responses to broadcasts quickly decline. Furthermore, broadcasting loud calls from a vehicle can hinder sound propagation and deafen observers. Instead, speakers should be disguised with foliage or hidden in vegetation a short distance away from the research vehicle. Speaker placement outside the vehicle presents its own challenges; our subjects may flee if they see humans exit a vehicle, and their strong jaws threaten any equipment on the ground.

A novel technology with which we have been experimenting involves deploying GPS radio collars with built-in microphones and sound cards. Each microphone must be tightly covered with sound-transparent fabric, to which mud and blood cannot stick. Because fitting hyenas with radio collars involves immobilizing them, we use collars (produced by Tellus, Lindesberg, Sweden) that drop off the hyena when triggered by a radio signal. The sound files stored on the collars are huge and cannot currently be offloaded without retrieving the collars, but they contain an immense wealth of hyena vocalizations.

Collection and Use of Olfactory Data

Paste samples must be collected from the scent glands of immobilized hyenas and stored frozen until used. Cubs and subadults produce little or no paste, but adult anal

Table 11.1. Essential experimental tools required to study hyenas and their function.

Tool	Function
Flashlight or spotlight	Powerful enough to identify hyenas at night
Digital voice recorder	Record behavioural data for later transcription
DSLR camera with telephoto lens	Taking hyena ID photos, two lenses are best: a telephoto lens for photographing distant hyenas during the daytime (at least 100 mm), and wide angle lens for low-light conditions (< 20 mm). Many DSLR zoom lenses can accommodate both ranges. A good point-and-shoot camera with a superzoom lens is acceptable, if one has budget constraints, but is inadequate at capturing spots for identifying hyenas in low-light and night conditions
Good camcorder	Filming busy events like carcass sessions, hunts, mating and lion–hyena interactions, or recording behaviour during experimental trials
Computer	A computer with a good battery life and durable hardware (with a dustproof keyboard cover) works better in field conditions. MacBook Pros and Airs seem superior to PCs on these two factors
Printer	To print hyena ID photos
Speakers	For playback experiments
MP3 player	To store and playback sounds
Recording equipment	For recording vocalizations
Binoculars	For finding and identifying hyenas and other animals, at least 8 × 40 (wide angle is better)
Hyena ID photo album	Necessary to confirm the identities of all hyenas present
GPS	Navigating study site, marking locations of dens, landmarks and hyenas
Charging cords for all equipment	Ideally, all electronics can run off the car battery, so that equipment does not lose power at inopportune moments
Extra batteries	For equipment that does not run off the car battery (e.g. DVRs, cameras)
Window tripod	For camcorders and/or cameras, to keep your hands free during filming and photography, so that you can manage DVRs, vocalization equipment, etc.
Four-wheel drive vehicle	Necessary for navigating off-road terrain
Vehicle supplies	For fixing flats and getting unstuck from mud or rocks, fluids for leaks/overheating
Water	Large amount to add to radiator in case of overheating, and for drinking if car breaks down and you are stuck somewhere for a long time
Buff, scarf or bandana	Cover your mouth and nose from the smell of rotting meat, to make handling stinky bait much more tolerable
A large supply of latex gloves	Careful handling of bait is necessary to avoid getting fluids on yourself and the inside of the vehicle
Non-nylon clothing	Hyenas can be startled by your movement within the vehicle if your clothing makes scratching noises when you move

glands reliably contain 2–3 g that can be collected with a sterile spatula. Theis (2008) presented paired paste samples to spotted hyenas at dens, on synthetic grass stalks made of stiff plastic-coated wire embedded in the ground. He spent many nights at dens wearing night-vision goggles to collect data on olfactory discrimination, using time spent sniffing each synthetic stalk as the dependent measure. Hyenas readily investigated and pasted over previously frozen paste samples presented in this way. Paste can also be collected from grass stalks immediately after an individual has pasted on them and stored frozen. Burgener and colleagues (2009) used gas chromatography–mass spectrometry to examine the chemical composition of paste samples collected in this way. Variation in chemical composition can be used to identify scent profiles of individual hyenas.

Presenting Test Apparatuses to Hyenas

We strive to deploy cognitive test apparatuses without our subjects associating them with humans, but situated such that each subject can see the apparatus when we want it to. In our study area, we also need to avoid tourists and other animals while ensuring that the apparatus is observable so that subjects' responses can be recorded. In addition to our vehicle serving as a mobile blind from which we record observations, it also functions as a sight barrier while we set up an apparatus.

Unbaited Test Apparatuses

Lifesize foam model hyenas can be used to test boldness (Figure 11.6A): subjects appear to believe it is a real hyena until they get close enough to use olfactory or tactile cues, at which point they explore it further, lose interest, or bite it. A surprising array of foam models are produced as life-size animals, including many of the ungulates on which hyenas prey. The models weigh little and come in multiple pieces, so they are easy to transport. However, the base pegs on the feet are designed to be pounded into the ground, so when preparing the model for easy deployment, we instead mount it on a stable wooden stand that can quickly be placed on the ground, without drawing unwanted attention from test subjects.

Having identified a lone untested hyena with binoculars, we usually back up, set the model on the ground, and then drive to a position roughly 40 m away, oriented parallel to the line between the approaching hyena and the model. We then set up one camera at full wide angle on a window-mounted tripod, to track distances between subject and model, and a second hand-operated camera zoomed in on the subject, to record its specific behaviours. Once the subject has moved off, we retrieve the model, using our vehicle as a visual barrier between model and subject.

We use similar methods in novel object trials with cubs at dens (Figure 11.6B,C), where we deploy cheap novel disposable items such as umbrellas, buckets, plastic thermoses and plastic stools. Objects are placed 15 m from the den, and trials start when one or more cubs approach within 10 m of the object. Here we must control statistically for rank, number of other individuals present and the behaviour of those animals.

Baited Apparatuses

Baited test apparatuses present two new difficulties over unbaited apparatuses. First, the bait used in testing affects the motivation of the hyena. Second, obtaining the bait from inside an apparatus requires active participation by hyena subjects. Although captive hyenas usually participate readily in most types of cognitive trials, participation by wild

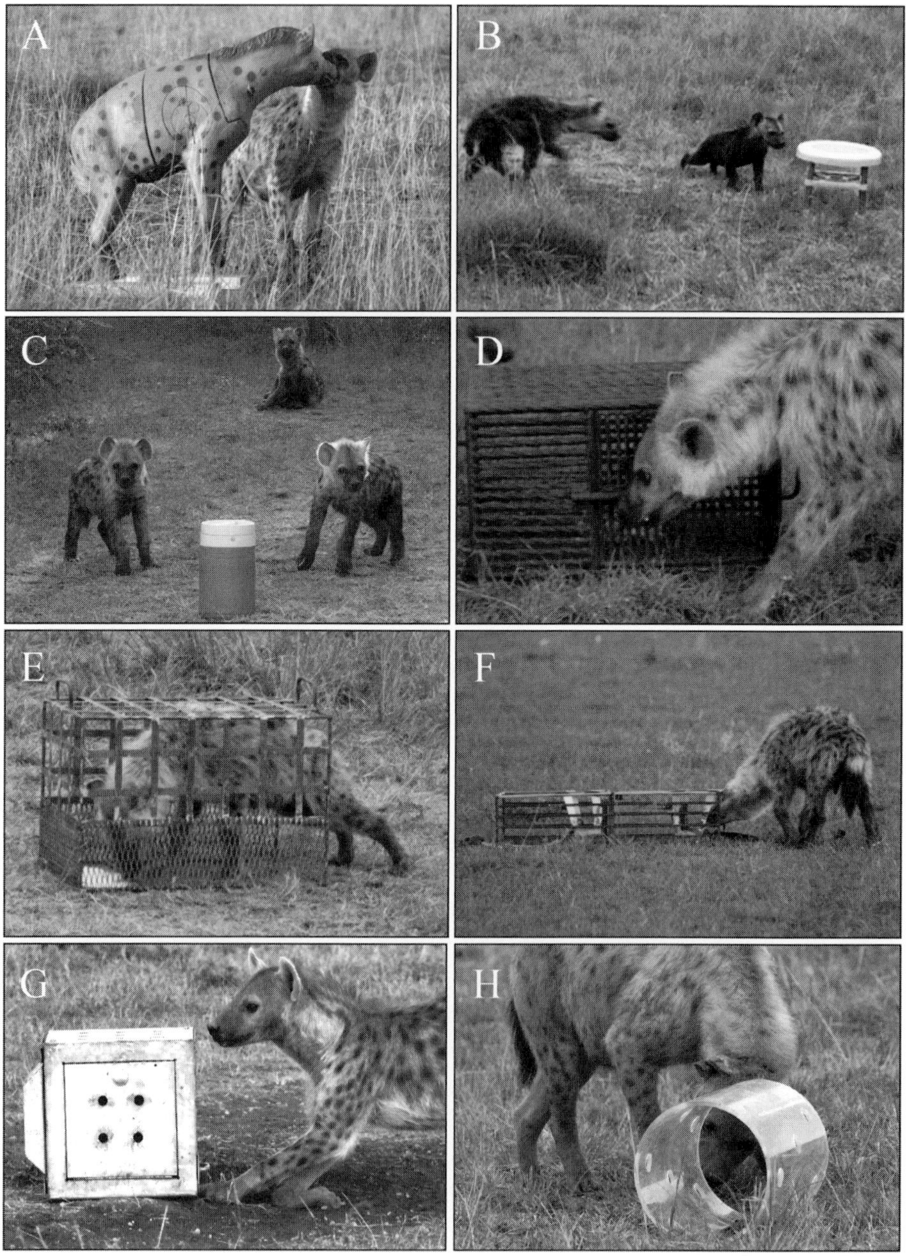

Figure 11.6. Test apparatuses presented to wild spotted hyenas. (A) Mock intruder, photo credit: J. W. Turner. (B) Novel object, photo credit: J. R. Greenberg. (C) Novel object, photo credit: J.R. Greenberg. (D) Puzzle box, photo credit: S. Benson-Amram. (E) Boldness box, photo credit: J. R. Greenberg. (F) Reversal-learning box, photo credit: A. Laurence. (G) Multi-access box, photo credit: L. Johnson-Ulrich. (H) Inhibitory control cylinder.
Photo by L. Johnson-Ulrich.

hyenas is uncertain and may be influenced by myriad factors. We have used several baited cognitive test apparatuses with wild hyenas to date (Figure 11.6D–H), including puzzle boxes to be opened with mouth/paw, metal mesh boxes to be entered by cubs, rebar reversal learning boxes with 2-cm-diameter ropes to be pulled, stainless steel multi-access boxes with four doors that can only be opened via different behaviours, PVC tubes in an inhibitory control detour-reaching-task, and lidded metal bucket-within-bucket arrays to test learning and memory in hyenas. Test apparatuses with which spotted hyenas interact to get food must either be disposable, easily repairable or tough enough to withstand the hyena's bite forces. They also must be sufficiently light and wieldy for the experimenter to lift, carry and set them up easily. Rebar is generally strong enough for building puzzle boxes but rusts rapidly if used outdoors, so we have also used galvanized and stainless steel apparatuses. Steel thinner than 1/8″ thick can be bent by the hyena's jaws, but the use of heavier, thicker steel reduces our ability to lift apparatuses in and out of vehicles. In our PVC and clear acrylic apparatuses, we use 3/8″ thick walls. We recommend cast acrylic over extruded acrylic, because it is stronger and has greater clarity, and we keep plastic polish on hand, as it scratches easily. Importantly, test apparatuses need to be manipulatable by hyenas' jaws or paws. Hyenas dig or slap at apparatuses with their paws, but primarily use their mouths for manipulation and, if motivated, readily bite and pull on protruding parts of an apparatus.

Bait

Spotted hyenas are extremely fond of fresh meat and clearly prefer it to rancid meat, although the stronger scent of rotting meat appears to be a more powerful attractant, because it is detectable from farther away. Skin and lungs are the only body parts hyenas may disdain. Raw eggs can be used as bait, but they have little scent and may be unattractive to hyenas who have never tasted them. By contrast, raw eggs coated in bacon grease are attractive to all subjects. However, the most effective bait is often full-cream powdered milk. In familiarization trials, milk powder sprinkled on the ground near the apparatus forces the subject to remain in extended proximity to the apparatus, whereas meat scraps are snatched and quickly carried away. On the other hand, during test trials, using milk powder as bait causes a much longer delay between trials, because subjects invariably attempt to lick up every last molecule of powder. It often helps to familiarize hyenas with milk powder before any testing begins, by leaving small piles of it near the communal den. We use a fist-sized piece of meat, one egg or a cup of milk powder to bait our test apparatuses, and these motivate our subjects quite vigorously. If more hyenas are present in a particular trial, we often put more food in the apparatus, so that multiple hyenas can feed. For a single hyena requiring substantial motivation, three fist-sized pieces of meat suffice. Captive hyenas are more highly motivated to participate in cognitive tests than wild hyenas, and their bait need be nothing other than their regular diet, with testing timed to coincide with regular feeding times.

Multiple Trials

If a cognitive experiment requires administering multiple trials to each subject, we recommend running multiple trials in quick succession, to avoid the difficulty of relocating the subject within a few days of initial testing. Administering several successive trials does not appear to decrease motivation and may in fact enhance learning. Hyenas can eat up to 20 per cent of their own body mass in one meal (Kruuk, 1972), and they never appear to lose motivation due to satiation. Even obese hyenas readily participate in cognitive trials for food rewards. To assess a hyena's willingness to work to obtain our chosen bait, we toss a piece of bait roughly 5 m from the animal, and note whether it approaches and consumes the meat before we undertake any further testing. If the animal ignores the meat, it will seldom work to obtain bait from a test apparatus. Regardless, it is critical to record the amount of time that passes between trials, so this can be controlled in statistical analyses.

Familiarization Trials

Spotted hyenas do not need familiarization trials to associate an apparatus with food, because the scent of food inside is enough to attract them. However, most individuals do require at least one familiarization trial to overcome any neophobia and become accustomed to reaching inside the apparatus to retrieve food. Although we recommend giving multiple test trials in a row, we do not recommend administering multiple familiarization trials or giving a test trial immediately after a familiarization trial. After a familiarization trial, many hyenas associate the test apparatus with free food, and will not work to get more. Thus, familiarization trials decrease neophobia, but may also decrease motivation.

The Umwelt of the Spotted Hyena and its Effects on Cognitive Tests

A stronger-smelling bait can provide a more powerful incentive to hyenas, and bait should be placed upwind of subjects. Presenting an apparatus at a carcass or a den is frequently more successful than elsewhere, as there are often multiple active and hungry hyenas. Multiple hyenas also permit socially facilitated interaction with the test apparatus, which may or may not be desirable.

Although spotted hyenas are excellent hunters, they are also scavengers, and when scavenging, hyenas exhibit remarkable patience and are highly tolerant of delayed gratification. For instance, we have seen multiple hyenas lie down and wait for several hours near a mother giraffe guarding her stillborn calf. Hyenas also often wait hours for lions to finish consuming a carcass and move away. During test trials with a puzzle box immediately after a familiarization trial, a hyena may walk off a few metres and simply lie down to wait for the situation to improve. In many of our test protocols, subjects time out if they remain more than 5 m from an apparatus for over 5 min, but this criterion fails if the hyena is waiting strategically rather than giving up. To foil a hyena's waiting strategy, we now remove the apparatus without food reward or subsequent testing if the subject lies down near the apparatus, so it learns that its waiting strategy fails in this situation. However, during cognitive tests in which only a single trial is administered, there is no way to control for potentially strategic waiting.

Spotted hyenas are far more likely to investigate a test apparatus when conspecifics are present than when they are alone. This is especially useful for reducing neophobia in hyenas. We control for group size statistically, and the larger number of hyenas participating greatly increases our sample size. Possibly, testing animals in isolation is unnatural for gregarious carnivores like hyenas and thus yields less-accurate data about their cognitive abilities than group testing.

Resources

Research groups:

- Dr Kay Holekamp, Mara Hyena Project: www.holekamplab.org
- Dr Oliver Höner, Ngorogoro Crater Hyena Project: hyena-project.com
- Dr Emma Stone, Carnivore Research Malawai: www.carnivoreresearchmalawi.org
- Dr Scott Creel, Zambian Carnivore Project: www.zambiacarnivores.org

Websites:

- MSU Hyena Blog: msuhyenas.blogspot.com
- IUCN Hyena Specialist Group: www.hyaenidae.org

Books:

- Kruuk, H. (1972). *The spotted hyena: a study of predation and social behaviour.* Chicago, IL: University of Chicago Press.
- Mills, M. G. L. (1990). *Kalahari hyaenas.* London: Unwin Hyman.

Documentaries:

- *Night of the hyena* (2008). Austin Stevens Adventures, Discovery Channel.
- *Killer IQ: Lion vs. hyena* (2015). Smithsonian Channel.

Profile

Lily Johnson-Ulrich, Kenna D. S. Lehman and Julie W. Turner are senior graduate students at Michigan State University, working with Dr Kay Holekamp. Lily studies physical cognition in spotted hyenas, comparing performance of hyenas in the Maasai Mara, Kenya with that of fully urbanized hyenas in Mekelle, Ethiopia. Spotted hyenas are excellent subjects for understanding the socio-ecological factors that shape the evolution of intelligence due to their social complexity and their generalist tendencies. Kenna studies the vocal signalling of spotted hyenas. Their extensive vocal repertoire makes hyenas ideal for asking questions about the evolution of complex signals in the context of fission–fusion sociality. Julie studies hyena personality development in the context of social network analysis. The unambiguous life-history milestones in this species make it a good model for studies of personality development. Kay Holekamp is an evolutionary behavioural ecologist who has been studying spotted hyenas in Kenya since the 1980s.

References

Abay, G. Y., Bauer, H., Gebrihiwot, K., and Deckers, J. (2011). Peri-urban spotted hyena (*Crocuta crocuta*) in northern Ethiopia: diet, economic impact, and abundance. *European Journal of Wildlife Research*, **57**, 759–765.

Arsznov, B. M., Lundrigan, B. L., Holekamp, K. E., and Sakai, S. T. (2010). Sex and the frontal cortex: a developmental CT study in the spotted hyena. *Brain, Behaviour and Evolution*, **76**, 185–197.

Benson-Amram, S., and Holekamp, K. E. (2012). Innovative problem solving by wild spotted hyenas. *Proceedings of the Royal Society of London B: Biological Sciences*, **279**, 4087–4095.

Benson-Amram, S., Heinen, V. K., Dryer, S. L., and Holekamp, K. E. (2011). Numerical assessment and individual call discrimination by wild spotted hyaenas, *Crocuta crocuta*. *Animal Behaviour*, **82**, 743–752.

Benson-Amram, S., Weldele, M. L., and Holekamp, K. E. (2013). A comparison of innovative problem-solving abilities between wild and captive spotted hyaenas, *Crocuta crocuta*. *Animal Behaviour*, **85**, 349–356.

Benson-Amram, S., Heinen, V. K., Gessner, A., Weldele, M. L., and Holekamp, K. E. (2014). Limited social learning of a novel technical problem by spotted hyenas. *Behavioural Processes*, **109**, 111–120.

Booms, A. S., Montgomery, T. M., and Holekamp, K. E. (2017). Global positioning system (GPS) data collected from collars deployed on dispersing male hyenas. Unpublished raw data.

Boydston, E. E., Morelli, T. L., and Holekamp, K. E. (2001). Sex differences in territorial behaviour exhibited by the spotted hyena (Hyaenidae, *Crocuta crocuta*). *Ethology*, **107**, 369–385.

Burgener, N., Dehnhard, M., Hofer, H., and East, M. L. (2009). Does anal gland scent signal identity in the spotted hyaena? *Animal Behaviour*, **77**, 707–715.

Calderone, J., Reese, B., and Jacobs, G. (2003). Topography of photoreceptors and retinal ganglion cells in the spotted hyena (*Crocuta crocuta*). *Brain Behaviour and Evolution*, **62**, 182–192.

Curren, L. J. (2012). *Competition and cooperation among males in a sex-role reversed mammal, the spotted hyena (Crocuta crocuta)*. PhD thesis, Michigan State University.

Curren, L. J., Linden, D. W., Heinen, V. K., McGuire, M. C., and Holekamp, K. E. (2015). The functions of male–male aggression in a female-dominated mammalian society. *Animal Behaviour*, **100**, 208–216.

Drea, C. M., and Carter, A. N. (2009). Cooperative problem solving in a social carnivore. *Animal Behaviour*, **78**, 967–977.

Drea, C. M., and Frank, L. G. (2003). The social complexity of spotted hyenas. In *Animal social complexity: intelligence, culture, and individualized societies* (pp. 121–148). Cambridge, MA: Harvard University Press.

Drea, C. M., Vignieri, S. N., Cunningham, S. B., and Glickman, S. E. (2002a). Responses to olfactory stimuli in spotted hyenas (*Crocuta crocuta*): I. Investigation of environmental odours and the function of rolling. *Journal of Comparative Psychology*, **116**, 331.

Drea, C. M., Vignieri, S. N., Kim, H. S., Weldele, M. L., and Glickman, S. E. (2002b). Responses to olfactory stimuli in spotted hyenas (*Crocuta crocuta*): II. Discrimination of conspecific scent. *Journal of Comparative Psychology*, **116**, 342.

East, M. L., Hofer, H., and Wickler, W. (1993). The erect "penis" is a flag of submission in a female-dominated society: greetings in Serengeti spotted hyenas. *Behavioural Ecology and Sociobiology*, **33**, 355–370.

East, M. L., Burke, T., Wilhelm, K., Greig, C., and Hofer, H. (2003). Sexual conflicts in spotted hyenas: male and female mating tactics and their reproductive outcome with respect to age, social status and tenure. *Proceedings of the Royal Society of London B: Biological Sciences*, **270**, 1247–1254.

Engh, A., Esch, K., Smale, L., and Holekamp, K. E. (2000). Mechanisms of maternal rank "inheritance" in the spotted hyaena, *Crocuta crocuta*. *Animal Behaviour*, **60**, 323–332.

Engh, A. L., Funk, S. M., Van Horn, R. C., *et al.* (2002). Reproductive skew among males in a female-dominated mammalian society. *Behavioural Ecology*, **13**, 193–200.

Engh, A. L., Siebert, E. R., Greenberg, D. A., and Holekamp, K. E. (2005). Patterns of alliance formation and postconflict aggression indicate spotted hyaenas recognize third-party relationships. *Animal Behaviour*, **69**, 209–217.

Frank, L. G., Glickman, S. E., and Powch, I. (1990). Sexual dimorphism in the spotted hyaena (*Crocuta crocuta*). *Journal of Zoology*, **221**, 308–313.

Gersick, A. S., Cheney, D. L., Schneider, J. M., Seyfarth, R. M., and Holekamp, K. E. (2015). Long-distance communication facilitates cooperation among wild spotted hyaenas, *Crocuta crocuta*. *Animal Behaviour*, **103**, 107–116.

Glickman, S. E., Zabel, C. J., Yoerg, S. I., Weldele, M. L., Drea, C. M., and Frank, L. G. (1997). Social facilitation, affiliation, and dominance in the social life of spotted hyenas. *Annals of the New York Academy of Sciences*, **807**, 175–184.

Gosling, S. D. (1998). Personality dimensions in spotted hyenas (*Crocuta crocuta*). *Journal of Comparative Psychology*, **112**, 107–118.

Greenberg, J. R., and Holekamp, K. E. (2017). Human disturbance affects personality development in a wild carnivore. *Animal Behaviour*, **132**, 303–312.

Henschel, J. R., and Skinner, J. D. (1991). Territorial behaviour by a clan of spotted hyaenas *Crocuta crocuta*. *Ethology*, **88**, 223–235.

Hofer, H., and East, M. L. (1993a). The commuting system of Serengeti spotted hyaenas: how a predator copes with migratory prey. I. Social organization. *Animal Behaviour*, **46**, 547–557.

Hofer, H., and East, M. L. (1993b). The commuting system of Serengeti spotted hyaenas: how a predator copes with migratory prey. II. Intrusion pressure and commuters' space use. *Animal Behaviour*, **46**, 559–574.

Hofer, H., and East, M. L. (1995). Population dynamics, population size, and the commuting system of Serengeti spotted hyenas. In *Serengeti II: dynamics, management, and conservation of an ecosystem* (pp. 332–363). Chicago, IL: University of Chicago Press.

Holekamp, K. E., and Dloniak, S. M. (2010). Intraspecific variation in the behavioural ecology of a tropical carnivore, the spotted hyena. In *Advances in the study of behaviour: behavioural ecology of tropical animals* (pp. 189–229). Burlington, MA: Academic Press.

Holekamp, K. E., and Engh, A. (2009). Reproductive skew in female-dominated mammalian societies. In *Reproductive skew in vertebrates: proximate and ultimate causes* (pp. 53–83). New York, NY: Cambridge University Press.

Holekamp, K. E., and Smale, L. (1991). Dominance acquisition during mammalian social development: the "inheritance" of maternal rank. *American Zoologist*, **31**, 306–317.

Holekamp, K. E., and Smale, L. (1993). Ontogeny of dominance in free-living spotted hyaenas: juvenile rank relations with other immature individuals. *Animal Behaviour*, **46**, 451–466.

Holekamp, K. E., Ogutu, J. O., Dublin, H. T., Frank, L. G., and Smale, L. (1993). Fission of a spotted hyena clan: consequences of prolonged female absenteeism and causes of female emigration. *Ethology*, **93**, 285–299.

Holekamp, K. E., Smale, L., and Szykman, M. (1996). Rank and reproduction in the female spotted hyaena. *Journal of Reproduction and Fertility*, **108**, 229–237.

Holekamp, K. E., Smale, L., Berg, R., and Cooper, S. M. (1997). Hunting rates and hunting success in the spotted hyena (*Crocuta crocuta*). *Journal of Zoology*, **242**, 1–15.

Holekamp, K. E., Boyd, E. E., Szykman, M., *et al.* (1999). Vocal recognition in the spotted hyaena and its possible implications regarding the evolution of intelligence. *Animal Behaviour*, **58**, 383–395.

Holekamp, K. E., Sakai, S., and Lundrigan, B. (2007). The spotted hyena (*Crocuta crocuta*) as a model system for study of the evolution of intelligence. *Journal of Mammalogy*, **88**, 545–554.

Holekamp, K. E., Smith, J. E., Strelioff, C. C., Van Horn, R. C., and Watts, H. E. (2012). Society, demography and genetic structure in the spotted hyena. *Molecular Ecology*, **21**, 613–632.

Holekamp, K. E., Swanson, E. M., and Van Meter, P. E. (2013). Developmental constraints on behavioural flexibility. *Philosophical Transactions of the Royal Society B: Biological Sciences*, **368**, 20120350.

Holekamp, K. E., Dantzer, B., Stricker, G., Shaw Yoshida, K. C., and Benson-Amram, S. (2015). Brains, brawn and sociality: a hyaena's tale. *Animal behaviour*, **103**, 237–248.

Jacobs, G. (1993). The distribution and nature of colour vision among the mammals. *Biological Reviews*, **68**, 413–471.

Kruuk, H. (1972). *The spotted hyena: a study of predation and social behaviour*. Chicago, IL: University of Chicago Press.

Lehmann, K. D. S., Montgomery, T. M., Maclachlan, S. M., *et al.* (2017). Lions, hyenas and mobs (Oh my!). *Current Zoology*, **63**, 313–322.

Mills, M. G. L. (1990). *Kalahari hyaenas*. London: Unwin Hyman.

Reader, S. M., and Laland, K. N. (2003). *Animal innovation*. Oxford: Oxford University Press.

Smale, L., Frank, L. G., and Holekamp, K. E. (1993). Ontogeny of dominance in free-living spotted hyaenas: juvenile rank relations with adult females and immigrant males. *Animal Behaviour*, **46**, 467–477.

Smith, J. E., Memenis, S. K., and Holekamp, K. E. (2007). Rank-related partner choice in the fission–fusion society of the spotted hyena (*Crocuta crocuta*). *Behavioural Ecology and Sociobiology*, **61**, 753–765.

Smith, J. E., Kolowski, J. M., Graham, K. E., Dawes, S. E., and Holekamp, K. E. (2008). Social and ecological determinants of fission–fusion dynamics in the spotted hyaena. *Animal Behaviour*, **76**, 619–636.

Smith, J. E., Van Horn, R. C., Powning, K. S., *et al.* (2010). Evolutionary forces favoring intragroup coalitions among spotted hyenas and other animals. *Behavioural Ecology*, **21**, 284–303.

Smith, J. E., Powning, K. S., Dawes, S. E., *et al.* (2011). Greetings promote cooperation and reinforce social bonds among spotted hyaenas. *Animal Behaviour*, **81**, 401–415.

Szykman, M., Engh, A. L., Van Horn, R. C., Boydston, E. E., Scribner, K. T., and Holekamp, K. E. (2003). Rare male aggression directed toward females in a female-dominated society: baiting behaviour in the spotted hyena. *Aggressive Behaviour*, **29**, 457–474.

Tanner, J. B., Dumont, E. R., Sakai, S. T., Lundrigan, B. L., and Holekamp, K. E. (2008). Of arcs and vaults: the biomechanics of bone-cracking in spotted hyenas (*Crocuta crocuta*). *Biological Journal of the Linnean Society*, **95**, 246–255.

Tanner, J. B., Zelditch, M. L., Lundrigan, B. L., and Holekamp, K. E. (2010). Ontogenetic change in skull morphology and mechanical advantage in the spotted hyena. *Journal of Morphology*, **271**, 353–365.

Theis, K. R. (2008). *Scent marking in a highly social mammalian species, the spotted hyena, Crocuta crocuta*. PhD thesis, Michigan State University.

Theis, K. R., Schmidt, T. M., and Holekamp, K. E. (2012). Evidence for a bacterial mechanism for group-specific social odours among hyenas. *Scientific Reports*, **2**, 615.

Trinkel, M., Fleischmann, P. H., and Kastberger, G. (2006). Comparison of land-use strategies of spotted hyenas (*Crocuta crocuta*, Erxleben) in different ecosystems. *African Journal of Ecology*, **44**, 537.

Turner, J. W. (2018). *Social development and its influence on adult traits in the spotted hyena*. Michigan State University.

Van Horn, R. C., McElhinny, T. L., and Holekamp, K. E. (2003). Age estimation and dispersal in the spotted hyena (*Crocuta crocuta*). *Journal of Mammalogy*, **84**, 1019–1030.

Van Horn, R. C., Engh, A. L., Scribner, K. T., Funk, S. M., and Holekamp, K. E. (2004a). Behavioural structuring of relatedness in the spotted hyena (*Crocuta crocuta*) suggests direct fitness benefits of clan-level cooperation. *Molecular Ecology*, **13**, 449–458.

Van Horn, R. C., Wahaj, S. A., and Holekamp, K. E. (2004b). Role-reversed nepotistic interactions between sires and offspring in the spotted hyena. *Ethology*, **110**, 1–14.

Wahaj, S. A., Guse, K. R., and Holekamp, K. E. (2001). Reconciliation in the spotted hyena (*Crocuta crocuta*). *Ethology*, **107**, 1057–1074.

Wahaj, S. A., Van Horn, R. C., Van Horn, T. L., *et al.* (2004). Kin discrimination in the spotted hyena (*Crocuta crocuta*): nepotism among siblings. *Behavioural Ecology and Sociobiology*, **56**, 237–247.

Watts, H. E., Tanner, J. B., Lundrigan, B. L., and Holekamp, K. E. (2009). Post-weaning maternal effects and the evolution of female dominance in the spotted hyena. *Proceedings of the Royal Society of London B: Biological Sciences*, **276**, 2291–2298.

12 Lizards – Measuring Cognition: Practical Challenges and the Influence of Ecology and Social Behaviour

Martin J. Whiting and Daniel W. A. Noble

Species Description

Anatomy

While lizards span a great variety of body shapes, sizes and anatomical features, the majority of species are relatively small and of a size that is amenable to maintaining in the lab. Lizards on the small end of the scale can perch on the tip of a matchstick (e.g. leaf chameleons), while the largest are the varanids (e.g. Komodo dragon), which can be 3 m in length. Their anatomy is strongly indicative of their ecology and behaviour. For example, many lineages have experienced limb reduction and retain only vestiges of their appendages that are non-functional. These species are often sand-swimmers, living in fine sands just below the surface, in desert or coastal areas. Similarly, other species live in grasslands, where a serpentine form improves locomotor performance. These species move more like a snake, and also frequently have tails much longer than their body. Conversely, arboreal lizards have digits capable of greater traction on vertical surfaces (e.g. geckos), or long hind-limbs that allow them to sprint faster on broad surfaces or short stubby limbs for grasping thin perches such as bushes (e.g. bush anoles). A wide range of species live on rock surfaces and are either dorso-ventrally flattened, to allow them to squeeze into narrow crevices to escape from predators, or they may have digits and limbs that facilitate grip or adhesion to rocky surfaces (e.g. geckos). As we would predict, lizards exhibit a tight link between morphology and habitat use, and this needs to be taken into account in cognition studies. Species that are secretive and/or highly specialized may be more challenging to study in the wild, and will require a set-up in the lab that caters for their specific habitat requirements. For example, some active foragers have high rates of movement and high field body temperatures. These species are particularly challenging to keep in the lab and equally challenging to study in the field. For an excellent overview of lizard diversity that documents links between morphology, ecology and behaviour, see Pianka and Vitt (2003).

The vast range of body sizes in lizards also presents a practical challenge. No studies have been attempted on 'miniature' species, such as some of the leaf chameleons or dwarf geckos. However, we have conducted learning trials with small baby skinks (*Bassiana duperreyi*, snout–vent length, SVL = about 25 mm; Clark *et al.*, 2014), training them to move coloured caps from food wells. For other small species, an alternative is to position a cue behind a food well sunk into a block of wood, which would require the lizard to make an active choice by approaching and looking into a well. Larger lizards such as varanids (monitor lizards) are challenging for the opposite reason – many species are quite large and therefore difficult to keep in the lab. However, many zoos have captive animals and they are frequently amenable to collaborative studies of their learning ability. There are many anecdotal reports of monitor lizards being particularly 'intelligent', but besides a single study (Manrod *et al.*, 2008), in which eight individuals rapidly solved a motor task, this is largely unsubstantiated. In Australia, monitor lizards frequently occur near picnic areas, where they are habituated to people. These individuals could be suitable candidates for cognition studies in the wild.

Perception

Visual and chemosensory modalities are strongly developed in lizards, and are the primary means by which individuals perceive stimuli from their environment. Hearing in lizards is generally not well understood, and is thought to be less important, although some geckos use acoustic communication (Marcellini, 1977). In terms of vision, lizards are tetrachromatic and can rely on a broad spectrum of colour-based visual cues (Fleischman *et al.*, 1993, 2011). In addition, lizards tongue-flick to sample chemicals from their environment, and this information is extracted in the vomero-nasal organ in the roof of the mouth, before being processed in the brain (Halpern, 1992; Cooper, 1994a). Ambush foragers rarely tongue-flick in the absence of social cues and typically rush out from an ambush post to capture prey, being far more visually oriented than actively foraging species. Conversely, active foragers will move through the landscape, repeatedly tongue-flicking the ground in search of hidden prey (Cooper, 1994b). Active foragers use their forelimbs to move aside leaves and debris that might be sheltering arthropod prey. They also dig up arthropods that are buried below the surface (Reilly *et al.*, 2007).

Cognitive studies to date have taken advantage of lizards' well-developed visual and chemosensory modalities in designing cognitive tasks. Cognitive tasks using chemosensory modalities can be quite difficult to design for certain species, as they require a greater degree of control and a basic understanding on the chemical composition of cues that are likely to elicit behavioural responses. Nonetheless, creative experimentation has been shown to be powerful in understanding, for example, individual recognition (Carazo *et al.*, 2008). Given these difficulties, it is therefore not surprising that most cognitive tasks make use of visual stimuli for training and learning. However, in reality, lizards most likely use a combination of cues, and there are studies that nicely illustrate this. For instance, Pérez-Cembranos and Pérez-Mellado (2015) make use of both visual and chemosensory modalities in the design of experiments. It is therefore important to think carefully about the specific cues in any cognitive task early in the design stages (see below for more details).

Life Cycle

With respect to life cycle, lizards are either oviparous (egg-laying) or viviparous (live-bearing), and this is commonly linked to climate, where colder areas favour viviparity

(Shine, 2014). For the majority of species, there is no parental care, and offspring either disperse after birth or hatching. However, there are species that brood their eggs and protect them from predators (e.g. *Mabuya longicaudata*; Huang, 2006), and in many family-living species there is parental care through association with parents, whereby the risk of infanticide is significantly lowered (While *et al.*, 2014). Age, sex and reproductive state can also influence cognitive ability. Sexual selection can be intense in many species of lizards (Stamps, 1983), and this is reflected in hormone profiles that are dependent on social status and season (Husak *et al.*, 2009). In spring, males are frequently establishing territories or searching for mates, and they typically have higher levels of testosterone than at other times of the year (Moore, 1988; Wack *et al.*, 2008). Likewise, females become receptive and later pregnant, resulting in significant changes in oestrogen and progesterone levels (Jones, 2011). Furthermore, some females become more aggressive during pregnancy (Sinn *et al.*, 2008). Changes in hormone profiles could impact performance in cognition tests, and for studies incorporating sex differences, timing could play a significant role. For these species, it may be prudent to conduct cognitive experiments outside of the breeding season, unless the study question links to some aspect of reproductive biology or breeding behaviour.

Longevity in lizards is quite variable and ranges from being seasonal to long-lived. In the case of the annual chameleon *Furcifer labordi*, there is a point in their life cycle where all individuals exist as eggs beneath the ground, following the death of the adult stage after only a 4–5-month life span (Karsten *et al.*, 2008). Conversely, the sleepy lizard and members of the *Egernia* group, such as the Cunningham's skink, live to at least their fifties (Whiting and While, 2017). Longevity is linked to a range of covarying life-history traits, such as length of activity season, age at first reproduction, foraging mode, growth rate and frequency of reproduction (Dunham *et al.*, 1988). Collectively, these life-history traits are under strong selection and likely influence constraints on cognition.

Social Characteristics

Lizard social systems can be viewed as components of three broad categories: social organization, social structure and mating systems (Whiting and While, 2017). The majority of what we know about sociality has come from studies of social structure and mating systems (e.g. on aggression, dominance and territoriality), largely because many species are easy to observe and frequently interact. Furthermore, dyadic contests can easily be staged in the lab. Relative dominance is thought to influence information use. For example, subadult but not adult male eastern water skinks (*Eulamprus quoyii*) use social information to solve a task, and although this was hypothesized to be the result of social feedback (Noble *et al.*, 2014), subsequent tests of this hypothesis found no effect of dominance on social learning ability (Kar *et al.*, 2017). Some species of lizards also live in family groups, and this system of complex sociality offers a unique opportunity for understanding how complex sociality may influence cognition. Social learning, for instance, has been documented in female adult tree skinks (*Egernia striolata*; Whiting *et al.*, in review), and studies on related species with different levels of sociality are currently underway in our lab.

State of the Art

Cognitive studies using lizards have experienced a resurgence over the last 10 years, owing to the need for a greater understanding of the degree of behavioural flexibility and underlying cognitive mechanisms across taxonomically diverse groups (Wilkinson and Huber, 2012). Despite this, studies using lizards are still relatively rare compared to work with mammals and birds, and mainly attempt to address three major types of questions: (1) Can lizards learn novel cognitive tasks? (2) What is the diversity of cognitive tasks that can be undertaken and the mechanisms through which individuals learn? (3) What drives variability in learning among individuals, populations and species? Lizard cognition studies have applied both well-established protocols, developed in the bird and mammal literature (e.g. radial arm, Barnes and T-mazes: Mueller-Paul *et al.*, 2012; Bezzina *et al.*, 2014; LaDage *et al.*, 2017), or have adopted modified and/or species-specific operant or associative learning tasks, which attempt to quantify learning under more ecologically relevant contexts for a given species (e.g. spatial associative learning: Noble *et al.*, 2012; Carazo *et al.*, 2014; Dayananda and Webb, 2017). Much of this work has focused on quantifying cognitive abilities of species through changes in behaviour (e.g. proportion of incorrect choices, latency, etc.); however, a number of studies have quantified brain structure across individuals, populations or species, as a more indirect measure of cognitive capacity (Day *et al.*, 2001; Striedter, 2015; LaDage *et al.*, 2016; Hoops *et al.*, 2017).

Despite the different approaches across studies, much of the early lizard cognition research has been focused on characterizing the extent and variability of learning in lizards (Alkov and Crawford, 1965; Krekorian *et al.*, 1968; Davidson and Richardson, 1970; Powell and Peck, 1970; Garzanit and Richardson, 1974; Loop, 1976; Kirkish *et al.*, 1979; Wilkinson and Huber, 2012). This important research continues today, owing to the difficulty in quantifying, and the general lack of understanding of, lizard cognitive ability across species (Manrod *et al.*, 2008; Gaalema, 2011; LaDage *et al.*, 2012; Leal and Powell, 2012; Noble *et al.*, 2012). Until recently, lizards (and reptiles more generally) were considered to have limited capacity to learn novel problems (LaDage *et al.*, 2012; Leal and Powell, 2012; Noble *et al.*, 2012; Kis *et al.*, 2015). However, this has largely stemmed from the application of inadequate cognitive tasks, contrived situations or a poor understanding of the ecology for a given species. For example, it is not always clear what a useful reward-based stimulus is for ectotherms – one that both stimulates learning in standardized tasks and maintains motivation throughout a task. Indeed, these factors can be dependent on the test temperatures (Krekorian *et al.*, 1968). For food-based rewards, this can also depend on a species' foraging mode, with active foragers often responding more strongly to food rewards and more readily removing a lid from a dish than an ambush forager. Furthermore, active foragers will use prey/food chemicals to detect food rewards hidden from view, so that chemical cues need to be controlled for in an experiment. Nevertheless, many lizards will simply use their snout to manipulate a simple task, such as a lid covering a well (Leal and Powell, 2012; Clark *et al.*, 2014; Noble *et al.*, 2014) or even a sliding door (Kis *et al.*, 2015). Lack of learning may also be related to the artificial nature or ecological relevance of a task (Day *et al.*, 1999a; Noble *et al.*, 2012). Indeed, many preconceived ideas, such as the limited use of social learning in lizards due to their 'non-social' nature, have recently been shown to be wrong (Noble *et al.*, 2014; Kis *et al.*, 2015; Pérez-Cembranos and Pérez-Mellado, 2015). When considering the ectothermic nature, ecology and motivational differences among species, tasks that attempt to quantify cognitive ability can be more easily designed. Researchers can then begin to address the mechanistic processes underlying learning and memory, the drivers of cognitive differences among individuals and their relationship to fitness.

Mechanistically, lizards have been shown to use a variety of visual cues when learning and navigating environments, with most studies testing animals under a spatial learning paradigm (Day *et al.*, 2003; Paulissen, 2008, 2014; Leal and Powell, 2012; Wilkinson and Huber, 2012; Carazo *et al.*, 2014; Clark *et al.*, 2014; Riley *et al.*, 2017). Selection on spatial learning is thought to be strong in lizards because of the need to locate food or prey patches, safe refuges or mates. Compared to sit-and-wait foragers that are mostly immobile, active foragers move through the landscape in search of food and are required to have knowledge of key resources over a potentially greater area, and should thus perform better in spatial tasks. This was tested in two closely related species: *Acanthodactylus boskianus*, an active forager, and *A. scutellatus*, an ambush forager (Day *et al.*, 1999a). Surprisingly, there was no difference between the two species in their performance on a spatial memory task. However, the active forager performed better in a visual discrimination task, which was a non-spatial task reversal. This result was counter to the predicted spatial adaptation model for vertebrates and led to the development of the pliancy model: active foragers experience selection for behavioural flexibility, which favours complex associations between unpredictably changing stimuli and reinforcers (Day *et al.*, 1999a). Interestingly, when the authors examined the brains of these two species, they found a larger dorsal (DC) and medial cortex (MC), two putative reptilian hippocampal homologues, in the active forager. This is consistent with the prediction for selection on brain regions in relation to demand, but was not borne out in the spatial learning trials (Day *et al.*, 1999b).

In many lizard species, males may defend territories or adopt alternate reproductive tactics, whereby they search for females and sneak copulations (Noble *et al.*, 2013). This is thought to create a greater selective pressure on spatial memory in males than females. Indeed, in the eastern water skink (*Eulamprus quoyii*), males performed better than females in a spatial task (Carazo *et al.*, 2014). In the side-blotched lizard (*Uta stansburiana*), the size of the DC and MC is correlated with spatial demands, such that strongly territorial male morphs have the largest DC and MC, followed by those that defend small territories, and finally, individuals that are floaters and do not defend territories (LaDage *et al.*, 2009). Side-blotched lizards have also been used to confirm the existence of spatial memory, using a Barnes maze, a common test for mammals (LaDage *et al.*, 2012). Finally, the size of the MC and DC are strongly dependent on the environment in which the animals develop, and their development is constrained by simplified environments, such as those in a captive setting (LaDage *et al.*, 2016).

Interestingly, territorial males in *Uta stansburiana* appear to be more sensitive to changes in their environment and experience greater levels of neurogenesis when shifting to more complex environments, highlighting the importance of the environment for brain development (LaDage *et al.*, 2013, 2016).

Behavioural flexibility (i.e. the ability of animals to solve novel problems or use different methods to solve the same problem) was recently demonstrated in lizards, which solved multiple tests across different cognitive domains, including reversal learning (Leal and Powell, 2012). Since then, other studies have commonly demonstrated reversal learning and an ability to solve a multitude of tasks, although they might not specifically reference behavioural flexibility. We are currently using a set-shifting paradigm to test for behavioural flexibility in the *Egernia* group of lizards, which have a wide range of sociality (solitary to family living) and mating systems (monogamy to promiscuity). Set-shifting, or task-switching, is an executive function and a form of cognitive flexibility that involves the ability to shift attention between one task and another, and has been successfully used across taxa (e. g. Roberts *et al.*, 1988; Birrell and Brown, 2000; Colacicco *et al.*, 2002; Weed *et al.*, 2008; Titulaer *et al.*, 2012). One constraint for lizard studies is the length of time required to conduct set-shifting experiments, because lizards are hard-pressed to do more than two trials a day because of their energetic needs. Nevertheless, these experiments are likely to be highly informative and will allow a comparison across a diversity of taxa.

Lizards are also an ideal model to study the role of cognitive processes and brain structure in fitness, and whether these traits are heritable (Croston *et al.*, 2015), because they typically show a range of variation necessary for natural selection, and they can be brought into the lab for measurement of cognitive traits and then released back into a population in which they can be tracked. Unfortunately, we are only aware of one study that has explicitly linked cognitive performance to fitness in the wild (Dayananda and Webb, 2017). In this study, velvet gecko (*Amalosia lesueurii*) eggs were incubated at hot or cold temperatures, and offspring from the colder temperature had higher learning scores and higher survival in the wild.

All for One and One for All

Box 12.1 Snake Cognitive Abilities

Michael S. Grace

The cognitive abilities of snakes are poorly understood relative to those of other reptiles, in part because snake anatomical and physiological adaptations may be incompatible with some of the traditional methods used to study cognition in other reptilian and vertebrate taxa. However, these same adaptations (including limblessness, poor visual accommodative ability, lack of eyelids and external ear openings and, in many snake species, the infrequent consumption of massive meals) make snakes fascinating subjects for the study of sensory biology, behaviour and evolution.

(*cont.*)

Early studies of snake cognition yielded mixed results. Takemasa and Nakamura (1935) found that snakes could learn to efficiently escape confinement, and Kellogg and Pomeroy (1936) found that watersnakes (*Nerodia fasciata*) demonstrated learning capability in a water maze using heat as a positive reinforcer. Conversely, Wolfe and Browne (1940) saw no evidence of diamondback watersnake (*Nerodia rhombifera*) learning in a terrestrial environment, using potentially noxious heat as a goal or electric shock as an aversive stimulus. Crawford and Bartlett (1966) found no evidence that grey ratsnakes (*Pantherophis obsoletus*) learn to locate food and water following 7 days of food and water deprivation. The methods used in many of these studies suggest the importance of employing experimental paradigms and conditioning stimuli that are appropriate to snake physiology and behaviour. Thermal targets beyond the preferred temperature range of a given species likely make poor goals; aquatic and semi-aquatic snakes may perform more poorly in terrestrial versus aquatic set-ups; and short-term food and water deprivation may have little motivating effect in snakes that efficiently conserve water and may go months without eating.

However, more recent studies employing conditions and testing paradigms more appropriate to snake physiology and behaviour clearly demonstrate that snakes have the ability to learn, and in some cases to perform complex series of novel tasks. Plains garter snakes (*Thamnophis sirtalis*), for example, used novel airborne odorants as cues to learn to navigate a simple maze, in order to gain access to food rewards (Begun *et al.*, 1988). Corn snakes (red ratsnakes, *Pantherophis guttata*), like many snake species, actively seek out shelter in the form of holes and crevices. Holtzman and colleagues (1999) took advantage of this behaviour by setting up a spatial learning arena, in which one of eight hide holes was open and thus available as a retreat. These snakes rapidly learned to navigate the arena, significantly decreasing the latency to find the goal and the distance travelled to reach the goal over the course of only 4 days of trials. In the most complex behavioural challenge yet, Emer and colleagues (2015) trained wild-caught Burmese pythons to accept much smaller food items than would normally be consumed and then used very small food rewards to condition snakes to reliably depress an illuminated button in order to gain access to hidden food rewards. These studies demonstrate that snakes can learn even unnatural and somewhat complex tasks. Taken together, they show that in order for learning to be demonstrable, environmental conditions, tasks and rewards must be appropriate to snake anatomy, physiology and behaviour.

References

Begun, D., Kubie, J. L., Plough O'Keefe, M., and Halpern, M. (1988). Conditioned discrimination of airborne odorants by garter snakes. *Journal of Comparative Psychology*, **102**, 35–43.

(*cont.*)

Crawford, F., and Bartlett, C. (1966). Runway behavior of the gray rat snake with food and water reinforcement. *Psychonomic Science*, **4**, 99–100.
Emer, S. A., Mora, C. V., Harvey, M. T., and Grace, M. S. (2015). Predators in training: operant conditioning of novel behavior in wild Burmese pythons (*Python molurus bivitattus*). *Animal Cognition*, **18**, 269–278.
Holtzman, D., Harris, T. W., Aranguren, G., and Bostock, E. (1999). Spatial learning of an escape task by young corn snakes (*Elaphe guttata guttata*). *Animal Behaviour*, **57**, 51–60.
Kellogg, W., and Pomeroy, W. (1936). Maze learning in water snakes. *Journal of Comparative Psychology*, **21**, 275–295.
Takemasa, T., and Nakamura, K. (1935). A study of learning using snakes. *Kyoiku Shinri Kenkyu*, **10**, 575–581.
Wolfe, D., and Browne, C. (1940). A learning experiment with snakes. *Copeia*, **1940**, 134.

Field Guide

Experimental Set-up and Practical Considerations

A major challenge in cognition studies is ensuring rigorous experimental procedures in the face of logistical constraints. In a captive setting, many cognition tests are food-based, and lizards anticipate a feeding opportunity. While there are no data on lizards that suggest a 'clever Hans' effect, whereby the experimenter inadvertently cues the animal to the reward, it is best practice to eliminate this possibility. Ideally, one experimenter would set up the apparatus and another would place it in the animal's enclosure or testing arena ('blind experimentation'). If this is not possible, a simple alternative is to either usher a lizard into its refuge, and then place the apparatus in the enclosure (with trials beginning when the lizard emerges), or have a separate chamber connected to the animal's enclosure, which can be opened once the apparatus has been inserted. Both alternatives have the advantage of starting the animal at a constant distance from the experimental apparatus.

For all cognition tests in the lab, we advocate using a camera system (e.g. CCTV) to remotely record the animal's behaviour and performance in all trials (Figure 12.1). By doing so, lizards are not distracted or influenced by the presence of an investigator. In field studies, depending on the circumstances, this may not always be possible. If this is the case, the investigators should first habituate animals to their presence, wear bland clothing and move as little as possible during a trial. If possible, we suggest using a camera that links to a remote monitor and thereby removes the experimenter. In the event that an investigator is present, it may be best not to include measures of latency, in case it is influenced by the experimenter's presence. Video scoring usually involves collecting data on the choices (i.e. whether the lizard chooses correctly/number of incorrect choices or mistakes) and the latency to choose (i.e. the time from the start of the trial to the execution of the task). Videos should be scored blind when possible

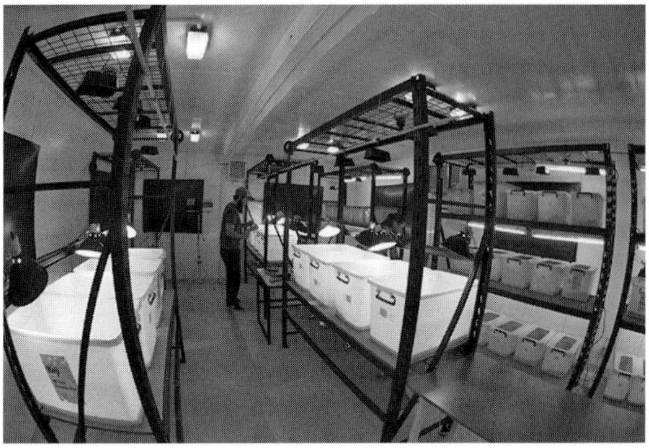

Figure 12.1. A typical set-up for cognitive studies, in which lizards perform trials in their home enclosures in plastic tubs. CCTV cameras are mounted on bars to the side of each rack (between two lights), allowing the filming of trials (multiple tubs can be filmed by one camera). We create a thermal gradient using heat tape below the tubs (not pictured). Additional warmth is provided by a spot lamp, which also illuminates the enclosure for CCTV filming. For husbandry purposes, lights and heat cables can be connected to a timer and turned off at night. Each camera connects to a DVR and a monitor for remote viewing. At the end of each trial or at the end of the day, all trials can be backed up to an external USB drive that connects to the DVR. More sophisticated systems allow a connection via Wi-Fi and remote back-ups.

('blind scoring'), even if 'choice' for many tasks is rather unambiguous (e.g. removing a lid from a well), or at least partially recoded by a second observer.

Two well-known constraints in cognition studies are colour preference and lateralization, which may result in a side bias. For example, lizards may have a preference for red, because it is the colour of ripe fruit (Whiting and Greeff, 1997). This is not necessarily a problem if the question of interest is a comparison across treatments (e.g. social learners versus a control with the same stimulus). However, it is always better to split the treatment group in half and use two different colours. Another option is to test lizards a priori for a colour preference, by placing equal amounts of food in two coloured dishes and presenting them over a set number of trials (e.g. 20), alternating between left and right sides. As lizards are tetrachromats with good visual acuity and can cue in on either luminance or hue, it is important to use the same source of paint to ensure that colour cue cards are identical, manipulating hue and luminance with an optic spectrophotometer, if needed (Kemp *et al.*, 2015). Because lateralization may be common in lizards, it is possible that some species or individuals may have a side bias. This can be tested before the start of any cognitive trial by presenting two equal dishes/food rewards on the left and right side of the test arena. Depending on the proportion of individuals with evidence of a side bias, we see three viable options. First, if the proportion of animals is small (e.g. $<$ 5–10 per cent), these animals could be excluded and a clear statement about this made within the study. Second, if the proportion of animals is moderate (~50 per cent), then this could be dealt with in the analysis stages: assuming sufficient numbers are present across treatments, individuals could be dummy-coded ('1' – left bias; '0' – right bias; see below). Lastly, if a high proportion of animals exhibit a side bias, they could first be trained to learn the reward from the opposite of their preferred side. However, care should be taken when interpreting these data, and it should also be made explicit that such biases exist. This will also affect the interpretation of any reversal tasks that should also be discussed. Indeed, it may be the case that the real cognitive question involves understanding laterality itself, if the proportion of individuals with a side bias is high (i.e. decide a priori the proportion of animals with a particular side bias that is acceptable).

Quantifying Learning

Learning in lizards is usually quantified by testing for a change in behaviour across time, in response to an unconditioned stimulus. Ideally, data should be collected consistently during the learning period on all lizards and within each treatment. However, this may be logistically challenging, and one may need to either compare groups of individuals through time (i.e. across every trial) and estimate their learning rates, or to compare individuals exposed to different stimuli at two time points. Our experiments, for example, usually take 2–3 months to complete, and one experiment took 9 months (Szabo *et al.*, unpubl. data). Our tasks generally involve running trials in the morning and afternoon (i.e. twice per day, 10/week). We suggest running trials in 5-day blocks and scoring videos on the same day, once trials are complete, to avoid trial 'fatigue' and also because lizards are ectotherms, and thus have lower food intake requirements.

For studies of social learning, treatments often involve quantifying the change in behaviour for a group of individuals that are able to observe or interact with conspecifics, as compared to a control group of experimental lizards that do not observe conspecifics performing the tasks (Noble *et al.*, 2014; Kis *et al.*, 2015; Pérez-Cembranos and Pérez-Mellado, 2015; Kar *et al.*, 2017). The control group is essential in disassociating any effects of social feedback on learning (Noble *et al.*, 2014; Kar *et al.*, 2017). Depending on the question of interest, one can allow observers or experimental animals to interact with conspecifics (i.e. obtain visual, chemosensory and social feedback), or restrict experimental lizards to particular sensory modalities (e.g. visual or chemosensory only). Depending on the experimental design chosen, any inferences drawn from such studies need to be related to the specific sensory domain being tested. However, practically speaking, it will almost always be necessary to separate demonstrating and experimental lizards. As lizards are extremely visual, this can be done using video stimuli or trained demonstrators that are viewed behind a transparent divider (Noble *et al.*, 2014; Kis *et al.*, 2015; Pérez-Cembranos and Pérez-Mellado, 2015; Kar *et al.*, 2017; Figure 12.2). For example, in the bearded dragon (*Pogona vitticeps*), lizards observed a video demonstrating the bidirectional opening of a sliding door (opening either left or right, but not both ways) or a control video consisting of a blank screen. This is a highly effective design, because it tests for imitation and excludes the possibility of goal emulation or local enhancement (Kis *et al.*, 2015).

The incubation environment also has major effects on reptile learning and other cognitive traits (Amiel and Shine, 2012; Amiel *et al.*, 2014, 2017; Clark *et al.*, 2014;

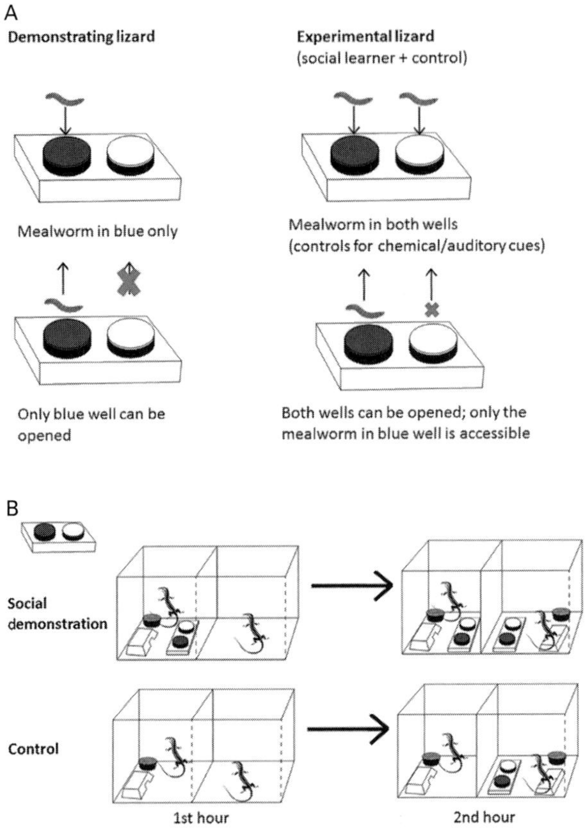

Figure 12.2. Social learning experimental set-up, involving a demonstrator with a social learning treatment compared to a control. (A) The reward (in this case a mealworm) is only available to the demonstrator in the correct well. The lid on the incorrect well is sealed to the well. In the treatment and control groups, the reward is in both wells; however, while both lids can be removed, the reward in the incorrect well is covered by mesh and not accessible to the lizard. (B) The first hour is an observational period, during which the 'learner' watches a demonstrator extract a food reward from the correct dish, while the control 'learner' observes another lizard in the absence of the task. In the second hour, an opaque divider is inserted and the focal lizards are given the task. We suggest two trials per day with at least 1.5 h between trials. For more details, see Noble and colleagues (2014).

Dayananda and Webb, 2017) and is likely a key source of environmental variation driving cognitive differences among individuals (Noble *et al.*, 2018). Comparing learnt behaviour for multiple tasks can be done for multiple treatment groups (i.e. different incubation temperatures: 20°C versus 27°C; social environments: small versus large social groups) to ascertain how the developmental environment impacts cognitive ability. There are now excellent protocols developed for combining an understanding of changes in brain structure (e.g. Herculano-Houzel *et al.*, 2015; Hoops, 2015), with detailed behavioural experiments for lizards that are likely to pave the way for a more integrative examination of environmental effects on cognition in reptiles.

Practical Considerations for Analysis: Learning Curves, Learning Criteria and Statistical Power

Analysing data collected from learning experiments is by far one of the most challenging aspects of any cognitive experiment, depending on the question at hand, the sample size and the intended power of an experiment (Nakagawa and Foster, 2004). This is especially problematic for most lizard cognition experiments, given that there are often major logistical constraints in measuring large numbers of individuals (Nakagawa and Hauber, 2011). Power analyses prior to experimental design can be conducted using published estimates taken from similar studies in the literature, which can help guide the sample size required while planning an experiment. Moreover, expert advice and pilot studies can inform in this area.

In addition, it is often important to control for covariates such as sex (Carazo *et al.*, 2014), body size (Clark *et al.*, 2014) and temperature (Krekorian *et al.*, 1968), as these factors can impact learning. Experimental designs should carefully balance these factors, and we suggest pseudo-randomizing levels of a covariate to each treatment in as balanced a manner as possible. For example, if both male and female lizards will be collected for a social learning experiment, then it is important to balance the sex of the observers across control and social learning treatments as evenly as possible, but also in a randomized fashion. This ensures that sufficient sample sizes are present in each treatment to test for sex effects and that covariates are not confounded by treatment effects. Confounding effects can be problematic for experiments involving incubation temperature, as sex is often affected by temperature in many lizards (Clark *et al.*, 2014). The need to control for covariates, whether these be biological (sex, size, mass) or methodological (batch effects), requires careful planning during the experimental design stages, but also requires some foresight on how such data will be analysed. The low power of many cognition studies means that simplifying assumptions are often necessary. For example, testing treatment effects on a small sample of lizards, where males and females are likely to differ, means there may be a limited sample size for testing sex effects. In these circumstances, it may be better to increase the sample size of one sex, and only focus on one sex, to ensure there is sufficient power to test a given question (e.g. Noble *et al.*, 2012, 2014).

Data collected on all individuals for every trial, whether the individuals are part of multiple treatments or not, can be analysed in a number of different ways. Often, it is useful to organize these data in an easy to view format, which does not necessarily match formats needed for analysis. We provide a link with an example file of how we format our data while running experiments, and we have also written some simple functions (should this format be followed) that can then convert these files to analysis-ready format, saving a substantial amount of time. This can be downloaded (https://github.com/daniel1noble/cogdat) as a package that can be used in the free analysis software package R (R Core Team, 2017).

Theoretically, all these different analyses should support one another, but this will not always be the case, given the different assumptions inherent to the alternative statistical tests and their varying levels of precision. Therefore, care should be taken in establishing whether experimentalists have sufficient data for a given type of analysis, and

Table 12.1. Basic equipment used in the study of lizard cognition.

Equipment	Function
DVR and camera system	Remote filming of trials. Compared to stand-alone cameras, allows monitoring of many animals simultaneously
External hard drives	Used for daily backup from DVR
Camera and tripod	Used for field studies and lab studies requiring higher definition
Plastic tubs or reptile cages	Lizards can be maintained in large plastic tubs while doing trials, open top. Lizards need a refuge and water bowl, can be given objects for enrichment (e.g. bark, leaves, twigs)
Outdoor enclosures	Lizards can be maintained in outdoor enclosures, if species perform better in a more natural environment
Heating, lighting	Under-cage heating wire creates a thermal gradient. A spot lamp can be provided for basking in some species. UV lamps may be necessary for longer studies
Stimulus reward	Depending on species: mealworms, crickets, dog food or baby food (fruit). Wet dog food and baby food can be measured more accurately for quantity
Spray paint, plastic wells, black tape, fine mesh, wooden platforms, putty	For association trials, we use small Petri dishes and reduce the lip of the lid, to allow easier removal by the lizard. Dishes can be mounted on a wooden platform with putty, to allow easy removal. Lids are spray-painted and sides of dishes taped to render them opaque. Avoid painting lids red, because lizards have a strong preference for red. Mesh is used in control well and prevents lizards accessing food (controls for chemical cues). For some species, dishes can be left open, but placed atop a wooden ramp with a cue card
Wood, plastic, Perspex, spray paint, standard-sized cue cards	General materials necessary for constructing a maze, puzzle box, cognitive apparatus, set-shifting set-up

general power analyses can be used to assess this. Analyses largely fall into three different types that statistically compare: (1) group- or treatment-level differences in means, trials to criterion or latencies, preferably at two time points; (2) group- or treatment-level learning or survival curves (survival analysis); or (3) learning curves at both the within- and between-individual levels for different groups or treatments (multilevel, mixed models or generalized estimating equations).

Analyses often take means of a given statistic for a set of independent individuals (e.g. 'average' number of incorrect choices made, average number of trials to criterion for an individual). The binomial probability or simulations can be used to assess the probability of obtaining specific outcomes by chance, when testing learning. Individual choice data and latencies across trials can also be analysed, using powerful mixed-modelling or survival analysis approaches (Gallistel *et al.*, 2004; Noble *et al.*, 2012, 2014; Kar *et al.*, 2017; Riley *et al.*, 2017). These can explicitly account for within- and between-level variability in learning rates and make use of the maximal amount of data from a given experiment (Figure 12.3). Choice data can often be modelled assuming a

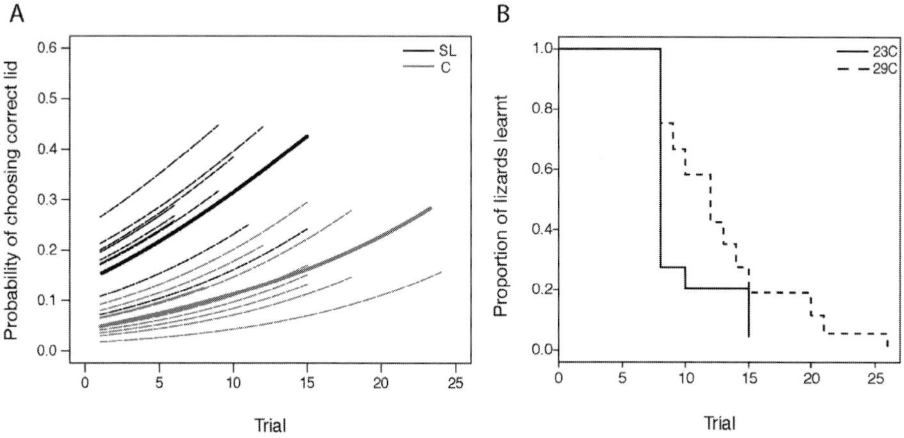

Figure 12.3. Example of presenting figures for cognitive analysis. (A) Modified from Noble and colleagues (2014) with kind permission of the Royal Society, an example of individual based-learning curves for two treatments (control versus social), for a social learning experiment on *E. quoyii*, which provides evidence for age-dependent social learning. Small solid lines are predictions of individual learning 'rates', whereas solid lines are population-average lines for the two treatment groups. (B) An example of a survival analysis for two groups of lizards, using time to event (in this case, time to learn or reach criterion).

Bernoulli or multinomial probability distribution, and, after log-transformation, latency data can often be modelled assuming normality. While there is some debate about whether learning curves are gradual or step-like (Gallistel *et al.*, 2004), we believe that this depends on the variable of interest and the type of task. In our experience, assuming fairly standard error distributions common to many statistical software packages is usually sufficient. Nonetheless, these models are data-hungry and rely on a sufficiently large number of independent animals for models to converge properly, so this should be considered in their use. In Resources, we further provide the link to some simulated data and analysis code that can be downloaded for learning.

Wild vs. Lab

Box 12.2 Cognition Outside the Box

David S. Steinberg and Manuel Leal

As referenced in the current chapter, the unique metabolic requirements and relatively low activity rates of ectotherms impose serious logistical constraints that often hamper laboratory studies of lizard cognition, by limiting sample size and the power of statistical analyses (Burghardt, 1977). These traits also often preclude the use of traditional cognitive paradigms (but see Leal and Powell, 2012), which have been developed largely for organisms with high activity rates. One way to alleviate some of the problems associated with lab-based research (see Shettleworth, 1998; Morand-

(cont.)

Ferron *et al.*, 2015) might be to investigate the cognitive abilities of lizards in nature. By studying free-ranging lizards in the wild, scientists can potentially evaluate many more individuals, without having to provide adequate or appropriate artificial testing conditions (e.g. in terms of space, temperature and humidity). Instead, researchers must simply transport a testing apparatus from individual to individual in their natural habitat. The most obvious and serious obstacle that must be overcome in this sort of field-based research of cognition is reliably relocating focal subjects over an extended period of time, because most studies of cognition are both long-term and serial. Studying species that are fiercely territorial or exhibit considerable site fidelity, which is common in lizards, can alleviate this problem. Alternatively, modern tracking technologies (e.g. Croston *et al.*, 2016; Morand-Ferron *et al.*, 2015), including satellite-based or radiotelemetry tags, might be useful in finding lizards that are non-territorial, wide-ranging, or simply cryptic and difficult to spot.

Field-based research of cognition in lizards, as well as in other taxa, has many benefits beyond simply avoiding the common husbandry-related drawbacks of laboratory investigations. First, studies of cognition in natural contexts avoid the need to place subjects in artificial and alien environments, which might generate stress responses that mask, alter or in any way distort cognitive function (Shettleworth, 1998; Toxopeus *et al.*, 2005; Jacobs and Menzel, 2014). Although the exact effects of displacement to a laboratory setting on cognition in lizards are unknown, behaviour in general and cognitive functions in particular are strongly influenced by external stimuli. Second, conducting an experiment within the natural habitat of a species requires the experimenter to consider the natural history of the organism in question (Leal and Losos, 2015), thereby allowing the experimenter to design the most appropriate tests or tasks for a given species. Furthermore, these experiments provide an opportunity to measure cognition under the conditions where the costs and benefits of these traits are normally experienced. Finally, studying individuals in the field can prevent the repeated use of the same individuals in multiple cognitive experiments. The repeated use of subjects is a problem common to many studies of cognition in vertebrates and assumes that experimental experience will not bias future experiments. Such an assumption is likely to be unfounded.

References

Burghardt, G. M. (1977). Learning processes in reptiles. In *Biology of the Reptilia: ecology and behaviour* (pp. 555–681). London: Academic Press.

Croston, R., Kozlovsky, D. Y., Branch, C. L., Parchman, T. L., Bridge, E. S., and Pravosudov, V. V. (2016). Individual variation in spatial memory performance in wild mountain chickadees from different elevations. *Animal Behavior*, **111**, 225–234.

Jacobs, L. F., and Menzel, R. (2014). Navigation outside of the box: what the lab can learn from the field and what the field can learn from the lab. *Movement Ecology*, **2**, 1–22.

(*cont.*)

Leal, M., and Losos, J. B. (2015). A naturalist's insight into the evolution of signal redundancy. *American Naturalist*, **186**, 2–4.

Leal M, and Powell, B. J. (2012). Behavioural flexibility and problem-solving in a tropical lizard. *Biology Letters*, **8**, 28–30.

Morand-Ferron, J., Hamblin, S., Cole, E. F., Aplin, L. M., and Quinn, J. L. (2015). Taking the operant paradigm into the field: associative learning in wild great tits. *PLoS ONE*, **10**(8), 16.

Shettleworth S. (1998). *Cognition, evolution, and behavior*. New York, NY: Oxford University Press.

Toxopeus, I. B., Sterck, E. H. M., Hooff, J. A. R. A. M., Spruijt, B. M., and Heeren, T. J. (2005). Effects of trait anxiety on performance of socially housed monkeys in a learning test. *Behaviour*, **142**, 1269–1287.

Resources

- Instructional video and PDF published by the *Journal of Visualized Experiments* on how to assess spatial learning and memory in small squamate (snake and lizard) reptiles, using a dry land Barnes maze (LaDage *et al.*, 2017). An empirical study by the authors was separately published (LaDage *et al.*, 2012): www.jove.com/video/55103/assessing-spatial-learning-and-memory-in-small-squamate-reptiles
- Video showing a social learning experimental set-up in the eastern water skink (*Eulamprus quoyii*): the lizard makes an incorrect choice and is not able to access the food reward (Noble *et al.*, 2014).
- Example data sheet for running cognitive experiments, and functions for helping reformat cognition data sheets to analysis-ready format: https://github.com/daniel1noble/cogdat
- Analysis code for running mixed models with individual choice data: https://github.com/daniel1noble/cogAnalysis

Profile

As a behavioural ecologist, Martin has been increasingly drawn to the influence of cognition on lizard behaviour and its potential role in fitness. He is particularly interested in links between sociality, social complexity, cognition and brain size. He is also interested in how a lizard's developmental environment, which is so dependent on environmental conditions such as temperature, can affect a lizard's learning ability and ultimately, survival and fitness.

Daniel is a behavioural ecologist interested in understanding how behavioural traits evolve and are shaped by the environment. He moved to Australia to do his PhD on the charismatic water skinks. They turned out to be an excellent model species for exploring the capacity of lizards to solve novel problems. Since then, Daniel has worked closely with Martin to explore behavioural flexibility across different lizard species, in an attempt to understand how the environment shapes variation in cognition.

References

Alkov, R. A., and Crawford, F. T. (1965). Runaway behaviour of lizards to heat and light reinforcement. *Psychological Reports*, **16**, 423–426.

Amiel, J. J., and Shine, R. (2012). Hotter nests produce smarter young lizards. *Biology Letters*, **8**, 372–374.

Amiel, J. J., Lindström, T., and Shine, R. (2014). Egg incubation effects generate positive correlations between size, speed and learning ability in young lizards. *Animal Cognition*, **17**, 337–347.

Amiel, J. J., Bao, S., and Shine, R. (2017). The effects of incubation temperature on the development of the cortical forebrain in a lizard. *Animal Cognition*, **20**, 117–125.

Bezzina, C. N., Amiel, J. J., and Shine, R. (2014). Does invasion success reflect superior cognitive ability? A case study of two congeneric lizard species (*Lampropholis*, Scincidae). *PLoS ONE*, **9**, e86271.

Birrell, J. M., and Brown, V. J. (2000). Medial frontal cortex mediates perceptual attentional set shifting in the rat. *The Journal of Neuroscience*, **20**, 4320–4324.

Carazo, P., Font, E., and Desfilis, E. (2008). Beyond 'nasty neighbours' and 'dear enemies'? Individual recognition by scent marks in a lizard (*Podarcis hispanica*). *Animal Behaviour*, **76**, 1953–1963.

Carazo, P., Noble, D. W. A., Chandrasoma, D., and Whiting, M. J. (2014). Sex and boldness explain individual differences in spatial learning in a lizard. *Proceedings of the Royal Society of London B: Biological Sciences*, **281**, 20133275.

Clark, B. F., Amiel, J. J., Noble, D. W. A., and Whiting, M. J. (2014). Colour discrimination and associative learning in hatchling lizards incubated at 'hot' and 'cold' temperatures. *Behavioral Ecology and Sociobiology*, **68**, 239–247.

Colacicco, G., Welzl, H., Lipp, H.-P., and Wuerbel, H. (2002). Attentional set-shifting in mice: modification of a rat paradigm, and evidence for strain-dependent variation. *Behavioural Brain Research*, **132**, 95–102.

Cooper, W. E. (1994a). Chemical discrimination by tongue-flicking in lizards – a review with hypotheses on its origin and its ecological and phylogenetic relationships. *Journal of Chemical Ecology*, **20**, 439–487.

Cooper, W. E. J. (1994b). Prey chemical discrimination, foraging mode, and phylogeny. In *Lizard ecology: historical and experimental perspectives* (pp. 95–116). Princeton, NJ: Princeton University Press.

Croston, R., Branch, C. L., Kozlovsky, D. Y., Dukas, R., and Pravosudov, V. V. (2015). Heritability and the evolution of cognitive traits. *Behavioral Ecology*, **26**, 1447–1459.

Davidson, R. E., and Richardson, A. M. (1970). Classical conditioning of skeletal and autonomic responses in the lizard (*Crotaphytus collaris*). *Physiology and Behavior*, **5**, 589–594.

Day, L. B., Crews, D., and Wilczynski, W. (1999b). Relative medial and dorsal cortex volume in relation to foraging ecology in congeneric lizards. *Brain, Behavior and Evolution*, **54**, 314–322.

Day, L. B., Crews, D., and Wilczynski, W. (1999a). Spatial and reversal learning in congeneric lizards with different foraging strategies. *Animal Behaviour*, **57**, 393–407.

Day, L. B., Crews, D., and Wilczynski, W. (2001). Effects of medial and dorsal cortex lesions on spatial memory in lizards. *Behavioural Brain Research*, **118**, 27–42.

Day, L. B., Ismail, N., and Wilczynski, W. (2003). Use of position and feature cues in discrimination learning by the whiptail lizard (*Cnemidophorus inornatus*). *Journal of Comparative Psychology*, **117**, 440–448.

Dayananda, B., and Webb, J. K. (2017). Incubation under climate warming affects learning ability and survival in hatchling lizards. *Biology Letters*, **13**(3), 20170002.

Dunham, A. E., Miles, D. B., and Reznick, D. N. (1988). Life history patterns in squamate reptiles. In *Biology of the Reptilia. Ecology B: defense and life history* (pp. 441–522). New York, NY: Alan R. Liss.

Fleishman, L. J., Loew, E. R., and Leal, M. (1993). Ultraviolet vision in lizards. *Nature*, **365**, 397.

Fleishman, L. J., Loew, E. R., and Whiting, M. J. (2011). High sensitivity to short wavelengths in a lizard and implications for understanding the evolution of visual systems in lizards. *Proceedings of the Royal Society of London B: Biological Sciences*, **278**, 2891–2899.

Gaalema, D. E. (2011). Visual discrimination and reversal learning in rough-necked monitor lizards (*Varanus rudicollis*). *Journal of Comparative Psychology*, **125**, 246–249.

Gallistel, C. R., Fairhurst, S., and Balsam, P. (2004). The learning curve: implications of a quantitative analysis. *Proceedings of the National Academy of Sciences*, **101**, 13124–13131.

Garzanit, F. S., and Richardson, A. M. (1974). Black–white discrimination and orienting behavior in the desert iguana (*Dipsosaurus dorsalis*). *Animal Learning and Behavior*, **2**, 126–128.

Halpern, M. (1992). Nasal chemical senses in reptiles: structure and function. In *Biology of the Reptilia: brain, hormones, and behavior* (pp. 423–522). Chicago, IL: University of Chicago Press.

Herculano-Houzel, S., Kaas, J. H., Miller, D., and Von Bartheld, C. S. (2015). How to count cells: the advantages and disadvantages of the isotropic fractionator compared with stereology. *Cell and Tissue Research*, **360**, 29–42.

Hoops, D. (2015). A perfusion protocol for lizards, including a method for brain removal. *MethodsX*, **2**, 165–173.

Hoops, D., Pullman, J. F. P., Janke, A. L., Vidal-Garcia, M., *et al.* (2017). Sexual selection predicts brain structure in dragon lizards. *Journal of Evolutionary Biology*, **30**, 244–256.

Huang, W. S. (2006). Parental care in the long-tailed skink, *Mabuya longicaudata*, on a tropical Asian island. *Animal Behaviour*, **72**, 791–795.

Husak, J. F., Irschick, D. J., Henningsen, J. P., Kirkbride, K. S., Lailvaux, S. P., and Moore, I. T. (2009). Hormonal response of male green anole lizards (*Anolis carolinensis*) to GnRH challenge. *Journal of Experimental Zoology A*, **311**, 105–114.

Jones, S. M. (2011). Hormonal regulation of ovarian function in reptiles. In *Hormones and reproduction of vertebrates* (pp. 89–115). London: Elsevier.

Kar, F., Whiting, M. J., and Noble, D. W. A. (2017). Dominance and social information use in a lizard. *Animal Cognition*, **20**, 805–812.

Karsten, K. B., Andriamandimbiarisoa, L. N., Fox, S. F., and Raxworthy, C. J. (2008). A unique life history among tetrapods: an annual chameleon living mostly as an egg. *Proceedings of the National Academy of Sciences*, **105**, 8980–8984.

Kemp, D. J., Herberstein, M. E., Fleishman, L. J., *et al.* (2015). An integrative framework for the appraisal of colouration in nature. *The American Naturalist*, **185**, 705–724.

Kirkish, P. M., Fobes, J. L., and Richardson, A. M. (1979). Spatial reversal learning in the lizard *Coleonyx variegatus*. *Bulletin of Psychonomic Science*, **13**, 265–267.

Kis, A., Huber, L., and Wilkinson, A. (2015). Social learning by imitation in a reptile (*Pogona vitticeps*). *Animal Cognition*, **18**, 325–331.

Krekorian, C. O., Vance, V. J., and Richardson, A. M. (1968). Temperature-dependent maze learning in the desert iguana *Dipsosaurus dorsalis*. *Animal Behaviour*, **16**, 429–436.

LaDage, L. D., Riggs, B. J., Sinervo, B., and Pravosudov, V. V. (2009). Dorsal cortex volume in male side-blotched lizards, *Uta stansburiana*, is associated with different space use strategies. *Animal Behaviour*, **78**, 91–96.

LaDage, L. D., Roth, T. C., Cerjanic, A. M., Sinervo, B., and Pravosudov, V. V. (2012). Spatial memory: are lizards really deficient? *Biology Letters*, **8**, 939–941.

LaDage, L. D., Roth II, T. C., Sinervo, B., and Pravosudov, V. V. (2013). Interaction between territoriality, spatial environment, and hippocampal neurogenesis in male side-blotched lizards. *Behavioral Neuroscience*, **127**, 555–565.

LaDage, L. D., Roth II, T. C., Sinervo, B., and Pravosudov, V. V. (2016). Environmental experiences influence cortical volume in territorial and nonterritorial side-blotched lizards, *Uta stansburiana*. *Animal Behaviour*, **115**, 11–18.

LaDage, L. D., Cobb Irvin, T. E., and Gould, V. A. (2017). Assessing spatial learning and memory in small squamate reptiles. *Journal of Visual Experiments*, **119**, e55103.

Leal, M., and Powell, B. J. (2012). Behavioural flexibility and problem-solving in a tropical lizard. *Biology Letters*, **8**, 28–30.

Loop, M. S. (1976). Autoshaping a simple technique for teaching a lizard to perform a visual discrimination task. *Copeia*, **3**, 574–576.

Manrod, J. D., Hartdegen, R., and Burghardt, G. M. (2008). Rapid solving of a problem apparatus by juvenile black-throated monitor lizards (*Varanus albigularis albigularis*). *Animal Cognition*, **11**, 267–273.

Marcellini, D. (1977). Acoustic and visual display behavior of gekkonid lizards. *Integrative and Comparative Biology*, **17**, 251–260.

Moore, M. C. (1988). Testosterone control of territorial behavior: tonic-release implants fully restore seasonal and short-term aggressive responses in free-living castrated lizards. *General and Comparative Endocrinology*, **70**, 450–459.

Mueller-Paul, J., Wilkinson, A., Hall, G., and Huber, L. (2012). Response-stereotypy in the jewelled lizard (*Timon lepidus*) in a radial-arm maze. *Herpetology Notes*, **5**, 243–246.

Nakagawa, S., and Foster, T. M. (2004). The case against retrospective power analyses with an introduction to power analysis. *Acta Ethologica*, **7**, 103–108.

Nakagawa, S., and Hauber, M. E. (2011). Great challenges with few subjects: statistical strategies for neuroscientists. *Neuroscience and Biobehavioral Reviews*, **35**, 462–473.

Noble, D. W. A., Carazo, P., and Whiting, M. J. (2012). Learning outdoors: male lizards show flexible spatial learning under semi-natural conditions. *Biology Letters*, **8**, 946–948.

Noble, D. W. A., Wechmann, K., Keogh, J. S., and Whiting, M. J. (2013). Behavioral and morphological traits interact to promote the evolution of alternative reproductive tactics in a lizard. *American Naturalist*, **182**, 726–742.

Noble, D. W. A., Byrne, R. W., and Whiting, M. J. (2014). Age-dependent social learning in a lizard. *Biology Letters*, **10**, 20140430.

Noble, D. W. A., Stenhouse, V., and Schwanz, L. E. (2018). Developmental temperatures and phenotypic plasticty in reptiles: a systematic review and meta-analysis. *Biological Reviews*, **93**, 72–97.

Paulissen, M. A. (2008). Spatial learning in the little brown skink, *Scincella lateralis*: the importance of experience. *Animal Behaviour*, **76**, 135–141.

Paulisson, M. A. (2014). The role of visual cues in learning escape behaviour in the little brown skink (*Scincella lateralis*). *Behaviour*, **151**, 2015–2028.

Pérez-Cembranos, A., and Pérez-Mellado, V. (2015). Local enhancement and social foraging in a non-social insular lizard. *Animal Cognition*, **18**, 629–637.

Pianka, E. R., and Vitt, L. J. (2003). *Lizards: windows to the evolution of diversity*. Berkeley, CA: University of California Press.

Powell, R. W., and Peck, K. (1970). Instrumental aversive conditioning in the skink *Eumeces inexpectatus* studied with two test chambers. *Psychonomic Science*, **18**, 263–264.

Reilly, S. M., McBrayer, L. B., and Miles, D. B. (2007). *Lizard ecology: the evolutionary consequences of foraging mode*. Cambridge: Cambridge University Press.

Riley, J. L., Noble, D. W. A., Bryne, R. W., and Whiting, M. J. (2017). Does social environment influence learning ability in a family-living lizard? *Animal Cognition*, **20**, 449–458.

Roberts, A. C., Robbins, T. W., and Everitt, B. J. (1988). The effects of intradimensional and extradimensional shifts on visual discrimination learning in humans and non-human primates. *The Quarterly Journal of Experimental Psychology Section B*, **40**, 321–341.

Shine, R. (2014). Evolution of an evolutionary hypothesis: a history of changing ideas about the adaptive significance of viviparity in reptiles. *Journal of Herpetology*, **48**, 147–161.

Sinn, D. L., While, G. M., and Wapstra, E. (2008). Maternal care in a social lizard: links between female aggression and offspring fitness. *Animal Behaviour*, **76**, 1249–1257.

Stamps, J. A. (1983). Sexual selection, sexual dimorphism and territoriality. In *Lizard ecology: studies of a model organism* (pp. 169–204). Cambridge, MA: Harvard University Press.

Striedter, G. F. (2015). Evolution of the hippocampus in reptiles and birds. *Journal of Comparative Neurology*, **524**, 496–517.

R Core Team. (2017). *R: a language and environment for statistical computing. Perfusion protocol for lizards, including a method for brain removal*. Vienna: Foundation for Statistical Computing.

Titulaer, M., van Oers, K., and Naguib, M. (2012). Personality affects learning performance in difficult tasks in a sex-dependent way. *Animal Behaviour*, **83**, 723–730.

Wack, C. L., Fox, S. F., Hellgren, E. C., and Lovern, M. B. (2008). Effects of sex, age, and season on plasma steroids in free-ranging Texas horned lizards (*Phrynosoma cornutum*). *General and Comparative Endocrinology*, **155**, 589–596.

Weed, M. R., Bryant, R., and Perry, S. (2008). Cognitive development in macaques: attentional set-shifting in juvenile and adult rhesus monkeys. *Neuroscience*, **157**, 22–28.

While, G. M., Halliwell, B., and Uller, T. (2014). The evolutionary ecology of parental care in lizards. In *Reproductive biology and phylogeny of lizards and tuatara* (pp. 590–619). Boca Raton, FL: CRC Press.

Whiting, M. J., and Greeff, J. M. (1997). Facultative frugivory in the cape flat lizard, *Platysaurus capensis* (Sauria: Cordylidae). *Copeia*, **1997**, 811–818.

Whiting, M. J., and While, G. M. (2017). Sociality in lizards. In *Comparative social evolution* (pp. 390–426). Cambridge: Cambridge University Press.

Whiting, M. J., Xu, F., Kar, F., Riley, J. L., Byrne, R. W., and Noble, D. W. A. (in review). Social learning in a family-living lizard.

Wilkinson, A., and Huber, L. (2012). Cold-blooded cognition: reptilian cognitive abilities. In *The Oxford handbook of comparative evolutionary psychology* (pp. 129–143). Oxford: Oxford University Press.

13 Meerkats – Identifying Cognitive Mechanisms Underlying Meerkat Coordination and Communication: Experimental Designs in Their Natural Habitat

Marta Manser

Species Description

Anatomy

Meerkats are small carnivores with an average adult mass of 700–800 g in their natural habitat. They are about 35 cm in height when standing up on their hind legs, which they do often in a range of behaviours, including sunning, bipedal vigilance and sentinel duty. Their tail enables them to stand bipedal for extended periods on the ground and also to balance when climbing up into shrubs or trees to act as sentinels. Digging is one of the main activities of meerkats to find prey in the sand (Doolan and MacDonald, 1996), to renovate their sleeping burrow entrances (Bousquet, 2011) or to clean out boltholes, which they use as shelter from predators (Manser and Bell, 2004). This has resulted in the evolution of strong forearms with elongated nails (up to 2 cm), enabling them to efficiently push away large amounts of sand.

Meerkats are well-camouflaged with the colour of their fur adjusted to the habitat they live in. They range from dark brown in the green scrubland (e.g. in Addo National Park) to light brown in the Kalahari (pers. obs.). The pattern of dark stripes on their back is unique and can be used for individual recognition. The belly is typically darker than other parts of the body and can be used to efficiently absorb heat from the sun. In the coldest times of the year, they stand with their belly directed towards the sun for up to an hour at the sleeping burrow entrances before they start foraging for the day. During the cold season, their hair grows much longer and denser. However, temperature regulation has its limitations during the hot periods of the year: meerkats stop foraging in the open when sand surface temperatures rise above 60°C and also stop foraging in the shade when air temperatures in shaded areas rise above 40°C.

Perception

Meerkats have evolved an elaborate vocal and olfactory communication system, and also use visual signals quite extensively. The range of frequencies in the different call types seems to be within the human hearing range (i.e. 20–20,000 Hz). Most of the tonal calls have a fundamental frequency of 200–300 Hz and a bandwidth of up to 4–8 kHz, while the noisiest broadband calls can range from low frequencies up to 20 kHz and potentially even above (Manser, 1998; Manser *et al.*, 2014). Currently, little is known about the hearing abilities of meerkats, including peak auditory sensitivity. Most calls likely have a transmission range between 10 and 30 m, although the noisiest broadband calls may carry further, with barks (Townsend *et al.*, 2014) potentially carrying up to 100 m, depending on environmental conditions.

Meerkats, like many mammals, rely heavily on smell, and in comparison to most other social mongoose species, their nose appears substantially elongated. This may be an adaptation to smelling in the digging holes for tunnels made by prey items, but may also allow them to perceive subtle vibrations when digging. Meerkats mark their territory with faeces, urine, scent marks and, to a lesser degree, saliva. Scent glands are located on their cheeks, along the side of their body and in the anal region. Olfactory signals and cues play a crucial role in meerkats, to which they may respond from several metres away, often recruiting others to the location by vocal and visual signals (e.g. recruitment calls or aroused body posture with tail up and hair erected; Manser *et al.*, 2001). Moreover, olfactory cues allow them to distinguish group members from non-group members (Mares *et al.*, 2011) and kin from non-kin (Leclaire *et al.*, 2013).

In regards to visual signals, little is known about colour or depth perception in detail (Moran *et al.*, 1983). However, based on our field observations, their eyesight is extremely adapted to detect and identify objects at far distances in the sky, and also in open and structured habitats. For example, meerkats will produce alarm signals in response to dangerous predators, such as a martial eagle, at distances over 1 km away (when they might not even be visible to humans with binoculars). However, they will not respond to a white-backed vulture of similar size and colours at the same distance (Kalahari Meerkat Project (KMP), unpublished long-term data). Meerkats can also look directly into the sun and still reliably detect objects in the sky. They appear to have poor visual perception of close objects and often fail to detect non-moving prey items at close distances if they do not stand out obviously against their background. However, meerkats seem to be very good at perceiving contrasts and can immediately detect anything moving, whether it is close by or at a far distance.

Life Cycle

Meerkats live in groups of 3–50 individuals, where mainly the dominant pair reproduces and the other group members help in raising their offspring (Clutton-Brock *et al.*, 2010). After birth, pups spend 3 weeks underground in their burrow, typically being looked after by one or two babysitters, while the rest of the group is foraging (Clutton-Brock *et al.*, 2001a). After having emerged, pups spend another week at the birth burrow and only then start to join in foraging with their group, being fed prey items by older group members (Brotherton *et al.*, 2001). They also start digging for prey themselves, and at the age of 3 months they find food rather independently, and pup feeding ceases completely (Thornton, 2008). When they are 6 months old, they have developed the behavioural repertoire of an adult meerkat, such as producing alarm calls (Hollén *et al.*, 2008), performing sentinel behaviour or also sometimes staying behind at the birth burrow as a babysitter. They usually become sexually mature around 1 year of age.

Males disperse voluntarily from their natal group when they are about 1.5–2 years old (Young *et al.*, 2007), while females do not leave unless they are forced out by the dominant female (Stephens *et al.*, 2004). These periods of conflicts provide very good opportunities to test their social knowledge and understanding of their social environment. Subordinate males, when starting to disperse, typically 'rove' for some weeks or months, temporarily leaving their natal group to explore other groups for mating opportunities or to immigrate. During this period, they seem to invest more into their own growth than performing cooperative tasks, as they are not able to maintain their energy expenditure with their limited foraging opportunities when by themselves on their roving excursions (Young *et al.*, 2007). Subordinate females are frequently attacked by the dominant female, especially in the second half of her pregnancy. During these periods, subordinate females try to either avoid the dominant female or show pronounced submission behaviour, including submission calls (Kutsukake and Clutton-Brock, 2006; Reber *et al.*, 2013). These behaviours seem to reduce the level of conflict and potentially delay the eviction by the dominant female.

Individual Identification

Each individual meerkat develops its own specific fur colouring with distinctly patterned dark stripes on their back, and the sexes are easy to distinguish due to the large testes in males. However, if wild individuals need to be distinguished in groups of more than five individuals from several metres away, excellent observation skills and memory are required. An effective solution is therefore to mark them with unique patterns of hair dye marks (which need to be reapplied every 2–3 weeks) at specific locations of their body (Jordan *et al.*, 2007; Figure 13.1). This ensures more reliable data collection, especially when several groups are studied by many different researchers. We also implant every meerkat with a transponder chip to ensure life-long identification (Jordan *et al.*, 2007); for example, if a meerkat is not seen for a long period of time due to dispersal or roving, and the hair dye mark disappears. Ear tags are not very effective, as meerkat ears are very small and tags get quickly lost. Similarly, we also tried freeze-branding, as done in other small mammals, such as ground squirrels (Waterman, 2002), but this is a rather invasive and unreliable method, which we do not use anymore. A skin sample is also collected from every meerkat captured from the population in order to determine the genetic relatedness of the different individuals (Griffin *et al.*, 2001).

Ecological Characteristics

Meerkats live in the dry semi-desert of the Kalahari in the southern part of Africa, including Botswana, Namibia, South Africa and the very southern tip of Angola. In the Kalahari, the climate includes the warm and wet season from October to April

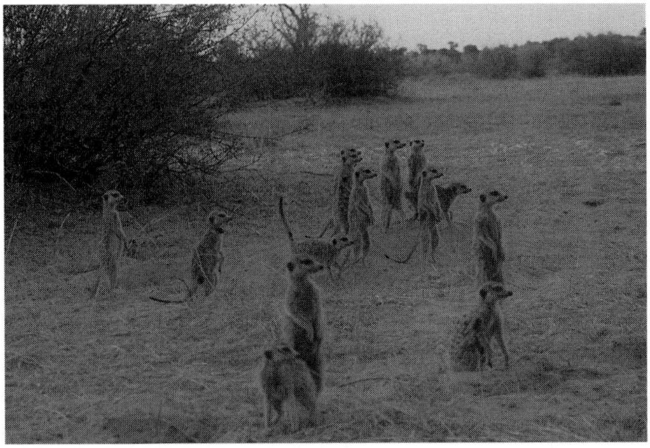

Figure 13.1. Meerkats in the southern Kalahari, being habituated to close observation, coordinate their group activities with vocal, olfactory and visual signal, and rely greatly on social learning. The second meerkat from the left carries a radio collar with a VHF transmitter, which allows finding the group at any stage. For individual recognition, meerkats are marked with hair dye at specific body parts (e.g. the one on the front to the right has a dark spot on the right shoulder). Photo taken by M. Manser.

(with little rain from October to December, and more rain from January to April) and the cold and dry season from May to September. During the warm season, and in particular from November to February, the meerkats get up with sunrise and start foraging more or less immediately until it gets too hot, then they rest under vegetation or in boltholes from around 10 AM to 6 PM, after which they forage for another hour until sunset, and finally disappear into their sleeping burrow. During the cold season, 20–60 minutes of sunning behaviour precedes foraging, which usually continues until sunset with a few short breaks in between.

At the study site of the KMP, the habitat consists of large, open, sandy areas, in particular along dry riverbeds, interspersed with large areas of bush (e.g. *Rhigozum* shrub). Meerkats prefer to forage in more open vegetation (i.e. below 1.5 m), where visual contact and call transmission are facilitated. Meerkats have many different aerial and terrestrial predators (Clutton-Brock *et al.*, 1999a), which have caused them to evolve a highly efficient anti-predator sentinel system (Clutton-Brock *et al.*, 1999b), which allows them to warn each other with alarm calls specific to the type and urgency of the threat (Manser, 2001).

The main food sources (including insect larvae, scorpions, spiders, barking geckos) need to be dug out of the sand, while some beetles and small reptiles are caught on the surface (Doolan and MacDonald, 1996). Large millipedes, tortoise eggs or pygmy mice can also be dug up, mainly from bolthole entrances, and lizards and small snakes can be caught and eaten. The majority of their active foraging time is spent palpating the soil surface, likely for entrances of animal tunnels or other disturbances of soil structure hinting towards prey location. Once they have located a promising spot, they then start to dig at this specific location and sometimes need up to 20 minutes to get the prey, creating holes down to

80 cm into the sand. Adults do not share food among each other, and pregnant or lactating dominant females often compete with subordinates for access to promising foraging holes (Flower, 2011b). However, food is shared with pups, until they have learned to forage independently by the age of 3 to 4 months (Brotherton *et al.*, 2001).

Social Characteristics

Meerkats are characterized by a clear dominance structure, with the dominant pair being the main breeders and other group members helping to raise their pups (Clutton-Brock *et al.*, 2001b). Within the subordinates, hierarchy is based on age, and in females on body size (Thavarajah *et al.*, 2014). Group members are typically highly related to each other, with the dominant pair, their offspring, and potentially one or a few unrelated immigrated males (Clutton-Brock *et al.*, 1998). Females are not accepted as immigrants into existing groups.

Except for roving males or subordinate females evicted by the dominant female, meerkats are always found in groups (Young and Monfort, 2009). Separation from the group is one of the most stressful situations for meerkats, and they have evolved an efficient vocal system to keep cohesion while foraging or to find each other when temporarily lost (Manser, 1998; Manser *et al.*, 2014; Gall and Manser, 2017).

During dominance competition, dominant individuals may evict same-sex subordinates that might threaten their position. In the wild, this occurs more frequently among females, with aggression increasing when the dominant female is pregnant (Young *et al.*, 2006). In males, it only occurs under specific group compositions, when the dominant male has a brother of similar age and weight, and both of them are immigrants and unrelated to the females in the group (KMP, long-term data).

State of the Art

Studies on meerkat cognition have addressed several aspects of physical and social cognition, with a special focus on group coordination (Bousquet *et al.*, 2011; Gall and Manser, 2017), vocal (Manser *et al.*, 2014) and olfactory (Leclaire *et al.*, 2013) communication, social learning and teaching (Thornton and Clutton-Brock, 2011). On the immediate level, group coordination in meerkats is largely achieved through vocal and visual communication. Vocal signals have been better investigated, because they are easier to identify and simulate, but also because meerkats have a large vocal repertoire, with more than 30 different discrete call types used for group cohesion, anti-predator behaviour, division of cooperative tasks and social interactions (Manser, 1998; Manser *et al.*, 2014).

Group Coordination and Communication

Meerkats forage as a cohesive unit throughout the day, and they emit several different call types to maintain group cohesion during their foraging excursions. ‘Lead’ and 'move' calls are given to coordinate departure from the sleeping burrow and to induce group members to switch foraging patches (Turbé, 2006). If more than three individuals are involved in emitting 'move' calls, the group moves to the next foraging area, but if just one or no individual replies to the call, the group usually continues to forage on the current foraging patch, suggesting that a quorum has not been reached (Bousquet *et al.*, 2011). While meerkats are foraging, they regularly emit soft 'close' calls, which are likely to maintain contact among the dispersed group members, and space themselves out to avoid frequent food competition (Manser, 1998; Engesser, 2011). Individuals that get separated from the group emit soft 'alert' calls, which turn into loud barks if they cannot see the group. Barking causes other group members to stand bipedally or to move in the direction of the lost animal (Manser, 1998).

Individual meerkats frequently stop foraging and move to a raised position where they scan the sky and surrounding area for predators (Clutton-Brock *et al.*, 1999b). Although there is no predictable rotation in sentinel behaviour, individuals alternate and typically avoid going on guard when another individual is already acting as a sentinel (Clutton-Brock *et al.*, 1999b; Manser, 1999). Individual contributions to sentinel duty vary and are positively associated with age, weight and foraging success, and are higher in males than females or after being artificially provisioned (Clutton-Brock *et al.*, 1999b). Average contributions to sentinel duty increase when the risk of predation is high, and also when pups are foraging with the group (Santema and Clutton-Brock, 2013).

When meerkats detect danger, they give alarm calls, which vary in their acoustic structure both in relation to the type of predator they have seen and to the urgency of the danger (Manser, 2001; Manser *et al.*, 2001, 2002). The likelihood of alarm-calling depends on whether other group members are close by (Townsend *et al.*, 2012). So far, we have no evidence that receivers adjust their response to the identity or reliability of the caller, possibly because the costs of ignoring alarm calls are too high (Schibler and Manser, 2007). However, receivers habituate to playbacks of alarm calls quite fast, and after the second or third playback they do not respond as intensively anymore if no actual predator approaches within a short period after having heard an alarm call (Karp *et al.*, 2014). Sentinels give regular high-pitched calls when they are on 'watch', which are perceived by other group members, allowing them to reduce their level of vigilance while foraging (Manser, 1999; Rauber and Manser, 2017).

Vocalizations also play an important role in regulating social relationships within groups. Meerkats express their affiliative or aggressive intentions when approaching each other with appropriate calls. Growls reflect aggression and are given by dominants to subordinate individuals, or during food competition by all individuals involved. Subordinates express their submission with higher-pitched, more tonal submission 'grovelling' calls (Kutsukake and Clutton-Brock, 2006). Furthermore, close calls are used to regulate (Gall and Manser, 2017) and monitor other individuals' movements (Townsend *et al.*, 2011). Responses to calls are adjusted to social circumstances. For example, subordinate females that experience aggression from the dominant female and are at risk of being evicted respond very strongly to aggressors' calls (Reber *et al.*, 2013).

Olfactory communication plays a role in inter- and intragroup communication, and several different types of media, including faeces, urine, gland secretions and even saliva are used to advertise the use of a territory (Jordan *et al.*, 2007). These signals include individual signatures, and allow the receivers to not only gain information on the identity of the territory owner, but also on kinship (Leclaire *et al.*, 2013). They are likely also used for intragroup communication. As for vocal communication, experiments suggest that receivers discriminate at the individual level and may maintain representations of the signal producer (Reber *et al.*, 2013).

Social Learning, Traditions and Teaching

As expected for cohesive living species with sharing cooperative tasks, meerkats rely on social learning. This is particularly obvious in the context of learning about foraging and likely also occurs in the context of predator recognition and spatial mapping of their home range. For animals relying on food which can vary depending on season or vegetation type and could even be poisonous, it is of advantage to learn early which food items are appropriate. In meerkats, young individuals follow the older group members and get fed in their first 2–3 months, while joining the foraging group. Thereby, they learn about edible food. Meerkats seem particularly neophobic to new food types and only eat what they have seen conspecifics eating (Thornton, 2008). However, we know less about how much they learn about predator recognition, shelter location or their territory in general. Current observations show that, when recognizing danger, pups up to 4–5 months largely rely on following older group members' responses (Hollén and Manser, 2006; Graw and Manser, 2007). Similarly, offspring seem to run independently to the shelter without prompting only after about 4–6 months of age (Manser and Bell, 2004), although we do not know how they learn about it.

In meerkats, there is evidence of tradition establishment. When specific individuals in a group are trained as demonstrators to be rewarded at landmarks characterized by a specific symbol, naïve individuals are more likely to approach landmarks of that type and obtain the rewards following encounters with demonstrators (Thornton and Malapert, 2009). However, individuals that learn that one type of landmark is profitable also begin to investigate the landmarks characterized with other symbols, and traditions to approach a specific symbol collapse over time. Other evidence for conservative traditions in meerkats is based on the observation that differences persist between neighbouring meerkat groups, in terms of emergence time from their sleeping burrow in the morning (Thornton *et al.*, 2010). Over an observation period of 11 years, some groups consistently emerged later in the morning than others, even when group membership changed (e.g. change in dominance or after immigration of males).

Moreover, meerkats show the different steps that are involved in animal teaching (Thornton and McAuliffe, 2006; Thornton and Raihani, 2010), according to the definition by Caro and Hauser (1992). When it comes to pup provisioning, group members adjust their behaviour to the age and experience of pups to enhance the pup's foraging skills. They feed the very young pups with dead or badly wounded prey and then gradually provide them with fully alive prey, which is able to escape or strike back (Thornton and McAuliffe, 2006). For example, scorpions are initially presented to pups when dead or wounded, with their stings removed, but as pups grow up, they are gradually presented with intact scorpions, which pups learn to kill after removing their sting. Experiments confirm that presenting pups with active prey improves the rate at which they learn handling skills at some cost to helpers, and consequently represents an example of teaching behaviour. In addition, helpers preferentially feed rarer food items to pups, which may help to broaden the range of food types they will eventually use (Thornton, 2008).

All for One and One for All

Box 13.1 Cooperative Breeding and Cognition

Judith M. Burkart

Like meerkats, callitrichid monkeys are cooperative breeders. They live in extended family groups, often complemented by immigrants, and all group members help raising the offspring (Erb and Porter, 2017). Also like meerkats, they have an elaborate vocal communication system (Snowdon, 2017) and are amenable to studies investigating cognitive mechanisms underlying vocal communication. Such efforts can build on rather solid knowledge of their perceptual capacities, including their hearing range (Osmanski and Wang, 2011) or colour vision system (Kawamura, 2016), and an increasing number of studies documenting their social and non-social cognitive skills (Schiel and Souto, 2017).

The breeding pair typically monopolizes reproduction (Yamamoto *et al.*, 2014), but behaviourally, this does not translate in marked dominance hierarchies. In fact, it is often not possible to establish clear dominance hierarchies within groups, because aggression is rare and interactions are highly tolerant (Schaffner and Caine, 2000). Accordingly, among primates, allomaternal care and thus cooperative breeding is associated with high social tolerance and proactive prosociality (i.e. a motivational concern for not only one's own but also others' welfare), as shown by comparative analyses over a large number of species (Burkart *et al.*, 2014). As a result of these predispositions, callitrichids tend to excel in socio-cognitive tasks, but perform just regularly in non-social cognitive tasks (Burkart and van Schaik, 2010, 2016). These results are highly relevant for biological anthropologists interested in human cognitive evolution (Hrdy, 2009; Burkart *et al.*, 2009; Tomasello and Gonzalez-Cabrera, 2017), because humans are the only other cooperative breeders among primates (even though some level of allomaternal care is widespread in this taxon).

A potential link between communicative complexity and cooperative breeding has been proposed by several researchers (e.g. Snowdon, 2001; Burkart *et al.*, 2009; Zuberbühler, 2011; Borjon and Ghazanfar, 2014; Leighton, 2017) and may be important to understand language evolution. Such a link may arise when proactive

(cont.)

prosociality is also expressed as information donation, when the coordination of cooperative care activities has to be fine-tuned via communicative signals, and when immatures use communicative signals to engage caregivers (Burkart *et al.*, in press).

Importantly, to systematically test for consequences of cooperative breeding, it is not enough to investigate cooperative breeders only. Rather, species with and without cooperative breeding need to be compared, while controlling for confounding factors such as brain size, ecology and phylogenetic relationship. Ideally, this is achieved with broad phylogenetic comparative analyses (Burkart *et al.*, 2014; MacLean *et al.*, 2014).

When broad phylogenetic comparisons are not possible, targeted contrasts provide a good approximation (MacLean *et al.*, 2012). Here, closely related taxa are compared that are as similar as possible to each other, but differ in their breeding system. In primates, this includes contrasts between the cooperatively breeding callitrichids versus their closely related but independently breeding sister taxa, the cebid monkeys; siamangs (high levels of allomaternal care) versus gibbons (low levels of allomaternal care); and humans (cooperative breeders) versus chimpanzees and bonobos (our closest related sister taxa, without cooperative breeding; Burkart and van Schaik, 2010). Variation in breeding system in mongoose species offers the opportunity to test additional contrasts outside primates.

References

Borjon, J. I., and Ghazanfar, A. A. (2014). Convergent evolution of vocal cooperation without convergent evolution of brain size. *Brain, Behavior and Evolution*, **84**, 93–102.

Burkart, J. M., and van Schaik, C. P. (2010). Cognitive consequences of cooperative breeding in primates? *Animal Cognition*, **13**, 1–19.

Burkart, J. M., and van Schaik, C. P. (2016). Revisiting the consequences of cooperative breeding. *Journal of Zoology*, **299**, 77–83.

Burkart, J. M., Hrdy, S. B., and van Schaik, C. P. (2009). Cooperative breeding and human cognitive evolution. *Evolutionary Anthropology: Issues, News, and Reviews*, **18**, 175–186.

Burkart, J. M., Allon, O., Amici, F., *et al.* (2014). The evolutionary origin of human hyper-cooperation. *Nature Communications*, **5**, 4747.

Burkart, J. M., *et al.* (in press). From sharing food to sharing information: cooperative breeding and language evolution. *Interaction Studies*.

Erb, W. M., and Porter, L. M. (2017). Mother's little helpers: what we know (and don't know) about cooperative infant care in callitrichines. *Evolutionary Anthropology: Issues, News, and Reviews*, **26**, 25–37.

Hrdy, S. B. (2009). *Mothers and others*. Cambridge, MA: Harvard University Press.

Kawamura, S. (2016). Color vision diversity and significance in primates inferred from genetic and field studies. *Genes and Genomics*, **38**, 779–791.

Leighton, G. M. (2017). Cooperative breeding influences the number and type of vocalizations in avian lineages. *Proceedings of the Royal Society B*, **284**(1868), 20171508.

(cont.)

MacLean, E. L., Matthews, L. J., Hare, B. A., *et al.* (2012). How does cognition evolve? Phylogenetic comparative psychology. *Animal Cognition*, **15**, 223–238.

MacLean, E. L., Hare B., Nunn, C. L., *et al.* (2014). The evolution of self-control. *Proceedings of the National Academy of Sciences*, **111**, 2140–2148.

Osmanski, M. S., and Wang, X. (2011) Measurement of absolute auditory thresholds in the common marmoset (*Callithrix jacchus*). *Hearing Research*, **277**, 127–133.

Schaffner, C. M., and Caine, N. G. (2000). The peacefulness of cooperatively breeding primates. In *Natural conflict resolution* (pp. 155–169). Berkeley, CA: University of California Press.

Schiel, N., and Souto, A. (2017). The common marmoset: an overview of its natural history, ecology and behavior. *Developmental Neurobiology*, **77**, 244–262.

Snowdon, C. T. (2001). Social processes in communication and cognition in callitrichid monkeys: a review. *Animal Cognition*, **4**, 247–257.

Snowdon, C. T. (2017). Vocal communication in family-living and pair-bonded primates. In *Primate hearing and communication* (pp. 141–174). Cham: Springer Cham.

Tomasello, M., and Gonzalez-Cabrera, I. (2017). The role of ontogeny in the evolution of human cooperation. *Human Nature*, **28**, 274–288.

Yamamoto, M. E., Araujo, A., de Fatima Arruda, M., Moreira Lima, A. K., de Oliveria Siqueira, J., and Hattori, W. T. (2014). Male and female breeding strategies in a cooperative primate. *Behavioural Processes*, **109**, 27–33.

Zuberbühler, K. (2011) Cooperative breeding and the evolution of vocal flexibility. In *The Oxford handbook of language evolution* (pp. 71–81). Oxford: Oxford University Press.

Field Guide

Habituation to Human Observers

Although observing the natural behaviour of a species can be informative about the potential of underlying cognitive mechanisms, experiments with controlled conditions are needed to disentangle potential alternative processes being involved. One requirement to experimentally test individuals is that subjects are relaxed and not distracted. This requires either remote-controlled experiments, which can also be observed and documented from a distance, or habituation to a level when the presence of an experimenter/observer no longer influences the animals' behaviour. Although remote-controlled experiments ensure that the test set-up is not influencing any aspect of the response, they do not facilitate spontaneously adjusting experimental set-ups to a given situation. This makes it particularly difficult for experiments in the wild, as the surroundings cannot be completely influenced and controlled during the experimental phase. These problems can be largely overcome by habituating meerkats to the presence of humans. In our KMP population, all group members are habituated to humans, walking behind them within a distance of 1 m and moving objects such as microphones even closer (Figure 13.2).

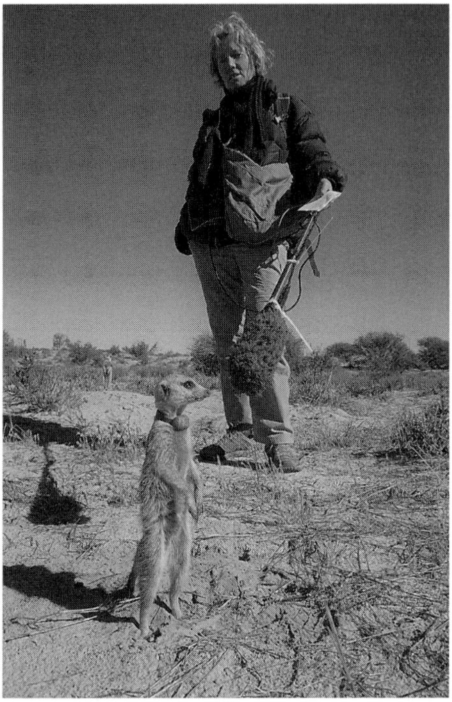

Figure 13.2. Observer recording habituated meerkat when guarding, while the rest of the group is foraging.
Photo taken by Jörg Niggli.

The process of habituating a completely wild group of meerkats can take up to 15 months, depending on their previous encounters with humans. Habituating meerkats in the Kgalagadi National Park, where people are not allowed to leave the car, often only took up to 3 months. In contrast, at the KMP (established on farm land about 200 km outside the park), it took up to 15 months. This can be explained by the fact that at the KMP the meerkats were often chased by humans, and wild groups run away as soon as they see us approaching from a distance as far as 300 m. The habituation process starts with sitting at a far distance (about 30–50 m) from their sleeping burrow, before they start to emerge in the morning. The wild meerkats will then watch us constantly from their safe burrow entrances for up to 2 hours, before leaving the burrow system from the most distant burrow entrance, where all of them run off at high speed to start foraging at some distance away. By more or less finding the group again at their sleeping burrows every day (at the beginning with the help of a local tracker, following their tracks to the sleeping burrow in the evening, later on by capturing an adult individual and putting on a VHF radio transmitter; Jordan *et al.*, 2007), we can slowly progress in sitting closer to the group and gently moving our body parts. Only once we can sit with most of them within 5–10 m, we start standing up and moving around slowly. This may happen after 6–8 months of habituation. The next large step is to try to follow the meerkats when they leave for foraging. For them, this means giving up the safety of the burrow entrances, and it takes quite a long time for them to trust us in this situation.

In general, meerkats are easily scared by abrupt movements and loud sounds. We repeatedly emit soft calming sounds when working with them, especially when we change our activity or move in their close surroundings. Also, when we approach a group, we produce these sounds, identifying us as non-dangerous humans. Individuals differ widely in how quickly they accept our presence and following behaviour. In a group of mainly habituated individuals, a less well-habituated meerkat can be approached quite closely by looking in the direction of another meerkat and moving slowly backwards towards the nervous individual: typically nervous meerkats seem to perceive this, as if the human's focus were on the other conspecific. The most important 'skill' in habituation is to observe the behaviour of each individual, and adjust our own movements and behaviour to the habituation level and response of the meerkats. Also, wild animals respond negatively to direct eye contact. However, this reaction appears to cease once meerkats are highly habituated.

Experiments

In their natural habitat, habituated groups of meerkats are most relaxed early in the morning or during summer time over lunch breaks. However, when they first emerge from their burrows, they look around nervously and scan their surroundings constantly. After some time, particularly when many other group members are up, they relax and still remain at the burrow, to warm themselves in the sun. During summer, these periods before foraging are typically short, but meerkats stop foraging for extended periods over the hot lunch periods. If they stay above ground, they lay in the shade and socialize, behaving very relaxed. These periods at the morning sleeping burrow or during lunch breaks are the times when it is best to perform problem-solving experiments, which take slightly more time (Thornton and Samson, 2012) than playback experiments or simple presentations of olfactory cues. Meerkats will be attentive and motivated, and not distracted by other group members' activities.

During foraging, in contrast, meerkats are constantly moving and strongly focused on finding prey items and maintaining group cohesion. Therefore, it is difficult to test meerkats individually for more than a minute, as target subjects become anxious and try to rejoin the group. However, it may be possible to test them by trying to predict their movement direction, as individuals may separate from the group for up to 5–10 m during foraging. A more active way to separate animals up to 30 m from the group is to lead them away with a scorpion, hanging it down on a fishing line in front of the meerkat's head (Zöttl, 2009). You can then present the test stimuli, although this brings up a general problem within experiments in relation to food rewards. Guiding meerkats to a certain location with food may strongly focus their attention on the food, rather than the intended test stimuli. Even during testing, if repeated food rewards are part of the experiments, subjects may focus more on the food than on the actual experimental stimuli presented.

In many ways, meerkats are ideal subjects for experiments that involve presentations of acoustic, olfactory or visual stimuli. We have performed many manipulations in the context of predator perception and responses, and more recently we have also experimentally tested the underlying cognitive mechanisms in spatial coordination and their social knowledge. As most of the vocalizations are soft and given over short distances, small loudspeakers (e.g. iHome rechargeable mini speaker, iHM79SC; Rauber and Manser, 2017) can be used, hiding them behind vegetation or otherwise easily camouflaging them. More recently, we often fix the loudspeaker to the leg of the experimenter, enabling broadcasting to occur at the height of a foraging or bipedal standing meerkat (Reber *et al.*, 2013; Figure 13.3). This allows fast adjustment to a changing context, which is particularly necessary during the constant movements of foraging meerkats. The presentation of olfactory cues, e.g. faeces or gland secretions, is best done by placing the stimulus next to (within 20–50 cm) a digging meerkat, without interrupting its activity (Leclaire *et al.*, 2013; Zöttl *et al.*, 2012). When the meerkat finishes digging, it will then likely attend to the sample, if it is of any interest to it. Visual stimuli, such as stuffed predators, kites or remote-controlled airplanes (to simulate raptors flying in), can be presented to meerkats at their morning sleeping burrows or also during foraging. Particular care has to be taken to do all the preparations before the group emerges, or to perform them in a calm manner if presentations will occur during foraging, to avoid meerkats associating these manipulations with us. Before testing occurs, any new objects that have to be brought in for the experiments (e.g. a hide for concealing a predator) must be shown to the meerkats in previous sessions, so that they can be habituated to the point where they do not respond to these objects anymore (this typically only takes one or few presentations).

Some caution needs to be taken with regards to habituation to experiments (i.e. not attending to them anymore), and also to how differences in their ecological and social environment can affect the responses to stimuli. We have experienced that the intensity of meerkat responses to presentations of acoustic, olfactory and visual stimuli decreases

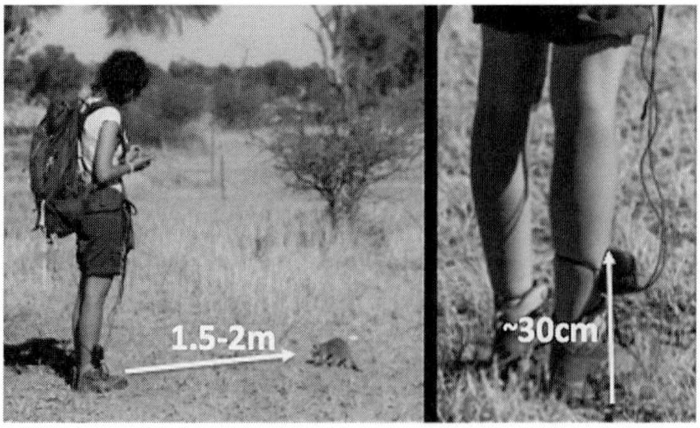

Figure 13.3. Playback set-up: experimenter following within a few metres of the test subject, with loudspeaker fixed to the leg at the height of a guarding meerkat.
Photo taken by Gabriela Gall.

quite fast if they are repeated more frequently than the natural occurrence rate of these situations in the wild (Schibler and Manser, 2007; Karp *et al.*, 2014; Voellmy *et al.*, 2014). We therefore have restrictions on how often such experiments can be performed in a group or to a specific individual, depending on the stimuli type, and also whether it induces a response from only the target subject or from the whole group. For example, close calls, the frequently emitted contact call produced every 4–20 s during foraging, can be played back more often than an alarm call, which potentially only occurs a few times per foraging session. In general, we limit experiments on the same group to every other day, and while close calls can be tested during each experimental trial, alarm calls can only be tested once per week, although within a session we may playback more than one alarm call or bout of alarm calls, depending on the experimental design and question. The same rules apply when deciding how frequently olfactory (Zöttl *et al.*, 2012) and visual stimuli (Thornton and Malapert, 2009) can be presented to a specific individual or group. These precautions are taken to avoid getting our groups used to experiments to the point where they no longer respond, or provide less-intense responses due to repeated exposure.

Moreover, it needs to be considered that even small differences in the context may trigger variation in their responses. In playback experiments during foraging, for instance, meerkats digging for a specific prey will be less responsive to the same call type than meerkats searching for prey or prey cues, such as tunnels (Amsler, 2008). This is also true when presenting olfactory or visual cues to meerkats. A meerkat digging for prey is focused on the task of obtaining that food item and is much less attentive to its environment. As a consequence, the stimuli should only be brought in to non-digging individuals, or in such a way that, when the target subject finishes digging, it will then be easily exposed to the well-placed stimuli. Also, meerkats close to shelter, such as sleeping burrow entrances or boltholes, will respond to stimuli more slowly or with less intensity than meerkats out in the open and far away from shelter options, particularly if predator-related stimuli are being tested (e.g. sentinels, typically located next to a bolthole, take longer to leave their position than foraging meerkats further away from shelters; Clutton-Brock *et al.*, 1999b). Furthermore, the social context in social species needs to be taken into account during testing: a group in a socially stable phase provides a rather different test environment than a group where social tension occurs (e.g. when the dominant female is pregnant). For example, subordinate females change their behaviour into submission when they hear that the dominant female is close by, but only during periods of ongoing social conflict between them (Reber *et al.*, 2013). These different conflict situations allow several opportunities to test cognition in different contexts.

As cooperative breeders, meerkats are a model species to investigate questions on prosociality and cooperation. By showing a high reproductive skew in favour of the dominant pair, they are prime examples to investigate others' motivation to help, although cooperation is largely limited towards pups and for common defence, and food sharing among adults does not exist. This competition for food may explain why so far we have failed to establish a convincing paradigm to test prosociality within a food sharing context (Amici *et al.*, 2017). The first attempts to apply existing methodological

Table 13.1. Key aspects relevant to the study of cognition in meerkats.

Key aspect	Natural habitat	Captive groups
Individual marking	Obvious dye marks, transponders	
Get attention to perform experiments	Only when sunning in the morning at sleeping burrow or when resting during the day	During non-feeding periods
Separating from group	Possible for a few minutes, luring away from group with food (e.g. with scorpion on fishing line)	Possible for a few minutes, separating in specific sections of enclosure or experimental cage
Playback experiments	At any time when individuals have emerged	
Habituation to manipulations (e.g. presentations of olfactory or audio stimuli)	Pay attention to context and do not conduct them too often (adjust to natural occurrence rate)	
Observation	If close by, ensure slow and calm movements, never run, make soft calming sounds	If in enclosure, ensure slow and calm movements, observe from outside enclosure or with video
Eye sight	Not very good at close distance, exceptional over far distance (predator recognition)	Not very good at close distance
To calm them down to close presence	Talking to them in soft voice and always move slowly	

set-ups requiring rope-pulling have failed on meerkats in captivity, as subjects only focused on the food reward, rather than the social partner or the experimental apparatus. Possibly, meerkats cannot pay attention to the environment while suppressing their own motivation to receive food, and end up maximizing their food income, regardless of other group members. Potentially, such an experiment should be repeated when pups are present, to see if they are more prosocial towards pups. As a side note, meerkats usually dig to find their food, so that even when being tested, they may end up digging with their paws, rather than pulling in a goal-directed way. If some pulling mechanism is required, it may be helpful to place it in front of the subjects, so that short-sighted meerkats can realize the presence of such a mechanism due to the contrast.

Meerkats also offer great opportunities to study individually based and social-based learning, as offspring pass through clearly defined phases in their lives. Their first 3 weeks are spent below the ground, with the protection of a babysitter, fully relying on them for food, thermoregulation and protection against predators. Once they emerge to the surface, they are exposed to a very different environment, and they learn the burrow entrance as their safe location, yet they already are exposed to additional ecological stimuli, such as approaching predators when above ground. Finally, as they join the group when foraging, they improve their spatial mapping abilities and have to quickly acquire knowledge on their physical and social environment. Because meerkats do not predominantly use only one sensory modality, but very much rely on acoustical, olfactory and visual stimuli, they also seem predisposed for tests on how they combine information from different modalities. This is typically done with cross-modal experiments (Proobs *et al.*, 2009), whereby subjects may be primed with information from one modality and then tested to assess whether they can correctly assign the according information from another modality (e.g. testing individual recognition from body odours and relating it to the matching vocalization from that individual). Because loudspeakers and olfactory cues such as faeces can be easily carried to a group, and specific individuals can be tested separately (easiest when the group is stationary at a burrow, but also with slightly more efforts while it forages, see above), such experiments seem feasible.

Other ideal experimental designs to test the knowledge of animals are violation-of-expectation experiments. Here the important point is to understand meerkats' natural behaviour and information processing in a specific situation, and then add the violating context. We have done this in a playback experiment, testing whether meerkats monitor other individuals' spatial location in the group (Townsend *et al.*, 2011). We presented the foraging test subject with a physically impossible situation by simulating the presence of the same group member in two different places within a few seconds, so that it was impossible for a meerkat to move from one place to the other in that time (Figure 13.4). The test subjects responded more strongly to this incongruent situation than during the control, congruent situation (i.e. the physically possible set-up of playing the calls of two different group members at the same two places and after the same time). Such experimental designs are promising to test specific aspects of information processes in situations where test subjects may not typically show a response, although they may have perceived the information (Reber *et al.*, 2013).

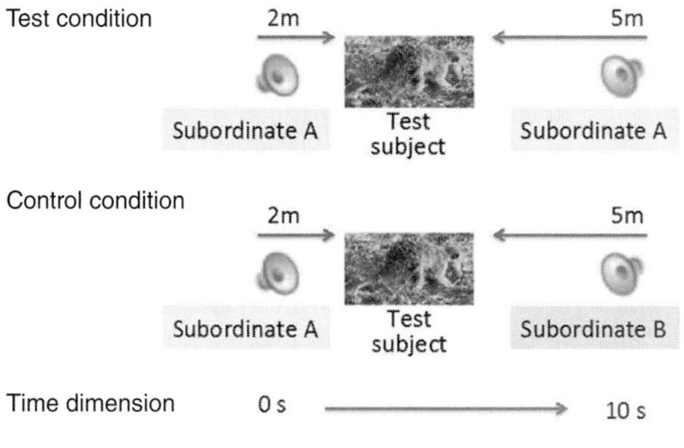

Figure 13.4. Schematic playback set-up of the violation of expectancy experiment, to test individual discrimination while meerkats are foraging. The test condition represents the incongruent set-up of playing the calls of the same subordinate individual, A, to a foraging test subject, from two different sites and within a short time period. The control condition represents the congruent set-up, in which the calls belonging to two different subordinate individuals A and B were played to the same test subject, from two different sites and within a short time period.

The Devil is in the Details

Box 13.2 Communication and Cognition in the Mongoose Family

Alex Thornton

The research described in the current chapter has not only helped to propel meerkats to animal super-stardom, with their fuzzy faces gracing TV screens and billboards around the world, but has also inspired work on other African mongoose species. Although closely related, these species show important ecological and social differences, ranging from solitary (slender mongooses, *Galerella sanguinea*) to facultatively social (yellow mongooses, *Cyncitis penicillata*) and cooperative systems that are either despotic (dwarf mongooses, *Helogale parvula*, and meerkats, *Suricata suricatta*) or egalitarian, with all females breeding synchronously (banded mongooses, *Mungos mungo*). These differences provide unique opportunities for comparative research, to understand the selective pressures driving behavioural and cognitive evolution (see Manser *et al.*, 2014). For instance, dwarf mongooses and meerkats use predator-specific alarm calls that elicit different responses, whereas the other species have a less-specific, urgency-based alarm call system. Manser and colleagues (2014) have speculated that differences in escape opportunities, linked to vegetation cover and predator strategies, may determine when functionally referential call systems provide adaptive benefits.

The methodological approaches used to study the different mongooses, including habituation to allow close observation, are broadly similar, but must of course be tailored to suit the requirements of the system. At the most basic level, habitat differences shape the logistics of data collection. In the southern Kalahari, hunting pressure has largely exterminated large predators, so researchers can follow meerkats and yellow and slender mongooses on foot for kilometres, whereas banded mongoose researchers in Uganda never stray too far from a vehicle, in case they need to beat a hasty retreat from assorted hostile megafauna.

On a more fundamental level, knowledge of each species' ecology shapes the design and execution of hypotheses and experiments. For example, Sharpe and colleagues (2013) took advantage of the fact that dwarf mongooses have a linear dominance hierarchy to use playback experiments and show that adults respond differentially to the calls of group members above or below them in rank. Banded mongoose societies are not hierarchical, but they do exhibit a unique form of offspring care in which pups form an exclusive bond with a single adult carer, known as 'escort'. This led Muller and Manser (2008) to hypothesize that escorts and their pups should have means for recognizing one another, and playback experiments suggest that this is in fact the case.

Knowledge of natural history also informs experiments testing animals' knowledge of their physical environments. Meerkats in the sparsely vegetated Kalahari, for example, have exquisite memory of the location of boltholes in their territories, as these provide means of escape from attacking predators (Manser and Bell, 2004).

(*cont.*)

Banded mongooses, in contrast, tend to dive into bushes when alarmed, but they do seem to remember the locations of hard objects such as rocks and trees, which they use as anvils to crack open encased food items like eggs (McAuliffe and Thornton, 2012). Reports of this behaviour have also led researchers to experimentally test their physical cognition: do mongooses discriminate between hard and soft, and choose anvils accordingly? In short, the answer is no – simple heuristics will do the trick, probably because solid objects in their environment are typically hard (Müller, 2010; McAuliffe and Thornton, 2012).

Truly comparative research remains unfortunately rare in the field of comparative cognition. Research on the mongoose family provides an excellent example of how good old-fashioned natural history can inform the design of elegant and rigorous experiments, to understand the cognitive challenges animals face in their natural environments.

References

Manser, M. B., and Bell, M. B. V. (2004). Spatial representation of shelter locations in meerkats, *Suricata suricatta*. *Animal Behaviour*, **68**, 151–157.

Manser, M. B., Jansen, D. A. W. A. M., Graw, B., *et al.* (2014). Vocal complexity in meerkats and other mongoose species. *Advances in the Study of Behavior*, **46**, 281–310.

McAuliffe, K., and Thornton, A. (2012). How do banded mongooses locate and select anvils for cracking encased food items? *Behavioural Processes*, **90**, 350–356.

Müller, C. A. (2010). Do anvil-using banded mongooses understand means-end relationships? A field experiment. *Animal Cognition*, **13**, 325–330.

Muller, C., and Manser, M. B. (2008). Mutual recognition of pups and providers in the cooperatively breeding banded mongoose. *Animal Behaviour*, **75**, 1683–1692.

Sharpe, L. L., Hill, A., and Cherry, M. I. (2013). Individual recognition in a wild cooperative mammal using contact calls. *Animal Behaviour*, **86**, 893–900.

Resources

Many film documentaries, including the TV series *Meerkat Manor*, describe the life of meerkats in amazing pictures and with more or less realistic comments about their behaviour. In the BBC documentary *Meerkats: Secrets of an Animal Superstar*, the background of the Kalahari Meerkat Project is presented, illustrating many of the experiments published and discussed above. National Geographic produced a 3D documentary in 2012. The German TV company BR produced two documentaries focusing on Manser's communication work: *Rufe aus der Kalahari* and *Vom Kuscheln, Träumen und Schmusen*. In addition, in many documentaries meerkats appear as short contributions, e.g. in BBC Earth *Africa*, where the interaction between drongos and meerkats is beautifully shown, based on the scientific publication by Flower and colleagues (Flower, 2011a) (see YouTube BBC drongo meerkat: www.youtube.com/watch?v=tEYCjJqr21A). The first documentary to make the meerkats famous was that by the BBC, called *Meerkat United* (1987).

The website of the Kalahari Research Centre provides much information on the species and also on the project and the habitat where meerkats occur. It also lists all the scientific publications and popular contributions (http://kalahari-meerkats.com/kmp/).

In a book written for the public with the same title as the TV series *Meerkat Manor*, Clutton-Brock (2010) describes the findings of our research over the first 10 years of the project, and gives a good introduction to the lives of meerkats for a popular audience. There are also several articles in popular science magazines (Milius, 2007) and on the Internet, such as a recent National Geographic blog 'Meerkats mysteriously know to outgrow rivals' (http://phenomena.nationalgeographic.com/2016/05/25/meerkats-adjust-their-growth-to-match-their-rivals/).

Profile

Marta's interest in meerkats began with her PhD under Tim Clutton-Brock's supervision on the evolution of vocal communication. Tim Clutton-Brock (Cambridge University, UK) founded the long-term Kalahari Meerkat Project, to investigate cooperative breeding in mammals. During Marta's PhD, it became obvious that meerkats coordinate their activities in similar ways to that described by Cheney and Seyfarth (1992) on vervet monkeys. Her research was very much influenced by a similar approach on understanding the function of alarm, contact and pup begging calls. During Marta's post-doc and in her later group leader positions, she became more interested in also trying to take into account meerkats' knowledge of their social and physical environment. The research of her group currently focuses on function and mechanisms of vocal and olfactory communication, collective behaviour, group decision-making and group movement. They are also investigating physiological aspects of vocal production and perception.

References

Amici, F, Colell, M., von Borell, C. and Bueno-Guerra, N. (2017). Meerkats (*Suricata suricatta*) fail to prosocially donate food in an experimental set-up. *Animal Cognition*, **20**, 1059–1066.

Amsler, V. (2008) *How urgency levels in alarm calls influence the forager's response in meerkats (Suricata suricatta)*. Zurich: University of Zurich.

Bousquet, C. A. (2011). *Group decision-making in meerkats (Suricata suricatta)*. Zurich: University of Zürich.

Bousquet, C. A., Sumpter, D. J., and Manser, M. B. (2011). Moving calls: a vocal mechanism underlying quorum decisions in cohesive groups. *Proceedings of the Royal Society of London B: Biological Sciences*, **278**, 1482–1488.

Brotherton, P. N. M., Clutton-Brock, T. H., O' Riain, M. J., *et al.* (2001). Offspring food allocation by parents and helpers in a cooperative mammal. *Behavioral Ecology*, **12**, 590–599.

Caro, T. M. and Hauser, M. D. (1992). Is there teaching in nonhuman animals? *The Quarterly Review of Biology*, **67**, 151–174.

Cheney, D. L., and Seyfarth, R. M. (1992). *How monkeys see the world: inside the mind of another species*. Chicago, IL: University of Chicago Press.

Clutton-Brock, T. (2010). *Meerkat manor: flower of the Kalahari*. London: Hachette UK.

Clutton-Brock, T. H., Gaynor, D., Kansky, R., *et al.* (1998). Costs of cooperative behaviour in suricates (Suricata suricatta). *Proceedings of the Royal Society of London B: Biological Sciences*, **265**, 185–190.

Clutton-Brock, T. H., Gaynor, D., McIlrath, G. M., *et al.* (1999a). Predation, group size and mortality in a cooperative mongoose, *Suricata suricatta. Journal of Animal Ecology*, **68**, 672–683.

Clutton-Brock, T. H., O'Riain, M. J., Brotherton, P. N. M., *et al.* (1999b). Selfish sentinels in cooperative mammals. *Science*, **284**, 1640–1644.

Clutton-Brock, T. H., Brotherton, P. N. M., O'Riain, M. J., *et al.* (2001a). Contributions to cooperative rearing in meerkats. *Animal Behaviour*, **61**, 705–710.

Clutton-Brock, T. H., Brotherton, P. N., Russell, A. F., *et al.* (2001b). Cooperation, control, and concession in meerkat groups. *Science*, **291**, 478–481.

Clutton-Brock, T. H., Hodge, S. J., Flower, T. P., Spong, G. F., and Young, A. J. (2010). Adaptive suppression of subordinate reproduction in cooperative mammals. *The American Naturalist*, **176**, 664–673.

Doolan, S. P., and MacDonald, D. W. (1996). Diet and foraging behaviour of group-living meerkats, *Suricata suricatta*, in the southern Kalahari. *Journal of Zoology*, **239**, 697–716.

Engesser, S. (2011). *Function of 'close' calls in a group foraging carnivore, Suricata suricatta*. Zurich: University of Zurich.

Flower, T. (2011a). Fork-tailed drongos use deceptive mimicked alarm calls to steal food. *Proceedings of the Royal Society of London B: Biological Sciences*, **278**, 1548–1555.

Flower, T. P. (2011b). *Competition for food in meerkats (Suricata suricatta)*. South Africa: University of Pretoria.

Gall, G. E., and Manser, M. B. (2017). Group cohesion in foraging meerkats: follow the moving 'vocal hot spot'. *Royal Society Open Science*, **4**, 170004.

Graw, B., and Manser, M. B. (2007). The function of mobbing in cooperative meerkats. *Animal Behaviour*, **74**, 507–517.

Griffin, A. S., Nürnberger, B., and Pemberton, J. M. (2001). A panel of microsatellites developed for meerkats (*Suricata suricatta*) by cross-species amplification and species-specific cloning. *Molecular Ecology Resources*, **1**, 83–85.

Hollén, L. I., and Manser, M. B. (2006). Ontogeny of alarm call responses in meerkats, *Suricata suricatta*: the roles of age, sex and nearby conspecifics. *Animal Behaviour*, **72**, 1345–1353.

Hollén, L. I., Clutton-Brock, T. and Manser, M. B. (2008). Ontogenetic changes in alarm-call production and usage in meerkats (*Suricata suricatta*): adaptations or constraints? *Behavioral Ecology and Sociobiology*, **62**, 821–829.

Jordan, N. R., Cherry, M. I., and Manser, M. B. (2007). The spatial and temporal distribution of meerkat latrines reflects intruder diversity and suggests a role of mate defence. *Animal Behaviour*, **73**, 613–622.

Karp, D., Manser, M. B., Wiley, E. M., and Townsend, S. W. (2014). Nonlinearities in meerkat alarm calls prevent receivers from habituating. *Ethology*, **120**, 189–196.

Kutsukake, N., and Clutton-Brock, T. H. (2006). Aggression and submission reflect reproductive conflict between females in cooperatively breeding meerkats *Suricata suricatta*. *Behavioral Ecology and Sociobiology*, **59**, 541–548.

Leclaire, S., Nielsen, J. F., Thavarajah, N. K., Manser, M. B., and Clutton-Brock, T. H. (2013). Odour-based kin discrimination in the cooperatively breeding meerkat. *Biology Letters*, **9**, 20121054.

Manser, M. B. (1998). *The evolution of auditory communication in suricates, Suricata suricatta*. Cambridge: University of Cambridge.

Manser, M. B. (1999). Response of foraging group members to sentinel calls in suricates, *Suricata suricatta*. *Proceedings of the Royal Society of London B: Biological Sciences*, **266**, 1013–1019.

Manser, M. B. (2001). The acoustic structure of suricates' alarm calls varies with predator type and the level of response urgency. *Proceedings of the Royal Society of London B: Biological Sciences*, **268**, 2315–2324.

Manser, M. B., and Bell, M. B. (2004). Spatial representation of shelter locations in meerkats, *Suricata suricatta*. *Animal Behaviour*, **68**, 151–157.

Manser, M. B., Bell, M. B., and Fletcher, L. B. (2001). The information that receivers extract from alarm calls in suricates. *Proceedings of the Royal Society of London B: Biological Sciences*, **268**, 2485–2491.

Manser, M. B., Seyfarth, R. M., and Cheney, D. L. (2002). Suricate alarm calls signal predator class and urgency. *Trends in Cognitive Sciences*, **6**, 55–57.

Manser, M. B., Jansen, D. A. W. A. M., Graw, B., *et al.* (2014). Vocal complexity in meerkats and other mongoose species. *Advances in the Study of Behavior*, **46**, 281–310.

Mares, R., Young, A. J., Levesque, D. L., Harrison, N., and Clutton-Brock, T. H. (2011). Responses to intruder scents in the cooperatively breeding meerkat: sex and social status differences and temporal variation. *Behavioral Ecology*, **22**, 594–600.

Milius, S. (2007). Science behind the soap opera: the cute and the shocking at meerkat manor. *Science News*, **171**, 138–140.

Moran, G., Timney, B., Sorensen, L., and Desrochers, B. (1983). Binocular depth perception in the meerkat (*Suricata suricatta*). *Vision Research*, **23**, 965–969.

Proops, L., McComb, K., and Reby, D. (2009). Cross-modal individual recognition in domestic horses (*Equus caballus*). *Proceedings of the National Academy of Sciences*, **106**, 947–951.

Rauber, R., and Manser, M. B. (2017). Discrete call types referring to predation risk enhance the efficiency of the meerkat sentinel system. *Scientific Reports*, **7**, 44436.

Reber, S. A., Townsend, S. W., and Manser, M. B. (2013). Social monitoring via close calls in meerkats. *Proceedings of the Royal Society of London B: Biological Sciences*, **280**, 20131013.

Santema, P., and Clutton-Brock, T. (2013). Meerkat helpers increase sentinel behaviour and bipedal vigilance in the presence of pups. *Animal Behaviour*, **85**, 655–661.

Schibler, F., and Manser, M. B. (2007). The irrelevance of individual discrimination in meerkat alarm calls. *Animal Behaviour*, **74**, 1259–1268.

Stephens, P. A., Russell, A. F., Young, A. J., Sutherland, W. J., and Clutton-Brock, T. H. (2004). Dispersal, eviction, and conflict in meerkats (*Suricata suricatta*): an evolutionarily stable strategy model. *The American Naturalist*, **165**, 120–135.

Thavarajah, N. K., Fenkes, M., and Clutton-Brock, T. H. (2014). The determinants of dominance relationships among subordinate females in the cooperatively breeding meerkat. *Behaviour*, **151**, 89–102.

Thornton, A. (2008). Social learning about novel foods in young meerkats. *Animal Behaviour*, **76**, 1411–1421.

Thornton, A., and Clutton-Brock, T. (2011). Social learning and the development of individual and group behaviour in mammal societies. *Philosophical Transactions of the Royal Society of London B: Biological Sciences*, **366**, 978–987.

Thornton, A., and Malapert, A. (2009). The rise and fall of an arbitrary tradition: an experiment with wild meerkats. *Proceedings of the Royal Society of London B: Biological Sciences*, **276**, 1269–1276.

Thornton, A., and McAuliffe, K. (2006). Teaching in wild meerkats. *Science*, **313**, 227–229.

Thornton, A., and Raihani, N. J. (2010). Identifying teaching in wild animals. *Learning and Behavior*, **38**, 297–309.

Thornton, A., and Samson, J. (2012). Innovative problem solving in wild meerkats. *Animal Behaviour*, **83**, 1459–1468.

Thornton, A., Samson, J., and Clutton-Brock, T. (2010). Multi-generational persistence of traditions in neighbouring meerkat groups. *Proceedings of the Royal Society of London B: Biological Sciences*, **277**, 3623–3629.

Townsend, S. W., Allen, C., and Manser, M. B. (2011). A simple test of vocal individual recognition in wild meerkats. *Biology Letters*, **8**, 179–182.

Townsend, S. W., Rasmussen, M., Clutton-Brock, T., and Manser, M. (2012). Flexible alarm calling in meerkats: the role of the social environment and predation urgency. *Behavioral Ecology*, **23**, 1360–1364.

Townsend, S. W., Charlton, B. D., and Manser, M. B. (2014). Acoustic cues to identity and predator context in meerkat barks. *Animal Behaviour*, **94**, 143–149.

Turbé, A. (2006). *Foraging decisions and space use in a social mammal, the meerkat*. Doctoral dissertation. University of Cambridge, Cambridge.

Voellmy, I. K., Goncalves, I. B., Barrette, M.-F., Monfort, S. L., and Manser, M. B. (2014). Mean fecal glucocorticoid metabolites are associated with vigilance, whereas immediate cortisol levels better reflect acute anti-predator responses in meerkats. *Hormones and Behavior*, **66**, 759–765.

Waterman, J. M. (2002). Delayed maturity, group fission and the limits of group size in female Cape ground squirrels (Sciuridae: Xerus inauris). *Journal of Zoology*, **256**, 113–120.

Young, A. J., and Monfort, S. L. (2009). Stress and the costs of extra-territorial movement in a social carnivore. *Biology Letters*, **5**, 439–441.

Young, A. J., Carlson, A. A., Monfort, S. L., Russell, A. F., Bennett, N. C., and Clutton-Brock, T. (2006). Stress and the suppression of subordinate reproduction in cooperatively breeding meerkats. *Proceedings of the National Academy of Sciences*, **103**, 12005–12010.

Young, A. J., Spong, G., and Clutton-Brock, T. (2007). Subordinate male meerkats' prospect for extra-group paternity: alternative reproductive tactics in a cooperative mammal. *Proceedings of the Royal Society of London B: Biological Sciences*, **274**, 1603–1609.

Zöttl, M. (2009). Benefits of secondary predator cue inspection and recruitment in a cooperative mammal (*Suricata suricatta*). Vienna: University of Vienna.

Zöttl, M., Lienert, R., Clutton-Brock, T., Millesi, E., and Manser, M. B. (2012). The effects of recruitment to direct predator cues on predator responses in meerkats. *Behavioral Ecology*, **24**, 198–204.

14 Octopuses – Mind in the Waters

Jennifer A. Mather and Michael J. Kuba

Species Description

Anatomy

Octopuses are molluscs by ancestry, which means that their ancestors probably resembled monoplacophorans. Their closest living relatives are clams and snails, definitely not animals with a great reach of intelligence (Giribet *et al.*, 2006). The cephalopods (i.e. 'head-foots', from the body arrangement) dominated the oceans in the Permian era, but most of those species, such as the ammonites and belemnoids, went extinct. About the time that the bony fishes were developing, a new branch of the cephalopods, the coleoids, also evolved. This may have been because the bony fishes, which now dominate the seas, were predators, prey and competition for the cephalopods (Packard, 1972). Coleoids lost the molluscan shell, and without this protection, began to specialize, increasing mobility and sense organs and evolving towards active predators. The family Octopodidae, with around 300 species, represents the near-shore flexible octopuses (Mather and Alupay, 2016). Like other groups of marine animals, the octopuses are still not well-known, and new species and genera are being named each year. That can be a problem if a researcher is ordering octopuses from a supplier, who might not know what species they are actually providing. Octopuses range in size from the few grams weight of pygmy octopuses to the giant Pacific octopus (GPO) that aquariums commonly keep, which weighs up to 40 kg (see Table 14.1 for a list of common species). Because of the boneless body, the only valid measure of size is weight.

Octopuses are unusual in the animal kingdom because they have muscular hydrostat movement systems (Kier and Smith, 1985). The characteristic of a muscular hydrostat is that it keeps the same volume regardless of its exact shape, so an arm can have a very small diameter and extend far, or contract to be very short with a large diameter. In theory, that gives them almost an unlimited number of degrees of freedom in action, although Flash and Hochner (2005) suggested instead that actions are reduced to 'motor primitives'. Moreover, octopuses have no bones; a complex set of muscles and cartilage provides the stiffening against which the other muscles contract. Movement is produced by jet propulsion due to contraction of the muscular mantle. In the cephalopods in general, this system is less efficient than the body bending of fish (O'Dor and Weber, 1986), although the combination of propulsion with arms and jetting by mantle contraction allows fine-tuning of locomotion in the octopuses. Jet propulsion is used to

Table 14.1. Scientific name, origin, size and some highlights about the most common species of octopuses.

Species	Origin	Size	Special notes
Abdopus aculeatus	East Pacific	Small	Social, diurnal, shallow
Eledone cirrhosa	North Atlantic	Medium	Very deep, inactive
Enteroctopus dofleini	North Pacific	Very large	Nocturnal, aquarium display
Hapalochlaena maculosa	Australia	Small	Shallow, deadly poisonous
Octopus bimaculoides	California	Medium	Nocturnal, genome sequenced
Octopus briareus	Caribbean	Medium	Nocturnal, shallow, active
Octopus cyanea	Pan-Pacific	Large	Shallow, diurnal, active
Octopus insularis	Caribbean	Medium	Formerly *vulgaris*
Octopus joubini (mercatorius)	Florida	Small	Nocturnal, inactive
Octopus rubescens	Washington	Small	Nocturnal, inactive, shallow
Octopus tetricus	Australia	Large	Deep
Octopus vulgaris	South Europe	Medium	Commonly used, active, adaptable

escape, capture visually sensed prey, repel scavengers and move items on the sea bottom (see Mather and Alupay 2016, for an ethogram of the Octopodidae).

Octopuses have a spectacular manipulation system in their arms: neurons abound more in the body than in the brain (Hanlon and Messenger, 1996). As the name octopus suggests, they have eight arms, each of which is equipped with one or two rows of grasping suckers all along its length, and all of which can act independently or in coordination. The suckers grasp and manipulate, as well as receive tactile and chemical information, and the arms, with longitudinal, radial, circular and oblique muscles, can both bend in two dimensions and twist at any location along their length. Control of a single arm is thus not simple, but coordination of all of them is even more complex. The arms are structurally similar, except for the third right one of males, which is modified for the passage of spermatophores during mating (Wells, 1978; Nixon and Young, 2003). The frontal four arms are usually used for exploration, and each octopus chooses a preferred arm for exploration tasks (Byrne *et al.*, 2006). The posterior arms are allocated to crawling; however, the octopus does not always proceed anterior-first, and arms are allocated flexibly according to the movement direction, with a suitable push–pull combination that has no discernible gait (Levy *et al.*, 2015).

Octopuses and many other cephalopods have a system that quickly alters their appearance in many different aspects (see Messenger, 2001; Mather and Kuba, 2013; Gutnick *et al.*, 2016). Chromatophores in the surface layer of the skin are elastic sacs containing yellow, red or black–brown pigments, which are pulled out by muscles under direct neural control. This fast control results in appearance changes within milliseconds and across areas as small as a square millimetre. Below the chromatophores, there is a layer of reflective leucophores, which reflect light of all wavelengths and thus facilitate matching the ambient wavelengths of light around the animals. In some areas of the skin, reflecting iridophores make the animal appear blue–green, although the light reflection from these structures depends also on the viewing angle (Mäthger *et al.*, 2009). Textural units assist appearance when the skin surface is raised in papillae in specific locations (Allen *et al.*, 2009), especially the ones above the eye bulb, which are often referred to as horns. Such appearance changes are complex and varied (see Hanlon and Messenger, 1988, for a repertoire of those by cuttlefish *Sepia officinalis*). Appearance is controlled at several levels (Mather and Alupay, 2016). First, reflexive responses, likely modulated by light and perhaps hormonally controlled, respond simply to luminance level, including those mentioned earlier, such as countershading (Ramirez and Oakley, 2015). Second, octopuses and cuttlefish that are benthic have excellent substrate-matching camouflage. These responses, which form startlingly good matches to texture, colour and unit size of the background structures, must be triggered by vision, but they may be open-loop, in that the octopus may not monitor the resulting pattern. Third, there are many voluntarily controlled patterns with communication function, such as deimatic startle and warnings addressed to predators, sexual signals to conspecifics, and patterns to startle potential prey.

Perception

Octopuses have excellent sensory capacities (Gutnick *et al.*, 2016), and the modality we know the most about is vision (see Gleadall and Shashar, 2004). Their lens-based eye is an example of convergent evolution, as it is structurally very similar to the mammalian eye. There are differences – octopuses examined thus far have only one photopigment with a peak sensitivity at 492 nm and thus are functionally colour blind, so will not perceive stimulus differences based on wavelengths of light (Messenger *et al.*, 1973; Mäthger *et al.*, 2005). Chromatic aberration caused by the off-axis pupils might allow them to receive spectral information, though (Stubbs and Stubbs, 2016). However, cuttlefish can discriminate the plane of light polarization (Shashar and Cronin, 1996), as they easily discriminate targets with a 90° polarization contrast. There is about a 10° frontal overlap in the fields of view of the two eyes, so octopuses are functionally monocular, and each individual has a preferred eye for viewing visual stimuli (Byrne *et al.*, 2004). Projection of information received by these eyes is crossed to the brain, so a discrimination learned with one eye seems to be initially stored in one half of the brain only, and is unavailable until the next day if the animal is tested with the other eye (Wells, 1978). Unlike in birds, however, the information is gradually accumulated in the optic lobes of the bilateral brain. Thus, a split brain octopus can be a good model for the lateralized use of visual stimuli. While visual information is processed in the optic lobes, and stimulation of these areas results in patterned output of skin displays (Liu and Chiao, 2017), the process of storage appears controlled by the vertical lobe, and damage to this area can block this process. In cuttlefish, there is some functional brain lateralization, which depends both on task and age (Graindorge *et al.*, 2006; Jozet-Alves *et al.*, 2012).

Octopuses have good visual acuity, measured at 9.7′ of arc (Muntz and Gwyther, 1988), so adequate-sized stimuli will be easy for them to see, although the lateralization of storage of visual information should be taken into account. Octopuses can learn to discriminate visual figures based on several different stimulus characteristics (Sutherland, 1969). Researchers have used the tremendous ability of cephalopods to control their skin appearance (see Hanlon and Messenger, 1988 for the possible patterns of cuttlefish) to test their visual perception. Placed on a visual surface, cuttlefish will usually attempt to match it, and characteristics of visual texture can be manipulated for the animal to match (Zylinsky and Ossorio, 2014). With three different skin patterns to produce (smooth, mottled and disruptive), cuttlefish use both the contrast between different parts of the pattern and the closure of visual features such as a circle, to evaluate the presence of visual form; however, they cannot match colours (Mäthger *et al.*, 2005). Using statistically well-defined stimuli is a promising approach, because it is non-invasive and an almost automatic adjustment to imitation of natural environments, although problems might arise, because we do not know the extent to which octopuses monitor the appearance of their skin (Gutnick *et al.*, 2016). Octopuses have an equal ability to match the background, and their camouflage ability could easily be tested with similar paradigms.

Little is known about other senses in octopuses. Their chemical sensitivity has so far only been tested with very primitive methods (Wells, 1978; Nixon and Young, 2003), with many chemical cues of potential food being important but understudied stimuli. Suckers on the arms have both chemical and tactile receptors for contact sensation (Wells, 1978). Octopuses also possess an olfactory organ, a ciliated pit below the eye, whose structural and physiological characteristics match those of chemoreceptors (Polese *et al.*, 2016). However, its use is unknown, though it may process information for reproductive behaviour (Polese *et al.*, 2015). Chemical cues are promising stimuli to study octopus behaviour, but the exact responses and chemicals are simply yet unknown.

Misunderstanding of comparative sensory systems has not yet allowed us to understand how octopuses and other cephalopods use distance mechanoreceptive cues. The word 'deaf' means inability to use the ear to process sounds, but the ear is a relatively recently evolved organ in vertebrates, which is specialized to receive and magnify mechanical vibration after it has passed through the air (Fay and Popper, 2000). Given the high density of water, special organs are not necessary to process this movement of molecules, so mechanical stimuli are processed without 'ears'. It is not surprising that water movements are received by a lateral line analogue in squid, similar to the lateral line of hair cells in fishes (Budelmann, 1995). Moynihan's (1985) comment that cephalopods might be 'deaf' overlooks the fundamental similarity in the mechanoreceptive cues used by animals that do/do not have ears (Hanlon and Budelmann, 1987); indeed, mammals that have returned to the marine habitat have radically modified their ears.

Mechanoreceptive responses to both angular and linear acceleration in octopuses are processed by a statocyst organ, described by Williamson and Chrachri (2007) as an excellent model, analogous to the vertebrate vestibular system. Cephalopods perceive acceleration in three different planes to monitor their movement in three dimensions. A statocyst also allows perception of linear acceleration, normally gravity, although such a receptor system would also be sensitive to disturbance in the water. Its level of behavioural control may be reflexive, as it receives orientation with relation to gravity, to control countershading of the skin appearance system (Ferguson and

Messenger, 1991), which is abolished by statocyst ablation. Stability of the visual image on the eyes by the oculomotor reflex (Budelmann and Tu, 1997) is also automatically controlled by the vestibular system. Still, little behavioural testing has been done for this sensory system.

Individual Identification

Octopuses are sometimes difficult to sex, as the main difference between male and female is a modified third right arm in males, which they are reluctant to let the researcher examine. Before maturity, there are few or no sex differences. As they approach maturity, males become more active and females more sedentary, although this has not been formally tested.

Life Cycle

In contrast to other highly intelligent mammals (but similar to rats), octopuses live very short lives, from 3 or 4 years for the GPO, to 6 months for many of the pygmy species. Researchers who buy a mature octopus may have only a few months to study it, so long-term studies in cephalopods have a different meaning depending on the species. Indeed, much effort is spent by aquaculture specialists to raise cephalopods for food (Iglesias *et al.*, 2014), but so far none has commercially succeeded. Some species that do not have a paralarva stage (e.g. *Octopus maya, O. bimaculoides* and *O. joubini*) have young which are easier to keep alive, and also have more or less the same lifestyle as adults. There is much potential for studying the development of behaviour in these species, although this has barely been done (Mather and Kuba, 2013). Cuttlefish, which also have relatively large eggs, have proven to be a model for early learning, even before hatching, using a paradigm of imprinting at the beginning of their lifespan (Darmaillacq *et al.*, 2014a).

At the beginning of octopuses' lives, eggs are very small and abundant (ranging from hundreds to tens of thousands), with the size of a grain of rice in the case of the GPO. At hatching, most octopuses float off into the open sea and lead a drifting life for a few weeks to months, until they are bigger and assume the normal octopus shape. At the end of the lifespan, males become senescent (Anderson *et al.*, 2008), making them a good model to study these physiological and behavioural changes, while females attend their eggs until they die, being semelparous (most of them reproduce all at once at the end of their lifespan; Mather, 2006).

Social Characteristics

Many octopuses are cannibalistic (Ibanez and Keyl, 2010). Some species, like *Abdopus aculeatus*, show mate guarding and male–male competition for females (Huffard *et al.*, 2008a). Few octopuses use visual sexual displays to conspecifics (but see Huffard *et al.*, 2008b, in *Abdopus aculeatus*). Chemical stimuli are likely involved in reproductive behaviour, as shown in other cephalopods such as *Sepia* cuttlefish and *Loligo* squid

(Boal *et al.*, 2010). Generally, octopuses are solitary, although males and females mate with several individuals, but they form dominance hierarchies in the laboratory (Mather 1980a). Recent studies on the lesser Pacific striped octopus (Caldwell *et al.*, 2015) and *Octopus tetricus* (Scheel *et al.*, 2016) have shown that at least some octopus species might have a more active and complex social life than previously assumed. Tricarico and colleagues (2011) suggested that individuals may habituate to the presence of neighbours.

Ecological Characteristics

Octopuses are strictly marine and mostly benthic predators, who shelter in protective 'homes', forage across the substrate in a saltatory search pattern (O'Brien *et al.*, 1990; Forsythe and Hanlon, 1997) and return for shelter. They are win-switch foragers (Mather, 1991), so *Octopus vulgaris*, for example, does not search in the same area during subsequent trips from the same location. Moreover, they return directly to their home after dislocation from their path of movement, suggesting that they may have a cognitive map and remember past trips.

Many octopuses are nocturnal, which makes behavioural observations difficult. Therefore, we tend to know more about the behaviour of diurnal or crepuscular species, such as *Octopus cyanea* (Figure 14.1), or species with much flexibility in their activity cycles, such as *Octopus vulgaris* (Meisel *et al.*, 2006). Octopuses are specializing generalist predators (Anderson *et al.*, 2008). They accept a wide variety of molluscan and crustacean prey, yet in the field each individual may learn to specialize on particular species, based on their availability (Leite *et al.*, 2016), ease of access or handling time (Anderson and Mather, 2007). They prefer living prey, but due to this adaptability they can be trained to accept thawed frozen food. Octopuses prefer crab prey (Onthank and Cowles, 2011) and are susceptible to a density effect when feeding on them – but not on

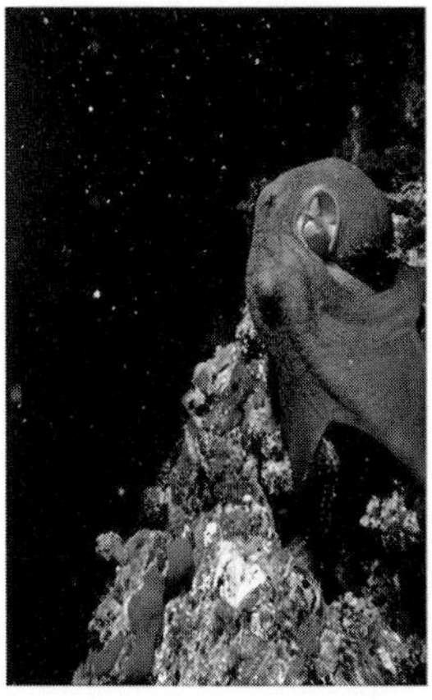

Figure 14.1. *Octopus cyanea* on a nocturnal hunting trip on the reef.

snails (Mather, 1980b). Over the long term, the baseline intake of an octopus will gradually increase as it grows larger. However, the daily *ad libitum* intake varies hugely, with no consistent pattern.

State of the Art

Years of testing with food rewards and minimal aversive shock (Wells, 1978) have shown that octopuses can discriminate visual stimuli based on vertical and horizontal projection, size, shape and even edge/area differences, leading Mackintosh (1965) to assume that these animals can 'learn what to learn' in terms of stimulus characteristics. Boal (1996) critically reviewed these procedures. In the same line, Hvoreckny and colleagues (2007) showed that octopuses can learn to conditionally discriminate when the correct choice between two figures depends on the situation. Although they used cuttlefish and not octopuses, Jozet-Alves and colleagues (2013) have shown that cephalopods can make an even more difficult discrimination, combining location, visual shape and timing to calculate which should be the rewarded stimulus. Recently, Bublitz and colleagues (2017) used a fully automated system to present stimuli for reversal learning, including a secondary reinforcement and no negative reinforcement for an incorrect choice. By controlling stimulus presentation, their set-up can overcome previous criticism. Bublitz and colleagues (2017) showed that octopuses can be trained to manage a reversal learning task. Pronk and colleagues (2010) have developed a video playback system, presenting footage of a water-filled aquarium, a conspecific and a crab. Octopuses were mostly attracted to the crab image and least to the image of a conspecific. Moreover, as cephalopods try to camouflage to blend into their surroundings, a well-designed and statistically defined virtual reality may open a unique window into how nervous systems compute a visual input into a neuromuscular output (chromatophore skin pattern). Hence, video projections and virtual reality settings for cephalopods will be one of the most interesting challenges in the next years.

Nesher and colleagues (2014) found that octopuses grasped amputated arms of their own with much less force than those of conspecifics, suggesting that there may be a chemical surface cue to designate the 'self'. This might be a primitive system of self-recognition, similar to the one found in cnidarians (Tidbal, 2012). However, as Gherardi and colleagues (2012) showed, chemical self-recognition can be quite complex in invertebrates, and thus further studies are needed to establish whether and how octopuses tell themselves from others. Still, the arm systems are not controlled completely separately, as recent research (Gutnick *et al.*, 2011) has demonstrated that octopus arm action can be guided by vision, and octopuses can learn tactile cues on a substrate to guide an arm in a T-maze (Gutnick, 2014; Gutnick *et al.*, pers. comm.). That is why the arm movement system appears somewhat independent of brain control. The brain may give only general commands to the arm, as the dorsal nerve cord consists of a chain of ganglia, and each sucker also has a ganglion directly above it. The arms may have subunits of control (Grasso and Basil, 2009). However, there is no system equivalent to a somatosensory homunculus in the higher motor centre of the brain (Zullo *et al.*, 2009).

T- or Y-mazes have also been used for testing chemoreception and navigational abilities. With regard to the former, distance chemoreception has been evaluated using changes in respiration rate (Boyle, 1983) and movement in a Y-maze (Boal and Marsh, 1998) in cuttlefish. Both responses to food odours and to water that had contained a conspecific were variable (Walderon *et al.*, 2011; Morse *et al.*, 2017). With regard to spatial cognition, Boal and colleagues (2000) used such a maze to test *O. bimaculoides*. Instead of a reward, they presented a situation familiar to the near-shore animals. They allowed the animal to explore a maze, which had deeper areas at the end of the two-end locations of the maze, and then reduced the water level, so that only these end points still contained water, and the octopuses learned to move to the deeper location. Such ability is also true for cuttlefish, and the two groups have parallel ability at goal-finding (Karson *et al.*, 2003). Studies on cuttlefish navigation have farther developed this paradigm. Jozet-Alvez and colleagues (2008) have tested for sex differences in *Sepia*. Male cuttlefish are more active in an open-field test and use different choice strategies than females in the T-maze. Lately, Scata and colleagues (2016) have adapted 2D-paradigms on path-finding in benthic animals to the more 3D world of cuttlefish. They found that cuttlefish preferred a benthic 2D route, but if more effort was required to go by a route along the sea bottom, they might switch to a more vertical route. Comparisons between these two groups in terms of spatial cognition (path-finding and neural control) surely deserve further attention.

One of the most striking features of cephalopods is their ability to resemble their background, both in terms of colour and texture. Adapting to backgrounds is under neuromuscular control by the central nervous system, which controls both the muscles around the chromatophores and the muscular hydrostat of the skin (Figure 14.2). Changes in appearance have also attracted researchers since Packard and Sanders (1971). Specific components of common patterns may be species identifiers (Packard and Hochberg, 1977), and similar patterns across groups (such as the black–white contrasts) may serve as similar anti-predator displays (Moynihan, 1975). The pattern of white blotches on the dorsal surface of *Wunderpus* allows humans individual

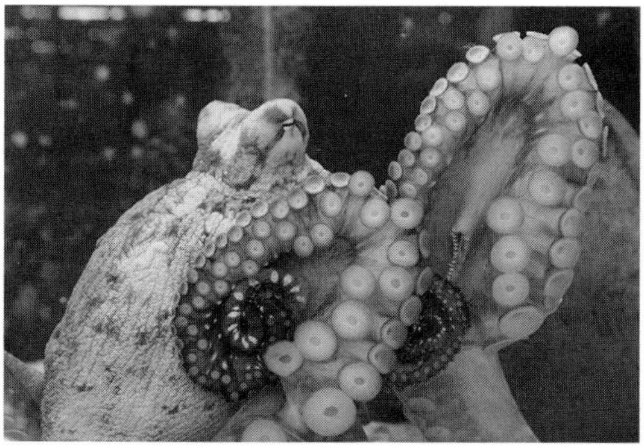

Figure 14.2. *Octopus cyanea* in the laboratory.
Photo taken by Kenji Togo.

identification (Huffard *et al.*, 2008), although we do not know whether conspecifics also do that. Individual identification of animals is very important in many research areas, although it has so far only been carried out in squid (Byrne *et al.*, 2010). Sophisticated camouflage is assumed to be directed to vertebrate predators, and although octopuses can discriminate the plane of light polarization, few studies of this capacity have been conducted (Shashar *et al.*, 1996). Cuttlefish learned to produce eye dots only to visual predators such as some fish (Langridge *et al.*, 2007), so control of skin displays may be learned. Both cuttlefish (Hall and Hanlon, 2002) and squid (Mather, 2016) have ritualized male–male visual contests, and tests with models would tell us much about their ability to perceive and discriminate in this ecologically relevant situation.

The flexibility and communicative capacity of the skin system is puzzling, as cephalopods do not have colour vision, although there are opsins in their skin (Mäthger *et al.*, 2010). In addition, octopuses out of their protective home and vulnerable to predators are not always camouflaged – see *Octopus cyanea* (Hanlon *et al.*, 1999). Instead, they may change their patterns unpredictably to confuse a predator dependent on a stable visual 'search image' of prey. Furthermore, it is not clear to what extent the octopuses can monitor the patterns they form. Stimulation of the optic lobe of the brain produces whole patterns of output (Boycott, 1954; Liu and Chiao, 2017), predominantly ipsilateral and on the mantle. Such stimulation showed that the representations were not organized somatotopically, and perhaps the lobe was a mosaic of pattern generators. Computerized display systems that can project images for octopuses will surely close some of the gaps in our understanding of this system.

All for One and One for All

Box 14.1 Independently Evolved Intelligence

Chuan-Chin Chiao

Cephalopods (octopus, squid and cuttlefish) are a unique group of animals in the phylum of Mollusca. Their visual system and brain organization are the most sophisticated among all invertebrates. They have been called vertebrates-in-honour and treated as vertebrates in Canada and Europe (Carere and Mather, in prep.). Cephalopods and vertebrates have been separated for more than 500 million years. Despite the seemingly similar intelligent behaviours, they have very different body plan and nervous system. Thus, it is of great interest to compare these two independently evolved intelligences on earth.

One prominent feature of studying cephalopod behaviour is individual differences (Huang and Chiao, 2013). Although it has been reported that cephalopods have personality, temperament and even consciousness (Mather and Anderson, 1993; Sinn *et al.*, 2001; Mather, 2008), the biological basis of individual differences is largely unknown. Nevertheless, this feature may also suggest that they have complex minds and perplexing behaviour. The other issue that has never been addressed is whether

(cont.)

cephalopods have emotions, and whether their moods affect decision-making. Studying the neural basis of cognition and emotion in cephalopods will help us understand their minds and eventually the origin of consciousness in animals.

While the wits of octopuses have fascinated people for centuries, squids and cuttlefish are also brilliant creatures in the ocean. Regardless of their body shape and form, these three groups of animals have one thing in common; that is, they have neurally controlled dynamic body patterns for camouflage and communication, and elaborate nervous systems for learning and memory. Octopuses and cuttlefish are benthic and solitary animals (but see the recent 'octopus city' study in Australia: Godfrey-Smith and Lawrence, 2012; Scheel *et al.*, 2017), while squids are pelagic and social animals. These differences in their lifestyle suggest that their cognitive abilities may have evolved as adaptation to different environments and challenges. Thus, when designing experiments to investigate their cognitive functions, it is crucial to take their natural behaviour into account. More importantly, some behavioural paradigms used in one group of animals may not be suitable for other groups.

Recent advances in display technology, such as computer screen or virtual reality, should be systematically explored to present visual stimuli to octopuses and cuttlefish (Pronk *et al.*, 2010; Orenstein *et al.*, 2016). However, their unique visual system (e.g. peculiar pupil shape, polarization sensitivity and seemingly colour-blindness) should be considered when applying display technology that is specifically designed for human vision. In addition, locomotion, arm manoeuvres and use of sensory modality differ in octopus, squid and cuttlefish, so that cognitive tasks and behavioural paradigms should be tailored to accommodate their specific needs. Nevertheless, some methods designed to study octopus' cognition, such as learning and memory, can be easily adapted to examine cuttlefish's cognition. On the other hand, the experimental paradigm developed to study visual perception and camouflage body patterns in cuttlefish (Chiao *et al.*, 2015) can be applied to investigate visual mechanisms and body coloration in octopuses.

Studying cephalopod cognition is a rewarding endeavour, but a challenging task. Unexpected findings can often teach us more than the experiment planned. Cephalopod minds await further exploration, with intellectual creativity and technological innovation.

References

Chiao, C. C., Chubb, C., and Hanlon R. T. (2015). A review of visual perception mechanisms that regulate rapid adaptive camouflage in cuttlefish. *Journal of Comparative Physiology*, **201**, 933–945.

Godfrey-Smith, P., and Lawrence, M. (2012). Long-term high-density occupation of a site by *Octopus tetricus* and possible site modification due to foraging behavior. *Marine and Freshwater Behaviour and Physiology*, **45**, 261–268.

(cont.)

Huang, K. L., and Chiao, C. C. (2013). Can cuttlefish learn by observing others? *Animal Cognition*, **16**, 313–320.
Mather, J. A. (2008). Cephalopod consciousness: behavioral evidence. *Consciousness and Cognition*, **17**, 37–48.
Mather, J. A., and Anderson, R. C. (1993). 'Personalities' of octopuses (*Octopus rubescens*). *Journal of Comparative Psychology*, **107**, 336–340.
Orenstein, E. C., Haaga, J. M., Gagnonc, Y. L., and Jaffe, J. S. (2016). Automated classification of camouflaging cuttlefish. *Methods in Oceanography*, **15**, 21–34.
Pronk, R., Wilson, D. R., and Harcourt, R. (2010). Video playback demonstrates episodic personality in the gloomy octopus. *The Journal of Experimental Biology*, **213**, 1035–1041.
Scheel, D., Chancellor, S., Hing, M., Lawrence, M., Linquist, S., and Godfrey-Smith, P. (2017). A second site occupied by *Octopus tetricus* at high densities, with notes on their ecology and behavior. *Marine and Freshwater Behaviour and Physiology*, **50**, 285–291.
Sinn, D. L., Perrin, N. A., Mather, J. A., and Anderson, R. C. (2001). Early temperamental traits in an octopus (*Octopus bimaculoides*). *Journal of Comparative Psychology*, **115**, 351–364.

Field Guide

One of the real challenges when working with octopuses is that nothing you know from other animals really prepares you for what is next – they are smart, but their world is so different from the one of 'standard' research animals that you will be surprised every day by what they will or will not do. Useful information on how to conduct experiments can be found in Table 14.2 as well as in a paper by Boal (2010), where several experiments that did not yield the desired results are described in detail. And yet, octopuses are eager learners and avid explorers, even if the exploration results in destruction of the testing apparatus. Their manipulative ability is so extensive that this capacity has not nearly been tested, and a simple change in conditions (Richter *et al.*, 2015) may radically alter an octopus' response. Most important of all, octopuses are problem-solvers, whether it means that they gain access to clamped-shut clams (Anderson and Mather, 2007), learn to push rather than pull to solve a puzzle problem (Richter *et al.*, 2016), or change techniques to outwit an approaching predator (Hanlon *et al.*, 1999).

Because an octopus consumes at least 5 per cent of its body weight per day, both the size and type of reward must be pre-tested. Octopuses often will not work for pieces of reward they consider too small or unacceptable. Early experimenters overcame this by feeding entire sardines to the animals at each test and testing them three times per day to a few times per week (Wells, 1978). In recent studies, octopuses were trained to perform 10–20 experimental trials per day (Gutnick *et al.*, 2011; Richter *et al.*, 2015, 2016). So far, only one study by Papini and Bitterman (1991) focused on the relation between learning speed and reward size. There is a minimal reward size (which might still be

Table 14.2. Essential experimental tools required to study octopuses, and their function.

Tool	Function
Large enriched enclosures (containing sand or pebbles as substrate, and bricks or rocks for den construction)	To keep animals active and healthy
Enclosure with an escape-proof cover	Octopuses are masters of escape – all openings have to be escape-proof and sturdy, to avoid losses of animals
Different dead food (crustaceans, molluscs and fish); if possible, live crustaceans and bivalves	To ensure nutrition and provide enrichment
Pilot animals	To establish if animals are in a good condition and reacting to food
Sturdy testing apparatus (to be used in home tank)	Octopuses can be very destructive. Testing in the home tank makes testing easier, as no extra acclimatization to novel arenas is needed
Coding sheet	To keep track of animals and tests they did
Video recording equipment	To document the experiment and ability, for detailed analysis

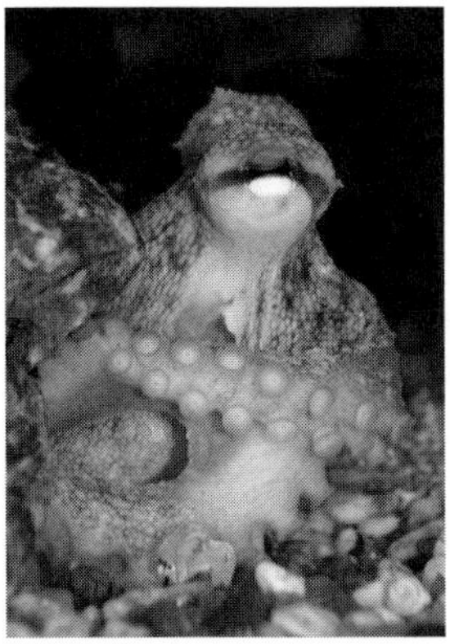

Figure 14.3. *Octopus vulgaris* in the laboratory, sitting in his den watching the human observer.

quite big) needed to motivate an animal to participate in an experiment. Shelter is very important to octopuses and can also be used as a reward. When using non-food-based rewards, however, attention needs to be paid to the fact that, being poikilotherm animals without fat deposits to draw energy from, cephalopods can tire easily. Moreover, they do not perform well when taken out of their shelter and moved to a testing tank, so they should rather be tested by taking the testing apparatus to the octopus' home tank, or moving them to the testing area while they are still hiding in a shelter (Figure 14.3). Pre-tests are needed to determine how many repetitions can be done per day/session and which intertrial interval is needed so as not to stress the animals.

Moreover, the disposition of the reward is relevant. Although octopuses are commonly tested with visual stimuli and visible rewards (Wells, 1978), their normal predatory behaviour consists of two stages (Mather *et al.*, 2014), one of them also including the use of chemical information. In a first stage, octopuses go to areas that, based on visual cues and learned information, likely contain prey. Once there, in a second stage, they extend their arms into crevices, around corners and under rocks to contact prey – the first contact with prey, as well as with conspecifics (Scheel *et al.*, 2016), is likely with an extended arm. Once food has been identified and located with the single arm, other arms contact it and it is moved under the arm web, out of sight. It is in this second stage when octopuses benefit from the chemical receptors on their arms. When Fiorito and colleagues (1998) presented octopuses with a crab confined to a glass jar, octopuses moved it under their arm web, but did not show the reduction in latency to remove the lid, which would indicate learning. It was when Anderson and Mather (2010) added chemical information on the sides of the jar that cued octopuses without visual information were able to do so. Thus, a situation mimicking the natural environment and giving a cue combination was most effective for learning the task.

Indeed, it is always important to use stimuli and contexts reflecting the animal's natural environment, but even when the octopuses learn to approach the visual stimuli for a reward, this is not an imitation of their natural behaviour. Recently, Bublitz and colleagues (2017) used a computerized presentation (solving the problem of the octopus having to relearn consequences of rewarded and shocked choices) and found that one octopus accomplished five reversals. Advances in technology and automated testing may thus help to improve testing procedures.

Observational field work with marine animals is difficult, although possible with diurnal and shallow-water species, such as *Abdopus aculeatus* (Huffard, 2007). For longer-term studies, tagging and relocation may be very useful. Scheel and Bisson (2010) used tagging studies to follow the large *Enteroctopus dofleini* (which is big enough to carry a substantial-sized tag), and similar studies have followed the large *Sepia apama* cuttlefish (Aitken *et al.*, 2005). However, such studies require a large investment of time and resources. To study nocturnal species, modern camera techniques can be of help. We recommend using either extreme low-light cameras, like the Canon ME20F-SH, which can record at a sensitivity setting of more than 4 million ISO, or cameras that can film in HD resolution using IR-sensitive sensors, which make recordings in almost complete darkness possible. In addition, 24-hour recordings are now possible, opening up a wide variety of studies on nocturnal species.

With regard to the testing apparatus, octopuses' manipulative capacity must be taken into account – force can be used to break it, so every apparatus for an octopus has to be built as stably as possible (see Dews, 1959). Perspex or similar materials usually provide a good structure, but it is a good idea to have several identical copies at hand to avoid delays if an animal damages an apparatus. Also, malleability and manipulation can allow an octopus to escape from its tank. Moreover, octopuses have distinct personalities (Mather and Anderson, 1993), so a procedure may be acceptable for most animals, but frighten others, and responsivity to a testing situation that most octopuses consider manageable may result in a jet of water in the face of the experimenter by others (Dews, 1959).

It is debated whether invertebrates suffer nociception (i.e. automatic reflexive response to unpleasant stimuli) or pain (i.e. with a cognitive and lasting component of reaction; Alupay *et al.*, 2014). Therefore, countries have begun to legislate for humane treatment of cephalopods. Canada was first, in 2000, but the passage of the welfare directive 2010/63/EU by the European Union had a much greater impact (Smith *et al.*, 2013). This directive has resulted in ongoing efforts to find out what a good quality of life for a cephalopod is (Fiorito *et al.*, 2014). As of 2017, countries like the USA or Japan do not require any ethical evaluation for research on invertebrates, but such concerns are likely to exist in the future. Meanwhile, some scholarly journals, such as *Animal Behaviour*, have begun to raise their level of scrutiny over invertebrate welfare. Unsurprisingly, with the rise of concern for animals' welfare and given the cephalopods' intelligence, questions have been raised about the welfare of octopuses in captivity (Mather and Anderson, 2007). Octopuses gain more weight and remain healthier when given some form of enrichment (Beigel and Boal, 2006; Yasumura and Ikeda, 2011), such as places to hide, items to manipulate and a varied substrate. Anderson and Wood (2001) have suggested ways to enrich the environment of octopuses in captivity, and Wood and Anderson (2004) have evaluated the tendency of different octopus species to escape. Moreover, the salinity and temperature of the water they are kept in has to be monitored closely. So do the nitrates, as octopuses excrete ammonia, which is toxic to them. In a closed system, denitrifying bacteria need to be cultivated in a biological filter system to remove the ammonia. In any system, the water needs to be changed often and extra air bubbled. In an open system (Figure 14.4), where water is pumped in from the ocean, supply and delivery have to be monitored. With all those arms, octopuses are great manipulators, so all the equipment has to be kept out of their reach. As they have a compressible body and great arm strength, they can easily move through very small openings and escape (Fiorito *et al.*, 2014).

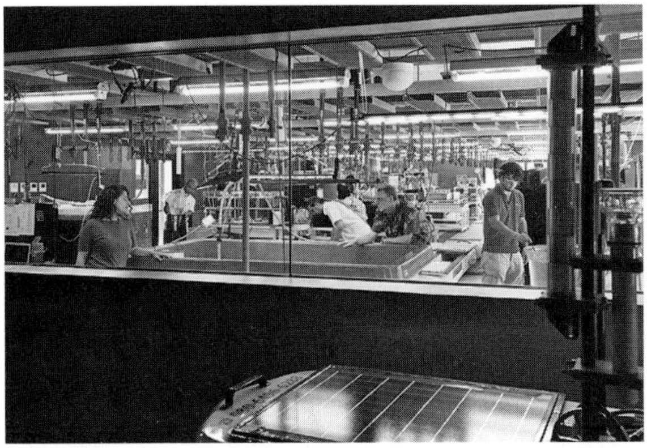

Figure 14.4. Marine laboratory in Seragaki, at the Okinawa Institute of Science and Technology. Note that the tank sizes vary between 4000 litres and a few litres, depending on the needs of the animal or experimenter.
Photo taken by Kenji Togo.

Resources

One useful collection of papers on octopuses and their relatives is *Cephalopod cognition* (2014), edited by Darmaillacq, Dickel and Mather. A recent chapter in the new edition of the classic *Molluscan physiology* specifically deals with the interplay of brain and behaviour, and it also introduces several new methodological approaches, from neurobiology to molecular techniques, which will increase our understanding of cephalopod behaviour and its underlying neuro-morphological structures (Gutnick *et al.*, 2016). A more general book is *Cephalopod behaviour* (1996), by Hanlon and Messenger, and one for the general public is *Octopus, the ocean's intelligent invertebrate* (2013), by Mather, Anderson and Wood.

Profile

Jennifer was born and raised in Victoria, BC, which partly fuelled her interest in sea animals, especially in octopus cognition and squid skin patterns and displays. She has dived with them in very different spots, from Bermuda to Hawaii or Bonaire. Discovering how intelligent they are, she has also felt very committed to promote discussion on invertebrates' rights. Jennifer's interests also extend to women in science and excellence in university teaching.

Michael is currently associated to the Okinawa Institute of Science and Technology. He feels passionate about cephalopods, especially octopuses. Within all the array of marvellous behaviours they can produce, he is particularly seduced by the study of their motor capacities, not only because it shows us how octopuses integrate information from different senses, but also because it has been inspirational for soft robotics architecture. Like Jennifer, he is also very concerned about cephalopod welfare.

References

Aitken, J. P., O'Dor, R. K., and Jackson, G. D. (2005). The secret life of the giant Australian cuttlefish *Sepia apama* (Cephalopoda): behaviour and energetics in nature revealed through radio acoustic positioning and telemetry (RAPT). *Journal of Experimental Marine Biology and Ecology*, **320**, 77–91.

Allen, J. J., Bell, G. G. R., Kuzirian, A. M., Velankar, S. S., and Hanlon, R. T. (2009). Comparative morphology of changeable skin papillae in octopus and cuttlefish. *Journal of Morphology*, **257**, 371–390.

Alupay, J. S., Hadjisolomou, S. P., and Crook, R. J. (2014). Arm injury produces long term behavioral and neural hypersensitivity in octopus. *Neuroscience Letters*, **558**, 137–142.

Anderson, J. A., Wood, J. B., and Mather, J. A. (2008). *Octopus vulgaris* in the Caribbean is a specializing generalist. *Marine Ecology Progress Series*, **371**, 199–202.

Anderson, R. C., and Mather, J. A. (2007). The packaging problem: bivalve mollusk prey selection and prey entry techniques of *Enteroctopus dofleini*. *Journal of Comparative Psychology*, **121**, 300–305.

Anderson, R. C., and Mather, J. A. (2010). It's all in the cues: octopuses learn to open jars. *Ferrantia*, **59**, 22–31.

Anderson, R. C., Mather, J. A., and Sinn, D. L. (2008). Octopus senescence: forgetting how to eat clams. *Festivus*, **15**, 55–56.

Anderson, R. T., and Wood, J. B. (2001). Enrichment for giant Pacific octopuses: happy as a clam? *Journal of Applied Animal Welfare Science*, **4**, 157–168.

Beigel, M., and Boal, J. G. (2006). The effect of habitat enrichment on the mudflat octopus. *The Shape of Enrichment*, **15**, 3–6.

Boal, J. G. (1996). A review of simultaneous visual discrimination as a method of training octopuses. *Biological Reviews*, **72**, 157–190.

Boal, J. G. (2010). Behavioral research methods for octopuses and cuttlefishes. *Vie et Milieu*, **61**, 203–210.

Boal, J. G., and Marsh, S. E. (1998). Social recognition using chemical cues in cuttlefish (*Sepia officinalis* Linnaeus, 1758). *Journal of Experimental Marine Biology and Ecology*, **230**, 183–192.

Boal, J. G., Dunham, A. W., Williams, K. T., and Hanlon, R. T. (2000). Experimental evidence for spatial learning in octopuses. *Journal of Comparative Psychology*, **114**, 246–252.

Boycott, B. B. (1954). Learning in *Octopus vulgaris* and other cephalopods. *Pubblicazione della Stazione Zoologica di Napoli*, **25**, 1–27.

Boyle, P. R. (1983). Ventilation rate and arousal in the octopus. *Journal of Experimental Marine Biology and Ecology*, **69**, 129–136.

Bublitz, A., Weinhold, S. R., Strobel, S., Dehnhardt, G., and Hanke, F. (2017). Reconsideration of serial visual reversal learning in octopus (*Octopus vulgaris*) from a methodological perspective. *Frontiers in Physiology*, **8**, 54.

Budelmann, B. U. (1995). The cephalopod nervous system: what evolution has made of the Molluscan design. In *The nervous system of invertebrates: an evolutionary approach* (pp. 115–138). Basel: Berkhauser Verlag.

Budelmann, B. U., and Tu, Y. (1997). The statocyst-oculomotor reflex of cephalopods and the vestibule-oculomotor reflex of vertebrates: a tabular comparison. *Vie et Milieu*, **47**, 95–99.

Byrne, R. A., Kuba, M. J., and Meisel, D. (2004). Lateral eye use in *Octopus vulgaris* shows an antisymmetric distribution. *Animal Behaviour*, **64**, 461–468.

Byrne, R. A., Kuba, M. J., Meisel, D., Greibel, U., and Mather, J. A. (2006). Does *Octopus vulgaris* have preferred arms? *Journal of Comparative Psychology*, **120**, 198–204.

Byrne, R. A., Wood, J. B., Anderson R. C., Greibel, U., and Mather, J. A. (2010). Non-invasive methods of identifying and tracking wild squid. *Ferrantia*, **59**, 22–31.

Caldwell, R. L., Ross, R., Rodanice, A., and Huffard, C. L. (2015). Behavior and body patterns of the larger Pacific striped octopus. *PLoS ONE*, **10**(8), e0134152.

Carere, C., and Mather, J. A. (In prep.). *The welfare of invertebrates*. Springer.

Darmaillacq, A.-S., Jozet-Alves, C., Bellanger, C., and Dickel, L. (2014a). Cuttlefish preschool, or how to learn in the pre-hatching period. In *Cephalopod cognition* (pp. 3–30). Cambridge: Cambridge University Press.

Darmaillacq, A.-S., Dickel, L., and Mather, J. A. (2014b). *Cephalopod cognition*. Cambridge: Cambridge University Press.

Dews, P. M. (1959). Some observations of an operant in the octopus. *Journal of the Experimental Analysis of Behavior*, **8**, 57–63.

Fay, R. R., and Popper, A. N. (2000). Evolution of hearing in vertebrates: the inner ear and processing. *Hearing Research*, **149**, 1–10.

Ferguson, G. P. A., and Messenger, J. B. (1991). A countershading reflex in cephalopods. *Proceedings of the Royal Society of London B: Biological Sciences*, **243**, 247–256.

Fiorito, G., Biederman, G. B., Davey, V. A., and Gherardi, F. (1998). The role of stimulus pre-exposure in problem solving by *Octopus vulgaris*. *Animal Cognition*, **1**, 107–112.

Fiorito, G., Affuso, A., Anderson, D. B., *et al.* (2014). Cephalopods in neuroscience: regulations, research and the 3Rs. *Invertebrate Neuroscience*, **14**, 13–36.

Flash, T., and Hochner, B. (2005). Motor primitives in vertebrates and invertebrates. *Current Opinion in Neurobiology*, **15**, 660–666.

Forsythe, J. W., and Hanlon, R. T. (1997). Foraging and associated behavior by *Octopus cyanea* Gray, 1849, on a coral atoll, French Polynesia. *Journal of Experimental Marine Biology and Ecology*, **209**, 15–31.

Gherardi, F., Aquilione, L., and Tricarico, E. (2012). Revisiting social recognition systems in invertebrates. *Animal Cognition*, **15**, 745–762.

Giribet, G., Okusu, A., Lindgren, A. R., Huff, S. W., Schrödl, M., and Nishiguchi, M. K. (2006). Evidence for a clade composed of molluscs with serially repeated structures: monoplacophorans are related to chitons. *Proceedings of the National Academy of Sciences*, **103**, 7723–7728.

Gleadall, I., and Shashar, N. (2004). *The octopus's garden: the visual world of cephalopods*. In *Complex worlds from simpler nervous systems* (pp. 269–308). Cambridge, MA: MIT Press.

Graindorge, N., Alves, C., Darmaillacq, A.-S., Chichery, R., Dickel, L., and Bellanger, C. (2006). Effect of dorsal and ventral vertical lobe lesions on spatial learning and locomotor activity in *Sepia officinalis*. *Behavioral Neuroscience*, **120**, 1151–1158.

Grasso, F. W., and Basil, J. (2009). The evolution of flexible behavioral repertoires in cephalopod mollusks. *Brain, Behavior and Evolution*, **74**, 231–245.

Gutnick, T. (2014). *Peripheral and central inputs in learning and navigation in Octopus vulgaris*. Doctoral thesis. Department of Life Science, Hebrew University, Jerusalem.

Gutnick, T., Byrne, R. A., Hochner, B., and Kuba, M. (2011). *Octopus vulgaris* uses visual information to determine the location of its arm. *Current Biology*, **21**, 460–462.

Gutnick, T., Shomrat, T., Mather, J. A., and Kuba, M. J. (2016). The cephalopod brain: motion control, learning, and cognition. In *Physiology of Mollusca* (pp. 139–177). Waretown: Apple Academic Press.

Hall, K., and Hanlon, R. (2002). Principal features of the mating system of a large spawning aggregation of the giant Australian cuttlefish *Sepia apama* (Mollusca: Cephalopoda). *Marine Biology*, **140**, 533–545.

Hanlon, R.T., and Budelmann, B. U. (1987). Why cephalopods are probably not 'deaf'. *American Naturalist*, **129**, 312–317.

Hanlon, R. T., and Messenger, J. B. (1988). Adaptive coloration in young cuttlefish (*Sepia officinalis L.*): the morphology and development of body patterns and their relation to behavior. *Philosophical Transactions of the Royal Society B: Biological Sciences*, **320**, 437–487.

Hanlon, R. T., and Messenger, J. B. (1996). *Cephalopod behaviour*. Cambridge: Cambridge University Press.

Hanlon, R. T., Forsythe, J. W., and Joneschild, D. E. (1999). Crypsis, conspicuousness, mimicry and polyphenism as antipredator defenses of foraging octopuses on Indo-Pacific coral reefs, with a method of quantifying crypsis from videotapes. *Biological Journal of the Linnean Society*, **66**, 1–22.

Huffard, C. L. (2007). Ethogram of *Abdopus aculeatus* (d'Orbigny, 1834) (Cephalopoda: Octopodidae): can behavioral characters inform octopodid taxonomy and systematics? *Journal of Molluscan Studies*, **73**, 185–193.

Huffard, C. L., Caldwell, R. L., and Boneka, F. (2008a). Mating behavior of *Abdopus aculeatus* (D'Orbigny, 1834) (Cephalopoda, Octopodidae) in the wild. *Marine Biology*, **154**, 353–362.

Huffard, C. L., Caldwell, R. L., DeLoach, N., Gentry, D. W., Humann, P., and MacDonald, B. (2008b). Individually unique body color patterns in octopus (*Wunderpus photogenicus*) allow for photoidentification. *PLoS ONE*, **3**, 1–5.

Hvoreckny, L. M., Grudowski, J. L., Blakeslee, C. J., *et al.* (2007). Octopuses (*Octopus bimaculoides*) and cuttlefish (*Sepia pharaonis, Sepia officinalis*) can conditionally discriminate. *Animal Cognition*, **10**, 449–459.

Ibanez, C. M., and Keyl, F. (2010). Cannibalism in cephalopods. *Review of Fish Biology and Fisheries*, **20**, 123–136.

Iglesias, J., Fuentes, L., and Villanueva, R. (eds.) (2014). *Cephalopod culture*. New York, NY: Springer.

Jozet-Alves, C., Moderan, J., and Dickel L. (2008). Sex differences in spatial cognition in an invertebrate: the cuttlefish. *Proceedings of the Royal Society of London B: Biological Sciences*, **275**, 2049–2054.

Jozet-Alves, C., Viblanc, V. A., Romagny, S., Dacher, M., Healy, S. D., and Dickel, L. (2012). Visual lateralization is task and age dependent in cuttlefish, *Sepia officinalis*. *Animal Behaviour*, **83**, 1313–1318.

Jozet-Alves, C., Bertin, M., and Clayton, N. (2013). Evidence of episodic-like memory in cuttlefish. *Current Biology*, **23**, 1033–1035.

Karson, M. A., Boal, J. G., and Hanlon R. T. (2003). Experimental evidence for spatial learning in cuttlefish (*Sepia officinalis*). *Journal of Comparative Psychology*, **17**, 149–155.

Kier, W. M., and Smith, K. K. (1985). Tongues, tentacles and trunks: the biomechanics of movement in muscular-hydrostats. *Zoological Journal of the Linnean Society*, **83**, 307–324.

Langridge, K. V., Broom, M., and Osorio, D. (2007). Selective signalling by cuttlefish to predators. *Current Biology*, **17**, 1044–1045.

Leite, T. S., Batista, A. T., Lima, F. D., Barbosa, J. C., and Mather, J. A. (2016). Geographic variability of *Octopus insularis* diet: from oceanic island to continental populations. *Aquatic Biology*, **25**, 17–27.

Levy, G., Flash, T., and Hochner, B. (2015). Arm coordination in crawling involves unique motor coordination strategies. *Current Biology*, **25**, 119501200.

Liu, T-H., and Chiao, C. C. (2017). Mosaic organization of body pattern control in the optic lobe of squids. *The Journal of Neuroscience*, **37**, 768–780.

Macintosh, N. J. (1965). Selective attention in animal discrimination learning. *Psychological Bulletin*, **64**, 124–150.

Mather, J. A. (1980a). Social organization and the use of space by *Octopus joubini* in a semi-natural situation. *Bulletin of Marine Science*, **30**, 848–857.

Mather, J. A. (1980b). Feeding and food intake in *Octopus joubini Robson*. *The Veliger*, **22**, 286–290.

Mather, J. A. (1991). Navigation by spatial memory and use of visual landmarks in octopuses. *Journal of Comparative Physiology A*, **168**, 491–497.

Mather, J. A. (2006). Behaviour development: a cephalopod perspective. *International Journal of Comparative Psychology*, **19**, 98–115.

Mather, J. A. (2008). Cephalopod consciousness: behavioral evidence. *Consciousness and Cognition*, **17**, 37–48.

Mather, J. A. (2016). Mating games squid play: reproductive behavior and sexual skin displays in Caribbean reef squid *Sepioteuthis sepioidea*. *Marine and Freshwater Behaviour and Physiology*, **49**, 359–373.

Mather, J. A., and Alupay, J. (2016). An ethogram for benthic octopods (Cephalopoda: Octopodidae). *Journal of Comparative Psychology*, **130**, 109–127.
Mather, J. A., and Anderson, R. C. (1993). "Personalities" of octopuses (*Octopus rubescens*). *Journal of Comparative Psychology*, **107**, 336–340.
Mather, J. A., and Anderson, R. C. (2007). Ethics and invertebrates: a cephalopod perspective. *Diseases of Aquatic Organisms*, **75**, 119–129
Mather, J. A., and Kuba, M. (2013). The cephalopod specialties: complex nervous system, learning and cognition. *Canadian Journal of Zoology*, **91**, 431–449.
Mather, J. A., Anderson, R. C., and Wood, J. B. (2013). *Octopus, the ocean's intelligent invertebrate*. Portland, OR: Timber Press.
Mather, J. A., Leite, T. S., Anderson, R. C., and Wood, J. B. (2014). Foraging and cognitive competence in octopuses. In *Cephalopod cognition* (pp. 125–149). Cambridge: Cambridge University Press.
Mäthger, L. M., Barbosa, A., Miner, S., and Hanlon, R. T. (2005). Color blindness and contrast perception in cuttlefish (*Sepia officinalis*) determined by a visual sensorimotor assay. *Vision Research*, **46**, 1746–1753.
Mäthger, L. M., Denton, E. J., Marshall, N. J., and Hanlon, R. T. (2009). Mechanisms and behavioural functions of structural coloration in cephalopods. *Journal of the Royal Society Interface*, **6**, 149–163.
Mäthger, L. M., Roberts, S. B., and Hanlon, R. T. (2010). Evidence for distributed light sensing in the skin of cuttlefish, *Sepia officinalis*. *Biology Letters*, **6**, 600–603.
Meisel, D. V., Byrne, R. A., Kuba, M. J., and Mather, J. A. (2006). Comparing the activity patterns of two Mediterranean octopus species. *Journal of Comparative Psychology*, **120**, 191–197.
Messenger, J. B. (2001). Cephalopod chromatophores: neurobiology and natural history. *Biological Reviews*, **76**, 473–518.
Messenger, J. B, Wilson, A. P., and Hedge, A. (1973). Some evidence for colour blindness in *Octopus*. *Journal of Experimental Biology*, **59**, 77–94.
Morse, P., Zenger, K. R., McCormick, M. I., Meekan, M. G., and Huffard, C. L. (2017). Chemical cues correlate with agonistic behavior and female mate choice in the southern blue-ringed octopus, *Hapalochlaena maculosa* (Hoyle, 1883) (Cephalopoda, Octopodidae). *Journal of Molluscan Studies*, **83**, 79–87.
Moynihan, M. (1975). Conservation of displays and comparable stereotyped patterns among cephalopods. In *Function and evolution of behavior: essays in honour of Professor Nico Tinbergen, F. R. S.* (pp. 276–291). Oxford: Oxford University Press.
Moynihan, M. (1985). Why are cephalopods deaf? *American Naturalist*, **125**, 465–469.
Muntz, R. A., and Gwyther, J. (1988). Visual acuity in *Octopus pallidus* and *Octopus australis*. *Journal of Experimental Biology*, **134**, 119–129.
Nesher, N., Levy, G., Grasso, F. W., and Hochner, B. (2014). Self-recognition mechanism between skin and suckers prevents octopus arms from interfering with each other. *Current Biology*, **24**, 1271–1275.
Nixon, M., and Young, J. Z. (2003). *The brains and lives of cephalopods*. Oxford: Oxford University Press.
O'Brien, W. J., Browman, H. I., and Evans, B. I. (1990). Search strategies of foraging animals. *American Scientist*, **78**, 152–160.
O'Dor, R. K., and Webber, D. M. (1986). The constraints on cephalopods: why squid aren't fish. *Canadian Journal of Zoology*, **64**, 1591–1605.

Onthank, K. L., and Cowles, D. L. (2011). Prey selection in *Octopus rubescens*: possible roles of energy budgeting and prey nutritional composition. *Marine Biology*, **158**, 2795–2804.

Packard, A. (1972). Cephalopods and fish: the limits of convergence. *Biological Reviews*, **47**, 241–307.

Packard, A., and Hochberg, F. G. (1977). Skin patterning in *Octopus* and other genera. In *The biology of cephalopods* (pp. 191–231). London: Academic Press.

Packard, A., and Sanders, G. (1971). Body patterns of *Octopus vulgaris* and maturation of the response to disturbance. *Animal Behaviour*, **19**, 780–790.

Papini, M. R., and Bitterman, M. E. (1991). Appetitive conditioning in *Octopus cyanea*. *Journal of Comparative Psychology*, **105**, 107–113.

Polese, G., Bertapelle, C., and Di Cosmo, A. (2015). Role of olfaction in *Octopus vulgaris* reproduction. *General and Comparative Endocrinology*, **210**, 55–62.

Polese, G., Bertapelle, C., and Di Cosmo, A. (2016). Olfactory organ of *Octopus vulgaris*: morphology, plasticity, turnover and sensory characterization. *Biology Open*, **5**, 611–619.

Pronk, R., Wilson, D. R., and Harcourt, R. (2010). Video playback demonstrates episodic personality in the gloomy octopus. *The Journal of Experimental Biology*, **213**, 1035–1041.

Ramirez, M. D., and Oakley, T. H. (2015). Eye-independent light-activated chromatophore expansion (LACE) and expression of phototransduction genes in the skin of *Octopus bimaculoides*. *Journal of Experimental Biology*, **218**, 1513–1520.

Richter, J. N., Hochner, B., and Kuba, M. J. (2015). Octopus arm movements under constrained conditions: adaptation, modification and plasticity of motor primitives. *Journal of Experimental Biology*, **218**, 1069–1076.

Richter, J. N., Hochner, B., and Kuba, M. J. (2016). Pull or push? Octopuses solve a puzzle problem. *PLoS ONE*, **11**(3), e0152048.

Scata, G., Jozet-Alves, C., Thomasse, C., Josef, N., and Shashar, N. (2016). Spatial learning in the cuttlefish *Sepia officinalis*: preference for vertical over horizontal information. *Journal of Experimental Biology*, **219**, 2928–2933.

Scheel, D., and Bisson, L. (2010). Movement patterns of giant Pacific octopuses, *Enteroctopus dofleini*. *Journal of Experimental Marine Biology and Ecology*, **416**, 21–31.

Scheel, D., Godfrey-Smith, P., and Lawrence, M. (2016). Signal use by octopuses in agonistic interactions. *Current Biology*, **26**, 377–382.

Shashar, N., and Cronin, T. W. (1996). Polarized contrast vision in *Octopus*. *The Journal of Experimental Biology*, **199**, 99–104.

Shashar, N., Rutledge, P. S., and Cronin, T. W. (1996). Polarization vision in cuttlefish – a concealed communication channel. *Journal of Experimental Biology*, **199**, 2077–2084.

Smith, J. A., Andrews, P. L. R., Hawkins, P., Louhimus, S., Ponte, G., and Dickel, L. (2013). Cephalopod research and EU Directive 2010 63 EU: requirements, impacts, and ethical reviews. *Journal of Experimental Marine Biology and Ecology*, **447**, 31–45.

Stubbs, A. L. and Stubbs, C. W. (2016). Spectral discrimination in color blind animals via chromatic aberration and pupil shape. *Proceedings of the National Academy of Sciences*, **113**, 8206–8211.

Sutherland, N. S. (1969). Shape discrimination in rat, octopus and goldfish: a comparative study. *Journal of Comparative and Physiological Psychology*, **67**, 160–176.

Tidbal, J. G. (2012). Cnidaria: secreted surface in biology of the integument. In *Biology of the integument: invertebrates* (pp. 69–76). Berlin: Springer.

Tricarico, E., Borelli, L., Gherardo, F., and Fiorito, G. (2011). I know my neighbour: individual recognition in *Octopus vulgaris*. *PLoS ONE*, **6**(4), e18710.

Walderon, M. D., Nolt, K. J., Haas, R. E., *et al.* (2011). Distance chemoreception and the detection of conspecifics in *Octopus bimaculoides*. *Journal of Molluscan Studies*, **77**, 309–311.

Wells, M. J. (1978). *Octopus: physiology and behaviour of an advanced invertebrate*. London: Chapman and Hall.

Williamson, R., and Chrachri, A. (2007). A model biological neural network: the cephalopod vestibular system. *Philosophical Transactions of the Royal Society B: Biological Sciences*, **362**, 473–481.

Wood, J. B., and Anderson, R. C. (2004). Interspecific evaluation of octopus escape behavior. *Journal of Applied Animal Welfare Science*, **7**, 95–106.

Yasumura, H., and Ikeda, Y. (2011). Effects of environmental enrichment on the behavior of the tropical octopus *Callistoctopus apiliosomaus*. *Marine and Freshwater Behaviour and Physiology*, **44**, 143–157.

Zullo, L., Sumbre, G., Agnisola, C., Flash, T., and Hochner, B. (2009). Nonsomatotopic organization of the higher motor centers in *Octopus*. *Current Biology*, **19**, 1632–1636.

Zylinski, S., and Osorio, D. (2014). Cuttlefish camouflage: vision and cognition. In *Cephalopod cognition* (pp. 197–222). Cambridge: Cambridge University Press.

15 Grey Parrots (*Psittacus erithacus*) – Cognitive and Communicative Abilities

Irene M. Pepperberg

Evaluating how methodology and physical, physiological, and behavioral characteristics affect avian cognition studies is daunting, even when restricting the topic to Grey parrots. This chapter, therefore, is meant as a reference source, not an exhaustive treatise nor detailed guide.

Species Description

Anatomy

Images of Grey parrot skeletal anatomy and its vascular system are available at www.avianstudios.com/the-grey-parrot-anatomy-project/images/ (Scott Echols, DVM). Particularly relevant for cognitive research are neural structures and vocal apparatus. The former clarify how creatures with walnut-sized brains demonstrate cognitive abilities comparable to (and occasionally more advanced than) those of great apes (see below). The latter explain Greys' ability to produce human speech sounds, which enables demonstration of certain advanced cognitive abilities. I discuss each in turn.

Early twentieth-century researchers suggested that different-looking brain areas mediated similar types of avian and mammalian intelligent behaviour (Kalischer, 1901), and that, as for mammals, relative sizes of these areas and learning capacities were correlated (e.g. Portmann, 1950; Cobb, 1960; Portmann and Stingelin, 1961; Stettner, 1967). Recently, specific functional homologies have been demonstrated between avian brain areas and the mammalian cerebral cortex (Jarvis *et al.*, 2005, 2013). For example, avian nidopallium caudolaterale (NCL) and dorsolateral corticoid (CDL) are likely homologues, respectively, of the posterior parietal cortex and parts of the prefrontal cortex (Butler *et al.*, 2005). Two studies are particularly relevant. One demonstrates that parrots such as Greys (and several corvids) have forebrain neuron counts equal to or greater than primates with much larger overall brains, suggesting that large numbers of neurons densely concentrated in the forebrain mediate advanced avian intelligence (Olkowicz *et al.*, 2016). The other examines brain structures involved in vocal (and possibly other forms of) learning (Chakraborty *et al.*, 2015). Certain avian species (sub-oscines such as North American flycatchers, members of pigeon and chicken families) lack specific neural structures responsible for vocal learning; their species-specific vocalizations thus develop innately. Vocal learning and the requisite neural structures characterize oscines, or songbirds. Greys are vocal learners, but their learning is open-ended and can include non-species-specific sounds; thus, unlike many (but not all) songbirds that may learn most of their repertoire early in life (e.g. dialects of natal territories) and then make few, if any, changes, parrots can constantly acquire new vocalizations. Most parrots thus have not only neural systems like those of songbirds and hummingbirds for conspecific vocal learning, but also a unique, separate 'shell' system, likely responsible for their open-ended abilities to learn and acquire even allospecific utterances. This shell system, larger in psittacids like Greys that exhibit extensive allospecific learning, may also be involved in non-vocal learning (Chakraborty *et al.*, 2015).

Grey parrot vocal mechanisms provide insight into their cognition. Because Greys *learn* to control their vocal tract – using cognitive processes (e.g. matching output to input) for such learning – their ability to acquire referential English speech not only facilitates studying their cognitive processing, but also such processing itself (Pepperberg, 1999, 2012b). But *how* do Greys produce human utterances? Brain structures and connectivity are necessary for vocal learning, but sound production also depends on the vocal tract. Parrots lack dentition and lips, and dramatic morphological differences exist

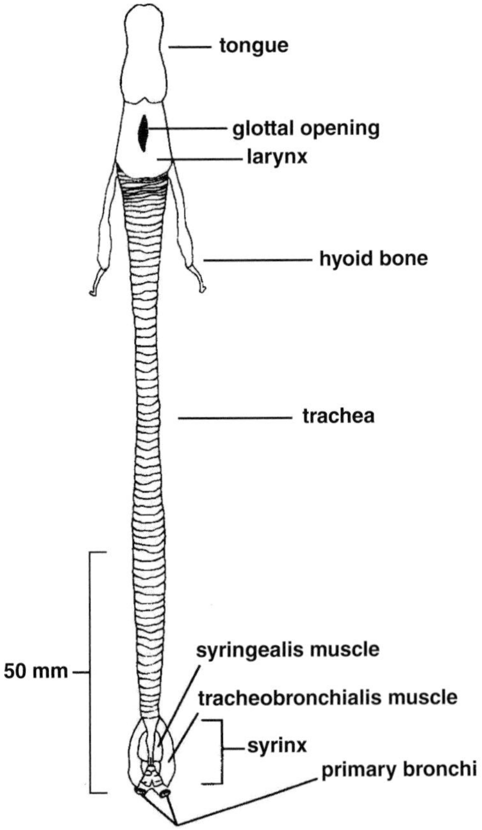

Figure 15.1. Dorsal view of Grey parrot vocal tract.
Illustration originally published in Warren *et al.*, 1996, reprinted with kind permission of the American Ornithological Society.

between other human and avian vocal structures, yet spectrograms of English labels produced by Greys and humans have striking similarities, including parrot and human formants (frequency bands that determine phonetic qualities of human speech; Patterson and Pepperberg, 1994, 1998; Bottoni *et al.*, 2009). Explaining these abilities requires examining the Grey parrot vocal tract (Figure 15.1).

Avian sound production originates in the syrinx (Greenewalt, 1968), where the trachea meets the bronchi. Parrot syringes, unlike those of many songbirds, produce only one sound at a time (Nottebohm, 1976; Gaunt and Gaunt, 1985; Patterson and Pepperberg, 1994). Grey parrot syringes may also be uniquely positioned ('further craniad than in all other parrot species studied') and shaped ('dorso-ventrally oriented cranial edges of the syringeal cartilages are straight, not semi-oval in outline'; Scanlan, 1988). These modifications may enable greater control of cartilages and membranes, possibly allowing Greys more precise regulation of vocalization periodicity and frequency than other psittacids (Scanlan, 1988; Warren *et al.*, 1996).

Suprasyringeal structures (trachea, glottis, larynx, tongue, nasal cavities, beak) also affect Greys' vocal production, probably more so than for songbirds, likely contributing to Greys' ability to reproduce human speech faithfully (Patterson *et al.*, 1997). I describe these structures, reviewing correlational evidence for their role in sound modification.

Tracheal length/configuration alteration could make this structure into a resonant chamber, modulating frequencies emanating from the syrinx. The Grey trachea (excised length, ~11 cm) is a series of ossified, complete rings, with minimal inter-ring intervals (Pepperberg *et al.*, 1998a). Rings can overlap, allowing length or configuration changes: protraction (i.e. bending) occurs for certain human vocalizations; lengthening is maximally ~10 per cent (Patterson and Pepperberg, 1994, 1998). Tracheal effects on Greys' human speech production are thus likely small, but a long tube, changing little in length, is an obvious candidate for psittacine first formant production (Warren *et al.*, 1996), which varies little across a Grey's vowels (Patterson and Pepperberg, 1994).

Greys' laryngeal anatomy (Homberger, 1979) differs from that of *Corvus* (Bock, 1978) and *Gallus* (White, 1968), but how these differences affect production is unknown. The avian larynx merely modifies sound produced by the syrinx (Riede and Goller, 2010). Back–front laryngeal movement could, however, quickly alter throat cavity resonant frequencies to achieve a targeted vocalization, by changing glottal opening position or size (Warren *et al.*, 1996; Homberger, 1999). The glottis, a slit exiting from the larynx, is between the trachea and the rest of the suprasyringeal areas (Warren *et al.*, 1996; Patterson *et al.*, 1997). Glottal size is also altered by intrinsic muscles (Homberger, 1979); thus, the glottis can cause considerable constriction, acting like the neck of a Helmholtz resonator, significantly affecting sounds produced by a Grey's vocal tract (Patterson and Pepperberg, 1998). Greys prepare to vocalize by transporting the larynx to a vocalizing position, then use synchronic movements during vocalization (Scanlan, 1988).

Among birds, psittacine tongues have a unique skeleton and musculature. Likely evolved for eating (Homberger, 1986), they also affect vocalizations. In Greys, three joints, six extrinsic and seven intrinsic pairs of lingual muscles affect tongue motion; the laryngeal glottal opening is just dorsal to the tongue (Homberger, 1986). This unique structure not only enables flexible laryngeal movements (Homberger, 1986; Scanlan,

1988), but also possible interconnectedness for certain tongue, laryngeal and tracheal movements; tongue movements may modify the shape and consequently resonant properties of the vocal tract (Nottebohm, 1976). Several studies implicate the tongue in second formant production in parrot speech (e.g. Patterson and Pepperberg, 1994; Beckers *et al.*, 2004; Ohms *et al.*, 2012).

Beak/lower mandible movement may serve both for visual display and to modify vocalization amplitude and frequency. Studies (e.g. X-ray video imaging) of how tongue, larynx positions and beak opening correlate suggest that by producing some vowels with a mostly closed beak, Greys form a slotted tube to extend throat cavity length and thereby additionally affect their second formants (Warren *et al.*, 1996; Patterson *et al.*, 1997).

Grey parrots, lacking lips and teeth, and with lungs, nasal cavities, trachea, bronchi, larynx and tongue differing considerably from human structures, produce sounds closely resembling English speech. Data suggest that Greys *learn* to control the various structures involved, and that such learning both reflects *and* affects how vocalizations can be used to investigate advanced cognitive processes (Pepperberg, 1999).

Perception

Functional brain similarities exist in parrot–human vocal learning areas, but not necessarily elsewhere, possibly causing divergence in various senses – hearing, vision, olfaction, taste, touch. Few Grey senses have been studied, but data from related species may provide insights.

Hearing would seem vital for a species that relies on vocal communication in nature. Dense forest often separates flock members and mates – for distance communication, vocal signals likely overshadow visual displays. The greatest auditory sensitivity in budgerigars, *Melopsittacus undulatus* (Dooling, 1986; Farabaugh and Dooling, 1996; Dooling *et al.*, 2000), cockatiels, *Nymphicus hollandicus* (Okanoya and Dooling, 1987), and orange-fronted conures, *Aratinga canicularis* (Wright *et al.*, 2003), is between 2 and 4 kHz; their thresholds are ~0.2–10 kHz. Humans' sensitivity is equivalent (Gelfand, 2016) and human thresholds greater. Given similarities among three parrots with differing ecological niches and humans, and Greys' abilities to reproduce human speech, Greys' ranges are likely comparable. Although a bird's hearing range provides little information about its sound characterization or categorization (e.g. Bregman *et al.*, 2014), Greys can, for example, distinguish labels varying in minimal pairs of English consonants (e.g. cork/corn; tea/pea; Patterson and Pepperberg, 1998), attaching appropriate referents to the different labels. Such data elucidate their auditory competence.

Avian vision is remarkable. Birds, more than humans, navigate in three dimensions, identify and respond quickly to obstacles and predators – demands matching or exceeding those placed on human visual systems, requiring considerable allocation of processing resources to vision. How do avian brains – smaller and somewhat differently organized from, but evolutionarily similar to, those of primates (e.g. Jarvis *et al.*, 2005) – function?

Two major visual pathways – lemnothalamic and collothalamic – exist in reptiles, birds and mammals, but similarities end there. Humans' lemnothalamic pathway is the more highly developed; in at least one bird, the pigeon (*Columba livia*), the collothalamic is more developed (Nguyen *et al.*, 2004). Chicks (*Gallus gallus*), however, are more human-like, using the lemnothalamic system for frontal viewing, showing more balanced/complementary use of both eyes, assisting their more global systems of visual analysis (Regolin *et al.*, 2004; but see Tommasi and Vallortigara, 2001). Parrots likely resemble chicks more than pigeons (G. Harrison, pers. comm.). For parrots, only the Senegal (*Poicephalus senegalus*) visual range is known (e.g. binocular overlap of ~30 per cent): if Greys resemble Senegals, they primarily use monocular vision with some binocular overlap (Demery *et al.*, 2011); sight should extend just below the bill tip and, by pitching their head and/or bringing items up to their heads with their feet, Greys should be able to see most of their environment. A visual acuity test, requiring a Grey to vocally identify variously sized numerals, showed full accuracy down to 6.3 mm, at distances between 10 and 15 cm (Pepperberg *et al.*, 2008). All studies should thus take into account avian–human visual field differences.

Human–avian flicker-fusion differences affect outcomes if studies use CRT screens for video stimuli (Ikebuchi and Okanoya, 1999). Flicker-fusion refers to the lowest frequency of flashing, at which a flickering light source is perceived as constant: continuous motion on CRT screens for humans appears as a series of single frames to most birds. Notably, Greys respond to images on LCD but not CRT screens (Pepperberg and Wilkes, 2004).

Grey parrots see in the ultraviolet range (Bowmaker *et al.*, 1994, 1996; Wilkie *et al.*, 1998; Cuthill *et al.*, 2000; Goldsmith and Butler, 2005; Carvalho *et al.*, 2011). Thus, parrot and human colour perception may differ for particular hues, and must be considered when tests involve colour discriminations and identifications (e.g. Pepperberg, 1999; Pepperberg *et al.*, 2008).

Little is known about Greys' olfaction, but Echols (www.avianstudios.com/the-grey-parrot-anatomy-project/images/) detected a large blood supply to the nares (nostrils), suggesting an olfactory role in nature. In laboratory studies, Greys do not use olfaction to locate hidden rewards or distinguish hidden foods separated by a few centimetres (e.g. Pepperberg *et al.*, 2013). Thus, olfactory cuing is unlikely in carefully designed research studies.

Similarly, Greys' taste has not been studied specifically. Parrots in general, with fewer taste buds than humans, are nevertheless sensitive to sweet, sour, bitter and salt (Berkhoudt, 1985). How taste might affect research is unclear, except possibly when using food rewards.

Parrots must have touch receptors (Necker, 2000), although no formal studies exist for Greys. Use of beak, tongue and feet to manipulate food and preen feathers involve touch; flight is affected by sensitivity to air stream patterns (air pressure, wind speed, etc.); all body parts respond to pain. Certain textures might be more or less appealing, which could affect responses to experimental stimuli.

Life Cycle

Grey parrots are K-selected, meaning they are long-lived (one captive bird is over 90 years old; J. Hooimeijer, pers. comm.), produce relatively few offspring per clutch (can lay up to five eggs; chick survival rate unknown) and have a fairly long juvenile period, not reaching sexual maturity until ~5 years old (Juniper and Parr, 1998). Few cognitive or physical developmental studies exist, other than one tracking the emergence of full Piagetian object permanence (Pepperberg *et al.*, 1997). Extrapolating from this study, attention to experimental apparatus develops over time, maturing around a year post-hatch (see also Pepperberg *et al.*, 2017).

Determining Grey parrot age is difficult. Eyes are completely black at hatching; irises lighten to straw-coloured after about 1 year. No other obvious colouration changes accompany ageing, although pink–red feathers may develop in extreme old age – like human hair going white, from decreasing melatonin. Occasionally, feather-bed damage causes this colour change in youth.

Repertoire size cannot determine age post-fledging. Greys, like most psittacids, are open-ended vocal learners (see above); new vocalizations may be acquired throughout life. Such knowledge is important when examining vocal communication (e.g. do flocks have vocal dialects; if so, do birds alter dialects to communicate across flocks, or if changing flocks?). Whether vocal learning flexibility translates into flexibility for other learning is unknown; concept-learning continues throughout life (e.g. Pepperberg and Carey, 2012; see below).

Individual Identification

Humans see Greys as sexually monomorphic. Claims of males being larger, having 'pointed' eye patches, etc. likely involve individual, not sexual, differences. However, given Greys' ultraviolet vision, and that other parrots (e.g. blue-fronted Amazons, *Amazona aestiva*) demonstrate visible sexual differences under UV light (Santos *et al.*, 2006), that possibility is being tested in Greys (von Bayern, pers. comm.). Although physical similarity makes widespread conspecific individual visual recognition unlikely in large flocks (e.g. night roosts of ~100 birds), variation in feather darkness, head and beak shape, neck length, foot size, etc., could enable individual recognition within small groups (e.g. 3–5 birds).

Greys may, however, recognize individuals vocally. Duets used for nest defence have parts unique to the resident pair (see below; May, 2004), which may be their signature. Spectacled parrotlets (*Forpus conspicillatus*) may have specific calls for family members (Wanker *et al.*, 2005); green-rumped parrotlets (*Forpus passerinus*) use individual contact calls for mate recognition (Berg *et al.*, 2011, 2012). Male budgerigars (*Melopsittacus undulatus*) imitate female contact calls to promote pair bonding and maintenance (Hile *et al.*, 2000, 2005), implying individual recognition. Contact calls serve as labelling mechanisms in female budgerigars (Dahlin *et al.*, 2014) and possibly Bahama Amazon parrots (*Amazona leucocephala bahamensis*; Gnam, 1988). Greys may behave similarly: although appropriate studies are lacking, May (2004) provides details of their vocal behaviour in the Congo basin, expanding the work of Cruickshank and colleagues (1993), who document only heterospecific vocal imitation.

Ecological and Social Characteristics

Greys were once endemic through central African forests and savannas (Ivory Coast and Cameroon, to Kenya and Uganda). Night-time roosts, sometimes encompassing 1000 birds, would split into daytime foraging groups of 5–30 birds (Juniper and Parr, 1998). A few hundred birds might congregate at water holes, eating greens and possibly clay on the ground, nuts and fruit in trees (Tamungang *et al.*, 2001; May, 2004). Greys, now almost extinct in east Africa, have declined precipitously in central and west Africa, and as of 2016, they are on CITES Appendix I (signifying most severely endangered; Bird Life International, 2016).

Few studies of wild Greys exist; the following information is based on small samples (Tamungang *et al.*, 2001; May, 2004). Greys are secondary cavity nesters: unable to excavate nest holes (Tamungang and Cheke, 2012), they instead alter existing cavities in old-growth trees. A dominance hierarchy likely exists, with competition for these nesting sites. In captive aviaries or breeding farms, lifelong monogamous bonds begin at sexual maturity, around 5 years of age (see www.proaviculture.com/africanparrotobservations.htm). Wild breeding occurs in loose colonies, each pair occupying its own tree; pairs defend nests from other pairs with vocal duets and display flights (Juniper and Parr, 1998; May, 2004). Little is known about courtship in nature; May (2004) recorded display flights around nest holes. Greys incubate for approximately a month. Males assist in feeding the young (Wilson, 2006).

How long post-fledging juveniles remain with parents is unknown, although small foraging groups may consist of families. Alternatively, such groups could be birds too young to mate, with older birds modelling behaviour for younger ones; both ideas are supposition. When not mating, Greys move in fission–fusion groups, foraging up to 60 km/day (May, 2004). Their system suggests that survival may depend upon knowledge about flock-mates: during ground feeding, for example, sentinels alarm call to predators (May, 2004); birds must recognize if this sentinel is trustworthy. Unlike some *Amazona* parrots (e.g. Brightsmith and Villalobos, 2011), Greys do not routinely congregate with other species (May, 2004).

Greys are endangered for many reasons. Human poaching (e.g. Tamungang and Cheke, 2012) and deforestation cause 63 per cent of losses (Tamungang *et al.*, 2014). Greys may be chased (but not hunted) by palm-nut vultures (*Gypohierax angolensis*), during competition for similar food (Thompson and Moreau, 1957). Greys suffer from aerial and terrestrial attacks (May, 2004; Tamungang *et al.*, 2014): black sparrowhawks (*Accipiter melanoleucus*) and Madagascar gymnogenes (*Polyboroides radiatus*) may hunt young Greys (Fotso, 1998); tree-dwelling animals may take eggs and nestlings (Juniper and Parr, 1998).

State of the Art

Grey parrot cognition has been studied since the 1950s, primarily in the non-social domain. Greys' abilities compare favourably with those of young children, non-human primates and marine mammals (e.g. Pepperberg, 1999, 2012b, in press). Here I summarize various capacities.

Greys' vocal flexibility enables acquisition and use of English speech for referential communication, which can be exploited to examine their cognition. Training involves observational learning – the model/rival (M/R) technique (see below), based on experiments by Bandura (1971) and Todt (1975) – and knowledge of their naturally complex communication system (see above). My oldest subject, Alex, used vocal labels to identify numerous objects, foods, quantities, materials, colours and shapes, and employed 'I want X' and 'Wanna go Y' to request items or changes of location; other Greys, particularly Griffin, have similar abilities (Pepperberg, 1981, 1988a, 1999). Greys learn in ways not unlike young children, and somewhat like adults acquiring a second language, heavily dependent upon social interaction and one-to-one connections between using an utterance and receiving the object or action to which it refers (Pepperberg, 1994b; Pepperberg and McLaughlin, 1996; Pepperberg *et al.*, 1998b, 1999, 2000; Pepperberg and Wilkes, 2004). Comprehension matches production, even for complicated queries involving multiple dimensions (e.g. 'What object is green and three-cornered?'; Pepperberg, 1990a, 1992). These data suggest that many cognitive abilities are not dependent on primate or even mammalian brains (Pepperberg, 2012b; Olkowicz *et al.*, 2016).

Like children, parrots also spontaneously acquire new labels, via both solitary sound play and by producing novel phonemic combinations, actively recombining parts of existing utterances to form labels that can be referentially mapped onto novel objects (e.g. Alex: 'grey' to 'grape', 'grain', 'chain', 'cane'; Kuczaj, 1983; Pepperberg, 1990b, 2007; Pepperberg *et al.*, 1991); they also transfer use from known to novel referents (e.g. Alex: 'paper' from index cards to computer printout; Arthur: 'wool' from woollen pompon to experimenter's shirt; Pepperberg, 1999, 2002). They demonstrate aspects of mutual exclusivity – temporarily rejecting a second label (e.g. a colour) for an object they can already label – and combine labels only after they can physically combine objects (Griffin: Pepperberg and Wilcox, 2000; Pepperberg and Shive, 2001).

Alex and Griffin acquired categorical concepts – for the same item, responding to different categorical queries ('What matter?', 'What colour?', 'What shape?', 'What toy?') with the appropriate label (e.g. 'wood', 'green', '4-corner' and 'block'). Such behaviour shows higher-order, hierarchical understanding of class concepts (Pepperberg, 1983, 1996): each colour, shape, material or object label is subsumed under specific, different category labels, and category labels have no intrinsic connection to individual labels constituting the categories.

Alex understood the abstract concept of same–different (Premack, 1983): not the far simpler concepts of identity/non-identity or homogeneity/non-homogeneity, demonstrated by other non-humans, but knowledge that two objects can simultaneously be 'same' with respect to certain dimensions and 'different' with respect to others, plus the ability to encode such information symbolically (Premack, 1983; Pepperberg, 1987a). Shown any two items and queried 'What's same?'/'What's different?' (e.g. Figure 15.2), Alex appropriately replied 'colour', 'shape' or 'mah-mah' (matter). After learning the concept of absence, he vocally stated 'none' if nothing were same or different for a pair (Pepperberg, 1988b).

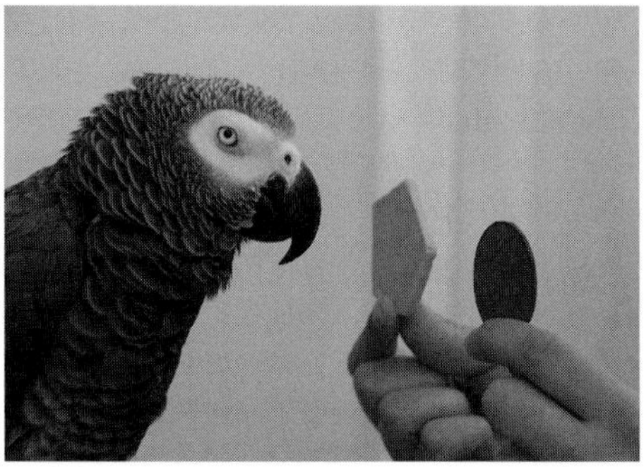

Figure 15.2. Alex being queried 'What's same?' to objects of different shapes and colours, but same material.
Photo by I. M. Pepperberg.

Another abstract concept that Alex acquired, and Griffin is learning, involves relative size – understanding not simply that 'A' is big and 'B' small, but that 'A' can be bigger than 'B' and simultaneously smaller than 'C' (Pepperberg and Brezinsky, 1991). Significantly, without training, Alex transferred his concept of absence from same–different to absence of a size differential, stating 'none' if two objects were equally sized.

Alex's most complicated series of experiments involved numerical concepts. Prior studies showed Greys could perform complex matching of numerical quantities (Koehler, 1950, 1953; Braun, 1952; Lögler, 1959). However, these abilities differ from exact human counting; could a non-human match human abilities?

Alex first learned to quantify various homogeneous object sets using standard vocal number labels 'one' to 'six', then expanded to heterogeneous sets – e.g. quantifying keys in a collection of corks and keys, something with which young children struggle (Pepperberg, 1987b). Next was a task used to disambiguate subitizing (a fast, approximate system for quantifying collections; for humans, generally of 1–4 items) from actual counting (Pepperberg, 1994a). Exactly enumerating a set of objects embedded within two different types of distractors requires counting (Trick and Pylyshyn, 1989, 1994). For Alex, we used colour and shape; for example, he successfully labelled the number of red balls in a mix of red and green balls and blocks. Thus, unlike most other non-humans, he demonstrated symbolic understanding of exact, not approximate, number (Carey, 2009). A subsequent study showed his comprehension was more accurate than production. He did not respond based on mass, contour or density; those aspects were controlled. Notably, without training, Alex again transferred use of 'none', to absence of a numerical set (a zero-like concept); he also manipulated trainers into asking the question that led to his demonstrating this ability (Pepperberg and Gordon, 2005).

Alex added small numerical sets, of different masses and sizes. He was shown a tray containing two upside-down cups, under which trainers had earlier hidden randomly shaped nut pieces, bits of cracker, candies or differently sized jelly beans. Each cup was lifted and replaced in turn, then Alex was asked 'How many total?' All possible sets of addends were tested, totalling from zero to six. He succeeded on all sets unless nothing was under both cups (then he refused to answer or said 'one'; Pepperberg, 2006a). Interestingly, he labelled 5 + 0 as 'six' if given only 2–3 seconds to respond; if given ~10 seconds, accuracy was 100 per cent. These results, compared with human subitizing data, provide evidence for actual counting: like humans, when beyond the subitizing limit of 4, he needed time to label the set exactly (Pepperberg, 2006a). After learning 'seven' and 'eight' and understanding that labels for sets could also be used for Arabic numerals (see below), he showed he could, like apes, sum three separate hidden sets or two hidden Arabic numerals (Pepperberg, 2012a). His death precluded testing all possible sums, combinations of addends or repeating most queries. Results, however, were statistically significant.

Another important numerical concept is ordinality – not simply acquiring a number line, but understanding that each number in the line is *exactly* one more in value than the preceding number. Children usually infer ordinality without training, albeit slowly (Carey, 2009), but ordinality must be trained extensively in non-human primates, even if they use symbolic numerical representation (reviewed in Pepperberg and Carey, 2012). Could Alex respond like children? Could he, after learning English labels for Arabic numerals (production and comprehension) in the absence of the physical quantities to which they refer, use the commonality of these English labels to equate quantities of physical objects and Arabic numerals, by labelling the colour of the numeral in a pair that was numerically the bigger or smaller (Pepperberg, 2006b; Figure 15.3)? He succeeded, including stating 'none' if numerals were the same value. He also responded correctly to Arabic numerals paired with sets of objects, unless the set had a single object. Then he responded on the physical, not the symbolic, basis.

Alex responded on number tasks more like children than like other non-humans but, unlike children, did not demonstrate a time saving when acquiring larger numbers.

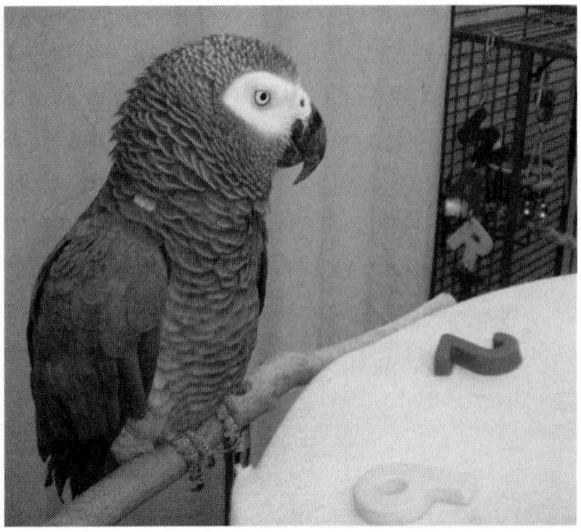

Figure 15.3. Alex being tested on ordinality: 'What colour number [is] bigger/smaller?'. Photo by I. M. Pepperberg.

Children, after slowly learning 'one' to 'four' and their number line over several years, relatively quickly intuit the meaning of numerals 'five' and above (Carey, 2009). Might a dissociation between vocal and conceptual learning have caused Alex's delays? Acquiring English number labels required that he not only learn their meaning, but also coordinate syrinx, tracheal muscles, glottis, larynx, tongue height and protrusion, beak opening, and even his oesophagus (see above; Patterson and Pepperberg, 1994, 1998).

To test this idea, Alex was taught to vocally label Arabic numerals 7 and 8 apart from their respective numerical sets, trained that $6 < 7 < 8$, then tested on relationships among 7 and 8 and his other Arabic numerals (Pepperberg and Carey, 2012). He inferred the new number line in its totality, but that did not address exact understanding of 7 and 8. Could he, like children ($\geq$ 4 years old), *spontaneously* understand that 'seven' represented exactly one more than 'six' and 'eight' two more than 'six' and one more than 'seven', by labelling appropriate physical sets on first trials (Pepperberg and Carey, 2012)? He not only induced cardinal meanings of 'seven' and 'eight' from their ordinal positions on a count list, but also showed that his representation of these and other numerals was exact: if the targeted set was missing from the testing display consisting of various numerical sets, he did not label the set closest in value, but said 'none' (Pepperberg and Carey, 2012). Symbolic communication, therefore, enabled a parrot, separated from the mammalian line by ~300 million years (e.g. Hedges *et al.*, 1996), to demonstrate numerical competency comparable to children who understand cardinal principles, something not yet achieved by phylogenetically closer apes.

Greys' referential speech also facilitates studying how they literally view the world, including optical illusions. As described earlier, parrots' and primates' visual systems differ considerably, but both function in the same environment. Parrots who can report exactly what they see enable detailed avian–primate comparisons in ways impossible with other non-humans.

Study of the Müller-Lyer illusion used the Brentano version (Pepperberg *et al.*, 2008), with white or black arrows (depending on the background) and two differently coloured shafts. Because Alex responded to 'What colour bigger/smaller?' and stated 'none' if objects appeared the same size (Pepperberg and Brezinsky, 1991), he was queried about permutations of shaft width and angle slant (including a 90° option in which the illusion would disappear for humans). Overall, he saw the illusion much as do humans, reporting it (or not) in appropriate circumstances.

Griffin's responses to two-dimensional representations of occluded and Kanizsa figures (Figure 15.4) were tested after he was trained to label vocally shapes and colours of three-dimensional (solid, non-occluded) polygons exclusively (Pepperberg and Nakayama, 2016). He responded much like adult humans, showing not only abilities difficult to demonstrate conclusively in other non-humans, but also spontaneous transfer from three-dimensional objects to their two-dimensional representations.

Greys succeed on tasks not requiring vocal responses. They show Stage 6 Piagetian object permanence (Pepperberg and Kozak, 1986; Pepperberg and Funk, 1990; Pepperberg *et al.*, 1997; Pepperberg, 2015), liquid conservation (Pepperberg *et al.*, 2017) and some understanding of mirror use, if not mirror self-recognition (Pepperberg *et al.*, 1995). They follow steady human gaze/head orientation and distal pointing if

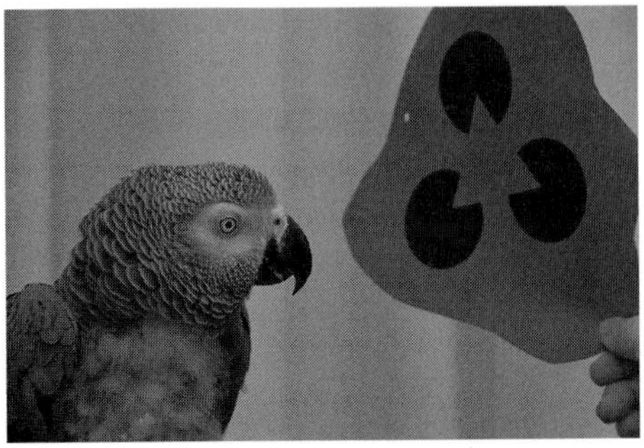

Figure 15.4. Griffin being shown a Kanisza figure and being questioned 'What shape [is] rose?' Photo by I. M. Pepperberg.

objects are at least 20 cm away and separated by 1.6 m, but not momentary cues when objects are closer to the human and each other (Giret *et al.*, 2009). In the laboratory, they engage in limited cooperative problem-solving (a string-pulling task, Péron *et al.*, 2011). They learn to work with another parrot to some extent in a tit-for-tat situation, but dominance issues affect results; they work more appropriately with a human (Péron *et al.*, 2013, 2014).

Greys have been tested on delayed gratification. Assessed for delay maintenance in an accumulation task, one of three Greys waited 2–3 seconds to access more seeds (Vick *et al.*, 2010). The aforementioned Griffin, however, responded to the label 'wait' for up to 15 minutes for a better-quality reward, in a task like those used with young children, whether or not the better quality reward or the experimenter was in view (Koepke *et al.*, 2015). Interestingly, for quality-based exchanges, various avian species and primates act similarly (see Hillemann *et al.*, 2014). Whether Griffin succeeds in a quantity-based paradigm remains to be seen.

Greys understand inferential reasoning by exclusion—deciding where a reward exists based on information about its absence. Mikolasch and colleagues (2011) replicated an experiment with apes (Premack and Premack, 1994), using tasks such as searching for food under one of two hiding sites after being shown the other is empty. They ruled out many alternative explanations (e.g. subjects simply avoiding the empty cup, being distracted by handling of the cups). The task is exquisitely sensitive to experimental design. For example, Greys responded to auditory clues about fullness or emptiness of a closed container, but only after horizontal, not vertical, shaking (Schloegl *et al.*, 2012), vertical action possibly being reminiscent of adults' feeding chicks, thus triggering a food-based response. Replication of Mikolasch *et al.* (2011), using two differently coloured cups instead of identical silver ones, helped birds remember where food had been removed and thus increased success (Pepperberg *et al.*, 2013). When food pairs of varying quality were used in some trials, birds would switch strategies, not necessarily avoiding the cup from which an item was removed – one high-quality reward is preferable to two much lower-quality rewards (Pepperberg *et al.*, 2013). Griffin (Carey *et al.*, in prep.) succeeded on complicated four-cup exclusion tasks, demonstrating even stronger inferential abilities (see Mody and Carey, 2016).

In sum, Grey parrot cognition appears equal to, or beyond that, of non-human primates, often comparable to that of young children. Two questions thus arise: for what purpose were these abilities evolutionarily selected? Are their achievements dependent upon use of English speech?

It is likely that evolutionary pressures were important. Big complex brains are energetically expensive. Although a rich (nut-biased) diet and high metabolism render such large brains somewhat less costly (Connor, 2007), why might they be needed in Greys? First, like primates, they are, as noted above, K-selected – long-lived, with few offspring that mature slowly; they have complex societies with a daily fission–fusion pattern, and probably dominance hierarchies requiring updating during their lifetimes. Second, their ecological–ethological niche resembles that of non-human primates. They eat a variety of foods, requiring navigation to and memories about large tracts of both terrestrial and aerial habitat that, again, alter during their lives (May, 2004). Furthermore, they have extensive vocal repertoires and open-ended vocal learning (May, 2004). Thus, evolutionary pressures exerted on the primate–hominid line likely were also exerted on psittacine precursors.

The capacity for symbolic representation is likely responsible for Grey parrot cognitive achievement. Premack (1983) cogently argued that use of symbols, be they vocalizations or plastic chips, enables non-human subjects to organize, analyse and process information about their world in ways unavailable to those without such symbols. Only non-humans with symbolic representation succeed in the numerical studies described above. Vocal (and signed) communication may, however, raise such abilities to an additional level: not requiring the presence of human experimental apparatus, these formats provide additional means and opportunities to process information (Pepperberg, 1999).

All for One and One for All

Box 15.1 Vocal Labelling by Bottlenose Dolphins

Stephanie King

Vocal labelling, or naming of social companions, is one of the defining features of human language, thought to set us apart from other animals. We form individual bonds, maintain associations and make new acquaintances by learning people's names, and we use those names in social interactions, as a way of addressing and soliciting the attention of particular individuals. This has often been thought as a uniquely human trait. Indeed, this ability is rare in the animal kingdom and perhaps most notably absent in non-human primates (Janik and Slater, 1997).

In this chapter, Pepperberg clearly demonstrates the ability of Grey parrots to use learned vocal labels. This remarkable ability is also present in bottlenose dolphins: research in the laboratory shows they use novel, learned signals to referentially label objects (Richards *et al.*, 1984). The bottlenose dolphin (*Tursiops* spp.) is one of the best-studied cetaceans (whales, dolphins and porpoises), both under human care and in

(*cont.*)

the wild, allowing a number of cognitive questions to be addressed. Laboratory studies on the cognitive and communicative abilities of dolphins reveal some striking parallels with the cognitive studies described by Pepperberg: like parrots, dolphins can understand relative numerosities (Jaakkola *et al.*, 2005) and can succeed on visible displacement tasks (Jaakkola *et al.*, 2010). Bottlenose dolphins have also been shown to use learning and innovation to develop their own unique labels in the wild, which they then use to address each other (Janik *et al.*, 2006; King and Janik, 2013).

While dolphins and parrots have vastly different evolutionary histories, some of the cognitive and behavioural similarities between them are compelling. This is perhaps not surprising, given that both are open-ended vocal learners that form fission–fusion societies and likely face the same social pressures. For example, within their social systems, both taxa have high encounter rates with conspecifics, and are likely to develop an extensive network of vocal recognition. Moreover, identity is transmitted through the acoustic channel in both taxa, as vision is often restricted in their natural environments. Natural selection may, therefore, have favoured the development of vocal labels that facilitate accurate recognition in both parrots and dolphins (Tibbetts and Dale, 2007). As such, both taxa are particularly suitable study subjects for sound playback experiments – an experimental approach that can be employed both in the lab and in the field. Interactive playback is a powerful tool that has been used to shed light on the vocal prowess of dolphins (King, 2015), including the function of vocal imitation (Reiss and McCowen, 1993; King *et al.*, 2014; King and McGregor, 2016), and could easily be incorporated to standard playbacks currently used with parrots (Balsby *et al.*, 2012).

What is somewhat surprising is that we know more about the communicative abilities of wild dolphins than we do of wild parrots. Recent technological advances have allowed cetacean researchers to use arrays of underwater microphones and acoustic source localization to identify which dolphin and/or group of dolphins produced which call. This has led us to ascertain that vocal labels play a critical role in greeting sequences between dolphin groups that encounter each other in the wild (Quick and Janik, 2012). As Pepperberg highlights, the Grey parrot's deftness and propensity for removing telemetry tags and leg bands makes the study of communication in wild parrots challenging, but hopefully not insurmountable. Innovative designs by biologists and engineers mean we can now place telemetry tags on the deepest-diving whales, and ever-more compact devices are making deployment feasible on smaller and smaller species.

References

Balsby, T. J. S., Momberg, J. V., and Dabelsteen, T. (2012). Vocal imitation in parrots allows addressing of specific individuals in a dynamic communication network. *PLoS ONE*, **7**, e49747.

(*cont.*)

Jaakkola, K., Fellner, W., Erb, L., Rodriguez, M., and Guarino, E. (2005). Understanding of the concept of numerically 'less' by bottlenose dolphins (*Tursiops truncatus*). *Journal of Comparative Psychology*, **119**, 296–303.

Jaakkola, K., Guarino, E., Rodriguez, M., Erb, L., and Trone, M. (2010). What do dolphins (*Tursiops truncatus*) understand about hidden objects? *Animal Cognition*, **13**, 103–120.

Janik, V. M., and Slater, P. J. (1997). Vocal learning in mammals. *Advances in the Study of Behavior*, **26**, 59–99.

Janik, V. M., Sayigh, L. S., and Wells, R. S. (2006). Signature whistle shape conveys identity information to bottlenose dolphins. *Proceedings of the National Academy of Sciences*, **103**, 8293–8297.

King, S. L. (2015). You talkin' to me? Interactive playback is a powerful yet underused tool in animal communication research. *Biology Letters*, **11**, 20150403.

King, S. L., and Janik, V. M. (2013). Bottlenose dolphins use learned vocal labels to address each other. *Proceedings of the National Academy of Sciences*, **110**, 13216–13221.

King, S. L., and McGregor, P. K. (2016). Vocal matching: the what, the why and the how. *Biology Letters*, **12**, 20160666.

King, S. L., Harley, H. E., and Janik, V. M. (2014). The role of signature whistle matching in bottlenose dolphins (*Tursiops truncatus*). *Animal Behavior*, **96**, 79–86.

Quick, N. J., and Janik, V. M. (2012). Bottlenose dolphins exchange signature whistles when meeting at sea. *Proceedings of the Royal Society of London B: Biological Sciences*, **279**, 2539–2545.

Reiss, D., and McCowen, B. (1993). Spontaneous vocal mimicry and production by bottlenose dolphins (*Tursiops truncatus*). *Journal of Comparative Psychology*, **107**, 301–312.

Richards, D. G., Wolz, J. P., and Herman, L. M. (1984). Vocal mimicry of computer-generated sounds and vocal labeling of objects by a bottlenose dolphin, *Tursiops truncatus*. *Journal of Comparative Psychology*, **98**, 10–28.

Tibbetts, E. A., and Dale, J. (2007). Individual recognition: it is good to be different. *Trends in Ecology and Evolution*, **22**, 529–537.

Field Guide

Limited Practical Information in Nature

Greys are highly endangered across Africa (e.g. Dändliker, 1992; Annorbah *et al.*, 2016; see above; see http://tracybrighten.com/environment/african-grey-parrot-silenced-by-trap pingandlogging/). Many countries of origin are unstable politically; illegal poachers threaten researchers (May and Lynn, pers. comm.). Fieldwork can be extremely dangerous. Places previously accessible to foreigners with appropriate permits (e.g. Central African Republic, Cameroon) are now considerably less safe.

Other research problems abound. Grey parrots fly through the canopy, often covering 60 km/day (May, 2004), making them extremely difficult to follow. Their powerful beaks, used for allo- and auto-preening and nut-cracking, can destroy commonly used animal-tracking devices, as well as the types of coloured leg bands used on other species for individual identification. Plus, during perching, leg bands that survive their beaks are generally feather-covered and unreadable. They are intolerant of materials attached to their bodies. Thus, individual recognition by researchers is almost impossible (May, 2004). A brief report on feeding behaviour during the short-term fruiting of a particular tree also describes many problems involved in studying this species (Chapman *et al.*, 1993). Consequently, little has been published on Grey parrot ethology in nature and nothing directly relating to cognition. Additional information about their ethological and ecological niche would, however, allow testing of different theories about evolutionary pressures that may have selected for advanced cognition (e.g. the social group hypothesis; Jolly, 1966; Humphrey, 1976).

In conclusion, few details of Grey parrot life in Africa are known. Interestingly, Greys might now be migrating to urban environments (www.birdlife.org/worldwide/news/grey-parrot-fading-africas-rainforests); conceivably, their adaptation to living in small city parks will facilitate cognitive studies. Such studies would not, however, allow researchers to understand their use of cognitive abilities in forests and savannas.

Limited Guide to Laboratory Studies

Each Grey is an individual. Some are motivated by food (and each by a different food, which changes on a whim), others by toys. Some work for long stretches (up to an hour), others for only a few minutes at a time, and their proclivity to work changes from day to day. Researchers must determine characteristics of each bird to ensure success.

General requirements for these birds involve a healthy diet and both physical and mental exercise. The basic diet should consist of organic pellets and seasonally available fresh organic fruits and vegetables, cooked organic grains, limited nuts and seeds, and fresh water (preferably fluorinated). Some Greys like raw pasta and dry cereals. Some will need vitamin supplements (to be determined by each bird's veterinarian). Individual birds will favour particular aspects of the diet. Greys need to have cage space to exercise their wings (even if clipped) and many differently sized perches to exercise their foot muscles. They need to be challenged mentally with a number of simultaneous research projects or at least enrichment foraging toys.

Grey parrot juveniles are neophilic; neophobia increases with age. As with vocal learning (see below), observation is a powerful tool for habituating Greys to novelty. When introducing new objects to older birds, neophobia can be decreased if humans interact with the items and demonstrate their use. If humans eat new foods in the presence of a Grey, the bird is likely to consume it readily; they also often try new foods that other birds are already consuming.

M/R training to establish interspecific communication involves observational learning, i.e. three-way social interactions among two humans and a parrot, to demonstrate the targeted vocal behaviour (Pepperberg, 1981). The parrot watches and listens as one trainer presents objects and queries the other trainer about them (e.g. 'What's here?', 'What colour?'), giving praise and transferring the named object to the human partner to reward correct answers. Incorrect responses are punished by scolding and temporarily removing

Table 15.1. Essential experimental tools required to study Grey parrots and their function.

Tool	Function
Organic pellets, seasonally available fresh organic fruits and vegetables, cooked organic grains, limited nuts and seeds, fresh water (preferably fluorinated), raw pasta, cereals	Basic food for captive Greys. Choices need to be adapted to each individual due to interindividual preferences. Favourite items can be rewards
Big cage	Allows subjects to exercise/stretch wings
Variously sized perches	Allow subjects to exercise foot muscles
Enrichment foraging toys	Keep the subject mentally challenged
Two experimenters	Three-way social learning for interspecific communication training. One experimenter asks a question; the other one (the model) responds correctly (is rewarded) or wrongly (is scolded)
Label targets	For language learning, allow the parrot to link concepts with objects and later request objects
Strong materials for apparatus	To avoid allowing their powerful beaks to destroy research material
Coding sheet	To record the individual's responses
Camera/large hard drive on storage unit	To record the sessions and keep the progress of the subject on record
Microphone	To record the parrot's voice and sometimes that of the trainer
Audio editing programs	To record spectrograms and analyse vocalizations

items from sight. Thus the second human is both a model for the parrot's responses and its rival for the trainer's attention, and illustrates consequences of errors. The model must try again or talk more clearly if the response was deliberately incorrect or garbled; that is, the model is subject to corrective feedback, which the bird observes. Furthermore, the roles of trainer and model are exchanged, so that the parrot sees that either can be the questioner or the respondent. The parrot is included in interactions, being queried and rewarded for successive approximations to correct responses; training is adjusted to its performance level. If a bird is inattentive or accuracy regresses, trainers threaten to leave. Note that other training techniques (e.g. Pepperberg and McLaughlin, 1996; Pepperberg *et al.*, 1998b, 1999, 2000; Pepperberg and Wilkes, 2004) are considerably less successful.

To ensure the closest possible link between labels or concepts to be learned and their appropriate referent, M/R training uses only *intrinsic* reinforcers: reward for uttering 'X' is X, the object to which the label or concept refers. Earlier unsuccessful attempts to teach birds to communicate with humans used *extrinsic* rewards: a single food neither relating to, nor varying with, the label or concept being taught (see Pepperberg, 1999), which confounded the label of the targeted exemplar or concept with that of the food reward. Initial use of labels as requests also demonstrates that uttering labels has functionality; later, birds learned 'I want X', to separate requesting and labelling (Pepperberg, 1988a) and to enable them to request preferred rewards, while learning labels for items they had little interest in obtaining.

Although some countries prohibit solitary captivity, Greys learn human speech most readily when kept apart from each other: initial acquisition proceeds best if a single Grey is completely immersed in a human environment and communication with conspecifics is impossible. A young bird may learn labels from an older bird, but only if the older bird is already extremely proficient (Pepperberg *et al.*, 2000). Training young birds in groups is generally unsuccessful. When exposure is limited only to a few training sessions per day and birds spend the rest of their time communicating with conspecifics using native calls and whistles, little reason exists to learn to communicate with humans; human speech acquisition will fail or be extremely limited (e.g. Giret *et al.*, 2010).

Resources

Field studies by my students ended 20 years ago; the most recent detailed studies of Grey parrot habitat use, in Cameroon, are by Tamungang and colleagues (2016). Tamungang (Laboratory of Applied Ecology and Biology, Department of Animal Biology, University of Dschang, Cameroon) is probably the most knowledgeable source for information on field research on Greys. Simon Valle (Division of Biology and Conservation Ecology, School of Science and the Environment, Manchester Metropolitan University, Manchester, UK) also studies Greys on the Island of Principe.

French, Czech and Austrian laboratory studies on Greys have ended, but new cognitive studies at Loro Park, Tenerife, have begun, primarily under Auguste von Bayern (Max Planck Institute of Ornithology, Seeweisen, Germany). Preliminary studies on trap tubes and economic decision-making were presented at the 2017 International Ethological Congress in Portugal.

Profile

Irene received her SB (MIT, chemistry) and her PhD (Harvard, chemical physics). At Harvard, she realized her long-standing interest in animal behaviour was stronger than that in theoretical chemistry. While finishing her doctorate, she attended seminars and audited courses on communicative behaviours of animals in nature, avian biology, interspecific communication and human language acquisition. She subsequently switched fields completely, becoming involved in the then-novel studies on interspecific communication and animal cognition. She studied the Grey parrot because previous research had demonstrated these birds' cognitive abilities, brain capacity to support such abilities and, purportedly, the clearest speech of any non-human. At that date, few researchers studied avian cognition, mostly testing pigeons in operant chambers. The possibility of working with a non-human that could learn to talk and be tested exactly like a young child, so as to gain a window into its mind (Griffin, 1976), was the driving force behind the research.

References

Annorbah, N. N. D., Collar, N. J., and Marsden, S. J. (2016). Trade and habitat change virtually eliminate the Grey Parrot *Psittacus erithacus* from Ghana. *Ibis*, **158**, 82–91.

Bandura, A. (1971). Analysis of modeling processes. In *Psychological modeling* (pp. 1–62). Chicago, IL: Aldine-Atherton.

Beckers, G. J. L., Nelson, B. S., and Suthers, R. A. (2004). Vocal-tract filtering by lingual articulation in a parrot. *Current Biology*, **14**, 1592–1597.

Berg, K. S., Delgado, S., Okawa, R., Bessinger, S. R., and Bradbury, J. W. (2011). Contact calls are used for individual mate recognition in free-ranging green-rumped parrotlets, *Forpus passerinus*. *Animal Behaviour*, **81**, 241–248.

Berg, K. S., Delgado, S., Cortopassi, K. A., Bessiner, S. R., and Bradbury, J. W. (2012). Vertical transmission of learned signatures in a wild parrot. *Proceedings of the Royal Society of London B: Biological Sciences*, **279**, 585–591.

Berkhoudt, H. (1985). Structure and function of avian taste receptors. In *Form and function in birds* (pp. 463–496). New York, NY: Academic.

BirdLife International. (2016). *Psittacus erithacus*. The IUCN Red List of Threatened Species, 2016:e.T22724813A94879563.

Bock, W. J. (1978). Morphology of the larynx of *Corvus brachyrhynchos* (Passeriformes: Corvidae). *Wilson Bulletin*, **90**, 553–565.

Bottoni, L., Masin, S., and Lenti-Boero, D. (2009). Vowel-like sound structure in an African Grey parrot (*Psittacus erithacus*) vocal production. *The Open Behavioural Science Journal*, **3**, 1–16.

Bowmaker, J. K., Heath, L. A., Das, D., and Hunt, D. M. (1994). Spectral sensitivity and opsin structure of avian rod and cone visual pigments. *Investigative Ophthalmology and Visual Science*, **35**, 1708.

Bowmaker, J. K., Heath, L. A., Wilkie, S. E., Das, D., and Hunt, D. M. (1996). Middle-wave cone and rod visual pigments in birds: spectral sensitivity and opsin structure. *Investigative Ophthalmology and Visual Science*, **37**, 804.

Braun, H. (1952). Über das Unterscheidungsvermögen unbenannter Anzahlen bei Papageien [Concerning the ability of parrots to distinguish unnamed numbers]. *Zeitschrift für Tierpsychologie*, **9**, 40–91.

Bregman, M. R., Patel, A. D., and Gentner, T. Q. (2014). Songbirds use spectral shape, not pitch, for sound pattern recognition. *Proceedings of the National Academy of Sciences*, **113**, 1666–1671.

Brightsmith, D., and Villalobos, E. M. (2011). Parrot behaviour at a Peruvian clay lick. *Wilson Journal of Ornithology*, **123**, 595–602.

Butler, A. B., Manger, P. R., Lindahl, B. I. B., and Århem, P. (2005). Evolution of the neural basis of consciousness: a bird–mammal comparison. *BioEssays*, **27**, 923–936.

Carey, S. (2009). *The origin of concepts*. New York, NY: Oxford University Press.

Carey, S., Gray, S. L., Mody, S., Cornero, F., and Pepperberg, I. M. (in prep.). Inferential reasoning by a Grey parrot: three- and four-cup exclusion studies.

Carvalho, L. S., Knott, B., Berg, M. L., Bennett, A. T. D., and Hunt, D. M. (2011). Ultraviolet-sensitive vision in long-lived birds. *Proceedings of the Royal Society of London B: Biological Sciences*, **278**, 107–114.

Chakraborty, M., Walløe, S., Nedergaard, S., *et al.* (2015). Core and shell song systems unique to the parrot brain. *PLoS ONE*, **10**(6), e0118496.

Chapman, C. A., Chapman, L. J., and Wrangham, R. (1993). Observations on the feeding biology and population ecology of the Grey Parrot *Psittacus erithacus*. *Scopus*, **16**, 89–93.

Cobb, S. (1960). Observations on the comparative anatomy of the avian brain. In *Perspectives in biology and medicine* (pp. 383–408). Chicago, IL: University of Chicago Press.

Connor, R. C. (2007). Dolphin social intelligence: complex alliance relationships in bottlenose dolphins and a consideration of selective environments for extreme brain size evolution in mammals. *Philosophical Transactions of the Royal Society B: Biological Sciences*, **362**, 587–602.

Cruickshank, A. J., Gautier, J.-P., and Chappius, C. (1993). Vocal mimicry in wild African Grey parrots *Psittacus erithacus*. *Ibis*, **135**, 293–299.

Cuthill, I. C., Hart, N. S., Partridge, J. C., Bennett, A. T. D., Hunt, S., and Church, S. C. (2000). Avian colour vision and avian colour playback experiments. *Acta Ethologica*, **3**, 29–37.

Dahlin, C. R., Young, A. M., Cordier, B., Mundry, R., and Wright, T. F. (2014). A test of multiple hypotheses for the function of call sharing in female budgerigars, *Melopsittacus undulatus*. *Behavioural Ecology and Sociobiology*, **68**, 145–161.

Dändliker, G. (1992). *The Grey parrot in Ghana: a population survey, a contribution to the biology of the species, a study of its commercial exploitation and management recommendations*. A report on CITES project S-30. Lausanne, Switzerland: CITES Secretariat.

Demery, Z. P., Chappell, J., and Martin, G. R. (2011). Vision, touch and object manipulation in Senegal parrots, *Poicephalus senegalus*. *Proceedings of the Royal Society of London B: Biological Sciences*, **278**, 3687–3693.

Dooling, R. J. (1986). Perception of vocal signals by budgerigars (*Melopsittacus undulatus*). *Experimental Biology*, **45**, 195–218.

Dooling, R. J., Lohr, B., and Dent, M. L. (2000). Hearing in birds and reptiles. In *Comparative hearing in birds and reptiles* (pp. 308–359). New York, NY: Springer.

Farabaugh, S. M., and Dooling, R. J. (1996). Acoustic communication in parrots: laboratory and field studies of budgerigars, *Melopsittacus undulatus*. In *Ecology and evolution of acoustic communication in birds* (pp. 97–117). Ithaca, NY: Cornell University Press.

Fotso, R. (1998). *Survey status of the distribution and utilization of the Grey parrot (Psittacus erithacus) in Cameroon*. A report for the CITES Secretariat. Lausanne, Switzerland: CITES.

Gaunt, A. S., and Gaunt, S. L. L. (1985). Electromyographic studies of the syrinx in parrots (Aves: Psittacidae). *Zoomorphology*, **105**, 1–11.

Gelfand, S. (2016). *Essentials of audiology*. New York, NY: Thieme.

Giret, N., Miklósi, A., Kreutzer, M., and Bovet, D. (2009). Use of experimenter-given cues by African Grey parrots (*Psittacus erithacus*). *Animal Cognition*, **12**, 1–10.

Giret, N., Péron, F., Lindová, J., *et al.* (2010). Referential learning of French and Czech labels in African grey parrots (*Psittacus erithacus*): different methods yield contrasting results. *Behavioural Processes*, **85**, 90–98.

Goldsmith, T., and Butler, B. K. (2005). Colour vision of the budgerigar (*Melopsittacus undulatus*): hue matches, tetrachromacy, and intensity discrimination. *Journal of Comparative Physiology A*, **191**, 933–951.

Gnam, R. (1988). Preliminary results on the breeding biology of Bahama amazon. *Parrot Letter*, **1**, 23–26.

Greenewalt, C. H. (1968). *Bird song: acoustics and physiology*. Washington, DC: Smithsonian Institution Press.

Griffin, D. R. (1976). *The question of animal awareness: evolutionary continuity of mental experience*. New York, NY: Rockefeller University Press.

Hedges, S. B., Parker, P. H., Sibley, C. G., and Kumar, S. (1996). Continental breakup and the ordinal diversification of birds and mammals. *Nature*, **381**, 226–229.

Hile, A. G., Plummer, T. K., and Striedter, G. F. (2000). Male vocal imitation produces call convergence during pair bonding in budgerigars, *Melopsittacus undulatus*. *Animal Behaviour*, **59**, 1209–1218.

Hile, A. G., Burley, N. T., Coopersmith, C. B., Foster, V. S., and Striedter, G. F. (2005). Effects of male vocal learning on female behaviour in the budgerigar, *Melopsittacus undulatus*. *Ethology*, **111**, 901–923.

Hillemann, F., Bugnyar, T., Kotrschal, K., and Wascher, C. A. F. (2014). Waiting for better, not for more: corvids respond to quality in two delay maintenance tasks. *Animal Behaviour*, **90**, 1–10.

Homberger, D. G. (1979). Functional morphology of the larynx in the parrot *Psittacus erithacus*. Abstract of paper presented at the annual meeting of the American Society for Zoologists. *American Zoologist*, **19**, 988.

Homberger, D. G. (1986). The lingual apparatus of the African Grey parrot, *Psittacus erithacus* Linne (Aves: Psittacidae). Description and theoretical mechanical analysis. *Ornithological Monographs*, **39**.

Homberger, D. G. (1999). The avian linguo-buccal system: multiple functions in nutrition and vocalization. In *Proceedings of the XXIInd International Ornithological Congress* (pp. 94–113). Durban: University of Natal.

Humphrey, N. K. (1976). The social function of intellect. In *Growing points in ethology* (pp. 303–317). Cambridge: Cambridge University Press.

Ikebuchi, M., and Okanoya, K. (1999). Male zebra finches and Bengalese finches emit directed songs to the video images of conspecific females projected onto a TFT display. *Zoological Science*, **16**, 63–70.

Jarvis, E. D., Güntürkün, O., Bruce, L., *et al.* (2005). Avian brains and a new understanding of vertebrate evolution. *Nature Reviews Neuroscience*, **6**, 151–159.

Jarvis, E. D., Yu, J., Rivas, M. V., *et al.* (2013). Global view of the functional molecular organization of the avian cerebrum: mirror images and functional columns. *Journal of Comparative Neurology*, **521**, 3614–3665.

Jolly, A. (1966). Lemur social behaviour and primate intelligence. *Science*, **153**, 501–506.

Juniper, T., and Parr, M. (1998). *Parrots: a guide to parrots of the world*. New Haven, CT: Yale University Press.

Kalischer, O. (1901). Weitere Mittheilung zur Grosshirnlocalisation bei den Vogeln [Further information on cerebral lesions in birds]. *Preussian Akademie der Wissenschaften, Berlin*, **1**, 428–439.

Koehler, O. (1950). The ability of birds to 'count'. *Bulletin of the Animal Behaviour Society*, **9**, 41–45.

Koehler, O. (1953). Thinking without words. *Proceedings of the XIVth International Congress of Zoology*, 75–88.

Koepke, A., Gray, S. L., and Pepperberg, I. M. (2015). Delayed gratification: a Grey parrot (*Psittacus erithacus*) will wait for a better reward. *Journal of Comparative Psychology*, **129**, 339–346.

Kuczaj, S. A. (1983). *Crib speech and language play*. New York, NY: Springer.

Lögler, P. (1959). Versuche zur Frage des 'Zähl'-Vermögens an einem Graupapagei und Vergleichsversuche an Menschen [Studies on the question of 'number' sense in a Grey parrot and comparative studies on humans]. *Zeitschrift für Tierpsychologie*, **16**, 179–217.

May, D. L. (2004). *The vocal repertoire of Grey Parrots (Psittacus erithacus) living in the Congo Basin (Central African Republic, Cameroon)*. PhD thesis, University of Arizona.

Mikolasch, S., Kotrschal, K., and Schloegl, C. (2011). African Grey parrots (*Psittacus erithacus*) use inference by exclusion to find hidden food. *Biology Letters*, **7**, 875–877.

Mody, S., and Carey, S. (2016). The emergence of reasoning by the disjunctive syllogism in early childhood. *Cognition*, **154**, 40–48.

Necker, R. (2000). The somatosensory system. In *Sturkie's avian physiology* (pp. 57–69). San Diego, CA: Academic Press.

Nguyen, A. P, Spetch, M. L., Crowder, N. A., Winship, I. R., Hurd, P. L., and Wylie, D. R. W. (2004). A dissociation of motion and spatial-pattern vision in the avian telencephalon: implications for the evolution of 'visual streams'. *Journal of Neuroscience*, **24**, 4962–4970.

Nottebohm, F. (1976). Phonation in the orange-winged Amazon parrot. *Journal of Comparative Physiology A*, **108**, 157–170.

Ohms, V. R., Beckers, G. J. L., ten Cate, C., and Suthers, R. A. (2012). Vocal tract articulation revisited: the case of the monk parakeet. *The Journal of Experimental Biology*, **215**, 85–92.

Okanoya, K., and Dooling, R. J. (1987). Hearing in passerine and psittacine birds: a comparative study of absolute and masked thresholds. *Journal of Comparative Psychology*, **101**, 7–15.

Olkowicz, S., Kocourek, M., Lučan, R. K., *et al.* (2016). Birds have primate-like numbers of neurons in the forebrain. *Proceedings of the National Academy of Sciences*, **113**, 7255–7260.

Patterson, D. K., and Pepperberg, I. M. (1994). A comparative study of human and parrot phonation: I. Acoustic and articulatory correlates of vowels. *Journal of the Acoustical Society of America*, **96**, 634–648.

Patterson, D. K., and Pepperberg, I. M. (1998). A comparative study of human and Grey parrot phonation: II. Acoustic and articulatory correlates of stop consonants. *Journal of the Acoustical Society of America*, **103**, 2197–2213.

Patterson, D. K., Pepperberg, I. M., Story, B. H., and Hoffman, E. (1997). How parrots talk: insights based on CT scans, image processing, and mathematical models. In *SPIE proceedings: physiology and function from multidimensional images* (pp. 14–24). Washington, DC: Bellingham.

Pepperberg, I. M. (1981). Functional vocalizations by an African Grey parrot. *Zeitschrift für Tierpsychologie*, **55**, 139–160.

Pepperberg, I. M. (1983). Cognition in the African Grey parrot: preliminary evidence for auditory/vocal comprehension of the class concept. *Animal Learning & Behaviour*, **11**, 179–185.

Pepperberg, I. M. (1987a). Acquisition of the same/different concept by an African Grey parrot (*Psittacus erithacus*): learning with respect to categories of colour, shape, and material. *Animal Learning & Behaviour*, **15**, 423–432.

Pepperberg, I. M. (1987b). Evidence for conceptual quantitative abilities in the African Grey parrot: labeling of cardinal sets. *Ethology*, **75**, 37–61.

Pepperberg, I. M. (1988a). An interactive modeling technique for acquisition of communication skills: separation of 'labeling' and 'requesting' in a psittacine subject. *Applied Psycholinguistics*, **9**, 59–76.

Pepperberg, I. M. (1988b). Comprehension of 'absence' by an African Grey parrot: learning with respect to questions of same/different. *Journal of the Experimental Analysis of Behaviour*, **50**, 553–564.

Pepperberg, I. M. (1990a). Cognition in an African Grey parrot (*Psittacus erithacus*): further evidence for comprehension of categories and labels. *Journal of Comparative Psychology*, **104**, 41–52.

Pepperberg, I. M. (1990b). Referential mapping: attaching functional significance to the innovative utterances of an African Grey parrot. *Applied Psycholinguistics*, **11**, 23–44.

Pepperberg, I. M. (1992). Proficient performance of a conjunctive, recursive task by an African Grey parrot (*Psittacus erithacus*). *Journal of Comparative Psychology*, **106**, 295–305.

Pepperberg, I. M. (1994a). Evidence for numerical competence in an African Grey parrot (*Psittacus erithacus*). *Journal of Comparative Psychology*, **108**, 36–44.

Pepperberg, I. M. (1994b). Vocal learning in African Grey parrots: effects of social interaction, reference and context. *Auk*, **111**, 300–313.

Pepperberg, I. M. (1996). Categorical class formation by an African Grey parrot (*Psittacus erithacus*). In *Stimulus class formation in humans and animals* (pp. 71–90). Amsterdam: Elsevier.

Pepperberg, I. M. (1999). *The Alex studies*. Cambridge, MA: Harvard University Press.

Pepperberg, I. M. (2002). Allospecific referential speech acquisition in Grey parrots: evidence for multiple levels of avian vocal imitation. In *Imitation in animals and artifacts* (pp. 109–131). Cambridge, MA: MIT Press.

Pepperberg, I. M. (2006a). Addition by a Grey parrot (*Psittacus erithacus*), including absence of quantity. *Journal of Comparative Psychology*, **120**, 1–11.

Pepperberg, I. M. (2006b). Ordinality and inferential abilities of a Grey parrot (*Psittacus erithacus*). *Journal of Comparative Psychology*, **120**, 205–216.

Pepperberg, I. M. (2007). Grey parrots do not always 'parrot': roles of imitation and phonological awareness in the creation of new labels from existing vocalizations. *Language Sciences*, **29**, 1–13.

Pepperberg, I. M. (2012a). Further evidence for addition and numerical competence by a Grey parrot (*Psittacus erithacus*). *Animal Cognition*, **15**, 711–717.

Pepperberg, I. M. (2012b). Symbolic communication in the Grey parrot. In *The Oxford handbook of comparative evolutionary psychology* (pp. 297–319). New York, NY: Oxford University Press.

Pepperberg, I. M. (2015). Reply to Jaakkola (2014): 'Do animals understand invisible displacements? A critical review'. *Journal of Comparative Psychology*, **129**, 198–201.

Pepperberg, I. M. (in press). Human–Grey parrot comparisons in cognitive performance. In *Cambridge handbook of evolutionary perspectives on human behaviour*. Cambridge: Cambridge University Press.

Pepperberg, I. M., and Brezinsky, M. V. (1991). Acquisition of a relative class concept by an African Grey parrot (*Psittacus erithacus*): discriminations based on relative size. *Journal of Comparative Psychology*, **105**, 286–294.

Pepperberg, I. M., and Carey, S. (2012). Grey parrot number acquisition: the inference of cardinal value from ordinal position on the numeral list. *Cognition*, **125**, 219–232.

Pepperberg, I. M., and Funk, M. S. (1990). Object permanence in four species of psittacine birds. *Animal Learning & Behaviour*, **18**, 97–108.

Pepperberg, I. M., and Gordon, J. D. (2005). Number comprehension by a Grey parrot (*Psittacus erithacus*), including a zero-like concept. *Journal of Comparative Psychology*, **119**, 197–209.

Pepperberg, I. M., and Kozak, F. A. (1986). Object permanence in the African Grey parrot (*Psittacus erithacus*). *Animal Learning & Behaviour*, **14**, 322–330.

Pepperberg, I. M., and McLaughlin, M. A. (1996). Effect of avian–human joint attention on allospecific vocal learning by Grey parrots (*Psittacus erithacus*). *Journal of Comparative Psychology*, **110**, 286–297.

Pepperberg, I. M., and Nakayama, K. (2016). Robust representation of shape by a Grey parrot (*Psittacus erithacus*). *Cognition*, **153**, 146–160.

Pepperberg, I. M., and Shive, H. A. (2001). Simultaneous development of vocal and physical object combinations by a Grey parrot (*Psittacus erithacus*): bottle caps, lids, and labels. *Journal of Comparative Psychology*, **115**, 376–384.

Pepperberg, I. M., and Wilcox, S. E. (2000). Evidence for a form of mutual exclusivity during label acquisition by Grey parrots (*Psittacus erithacus*)? *Journal of Comparative Psychology*, **114**, 219–231.

Pepperberg, I. M., and Wilkes, S. (2004). Lack of referential vocal learning from LCD video by Grey parrots (*Psittacus erithacus*). *Interaction Studies*, **5**, 75–97.

Pepperberg, I. M., Brese, K. J., and Harris, B. J. (1991). Solitary sound play during acquisition of English vocalizations by an African Grey parrot (*Psittacus erithacus*): possible parallels with children's monologue speech. *Applied Psycholinguistics*, **12**, 151–177.

Pepperberg, I. M., Garcia, S. E., Jackson, E. C., and Marconi, S. (1995). Mirror use by African Grey parrots (*Psittacus erithacus*). *Journal of Comparative Psychology*, **109**, 182–195.

Pepperberg, I. M., Willner, M. R., and Gravitz, L. B. (1997). Development of Piagetian object permanence in a Grey parrot (*Psittacus erithacus*). *Journal of Comparative Psychology*, **111**, 63–75.

Pepperberg, I. M., Howell, K. S., Banta, P. A., Patterson, D. K., and Meister, M. (1998a). Measurement of the trachea of the Grey parrot (*Psittacus erithacus*) via magnetic resonance imaging, dissection, and electron beam computed tomography. *Journal of Morphology*, **238**, 81–91.

Pepperberg, I. M., Naughton, J. R., and Banta, P. A. (1998b). Allospecific vocal learning by Grey parrots (*Psittacus erithacus*): a failure of videotaped instruction under certain conditions. *Behavioural Processes*, **42**, 139–158.

Pepperberg, I. M., Gardiner, L. I., and Luttrell, L. J. (1999). Limited contextual vocal learning in the Grey parrot (*Psittacus erithacus*): the effect of co-viewers on videotaped instruction. *Journal of Comparative Psychology*, **113**, 158–172.

Pepperberg, I. M., Sandefer, R. M., Noel, D., and Ellsworth, C. P. (2000). Vocal learning in the Grey parrot (*Psittacus erithacus*): effect of species identity and number of trainers. *Journal of Comparative Psychology*, **114**, 371–380.

Pepperberg, I. M., Vicinay, J., and Cavanagh, P. (2008). The Müller-Lyer illusion is processed by a Grey parrot (*Psittacus erithacus*). *Perception*, **37**, 765–781.

Pepperberg, I. M., Koepke, A., Livingston, P., Girard, M., and Hartsfield, L. A. (2013). Reasoning by inference: further studies on exclusion in Grey parrots (*Psittacus erithacus*). *Journal of Comparative Psychology*, **127**, 272–281.

Pepperberg, I. M., Gray, S. L., Lesser, J. S., and Hartsfield, L. A. (2017). Piagetian liquid conservation in Grey parrots (*Psittacus erithacus*). *Journal of Comparative Psychology*, **131**, 370–383.

Péron, F., Rat-Fischer, L., Lalot, M., and Bovet, D. (2011). Cooperative problem solving in African Grey parrots (*Psittacus erithacus*). *Animal Cognition*, **14**, 545–553.

Péron, F., Johns, M., Sapowicz, S., Bovet, D., and Pepperberg, I. M. (2013). A study of reciprocity in Grey parrots (*Psittacus erithacus*). *Animal Cognition*, **16**, 197–210.

Péron, F., Thornburg, L., Gross, B., Gray, S., and Pepperberg, I. M. (2014). Further studies on Grey parrot reciprocity. *Animal Cognition*, **17**, 937–944.

Portmann, A. (1950). Système nerveux. In *Traité de Zoologie* (pp. 185–203). Paris: Masson.

Portmann, A., and Stingelin, W. (1961). The central nervous system. In *Biology and comparative physiology of birds* (pp. 1–36). New York, NY: Academic Press.

Premack, D. (1983). The codes of man and beast. *Behavioural and Brain Sciences*, **6**, 125–167.

Premack, D., and Premack, A. J. (1994). Levels of causal understanding in chimpanzees and children. *Cognition*, **50**, 347–362.

Regolin, L., Marconato, F., and Vallortigara, G. (2004). Hemispheric differences in the recognition of partly occluded objects by newly hatched domestic chicks (*Gallus gallus*). *Animal Cognition*, **7**, 162–170.

Riede, T., and Goller, F. (2010). Peripheral mechanisms for vocal production in birds – differences and similarities to human speech and singing. *Brain and Language*, **115**, 69–80.

Santos, S. I. C. O., Elward, B., and Lumeij, J. T. (2006). Sexual dichromatism in the blue-fronted Amazon parrot (*Amazona aestiva*) revealed by multiple-angle spectrometry. *Journal of Avian Medicine and Surgery*, **20**, 8–14.

Scanlan, J. (1988). *Analysis of avian 'speech': patterns and production.* London: University College London.

Schloegl, C., Schmidt, J., Boeckle, M., Weiss, B. M., and Kotrschal, K. (2012). Grey parrots use inferential reasoning based on acoustic cues alone. *Proceedings of the Royal Society of London B: Biological Sciences*, **279**, 4135–4142.

Stettner, L. J. (1967). Brain lesions in birds: effects on discrimination acquisition and reversal. *Science*, **155**, 1689–1692.

Tamungang, S. A., and Cheke, R. A. (2012). *Population status and management plan of the African Grey parrot (Psittacus erithacus) in Cameroon. Full report prepared by MINFOF for CITES Secretariat.* Geneva: CITES.

Tamungang, S. A., Ayodele, I. A., and Akum, Z. E. (2001). Basic home range characteristics for the conservation of the African Grey parrot (*Psittacus erithacus*) in the Korup National Park, Cameroon. *Journal of the Cameroon Academy of Sciences*, **1**, 155–158.

Tamungang, S. A., Cheke, R. A., Mofor, G. Z., Tamungang, R. N., and Oben, F. T. (2014). Conservation concern for the deteriorating geographical range of the Grey Parrot in Cameroon. *International Journal of Ecology*, article ID 753294.

Tamungang, S. A., Onabid, M. A., Awa, T. II, and Balinga, V. S. (2016). Habitat preferences of the Grey parrot in heterogeneous vegetation landscapes and their conservation implications. *International Journal of Biodiversity*, autide ID 7287563.

Thompson, A. M., and Moreau, R. E. (1957). Feeding habits of the palm-nut vulture *Gypohierax. Ibis*, **99**, 608–613.

Todt, D. (1975). Social learning of vocal patterns and modes of their application in Grey parrots. *Zeitschrift für Tierpsychologie*, **39**, 178–188.

Tommasi, L., and Vallortigara, G. (2001). Encoding of geometric and landmark information in the left and right hemispheres of the avian brain. *Behavioural Neurosciences*, **115**, 602–613.

Trick, L., and Pylyshyn, Z. (1989). *Subitizing and the FNST spatial index model.* Oshawa, ON: University of Ontario.

Trick, L., and Pylyshyn, Z. (1994). Why are small and large numbers enumerated differently? A limited-capacity preattentive stage in vision. *Psychological Review*, **101**, 80–102.

Vick, S. J., Bovet, D., and Anderson, J. R. (2010). How do African Grey parrots (*Psittacus erithacus*) perform on a delay of gratification task? *Animal Cognition*, **13**, 351–358.

Wanker, R., Sugama, Y., and Prinage, S. (2005). Vocal labeling of family members in spectacled parrotlets, *Forpus conspicillatus. Animal Behaviour*, **70**, 111–118.

Warren, D. K., Patterson, D. K., and Pepperberg, I. M. (1996). Mechanisms of American English vowel production in a Grey parrot (*Psittacus erithacus*). *Auk*, **113**, 41–58.

White, S. S. (1968). Movements of the larynx during crowing in the domestic cock. *Journal of Anatomy*, **103**, 390–392.

Wilkie, S. E., Vissers, P. M. A. M., Das, D., DeGrip, W. J., Bowmaker, J. K., and Hunt, D. M. (1998). The molecular basis for UV vision in birds: spectral characteristics, cDNA sequence and retinal localization of the UV-sensitive visual pigment of the budgerigar (*Melopsittacus undulatus*). *Biochemical Journal*, **330**, 541–547.

Wilson, G. H. (2006). Behaviour of captive psittacids in the breeding aviary. In *Manual of parrot behaviour* (pp. 281–290). Oxford: Blackwell.

Wright, T. F., Cortopassi, K. A., Bradbury, J. W., and Dooling, R. J. (2003). Hearing and vocalizations in the orange-fronted conure (*Aratinga canicularis*). *Journal of Comparative Psychology*, **117**, 87–95.

16 Sharks – Elasmobranch Cognition

Tristan L. Guttridge, Kara E. Yopak and Vera Schluessel

Species Description

Anatomy

Cartilaginous fishes (class: Chondrichthyes) hold an important basal position at the onset of gnathostomes (jawed vertebrates), with evidence in the fossil record dating back approximately 400 million years ago (see Grogan *et al.*, 2012). They share several distinctive features, including an internal skeleton comprised entirely of cartilage, paired fins, placoid dermal scales, external copulatory organs and internal fertilization, 5–7 paired gill slits, and a battery of highly developed senses (see Collin *et al.*, 2015). There are approximately 1200 extant species, which are divided into the Elasmobranchii (sharks, skates and rays), representing 96 per cent of described species, and the Holocephali (e.g. chimaeras and ratfishes). Taxonomic relationships within these groups remain partially unresolved (see Naylor *et al.*, 2012).

Furthermore, sharks have a remarkable diversity in terms of their morphological and physiological attributes, including body form, swimming mode, ventilation strategy and reproductive mode. Indeed, members of this group range from the smallest documented species, the dwarf lantern shark, *Etmopterus perryi* (180–212 mm), up to the largest fish in the sea, the whale shark, *Rhincodon typus* (up to 12 m). Although all swim with a form of lateral undulation, this can range from anguilliform (e.g. Orectolobiformes) to thunniform (e.g. Lamniformes) swimming. Many of the large-bodied carangiform and thunniform swimmers are also obligate ram ventilators, whereby they must swim continuously, thus expending the greatest amount of metabolic energy, while many less-active, benthic species ventilate via active buccal pumping (see Wegner, 2015).

Ecological Characteristics

Chondricthyans are one of the most speciose lineages of predators on earth, playing important functional roles in the top-down control of coastal and oceanic ecosystem structure and function (Ferretti *et al.*, 2010). They occupy nearly every aquatic niche, from coastal habitats, to coral reefs, to the open ocean, to deep water and freshwater. Within these habitats, feeding strategy can range from planktivores (e.g. *Rhincodon, Megachasma*) to apex predators (e.g. *Carcharodon*), from specialists (e.g. *Sphyrna tiburo*) to generalist feeders (e.g. *Galeocerdo*), with shifts in diet that occur ontogenetically (Wetherbee and Cortes, 2004). Further, many species are known to undertake long-range movements and therefore serve as important mobile link species between ecosystems, playing an important part in the structure and stability of these systems (Ferretti *et al.*, 2010).

Perception – Peripheral and Central Nervous System

As previously stated, sharks occupy nearly every aquatic niche and each species is adapted to a complex set of environmental conditions. Although all species possess the same sensory modalities, which include chemoreception (olfaction and gustation), vision, mechanoreception (both lateral line and cutaneous touch), audition and electroreception, the relative importance of different sensory systems likely varies both inter- and intraspecifically, in terms of size and morphology of the peripheral sense organs, detection thresholds and sensitivity (Gardiner *et al.*, 2012; Collin *et al.*, 2015).

Brain Anatomy

Gnathostomes possess a common brain 'bauplan', consisting of the forebrain (olfactory bulbs, telencephalon and diencephalon), midbrain (mesencephalon) and hindbrain (cerebellum and medulla; Striedter, 2005; Figure 16.1). The most rostral component of the brain is the paired olfactory bulbs (OBs), which are associated with processing olfactory information (Meredith and Kajiura, 2010). Olfactory information is sent from the OBs on to the telencephalon, which can comprise up to as much as 67 per cent of the brain in the great, hammerhead, *Sphryna mokarran* (Yopak *et al.*, 2007). This structure

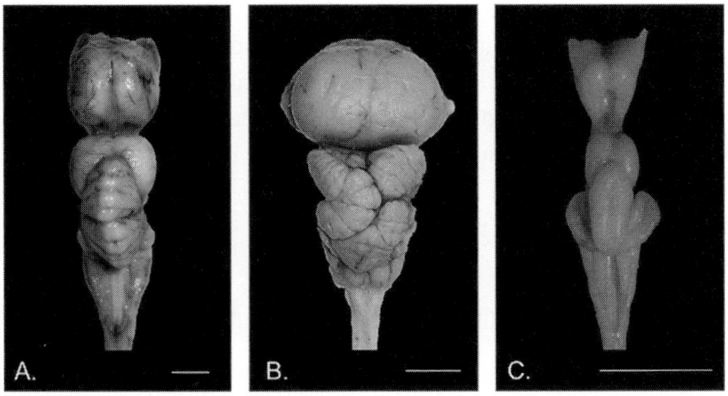

Figure 16.1. Photomicrographs of the brain of (A) the great white shark, *Carcharodon carcharias* (adapted from Yopak, 2012a, illustration reprinted with kind permission of John Wiley and Sons), (B) the smooth hammerhead, *Sphyrna zygaena* (adapted from Yopak *et al.*, 2007, © 2007 Karger Publishers, Basel, Switzerland), and (C) the blackbelly lanternshark, *Etmopterus lucifer* (adapted from Yopak and Montgomery, 2008, Copyright © 2008 Karger Publishers, Basel, Switzerland), in dorsal view, representing the dramatic differences in brain size and morphology across species. Scale bars correspond to 1 cm.

is implicated in a variety of functions (Hofmann and Northcutt, 2012), including multimodal sensory integration, complex behavioural control and higher cognitive functions, such as learning and memory, which likely occur in different subregions (Schluessel, 2015). The telencephalon is heavily interconnected with the diencephalon, which acts as an interface between the brain and the endocrine system (Smeets *et al.*, 1983). The midbrain is most readily associated with vision and visual processing (Graeber and Ebbesson, 1972), and is also involved in the processing of multisensory information (see Yopak, 2012a).

The function of the cerebellum has been an area of considerable speculation, although it is generally agreed that it is an effective regulator of motor control and adaptive motor learning (Montgomery *et al.*, 2012). Variation in size, convolution and symmetry of this structure across species (e.g. Puzdrowski and Gruber, 2009; Ari, 2011; Yopak *et al.*, 2016) likely reflects variation in cerebellar-dependent function and behavioural complexity (Yopak *et al.*, 2017). The medulla oblongata is the most caudal component of the hindbrain; it receives primary projections from the octavolateralis senses, which include the acoustic and vestibular system, electroreceptors and mechanoreceptive lateral line, and processes motor and sensory information (Smeets *et al.*, 1983). It also functions in sensory adaptive filtering, which effectively cancels out expected electroreceptive input (Bell *et al.*, 1997; Bodznick *et al.*, 1999), with implications for animals housed in captivity, who may habituate to continuous sensory signals.

Life History

Chondrichthyans tend to be long-lived, slow-growing species and possess the most diverse array of reproductive strategies of any vertebrate group, ranging from egg-laying to live-bearing with placental matrotrophy (e.g. Dulvy and Reynolds, 1997; Reynolds *et al.*, 2002). In many species, the developmental period is long (e.g. 6–10 months) and results in the production of small numbers of highly developed young. Chondrichthyans also exhibit direct development, where newborns resemble miniature versions of the adults (Helfman *et al.*, 1997). Most captive studies involve juveniles for practical purposes, due to size limitations of holding tanks and maintenance, although numerous characters can vary from juvenile to adult stages.

Ontogenetic Shifts in the Brain and Sensory Systems

Cartilaginous fishes experience indeterminate growth (Sebens, 1987), with brains (and other organs) that continue to grow throughout their lifespan (Gage, 2002), resulting in a highly plastic nervous system. The life histories of most sharks are characterized by ontogenetic shifts in habitat, movement patterns, diet and behaviour (e.g. Wetherbee and Cortés, 2004; Grubbs, 2010). Similarly, ontogenetic shifts in sensory systems have been documented, including response properties in the visual system (e.g. Litherland *et al.*, 2009a, b; Lisney *et al.*, 2012; Harahush *et al.*, 2014) and in the electroreceptive system (Sisneros and Tricas, 2002). These shifts in sensory organization may confer a functional shift in sensitivity and/or specialization, and suggest the peripheral nervous system may be highly susceptible to environmental conditions in a captive setting. In addition to post-parturition changes in peripheral sense organs, there is also evidence for varying sensory sensitivity in embryonic stages (Peters and Evers, 1985; Kempster *et al.*, 2013), with repeated exposure to sensory stimuli during the embryonic phase possibly impacting learning post-hatching, although the severity of the effects may vary across study species.

Although data are sparse, these ontogenetic shifts in habitat and sensory systems may have corresponding ontogenetic shifts in brain organization. For example, Lisney and colleagues (2007) demonstrated that, across seven species, the optic tectum is relatively enlarged in juveniles, while the olfactory bulbs were relatively enlarged in adults, suggestive of an ontogenetic shift in the importance of vision versus olfaction. Studies on the whale shark, *Rhincodon typus* (Yopak and Frank, 2009), and the blue spotted stingray, *Neotrygon kuhlii* (Lisney *et al.*, 2017), both showed an increase in the degree of folding of the cerebellum throughout life, which may reflect improved locomotor performance or the expansion of activity space. *N. kuhlii* also shows an increase in the size of the olfactory bulbs in mature individuals, although less than other species (Lisney *et al.*, 2007), which suggests that the degree of plasticity may be more pronounced in some species over others.

Given their functional implications, consideration of these ontogenetic shifts in peripheral and central organization is critical when undertaking behavioural studies. While juveniles are often easier to house in a laboratory setting, they may be more susceptible to plastic changes in the brain in relation to their rearing environment than adults. Although the brain continues to grow through adulthood, the steepest period of brain growth is often during the early juvenile stages (e.g. Lisney *et al.*, 2017), suggestive of a sensitive period before the onset of sexual maturity, where structural (and potentially functional) changes may be induced more rapidly.

Captive Rearing and Its Effects on the Brain

Having a brain that grows forever can have substantial implications for animals reared in captivity (see Gonda *et al.*, 2013). Although not studied extensively in cartilaginous fishes, work on bony fishes has shown that brain size and brain organization can vary between wild-caught and captive-reared populations (e.g. Marchetti and Nevitt, 2003; Lema *et al.*, 2005). Artificial selection studies in guppies have shown that large-brained individuals outperform small-brained individuals in a cognitive learning task, which suggests that an increase in brain size confers a cognitive advantage (e.g. Kotrschal *et al.*, 2013). Given this evidence in other species with indeterminate growth, captivity is likely to similarly induce plastic changes in the brain in cartilaginous fishes. Thus, consideration (and consistency) of rearing environment, learning opportunities and spatial structures across specimens, in addition to age class, are vital when selecting study species and designing cognitive studies in this group.

Sociality

Although the social characteristics of sharks and rays are not well understood, some species, such as the white shark (*Carcharodon carcharias*), are known to be solitary, while others, such as sphyrnid sharks and myliobatid rays, are considered social animals (Jacoby *et al.*, 2012a), which aggregate or form true schools, ranging in size from less than ten to thousands of individuals. These groupings are often segregated by sex or size, which may partly be the result of ontogenetic shifts in habitat and availability of resources (see Grubbs, 2010). There is also evidence of relatively complex social and reproductive behaviours, such as dominance hierarchies and courtship behaviour (see Jacoby *et al.*, 2012b). More recent studies have shown that some shark species organize into structured social networks, have preferred associations, recognize familiars and are able to learn from conspecifics (Jacoby *et al.*, 2012b; Mourier *et al.*, 2012; Guttridge *et al.*, 2013).

State of the Art

Information on cognitive skills in elasmobranchs is still limited (Guttridge *et al.*, 2009a; Yopak *et al.*, 2012a; Schluessel, 2015). Most behavioural studies conducted thus far have been on a few species that are easy to access, handle and keep, such as the lemon shark, *Negaprion brevirostris*, the grey or brown-banded bamboo shark, *Chiloscyllium punctautum*, the nurse shark, *Ginglymostoma cirratum*, or several *Potamotryon* species, as well as several marine stingrays from the Dasyatidae or Urotrygonidae families (e.g. *Urobatis jamaicensis*). There have also been studies on a few temperate-water species, such as the small-spotted catshark, *Scyliorhinus canicula* and the Port Jackson shark, *Heterodontus portusjacksoni*. Generally, warm-water species are easier to maintain in a laboratory setting than cold-water species, as the technical equipment is far more accessible and less expensive. Further, owing to their more sedentary lifestyle, benthic species are easier to keep than benthopelagic species. Due to the associated drawbacks in maintenance and handling, most studies are performed with small numbers of individuals (< 10), often limiting the power of statistical analyses.

Learning in elasmobranchs has usually been tested with reinforced operant conditioning, in which an animal is rewarded (e.g. with food or the company of conspecifics; see below) for performing a particular task. If punishment instead of reinforcement is used, sharks, like other animals, often become stressed and anxious, and usually terminate participation (e.g. Schwarze *et al.*, 2013).

Orientation

Most sharks move constantly in search for food, mates and shelter; many perform also daily, seasonal or annual migrations. To accomplish this, sharks use different orientation strategies, form spatial memories and maintain knowledge of spatial tasks for at least 12 weeks (Schluessel and Bleckmann 2005, 2012; Fuss *et al.*, 2014a–c). Ocellate freshwater stingrays, *Potamotrygon motoro* (Schluessel and Bleckmann, 2005) and bamboo sharks, *Chiloscyllium griseum* (Fuss *et al.*, 2014a,b), learn to locate a fixed food source by using either body-centred turns, a variety of landmarks or a combination of the two, possibly even by constructing cognitive spatial maps. Ocellate river stingrays generally place more importance on the overall environmental or geometric arrangement of an experimental arena than on the landmarks within it when memorizing the location of a food source (Schluessel *et al.*, 2015).

Tool Use

Fish manipulate objects to increase feeding efficiency, move objects or clean nests (Brown, 2012). In the only study on tool use in elasmobranchs, Kuba and colleagues (2010) investigated the ability of five subadult freshwater stingrays, *Potamotrygon castexi*, to use water as a tool to extract food from a tube. All rays accomplished the task, but applied different methods in the process, such as undulating fin movements, suction and/or a combination of both.

Social Cognition

While many shark species are solitary, juvenile lemon sharks prefer size-matched conspecifics over unmatched ones, and favour conspecifics over heterospecifics (Guttridge *et al.*, 2009b). Active partner preferences and differing leadership roles were also observed in lemon sharks (Guttridge *et al.*, 2011), in benthic wobbegong sharks, *Orectolobus maculatus* (Armansin *et al.*, 2016) and blacktip reef sharks, *Carcharhinus melanopterus* (Mourier *et al.*, 2012). The latter showed long-term associations and evidence for community structure driven by individual social preferences. Familiarity may be an important factor driving these preferences in small-spotted catsharks and lemon sharks (Jacoby *et al.*, 2012b; Keller *et al.*, 2017), with neonates hatching or being born in close temporal and spatial proximity developing familiarity and hence aggregating together. Results of a food-finding task, which tested for social learning abilities, indicated that test animals that had been allowed to watch conspecifics with previous experience completed more task-related behaviours and were faster than test animals that had been paired with naive conspecifics (Guttridge *et al.*, 2013; Thonhauser *et al.*, 2013).

Personality and Laterality

To date, only a handful of studies have investigated shark personality (see Finger *et al.*, 2017). In Port Jackson sharks, individuals vary greatly and reliably in terms of boldness and stress reactivity (Byrnes and Brown, 2016), with differences between males and females (Byrnes *et al.*, 2016b). They also show individual and sex-biased variation in laterality (i.e. the tendency for some neural functions of cognitive processes to be more dominant in one brain hemisphere than the other), which may be linked to stress reactivity (Byrnes *et al.*, 2016a). Moreover, Jacoby and colleagues (2014), working with juvenile small-spotted catsharks, found that individuals displayed consistent social interactions across varying habitat types. Finally, Finger and colleagues (2018) found that juvenile lemon sharks showed consistent individual differences in their social behaviours (e.g. following and paralleling), across short (4–18 days) and long (4 months) time scales. Habituation over consecutive trials largely varies across individuals, and habituation rate is negatively related to individual's movement behaviour in the very first open field trial (Finger *et al.*, 2016).

Object Recognition

Recognition and discrimination abilities are essential for a wide range of behaviours, such as the selection of food sources, identification of prey and predators, recognition of conspecifics, heterospecifics and potential partners, as well as recognition of territories and home ranges. Sharks show visual target discrimination (Tester and Kato, 1963; Aronson, 1967; Graeber *et al.*, 1972; Graeber and Ebbesson, 1973) and discriminate between symmetrical and asymmetrical shapes (Schluessel *et al.*, 2015), contrasts but not colours (Schluessel *et al.*, 2014a), stationary 2D objects (Schluessel and Duengen, 2015) and between moving objects, ranging from moving circles to differently moving organisms (Fuss *et al.*, 2017). In addition, sharks recognize some organisms based on their unique movement, but have difficulty recognizing familiar organisms shown from a new perspective (Fuss *et al.*, 2017). Bamboo sharks also successfully discriminate between various two-dimensional geometric stimuli and succeed in reversal tasks, likely retaining some information about previously learned stimuli, when progressing to new ones (Fuss *et al.*, 2014c). Finally, sharks show remarkable categorization abilities, i.e. using abstract stimuli (Schluessel, 2015) as well as 2D images of organisms (Schluessel and Duengen, 2015). Grey bamboo sharks were also tested for their ability to perceive a range of optical illusions (Fuss *et al.*, 2014d; Fuss and Schluessel, 2017), and were found to fall for Kanizsa figures (Figure 16.2) and subjective contours, but not Müller-Lyer or Ebbinghaus illusions.

Further, several studies have investigated electroreceptive discrimination abilities (Kimber *et al.*, 2011, 2014; Siciliano *et al.*, 2013). Small-spotted catsharks discriminate between prey-type electric fields; they prefer the stronger of two artificial fields with direct current (DC) and an alternative current (AC) over a DC current of the same magnitude, but not a natural DC current associated with a food reward over an artificial DC current of similar magnitude. Yellow stingrays, *Urobatis jamaicensis*, were successfully trained to bite either the anode or cathode, showing significant polarity discrimination (Siciliano *et al.*, 2013), and to associate a magnetic stimulus with a food reward, showing for the first time object discrimination based on magnetoreceptive cues (Newton and Kajiura, 2017).

Memory Retention

Memory windows vary greatly between species and tasks (Brown, 2001). In some cases, it may be advantageous for an animal to forget particular behaviours quickly to retain flexibility (Warburton, 2003), while others should be retained for longer periods

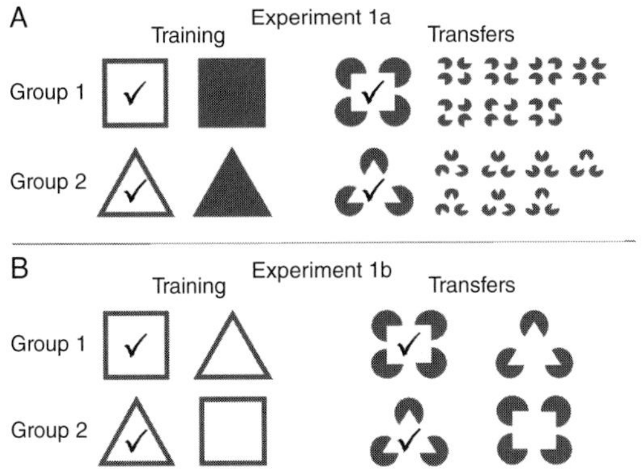

Figure 16.2. Shown are the stimuli that were presented to each group, during regular training and transfer test trials in experiments 1a and 1b. The positive, rewarded stimulus is indicated by a check mark. (A) In group 1, an empty square was the positive, rewarded stimulus; in group 2 it was an empty triangle. During the T1 transfer tests of experiment 1a, sharks were 'expected' to choose the correct Kanizsa figure. (B) During experiment 1b, group 1 was trained to recognize an empty square over an empty triangle, whereas group 2 was trained vice versa. During the T2 transfer tests, sharks were expected to choose the Kanizsa figure resembling the stimulus they had been trained on.
Adapted from Fuss *et al.*, 2014d, illustration under Creative Commons Attribution License.

of time or even indefinitely. Grey bamboo sharks were trained in two different spatial tasks and tested for their ability to solve them after an absence of reinforcement (Schluessel and Bleckmann, 2012). All sharks successfully remembered what they had been trained in, up to the maximally tested break period of 6 weeks. Sharks were also successful at remembering a two-alternative choice discrimination task, even after an absence of reinforcement of 50 weeks (Fuss and Schluessel, 2015). Similarly, Port Jackson sharks trained to pair an LED light or a stream of air bubbles with a food reward retained the learned associations for a period of at least 24 hours, and possibly up to 40 days (Guttridge and Brown, 2014). In addition, yellow stingrays solved a different task successfully after intervals of 90–180 days post-learning (Newton and Kajiura, 2017). Small-spotted catshark trained to associate a food reward with an artificial electric field, however, failed to retain the association after a 3-week interval, possibly because forgetting may be advantageous to species living in more variable environments (Kimber *et al.*, 2014). While feeding-related information may sometimes only be retained over short periods of time, life-threatening behaviour should preferentially be retained indefinitely. Mourier and colleagues (2017) found that blacktip reef sharks learned to avoid rod and line capture, which ultimately increased network robustness to experimental catch-and-release in a shark social network.

Brain and Cognition

While the link between a larger than expected brain for a given body size (encephalization) and enhanced cognitive capabilities continues to be highly contentious (Mitchell,

2016), there are documented patterns of encephalization across chondrichthyans, with cognitive implications. Indeed, the most encephalized species are chiefly found in reef-associated or oceanic habitats and/or often pursue more active predation strategies, such as *Sphyrna, Carcharhinus* and *Dasyatis* (see Yopak, 2012a), which may reflect higher cognitive demands. In particular, the cognitive requirements for learning the complex spatial organization of a coral reef, in addition to the complex social behaviours and intra- and interspecific interactions that are often prevalent in reef habitats, termed 'social intelligence' (Kotrschal *et al.*, 1998), might have influenced the evolution of brain size in these chondrichthyans.

Similarly, brain organization is often used as a neuroanatomical proxy for functional specialization. Reef-associated species have the largest telencephalons (which are associated to higher cognitive functions: Yopak *et al.*, 2007; Lisney *et al.*, 2007; Ari, 2011), large, highly foliated cerebellums (Yopak *et al.*, 2007), relatively small olfactory bulbs (Yopak *et al.*, 2015) and relatively large optic tectums (Yopak and Lisney, 2012), possibly reflecting the visual demands of complex reef habitats. In contrast, deep-sea chondrichthyan brains may reflect lower activity levels and a specialization of non-visual senses in bathyal environments, with small telencephalons (Yopak and Montgomery, 2008) and optic tectums (Yopak and Lisney, 2012), small, smooth cerebellums (Montgomery *et al.*, 2012), relatively enlarged olfactory bulbs (Yopak *et al.*, 2015) and a clear relative hypertrophy of the central termination sites for primary projections from the octavolateralis senses (Yopak and Montgomery, 2008). Therefore, the relative importance of different sensory systems likely varies across species (Collin *et al.*, 2015) and should always be considered when designing experiments. Finally, links between cognition and the relevant neural substrates are limited (Graeber *et al.*, 1978; Graeber 1978, 1980; Schwarze *et al.*, 2013; Fuss *et al.*, 2014a,b).

All for One and One for All

Box 16.1 Monotreme Cognition

Stewart Nicol

Just as sharks are not 'typical fish', monotremes are not typical mammals. Like sharks, the platypus (*Ornithorhynchus antinus*), the short-beaked echidna (*Tachyglossus aculeatus*) and the long-beaked echidnas (*Zaglossus* spp.) are often dismissed as being primitive, and this has influenced approaches to monotreme cognition. While egg-laying (a plesiomorphic feature) is a defining characteristic of the group, it is often not appreciated that monotremes have large brains. The echidnas have particularly large gyrified brains, equivalent in size to those of carnivores of the same mass, and because of their low metabolic rates, echidnas have brain size to basal metabolic rate relationships similar to those of primates (Nicol, 2017). This suggests that there must be very considerable fitness benefits for the echidnas to maintain such large brains, i.e. the cognitive benefits must outweigh the metabolic costs. But how should this be tested?

(cont.)

There have been four laboratory studies of echidna cognition. Saunders and colleagues (1971) tested the ability of echidnas to remember the position of a food reward in a T-maze. Gates (1978) used two-choice doors with a food reward to test the ability of echidnas to discriminate between symbols of different brightness, orientation and shape. Buchmann and Rhodes (1978) employed operant techniques: echidnas were trained to press a treadle for a food reward in response to visual, tactile and positional cues. Burke and colleagues (2002) attempted to study spatial memory performance of echidnas in terms of their foraging ecology, by testing their learning response to the positioning of food in two- and four-way mazes. All studies demonstrated cognitive performance at least equivalent to that by rats and cats.

Most of these studies preceded any systematic studies of behaviour in the field. Laboratory tests carry the risk of posing problems in an 'unfair' manner, particularly when done with very limited knowledge of normal behaviour. This must be particularly so for monotremes, whose sensory modalities, like those of sharks, include electroreception and a strong reliance on olfaction. While the semi-aquatic platypus has 40,000 mucous gland electroreceptors in the bill skin, short-beaked echidnas have only 400 (Pettigrew, 1999), and their predominant sensory input is olfactory: the echidna is the only mammal known to have a gyrified olfactory bulb, probably to expand the number of synaptic glomeruli available for the analysis of the odorant repertoire (Ashwell, 2013). We have identified a total of 186 compounds which are potentially used in olfactory communication by echidnas (Harris *et al.*, 2012), but testing how echidnas respond to subtle, probably unmeasurable changes in a complex suite of chemical signals is not practicable in the laboratory. By contrast, Manger and Pettigrew (1995) investigated how electroreception facilitates prey capture in platypuses by using an electrically shielded tank in which they could combine varying electrical stimuli with video recordings of feeding behaviour. Such a study is only practicable under laboratory conditions. In a very simple study, Augee and Gooden (1992) demonstrated that echidnas could detect buried 9-volt batteries in their normal environment, but the ecological significance of this is not clear.

References

Ashwell, K. W. S. (2013). Reflections: monotreme neurobiology in context. *Neurobiology of monotremes: brain evolution in our distant mammalian cousins* (pp. 285–298). Collingwood: CSIRO Publishing.

Augee, M. L., and Gooden, B. A. (1992). Evidence for electroreception from field studies of the echidna, *Tachyglossus aculeatus*. In *Platypus and echidnas* (pp. 211–215). Mosman: Royal Zoological Society of New South Wales.

Buchmann, O. L. K., and Rhodes, J. (1978). Instrumental learning in the echidna. *The Australian Zoologist*, **20**, 131–145.

(*cont.*)

Burke, D., Cieplucha, C., Cass, J., Russell, F., and Fry, G. (2002). Win-shift and win-stay learning in the short-beaked echidna (Tachyglossus aculeatus). *Animal Cognition*, **5**, 79–84.
Gates, G. R. (1978). Vision in the monotreme anteater. In: *Monotreme biology* (pp. 147–169). Mosman: Royal Zoological Society of New South Wales.
Harris, R. L., Davies, N. W., and Nicol, S. C. (2012). Chemical composition of odorous secretions in the Tasmanian short-beaked echidna (*Tachyglossus aculeatus setosus*). *Chemical Senses*, **37**, 819–836.
Manger, P. R., and Pettigrew, J. D. (1995). Electroreception and the feeding behaviour of platypus (*Ornithorhynchus anatinus*: Monotremata: Mammalia). *Philosophical Transactions of the Royal Society B: Biological Sciences*, **347**, 359–381.
Nicol, S. C. (2017). Energy homeostasis in monotremes. *Frontiers in Neuroscience*, **11**, 1–17.
Pettigrew, J. D. (1999). Electroreception in monotremes. *The Journal of Experimental Biology*, **202**, 1447–1454.
Saunders, J. C., Teague, J., Slonim, D., and Pridmore, P. A. (1971). A position habit in the monotreme *Tachyglossus aculeatus* (the spiny ant eater). *Australian Journal of Psychology*, **23**, 47–51.

Field Guide

Species Selection

How do you design cognition experiments for one of the earth's most revered predators? Firstly, not all sharks are large, apex predators; there is great diversity among this group (see above), ranging from small-bodied, tropical species (such as the bamboo shark), to giant, sluggish deep-ocean dwellers (such as the Greenland shark, *Somniosus microcephalus*, the longest-living vertebrate currently described (Nielsen *et al.*, 2016). Selecting the latter for cognition experiments would be rather challenging. However, the former is a useful model, with an egg-laying reproductive mode that allows for captive rearing, a preference for warm water (resulting in greater feeding motivation) and a small body size (facilitating capture, processing and replication). The decision to select a species will also depend on your research question, on their behaviour and biology, the availability of subjects, cost of capture and maintenance, accessibility, and ease of obtaining animal ethics approval and collection permits.

Sharks in Captivity

You cannot test an animal that you cannot catch, keep or maintain. An important first question is whether there is evidence of previous husbandry success. Small (< 1 m total length) benthic species like cat, bamboo and horn sharks are successfully kept in captivity. However, grey nurse, *Carcharias taurus*, sandbar, *Carcharhinus plumbeus*, sevengill, *Notorynchus cepedianus*, and scalloped hammerhead, *Sphyrna lewini*, sharks have also been successfully maintained in lab-based aquaria throughout the world, even though some of these species are almost 3 m in total length. Generally, large, pelagic species do very poorly in captivity (e.g. white shark, *Carcharodon carcharias*: Ezcurra *et al.*, 2012). Furthermore, the process to transition a large pelagic species from the wild to captivity is costly and time-consuming.

An alternative to laboratory testing is a semi-captive set-up, where sharks are kept in anchored ocean or shallow-water pens, or flow-through arena (Figure 16.3), with exposure to ambient conditions (e.g. water currents, temperature and tidal fluctuations). Such set-ups have been used effectively on juvenile nurse and lemon sharks in Bimini, Bahamas, with experiments exploring social preferences, learning (Guttridge *et al.*, 2009b, 2013) and personality (Finger *et al.*, 2017). Similarly, bonnethead, *S. tiburo*, scalloped hammerhead and sandbar sharks in Hawaii, USA, and small and large-spotted catsharks, *S. stellaris*, in Plymouth, UK, were housed successfully in comparable set-ups: a concrete tank (3–7 m diameter) with flow-through system.

A

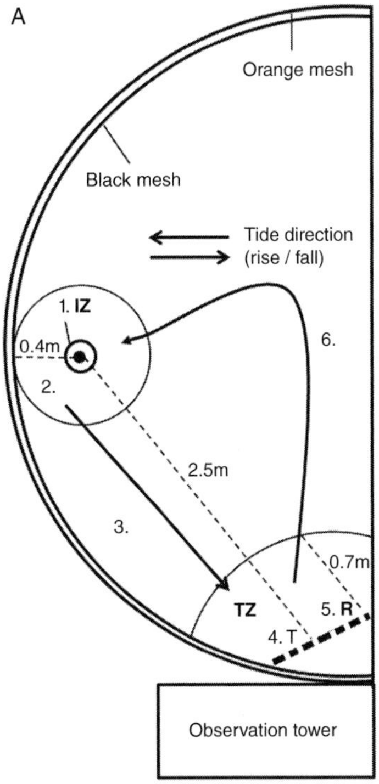

B

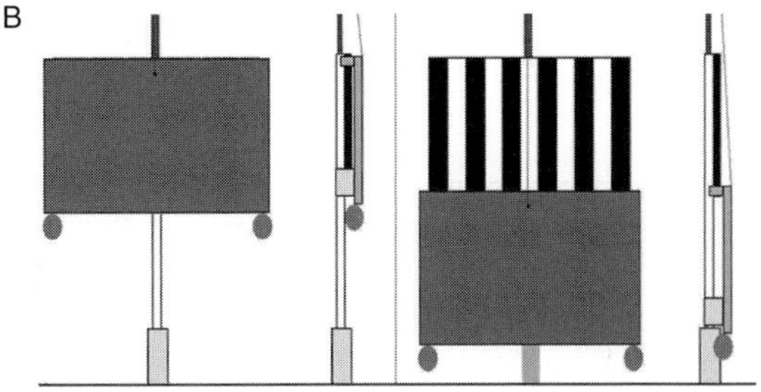

C

Step #	Description	Purpose
1	PVC cover pipe placed on bar in Indicator Zone (IZ)	Foraging task starts
2	Shark enters IZ	Target (T) exposed
3	Shark swims to Target Zone (TZ)	Enter TZ
4	Shark contacts T	Reward (R)
5	Consume R	T covered
6	Return to IZ	Restart task

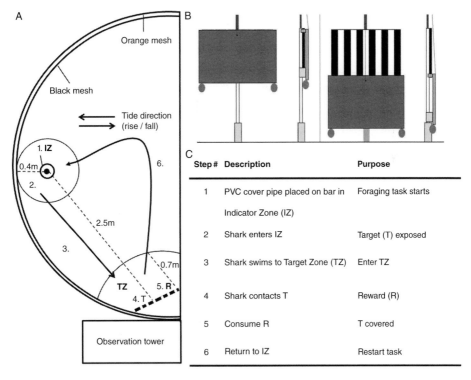

Figure 16.3. Semi-captive set-up of social learning experiments for juvenile lemon sharks in Bimini, Bahamas. (A) Positions and measurements of zones, target and reward. (B) Schematic representation of the target mechanism, showing covered and exposed position as well as side and front views. (C) Steps of the food task or trial.

Where are Sharks Sourced From?

Studies on shark cognition often use either captive-bred subjects or those that researchers capture on their own. Schluessel and colleagues have a long-term collaboration with *Haus des Meeres*, a public aquarium in Vienna, Austria, who breed and rear bamboo sharks (Schluessel, 2015). Researchers in Plymouth, UK, used 392 captive-reared small-spotted catsharks in experiments investigating social cognition (Jacoby *et al.*, 2012b) and trawl-captured adult small-spotted catsharks in learning and memory foraging tasks (Kimber *et al.*, 2014). Juvenile lemon and nurse sharks in Bimini, Bahamas, were captured via gillnetting and free-dive techniques, whereas scientists in Hawaii, USA, used simple rod and reel to obtain juvenile scalloped hammerhead or sandbar sharks. Sharks for all these experiments were transported by a small research vessel to nearby semi-captive pens, via aerated large tub or live-well (Kajiura, 2003; Guttridge *et al.*, 2009b, 2013). More recently, Guttridge and Brown (2014) working in Merimbula, Australia, obtained juvenile Port Jackson sharks from a commercial fisher who regularly caught the species as bycatch. Most studies on shark cognition suffer from a low sample size (Guttridge *et al.*, 2009a; Schluessel *et al.*, 2015), but often enough test subjects can be obtained or reared to make stronger conclusions about shark cognitive abilities.

How are Sharks Maintained in Captivity?

Successful maintenance begins with careful consideration of ecological, physiological and behavioural requirements of the species held. Tank size (horizontal and vertical) or shape will vary depending on the species. Circular tanks or pens are generally used, or rectangles with buffered corners; tanks with right-angle corners often cause stress, as sharks struggle to navigate out of them (Gruber *et al.*, 2001). For researchers choosing a semi-captive set-up, it is important to consider environmental factors, such as tidal changes, wave action or weather conditions, as these could impact space availability, water flow, visibility and temperature. We recommend the use of non-metal materials in tank and pen construction, specifically in behavioural experiments, as sharks can detect electric fields.

Adequate food as well as motivation to feed is essential. A diet similar to what the species naturally feeds on is optimal; as this may not be practical, a mixed diet of pre-frozen (to eliminate parasites) squid or fish, with mineral and vitamin supplements, is recommended (Kimber *et al.*, 2014; Schluessel, 2015). The amount and frequency of feeds depends on many factors (e.g. experiment, metabolism, age class, food type, tank size, water temperature). Daily rations for sharks have been estimated in the lab and captivity (Wetherbee and Cortes, 2004) and can range from 0.2 per cent body weight per day for the adult sevengill, to 4.34 per cent body weight per day for the bonnethead shark. During cognition experiments, test sharks are usually fed on a percentage just below the recommended daily ration (Kimber *et al.*, 2014). If test species' daily rations have not been calculated, we suggest trialling individuals before experimentation (Guttridge and Brown, 2014).

Prior to starting experiments, we recommend a captive acclimation period of 3–7 days. Knowledge of natural behaviours, sociobiology and physiology is important, as

Table 16.1. Considerations for elasmobranch cognitive experiments.

Species selection	
Sharks in captivity	Usually select small-bodied, benthic specialized species or juveniles, with history of successful husbandry and motivation to feed. Take into account cost of capture, transport and maintenance
Sharks in the wild	Select those that can be resighted or recaptured, resident to a habitat or area, or tagged with monitoring equipment (e.g. biotelemetry)
Sample size	For your study take enough sharks to be housed, tested or tracked for meaningful inference (power analysis). Take into account the possibility of using conspecifics, mixed sex but size-matched individuals
Provenance	Wild-caught (e.g. use of fishers, either recreational or commercial) or captive-bred; consider logistics and practicality of transport from capture site or breeding facility to experimental site
Housing	Lab-based housing (Figure 16.4); swimming pool or pen mesh fencing (Figure 16.3); flow-through system on the coast or similar penned area
Maintenance	Consider food type (squid, fish pieces) and amount (literature search, typically < 2 per cent daily ration); water flow, conductance, social and general tank environment; shark health (parasite load, weight loss, fin rot, blotches); euthanasia protocols (e.g. MS222)
Identification	External marker tags for ID (e.g. colour code, rototag), pattern discrimination (e.g. bamboo shark), biotelemetry or bio-logging techniques to track individuals for extensive periods
Permits	Implications of conservation status (use animals with low concern status in the IUCN red list); country of testing (Bahamas vs. Germany/UK – countries have very different requirements), Animal Ethics (IACUC)
Experimental design	
Lab methods	Traditional methods comprise: T-maze, force-two choice, classical or operant conditioning, shuttle-box
Materials	Use synthetic materials such as plastics (Perspex, PVC), because they are good for building compartments, arenas or targets for training; opaque barriers can be used to block off areas
Acclimation	Allow 2–3 days in captivity to ensure sharks exhibit normal behaviours, monitor stress signals (e.g. body blotching, not feeding, weight loss, wall leaning/thigmotaxis)
Stimulus selection	Prior to testing, control for detection and sensitivity to cues (e.g. visual, electrical, mechanical); during testing, ensure consistency of stimulus presentation (time of day, illumination)
Training paradigm	Control the number of feeding trials per day (linked to food quantity), intertrial time, ceiling time for trials, unintentional cueing, and mixing of water within set-up to avoid spatial biases; include further controls as needed
Feeding apparatus	Manually operated by experimenter, automated feeder
Moving between experimental compartments	Manually operated guillotine doors, ushering with net or mesh
Pre-training	Consisting of exposure to the experimental set-up and feeding protocol, use of food cues to attract sharks to areas within the set-up, set criterion for obtaining food rewards and once reached training commences
Ethogram	Develop an ethogram via observation of subjects prior to testing; some typical behaviours might include head shake, turn, swimming, bite or head contact with apparatus; if social, following, circling, or tactile resting

Table 16.1. *(cont.)*

Data analysis	
Information to be recorded	Latency to feed, side preference, search patterns, percentage of correct choices
Software and tools	For tracking individuals (image J, Mtrack J); overhead cameras (gopro, CCTV)
Statistics	Often non-parametric for traditional experiments (due to low sample size); exciting new tools available to analyse tracking data and bio-logging (network analysis, machine learning)

these norms can be compared to observations of reactions in captive situations. Some common parameters that could be used as indicators of stress for sharks include inappetence and anorexia, excessive resting, evasive or avoidance behaviour, and changes to any of the following: skin coloration (often blotches), ventilation rate or swimming behaviour (disorientation, obstacle contact, wall leaning or thigmotaxis). Having a detailed ethogram of behaviours for your test species is also useful when quantifying conditioned responses during learning trials, as often subtle movements can be important indicators (Guttridge and Brown, 2014).

Identification and Wild Observation

For some sharks, it is possible to identify individuals via pattern discrimination, fin markings or notches, as in captive bamboo sharks (Schluessel, 2015). However, tags are often needed to discriminate between individuals, attached either through the dorsal fin, and anchored or injected in the adjacent muscle via dart (plastic or stainless steel) or hypodermic needle. Tags can be colour-coded or numbered, microchip (PIT; Destron Fearing Inc.), fluorescent visible elastomer implant, T-bar, streamer, or plaque-shaped and of differing sizes, depending on the species (see below). Their use has been most effective for mark–recapture studies exploring life-history traits and movement (Casey and Natansen, 1992); however, studies on shark social cognition have also benefitted from using such tags (Guttridge *et al.*, 2013; Jacoby *et al.*, 2014; Keller *et al.*, 2017). For sharks, recent advances in remote monitoring devices, such as biotelemetry (satellite, radio and acoustic telemetry) and bio-logging (archival loggers), have revolutionized our capabilities for observation (Hussey *et al.*, 2015). Using these tools, it is now possible to reliably observe and relocate sharks, as well as record detailed information about their behaviour – an important pre-requisite for wild cognition experiments (Pritchard *et al.*, 2015).

Permits

Consideration should always be given to the conservation status and the requisite permits for collection and experimentation of a given species. The former can be found on the International Union for Conservation of Nature (IUCN) Red List of Threatened Species website (www.iucnredlist.org), while the latter are dependent on the jurisdiction and institute through which the research will be conducted. It is important to note that international journals will not consider reviewing a manuscript without evidence of collection and ethics permits.

Experimental Design

Designing an experiment investigating shark cognition should really be no different from that for any other animal, and includes determining how many animals to test, identifying which behaviours to quantify, which stimuli and set-up to use, and selecting a training protocol (Lieberman, 1990). Some classical approaches have been modified successfully to investigate cognitive processes in sharks. For example, the two-choice T-maze design was used effectively to examine spatial memory and orientation (Schluessel and Bleckmann, 2012), and classical or operant conditioning paradigms for exploring associative and social learning (Gruber and Schneiderman, 1975; Guttridge *et al.*, 2013; Schwarze *et al.*, 2013), as well as object categorization and symmetry perception (Fuss *et al.*, 2014c; Schluessel *et al.*, 2014b; Schluessel and Duengen, 2015; Figure 16.4). Below, we present tips and ideas gleaned from our personal experiences and discussed in the literature, to help overcome the challenges of designing an experiment investigating cognition in sharks.

Stimulus Selection and Presentation

Sharks exhibit great variation in their sensory systems, which suggests that the relative importance of sensory systems varies between species (see above). From experimental studies, Gardiner and colleagues (2014) found that, by blocking olfactory cues, nurse sharks were unable to detect food and subsequently feed, whereas blacktip sharks, *Carcharhinus limbatus*, and bonnethead sharks undergoing the same treatment detected prey at 1–2 m distance, using visual cues. Working with Port Jackson sharks, Guttridge and Brown (2014) found that individuals trained on a conditioning regime with air bubbles displayed significantly more anticipatory behaviours (e.g. turning towards the air bubbles and biting) than those trained on an underwater LED, possibly because the air bubble stimulus is more biologically relevant in this species. These examples emphasize how the perceptual ability of test subjects can impact task performance and thus should be an important factor to consider. Moreover, the spatial and/or temporal relationship between conditioning and food reward can influence the speed at which learning takes place, and the nature and intensity of the conditioned response (Lieberman, 1990). For example, Schluessel (2015) presented stimuli 3 cm from the tank base, due to the bottom-dwelling nature of their test subjects.

Most studies on shark cognition used positive reinforcement for conditioning, due to limited success of aversive stimuli (Tester and Kato, 1963; but see Gruber and Schneiderman, 1975). For example, Schwarze and colleagues (2013), using an electric shock paired with a green light, documented individual variation in avoidance responses,

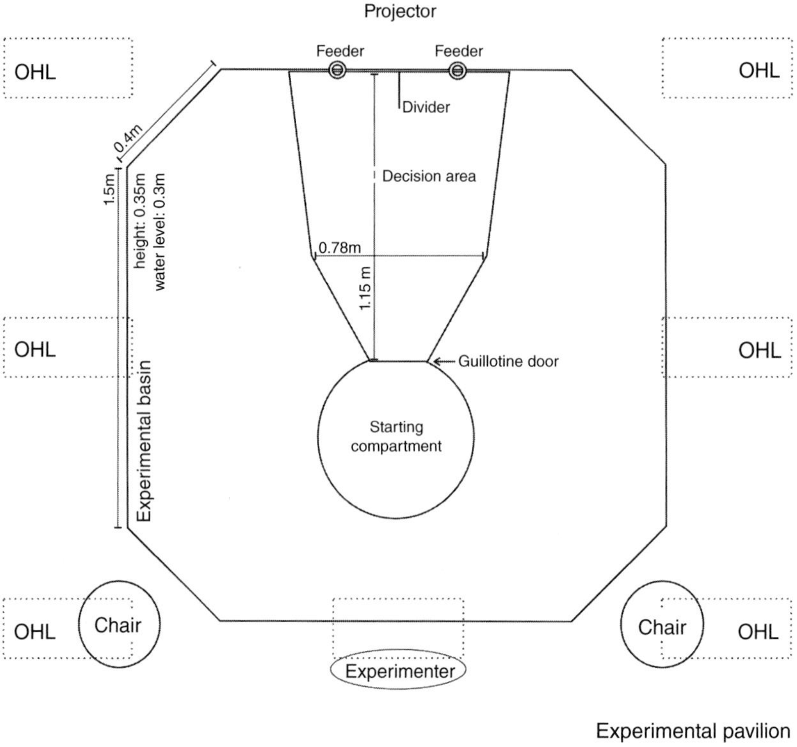

Figure 16.4. The experimental set-up within the experimental basin inside a white pavilion. The keyhole-shaped set-up consists of a starting compartment, a decision area and a frosted screen for projection, with a divider to allow the projection of two 2D objects at a time and to provoke a clear, unambiguous choice (left or right). For projection, an LED beamer is used. Sharks are placed within the SC at the start of each trial. OHL, overhead light.
Adapted with permission of Springer. This was original copyright in the article from *Zoology*, Visual discrimination abilities in the gray bamboo shark (*Chiloscyllium griseum*), **117** (2014), 104–111, Theodora Fuss, Horst Bleckmann, Vera Schluessel (Fuss *et al.*, 2014c).

including backwards swimming, side-to-side head and/or tail movements, making conclusions difficult to interpret. Furthermore, there was evidence that bamboo sharks habituated to an electric shock (Kimber *et al.*, 2014). Interestingly, during categorization learning, bamboo sharks learnt positive 'fish' images, but did not learn the unrewarded 'snail', unlike cichlids that learnt both negative and positive associations (Schluessel *et al.*, 2014b; Schluessel and Duengen, 2015). Finally, when presenting stimuli to sharks, it is essential to prevent any unintentional cueing, both through the experimenter and set-up environment (e.g. Schluessel, 2015).

Set-up Familiarity and Pre-training

Pre-exposure to the experimental set-up is important to avoid confounding effects of novelty and to eliminate unexpected problems with handling or feeding prior to testing. Previous studies have allowed test subjects to swim freely through the set-up, start box and doors, across a 1–3-day period (Guttridge and Brown, 2014; Kimber *et al.*, 2014; Schluessel, 2015). Some studies fed subjects in a pre-training phase to ensure that food rewards could be retrieved and to identify potential side-preferences (Schluessel *et al.*, 2012). Food should be delivered in a smooth and consistent manner, and arrive without delay in the appropriate location. For benthic species, rewards delivered close to the substrate (Fuss *et al.*, 2014c; Guttridge and Brown, 2014; Kimber *et al.*, 2014) were most effective, while feeding trials with lemon sharks had greater success at the surface (Guttridge *et al.*, 2013). Most studies used automated feeders or manually operated devices, varying from a syringe with plastic tubing to feeding rods to electronic or manually operated compartment feeders (Guttridge and Brown, 2014; Kimber *et al.*, 2014; Schluessel, 2015). The amount of food that test subjects receive daily should be enough to sustain them, but maintain motivation. The number of trials conducted per day, and the time between them (intertrial time), is important for any experiments using food rewards. During feeding, sharks tend to become 'switched-on' and participate eagerly; thus, we recommend short intertrial times and short daily experiment duration. For example, Schluessel and colleagues tested bamboo sharks once per day, with 10 trials per session. Guttridge and Brown (2014) conducted six trials per day with Port Jackson sharks, whereas Kimber and colleagues (2014) trained small-spotted catsharks in two trials per day. Intertrial time was similar (e.g. 60 s for Port Jackson sharks, 30–90 s for bamboo sharks and 300 s for small-spotted catsharks).

Recording Behaviours and Data Analyses

Probably, the best advice for any researcher is to first get to know their test subject, as many animals display subtle behavioural and/or physical changes in response to captivity, novelty, conspecifics, prey or predators. We suggest developing an ethogram of these behaviours, as well as recording their context, duration and whether one usually precedes another. This is particularly informative when deciding which behaviours to record during experiments. Most studies record the following information: latency to feed and/or respond with bite, left or right choice, percentage of correct choices in two-choice trials, trial duration, and behavioural information such as search patterns, body movements and type of swimming. These can be recorded by an observer and should be recorded by a camera for validation and reference, as subtle behaviours can be missed by an observer. Indeed, for some lab experiments, image tracking programs (e.g. image J, Mtrack J, Ctrax) have been used effectively to monitor interactions of schooling fish (Herbert-Read *et al.*, 2011), and these could be modified for sharks, given the right background and illumination. In a lab environment, conditions such as conductivity, pH and water temperature need to be maintained, but for semi-captive and/or wild studies it may be easier to record such environmental information and account for it in the analyses.

Wild vs. Lab

Box 16.2 Elasmobranch Cognition in the Wild

David M. P. Jacoby

Elasmobranchs are wonderfully diverse and extremely well-adapted, over a long evolutionary history, to the specific environments they occupy. As demonstrated throughout this chapter, elasmobranch cognitive abilities are intrinsically related to their lifestyle and, in particular, the relationship between their habitat and hunting strategies (e.g. ambush/pursuit predators, visual/olfactory). Thus, considerable variation in cognition exists between species (Yopak, 2012).

Advances in our understanding of cognition in sharks and rays has almost exclusively relied on controlled captive/semi-captive experiments (e.g. Guttridge and Brown, 2014). While such studies will undoubtedly continue to prove crucial for guiding progress in this field, translating some of this work to wild elasmobranchs is hugely challenging. However, technological innovations, e.g. animal-borne tags that are becoming increasingly smaller, cheaper and more sophisticated, continue to push the boundaries of animal ecology (Cooke *et al.*, 2013; Hussey *et al.*, 2015; Kays *et al.*, 2015), as do the techniques advancing analyses of large telemetry data sets (Krause *et al.*, 2013; Jacoby *et al.*, 2016). In fact, biotelemetry is already being employed to record fine-scale measurements on the activity of sharks, alongside visual observations in captive experiments on shark social behaviour (Jacoby *et al.*, 2010; Wilson *et al.*, 2015), hinting that the transition to fully wild data on cognitive function in elasmobranchs is imminent. Further, proximity logging two-way, acoustic transmitters have been shown to record social behaviour in wild sharks at very fine spatial scales (Guttridge *et al.*, 2010; Holland *et al.*, 2010). Using conventional tags (satellite/acoustic), the accuracy of determining the exact locations of individual sharks is still relatively low, unless the animal is at the surface. Animal-borne data loggers, such as accelerometers or depth-temperature recorders, however, can log at very high resolution, and this is facilitating exciting progress within the machine learning community in developing algorithms for pattern recognition and the detection of behavioural switching from raw telemetry data (Olden *et al.*, 2008; Krause *et al.*, 2013).

The use of electronic tags is, of course, costly and not always feasible. Therefore, observations and ethograms of wild shark behaviour at provisioning sites, where sharks are attracted to an area to feed for the benefit of paying tourists, actually offer an interesting compromise between captive and wild studies. Although careful interpretation is required to tease apart 'natural' and 'induced' behaviours, some studies have shown increased residency and aggression in sharks acclimatised to provisioning areas (e.g. Clua *et al.*, 2010).

Measuring and quantifying decision-making processes and repeatable behaviours in elasmobranchs may take many forms, including estimating consistency in navigation routes, feeding specializations, social network position or dominance.

(cont.)

However, all rely on the ability to monitor individuals over time and space and still retrieve the data. Moving forward, small benthic/demersal sharks will unquestionably continue to play an important role as model species; adult cat, lemon, bamboo and Port Jackson sharks (to name a few) are small enough to be housed and observed in captivity, yet large enough to carry logging or acoustic tags in the wild, allowing for repeated testing of individuals in both laboratory and wild contexts.

References

Clua, E., Buray, N., Legendre, P., Mourier, J., and Planes, S. (2010). Behavioural response of sicklefin lemon sharks *Negaprion acutidens* to underwater feeding for ecotourism purposes. *Marine Ecology Progress Series*, **414**, 257–266.

Cooke, S. J., Midwood, J. D., Thiem, J. D., *et al.* (2013). Tracking animals in freshwater with electronic tags: past, present and future. *Animal Biotelemetry*, **1**, 1–19.

Guttridge, T. L., and Brown, C. (2014). Learning and memory in the Port Jackson shark, *Heterodontus portusjacksoni*. *Animal Cognition*, **17**, 415–425.

Guttridge, T. L., Gruber, S. H., Krause, J., and Sims, D. W. (2010). Novel acoustic technology for studying free-ranging shark social behaviour by recording individuals' interactions. *PLoS ONE*, **5**, 1–8.

Holland, K. N., Meyer, C. G., and Dagorn, L. C. (2010). Inter-animal telemetry: results from first deployment of acoustic 'business card' tags. *Endangered Species Research*, **10**, 287–293.

Hussey, N. E., Kessel, S. T., Aarestrup, K., *et al.* (2015). Aquatic animal telemetry: a panoramic window into the underwater world. *Science*, **348**, 1255642.

Jacoby, D. M. P., Busawon, D. S., and Sims, D. W. (2010). Sex and social networking: the influence of male presence on social structure of female shark groups. *Behavioral Ecology*, **21**, 808–818.

Jacoby, D. M. P., Papastamatiou, Y. P., and Freeman, R. (2016). Inferring animal social networks and leadership: applications for passive monitoring arrays. *Journal of The Royal Society Interface*, **13**, 20160676.

Kays, R., Crofoot, M. C., Jetz, W., and Wikelski, M. (2015). Terrestrial animal tracking as an eye on life and planet. *Science*, **348**, aaa2478.

Krause, J., Krause, S., Arlinghaus, R., Psorakis, I., Roberts, S., and Rutz, C. (2013). Reality mining of animal social systems. *Trends in Ecology and Evolution*, **28**, 541–551.

Olden, J. D., Lawler, J. J., and Poff, N. L. (2008). Machine learning methods without tears: a primer for ecologists. *The Quarterly Review of Biology*, **83**, 171–193.

Wilson, A. D. M., Brownscombe, J. W., Krause, J., *et al.* (2015). Integrating network analysis, sensor tags, and observation to understand shark ecology and behavior. *Behavioral Ecology*, **26**, 1577–1586.

Yopak, K. E. (2012). Neuroecology of cartilaginous fishes: the functional implications of brain scaling. *Journal of Fish Biology*, **80**, 1968–2023.

Resources

Books:

- Smith, M., Warmolts, D., Thoney, D., and Hueter, R. (2017). *Elasmobranch husbandry manual II: captive care of sharks, rays and their relatives.* Ohio Biological Survey.
- Carrier, J. C., Musick, J. A., and Heithaus, M. R. (2012). *Biology of sharks and their relatives.* Boca Raton, FL: CRC Press.
- Brown, C., Laland, K., and Krause, J. (2011). *Fish cognition and behaviour.* Oxford: Wiley-Blackwell.

Websites:

- The Fish Lab: www.thefishlab.com
- Bimini Shark Lab: www.biminisharklab.com
- Elasmobranch Research Laboratory: www.science.fau.edu/sharklab/index.html
- Mote Marine Lab: www.mote.org
- Marine Biological Association: www.mba.ac.uk
- International Union for Conservation of Nature (IUCN) Redlist of Threatened Species: www.iucnredlist.org

Labs:

- Assistant Professor Christine Bedore; Georgia Southern University, USA; Elasmobranch Sensory Biology.
- Associate Professor Culum Brown; Macquarie University, Australia; Behavioral Ecology and Evolution of Fishes.
- Professor Shaun Collin; University of Western Australia, Australia; Neuroecology.
- Professor Samuel Gruber and Dr Tristan Guttridge; Bimini Biological Field Station Foundation, Bimini, Bahamas; Bimini Sharklab.
- Professor Kim Holland; Hawaii Institute of Marine Biology, USA; Shark and Reef Fish Research.
- Dr Robert Hueter; Mote Marine Lab, Sarasota, USA; Sharks and Rays Conservation Program.
- Dr Stephen Kajiura; Florida Atlantic University, USA; Elasmobranch Research Laboratory.
- Associate Professor Vera Schluessel; University of Bonn, Germany; Cognition in Elasmobranchs and Teleost Fishes.
- Professor David Sims; Marine Biological Association, Plymouth, UK; Movement Ecology and Conservation of Marine Predators.
- Assistant Professor Kara Yopak; University North Carolina Wilmington, USA; Evolutionary Neuroecology.

Tagging information:

- External marker tags: Floy Tags – www.floytag.com; Hallprint – www.hallprint.com
- Internal microchip tags: Biomark – www.biomark.com

- Acoustic tracking tags: Vemco – www.vemco.com; Sonotronics – www.sonotronics.com; Lotek – www.lotek.com
- Accelerometers: CEFAS – www.cefastechnology.co.uk; Gulf Coast Concepts – www.gcdataconcepts.com
- Satellite tags: Wildlife computers – www.wildlifecomputers.com; Microwave Telemetry – www.microwavetelemetry.com

Profile

Tristan is mesmerized by sharks. Being in the water with them is where he feels most inspired. His PhD at the Bimini Sharklab investigated the social organization of lemon sharks. In Australia he studied Port Jackson sharks. In 2012, Tristan returned to Bimini Sharklab as the Director to study sharks' personality.

Vera has been fascinated by sharks since a book she read at six. Her first hands-on experience came at the Bimini Sharklab. Then she studied stingray cognition and biology of white spotted eagle rays. Currently Vera works on cognition in sharks and stingrays (behaviour and anatomy) at Bonn University.

Kara has always been compelled to understand elasmobranchs' behaviour and sensory biology. Because her questions kept coming back to the brain, where all behaviours begin and end, her lab at the University of North Carolina Wilmington explores how the development of major brain areas (and behaviour) varies between species.

References

Ari, C. (2011). Encephalization and brain organization of mobulid rays (*Myliobatiformes, Elasmobranchii*) with ecological perspectives. *The Open Anatomy Journal*, **3**, 1–13.

Armansin, N. C., Lee, K. A., Huveneers, C., and Harcourt, R. G. (2016). Integrating social network analysis and fine-scale positioning to characterize the associations of a benthic shark. *Animal Behaviour*, **115**, 245–258.

Aronson, L. R., Aronson, F. R., and Clark, E. (1967). Instrumental conditioning and light-dark discrimination in young nurse sharks. *Bulletin of Marine Science*, **17**, 249–256.

Bell, C., Bodznick, D., Montgomery, J., and Bastian, J. (1997). The generation and subtraction of sensory experiments within cerebellar-like structures. *Brain, Behaviour and Evolution*, **50**, 17–31.

Bodznick, D., Montgomery, J., and Carey, M. (1999). Adaptive mechanisms in the elasmobranch hindbrain. *Journal of Experimental Biology*, **22**, 1357–1364.

Brown, C. (2001). Familiarity with the test environment improves the escape responses in the crimson spotted rainbowfish, *Melanotaenia duboulayi*. *Animal Cognition*, **4**, 109–113.

Brown, C. (2012). Tool use in fishes. *Fish Fisheries*, **13**, 105–115.

Byrnes, E. E., and Brown, C. (2016). Individual personality differences in Port Jackson sharks *Heterodontus portusjacksoni*. *Journal of Fish Biology*, **89**, 1142–1157.

Byrnes, E. E., Vila-Pouca, C., and Brown, C. (2016a). Laterality strength is linked to stress reactivity in Port Jackson sharks (*Heterodontus portusjacksoni*). *Behavioural Brain Research*, **305**, 239–246.

Byrnes, E. E., Pouca, C. V., Chambers, S. L., and Brown, C. (2016b). Into the wild: developing field tests to examine the link between elasmobranch personality and laterality. *Behaviour*, **153**, 1777–1793.

Casey, J. G., and Natanson, L. J. (1992). Revised estimates of age and growth of the sandbar shark (*Carcharhinus plumbeus*) from the western North Atlantic. *Canadian Journal of Fisheries and Aquatic Sciences*, **49**, 1474–1477.

Collin, S., Kempster, R., and Yopak, K. (2015). Sensing the environment. In *Physiology of elasmobranch fishes* (pp. 19–99). New York, NY: Elsevier.

Dulvy, N. K., and Reynolds, J. D. (1997). Evolutionary transitions among egg-laying, live-bearing, and maternal inputs in sharks and rays. *Proceedings of the Royal Society of London B: Biological Sciences*, **264**, 1309–1315.

Ezcurra, J. M., Lowe, C. G., Mollet, J. F., Ferry, L. A., and O'Sullivan, J. B. (2012). Captive feeding and growth of young-of-the-year white sharks, *Carcharodon carcharias*, at the Monterey Bay Aquarium. In *Global perspectives on the biology and life history of the great white shark research (Carcharodon carcharias)* (pp. 3–16). Boca Raton, FL: Taylor & Francis.

Ferretti, F., Worm, B., Britten, G. L., Heithaus, M. R., and Lotze, H. K. (2010). Patterns and ecosystem consequences of shark declines in the ocean. *Ecology Letters*, **13**, 1055–1071.

Finger, J. S., Dhellemmes, F., Guttridge, T. L., Kurvers, R. H. J. M., Gruber, S. H., and Krause, J. (2016). Rate of movements of juvenile lemon sharks in a novel open field, are we measuring activity or reaction to novelty? *Animal Behaviour*, **116**, 75–82.

Finger, J. S., Dhellemmes, F., and Guttridge, T. L. (2017). Personality in elasmobranchs with a focus on sharks: early evidence, challenges, and future directions. In *Personality in non-human animals* (pp. 129–152). Cham: Springer.

Finger, J. S., Guttridge, T. L., Wilson, A. D. M., Gruber, S. H., and Krause, J. (2018). Are some sharks more social than others? Short and long-term consistency in the social behaviour of juvenile lemon sharks. *Behavioural Ecology and Sociobiology*, **72**, 17.

Fuss, T., and Schluessel, V. (2015). Something worth remembering: Visual discrimination in sharks. *Animal Cognition*, **18**, 463–471.

Fuss, T., and Schluessel, V. (2017). The Ebbinghaus illusion in the gray bamboo shark (*Chiloscyllium griseum*) in comparison to the teleost damselfish (*Chromis chromis*). *Zoology*, **123**, 16–29.

Fuss, T., Bleckmann, H., and Schluessel, V. (2014a). Place learning prior to and after telencephalon ablation in bamboo and coral cat sharks (*Chiloscyllium griseum* and *Atelomycterus marmoratus*). *Journal of Comparative Physiology*, **200**, 37–52.

Fuss, T., Bleckmann, H., and Schluessel, V. (2014b). The shark *Chiloscyllium griseum* can orient using turn responses before and after partial telencephalon ablation. *Journal of Comparative Physiology*, **200**, 19–35.

Fuss, T., Bleckmann, H., and Schluessel, V. (2014c). Visual discrimination abilities in the gray bamboo shark (*Chiloscyllium griseum*). *Zoology*, **117**, 104–111.

Fuss, T., Bleckmann, H., and Schluessel, V. (2014d). The brain creates illusions not just for us: sharks (*Chiloscyllium griseum*) can "see the magic" as well. *Frontiers of Neural Circuits*, **8**, 24.

Fuss, T., Russnak, V., Stehr, K., and Schluessel, V. (2017). World in motion: perception and discrimination of movement in grey bamboo sharks (*Chiloscyllium griseum*). *Animal Behavior and Cognition*, **4**, 223–241.

Gage, F. (2002). Neurogenesis in the adult brain. *Journal of Neuroscience*, **22**, 612–613.

Gardiner, J. M., Hueter, R. E., Maruska, K. P., *et al.* (2012). Sensory physiology and behavior of elasmobranchs. In *Biology of sharks and their relatives* (pp. 349–402). New York, NY: CRC Press.

Gardiner, J. M., Atema, J., Hueter, R. E., and Motta, P. J. (2014). Multisensory integration and behavioral plasticity in sharks from different ecological niches. *PLoS ONE*, **9**(4), e93036.

Gonda, A. I., Herczeg, G. B., and Merila, J. (2013). Evolutionary ecology of intraspecific brain size variation: a review. *Ecology and Evolution*, **3**, 2751–2764.

Graeber, R. C. (1978). Behavioral studies correlated with central nervous system integration of vision in sharks. In *Sensory biology of sharks, skates, and rays* (pp. 195–225). Washington, DC: Government Printing Office.

Graeber, R. C. (1980). Telencephalic function in elasmobranchs. In: *Comparative neurology of the telencephalon* (pp. 17–39). Boston, MA: Springer.

Graeber, R. C., and Ebbesson, S. O. E. (1972). Visual discrimination learning in normal and tectal-ablated nurse sharks (*Ginglymostoma cirratum*). *Comparative Biochemistry and Physiology*, **42**, 131–139.

Graeber, R. C., Ebbesson, S. O. E., and Jane, J. A. (1973). Visual discrimination in sharks without optic tectum. *Science*, **180**, 413–415.

Graeber, R. C., Schroeder, D. M., Jane, J. A., and Ebbesson, S. O. E. (1978). Visual discrimination following partial telencephalic ablations in nurse sharks (*Ginglymostoma cirratum*). *Journal of Comparative Neurology*, **180**, 325–344.

Grogan, E. D., Lund, R., and Greenfest-Allen, E. (2012). The origin and relationships of early Chondrichthyans. In *Biology of sharks and their relatives* (pp. 3–29). Boca Raton, FL: CRC Press.

Grubbs, R. (2010). Ontogenetic shifts in movements and habitat use. In *Sharks and their relatives II: biodiversity, adaptive physiology, and conservation* (pp. 319–350). Boca Raton, FL: CRC Press.

Gruber, S. H., and Schneiderman, N. (1975). Classical conditioning of the nictitating membrane response of the lemon shark (*Negaprion brevirostris*). *Behavior Research Methods*, **7**, 430–434.

Gruber, S. H., De Marignac, J. R., and Hoenig, J. M. (2001). Survival of juvenile lemon sharks at Bimini, Bahamas, estimated by mark–depletion experiments. *Transactions of the American Fisheries Society*, **130**, 376–384.

Guttridge, T. L., and Brown, C. (2014). Learning and memory in the Port Jackson shark, *Heterodontus portusjacksoni*. *Animal Cognition*, **17**, 415–425.

Guttridge, T. L., Myrberg, A. A., Porcher, I. F., Sims, D. W., and Krause, J. (2009a). The role of learning in shark behavior. *Fish Fisheries*, **10**, 450–469.

Guttridge, T. L., Gruber, S. H., Gledhill, K. S., Croft, D. P., Sims, D. W., and Krause, J. (2009b). Social preferences of juvenile lemon sharks *Negaprion brevirostris*. *Animal Behaviour*, **78**, 543–548.

Guttridge, T. L., Gruber, S. H., DiBattista, J. D., *et al.* (2011). Assortative interactions and leadership in a free-ranging population of juvenile lemon shark *Negaprion brevirostris*. *Marine Ecology Progress Series*, **423**, 235–245.

Guttridge, T. L., van Dijk, S., Stamhuis, E. J., Krause, J., Gruber, S. H., and Brown, C. (2013). Social learning in juvenile lemon sharks *Negaprion brevirostris*. *Animal Cognition*, **16**, 55–64.

Harahush, B., Hart, N., and Collin, S. (2014). Ontogenetic changes in retinal ganglion cell distribution and spatial resolving power in the brown-banded bamboo shark *Chiloscyllium punctatum* (Elasmobranchii). *Brain Behavior and Evolution*, **83**, 286–300.

Helfman, G., Collette, B., and Facey, D. (1997). *The diversity of fishes*. Oxford: Blackwell Science.

Herbert-Read, J. E., Perna, A., Mann, R. P., Schaerf, T. M., Sumpter, D. J. T., and Ward, A. J. W. (2011). Inferring the rules of interaction of shoaling fish. *Proceedings of the National Academy of Sciences*, **108**, 18726–18731.

Hofmann, M. H., and Northcutt, R. G. (2012). Forebrain organization in elasmobranchs. *Brain, Behaviour and Evolution*, **80**, 142–151.

Hussey, N. E., Kessel, S. T., Aarestrup, K., *et al.* (2015). Aquatic animal telemetry: a panoramic window into the underwater world. *Science*, **348**, 1255642.

Jacoby, D. M., Croft, D. P., and Sims, D. W. (2012a). Social behaviour in sharks and rays: analysis, patterns and implications for conservation. *Fish and Fisheries*, **13**, 399–417.

Jacoby, D. M. P., Sims, D. W., and Croft, D. P. (2012b). The effect of familiarity on aggregation and social behaviour in juvenile small spotted catsharks *Scyliorhinus canicula*. *Journal of Fish Biology*, **81**, 1596–1610.

Jacoby, D. M. P., Fear, L. N., Sims, D. W., and Croft, D. P. (2014). Shark personalities? Repeatability of social network traits in a widely distributed predatory fish. *Behavioral Ecology and Sociobiology*, **68**, 1995–2003.

Kajiura, S. M. (2003). Electroreception in neonatal bonnethead sharks, *Sphyrna tiburo*. *Marine Biology*, **143**, 603–611.

Keller, B., Finger, J.-S., Gruber, S. H., Abel, D. C., and Guttridge, T. L. (2017). The effects of familiarity on the social interactions of juvenile lemon sharks, *Negaprion brevirostris*. *Journal of Experimental Marine Biology*, **489**, 24–31.

Kempster, R., Hart, N., and Collin, S. (2013). Survival of the stillest: predator avoidance in shark embryos. *PLoS ONE*, **8**, e52551.

Kimber, J. A., Sims, D. W., Bellamy, P. H., and Gill, A. B. (2011). The ability of a benthic elasmobranch to discriminate between biological and artificial electric fields. *Marine Biology*, **158**, 1–8.

Kimber, J. A., Sims, D. W., Bellamy, P. H., and Gill, A. B. (2014). Elasmobranch cognitive ability: using electroreceptive foraging behaviour to demonstrate learning, habituation and memory in a benthic shark. *Animal Cognition*, **17**, 55–65.

Kotrschal, A., van Staaden, M. J., and Huber, R. (1998). Fish brains: evolution and environmental relationships. *Reviews in Fish Biology and Fisheries*, **8**, 373–408.

Kotrschal, A., Rogell, B., Bundsen, A., *et al.* (2013). Artificial selection on relative brain size in the guppy reveals costs and benefits of evolving a larger brain. *Current Biology*, **23**, 168–171.

Kuba, M. J., Byrne, R. A., and Burghardt, G. M. (2010). A new method for studying problem solving and tool use in stingrays (*Potamotrygon castexi*). *Animal Cognition*, **13**, 507–513.

Lema, S. C., Hodges, M. J., Marchetti, M. P., and Nevitt, G. A. (2005). Proliferation zones in the salmon telencephalon and evidence for environmental influence on proliferation rate. *Comparative Biochemistry and Physiology A*, **141**, 327–335.

Lieberman, D. A. (1990). *Learning: behaviour and cognition*. Belmont, CA: Wadsworth.

Lisney, T. J., Bennett, M. B., and Collin, S. P. (2007). Volumetric analysis of sensory brain areas indicates ontogenetic shifts in the relative importance of sensory systems in elasmobranchs. *Raffles Bulletin of Zoology*, **14**, 7–15.

Lisney, T. J., Theiss, S. M., Collin, S. P., and Hart, N. S. (2012). Vision in elasmobranchs: 21st century advances. *Journal of Fish Biology*, **80**, 2024–2054.

Lisney, T. J., Yopak, E. E., Camilieri-Asch, V., and Collin, S. P. (2017). Ontogenetic shifts in brain organization in the bluespotted stingray *Neotrygon kuhlii* (Chondrichthyes: Dasyatidae). *Brain, Behaviour and Evolution*, **89**, 68–83.

Litherland, L., Collin, S., and Fritsches, K. (2009a). Eye growth in sharks: ecological implications for changes in retinal topography and visual resolution. *Visual Neuroscience*, **26**, 397–409.

Litherland, L., Collin, S., and Fritsches, K. (2009b). Visual optics and ecomorphology of the growing shark eye: a comparison between deep and shallow water species. *Journal of Experimental Biology*, **212**, 3583–3594.
Marchetti, M. P., and Nevitt, G. A. (2003). Effects of hatchery rearing on brain structures of rainbow trout, *Oncorhynchus mykiss*. *Environmental Biology of Fishes*, **66**, 9–14.
Meredith, T. L., and Kajiura, S. M. (2010). Olfactory morphology and physiology of elasmobranchs. *Journal of Experimental Biology*, **213**, 3449–3456.
Mitchell, C. (2016). The evolution of brains and cognitive abilities. In: *Evolutionary biology* (pp. 73–87). Cham: Springer.
Montgomery, J. C., Bodznick, D., and Yopak, K. E. (2012). The cerebellum and cerebellar-like structures of cartilaginous fishes. *Brain, Behaviour and Evolution*, **80**, 152–165.
Mourier, J., Vercelloni, J., and Planes, S. (2012). Evidence of social communities in a spatially structured network of a free-ranging shark species. *Animal Behavior*, **83**, 389–401.
Mourier, J., Brown, C., and Planes, S. (2017). Learning and robustness to catch-and-release fishing in a shark social network. *Biology Letters*, **13**, 20160824.
Naylor, G. J. P., Caira, J. N., Jensen, K., Rosana, K. A. M., Straube, N., and Lakner, C. (2012). Elasmobranch phylogeny: a mitochondrial estimate based on 595 species. In *Biology of sharks and their relatives* (pp. 31–56). New York, NY: CRC Press.
Newton, K. C., and Kajiura, S. M. (2017). Magnetic field discrimination, learning and memory in the yellow stingray (*Urobatis jamaicensis*). *Animal Cognition*, **20**, 603–614.
Nielsen, J., Hedeholm, R. B., Heinemeier, J., *et al.* (2016). Eye lens radiocarbon reveals centuries of longevity in the Greenland shark (*Somniosus microcephalus*). *Science*, **353**(6300), 702–704.
Peters, R., and Evers, H. (1985). Frequency selectivity in the ampullary system of an elasmobranch fish *Scyliorhinus canicula*. *Journal of Experimental Biology*, **118**, 99–109.
Pritchard, D. J., Hurly, T. A., Tello-Ramos, M. C., and Healy, S. D. (2016). Why study cognition in the wild (and how to test it)? *Journal of the Experimental Analysis of Behvior*, **105**, 41–55.
Puzdrowski, R. L., and Gruber, S. (2009). Morphologic features of the cerebellum of the Atlantic stingray, and their possible evolutionary significance. *Integrative Zoology*, **4**, 110–122.
Reynolds, J. D., Goodwin, N. B., and Freckleton, R. P. (2002). Evolutionary transitions in parental care and live bearing in vertebrates. *Philosophical Transactions of the Royal Society B: Biological*, **357**, 269–281.
Schluessel, V. (2015). Who would have thought that 'Jaws' also has brains? Cognitive functions in elasmobranchs. *Animal Cognition*, **18**, 19–37.
Schluessel, V., and Bleckmann, H. (2005). Spatial memory and orientation strategies in the elasmobranch *Potamotrygon motoro*. *Journal of Comparative Physiology A*, **191**, 695–706.
Schluessel, V., and Bleckmann, H. (2012). Spatial learning and memory retention in the grey bamboo shark (*Chiloscyllium griseum*). *Zoology*, **115**, 346–353.
Schluessel, V., and Duengen, D. (2015). Irrespective of size, scales, color or body shape, all fish are just fish: object categorization in the gray bamboo shark *Chiloscyllium griseum*. *Animal Cognition*, **18**, 497–507.
Schluessel, V., Beil, O., Weber, T., and Bleckmann, H. (2014a). Symmetry perception in bamboo sharks (*Chiloscyllium griseum*) and Malawi cichlids (*Pseudotropheus* sp.). *Animal Cognition*, **17**, 1187–1205.
Schluessel, V., Rick, I. P., and Plischke, K. (2014b). No rainbow for grey bamboo sharks: evidence for the absence of colour vision in sharks from behavioral discrimination experiments. *Journal of Comparative Physiology A*, **200**, 939–947.
Schluessel, V., Herzog, H., and Scherpenstein, M. (2015). Seeing the forest before the trees – spatial orientation in freshwater stingrays (*Potamotrygon motoro*) in a hole-board task. *Behavioural Processes*, **119**, 105–115.

Schwarze, S., Bleckmann, H., and Schluessel, V. (2013). Avoidance conditioning in bamboo sharks (*Chiloscyllium punctatum* and *C. griseum*): behavioural and neuroanatomical aspects. *Journal of Comparative Physiology A*, **199**, 843–856.

Sebens, K. P. (1987). The ecology of indeterminate growth in animals. *Annual Review of Ecology and Systematics*, **18**, 371–407.

Siciliano, A. M., Kajiura, S. M., Long Jr, J. H., and Porter, M. H. (2013). Are you positive? Electric dipole polarity discrimination in the yellow stingray *Urobatis jamaicensis*. *Biology Bulletin*, **225**, 85–89.

Sisneros, J. A., and Tricas, T. C. (2002). Neuroethology and life history adaptations of the elasmobranch electric sense. *Journal of Physiology*, **96**, 379–389.

Smeets, W. J. A. J., Nieuwenhuys, R., and Roberts, B. L. (1983). *The central nervous system of cartilaginous fishes: structural and functional correlations*. New York, NY: Springer.

Smith, M., Warmolts, D., Thoney, D., and Hueter, R. (2017). *Elasmobranch husbandry manual II: captive care of sharks, rays and their relatives*. Columbus, OH: Ohio Biological Survey.

Striedter, G. F. (2005). *Principles of brain evolution*. Sunderland, MA: Sinauer Associates.

Tester, A., and Kato, S. (1963). Visual target discrimination in blacktip sharks (*Carcharhinus melanopterus*) and grey sharks (*C. menisorrah*). *Pacific Science*, **20**, 461–471.

Thonhauser, K. E., Gutnick, T., Byrne, R. A., Kral, K., Burghardt, G. M., and Kuba, M. J. (2013). Social learning in cartilaginous fish (stingrays *Potamotrygon falkneri*). *Animal Cognition*, **16**, 927–932.

Warburton, K. (2003). Learning of foraging skills by fish. *Fish and Fisheries*, **4**, 203–215.

Wegner, N. (2015). Elasmobranch gill structure. *In Fish physiology. Physiology of Elasmobranch fishes*. (Vol. 34A, pp. 19–99). New York, NY: Elsevier.

Wetherbee, B., and Cortés, E. (2004). Food consumption and feeding habits. In *Biology of sharks and their relatives* (pp. 239–264). Boca Raton, FL: CRC Press.

Yopak, K. E. (2012a). Neuroecology in cartilaginous fishes: the functional implications of brain scaling. *Journal of Fish Biology*, **80**, 1968–2023.

Yopak, K. E. (2012b). The nervous system of cartilaginous fishes. *Brain, Behavior, and Evolution*, **80**, 77–79.

Yopak, K. E., and Frank, L. R. (2009). Brain size and brain organization of the whale shark, *Rhincodon typus*, using Magnetic Resonance Imaging. *Brain, Behavior, and Evolution*, **74**, 121–142.

Yopak, K. E., and Lisney, T. J. (2012). Allometric scaling of the optic tectum in cartilaginous fishes. *Brain, Behavior, and Evolution*, **80**, 108–126.

Yopak, K. E., and Montgomery, J. C. (2008). Brain organization and specialization in deep-sea chondrichthyans. *Brain, Behavior, and Evolution*, **71**, 287–304.

Yopak, K. E., Lisney, T. J., Collin, S. P., and Montgomery, J. C. (2007). Variation in brain organization and cerebellar foliation in chondrichthyans: sharks and holocephalans. *Brain, Behaviour and Research*, **69**, 280–300.

Yopak, K. E., Lisney, T. J., and Collin, S. P. (2015). Not all sharks are swimming noses: variation in olfactory bulb size in cartilaginous fishes. *Brain Structure and Function*, **220**, 1127–1143.

Yopak, K., Galinsky, V. L., Berquist, R. M., and Frank, L. R. (2016). Quantitative classification of cerebellar foliation in cartilaginous fishes (class: Chondrichthyes) using 3D shape analysis and its implications for evolutionary biology. *Brain, Behavior, and Evolution*, **87**, 252–264.

Yopak, K. E., Pakan, J., and Wylie, D. (2017). The cerebellum of non-mammalian vertebrates. In *Evolution of nervous systems* (Vol. 1, pp. 373–385). Kidlington, UK: Elsevier.

17 Spiders – Hints for Testing Cognition and Learning in Jumping Spiders

Elizabeth M. Jakob, Skye M. Long and Margaret Bruce

Species Description

The over 6000 jumping spider species (World Spider Catalog, 2017) vary considerably in size, morphology, behaviour and habitat (Maddison, 2015). Here, we will focus on the characteristics typical of most species, with a special emphasis on our primary subjects: *Phidippus audax, P. clarus* and *P. princeps*. While jumping spiders range in body length from 1 to 25 mm, *Phidippus* is larger, and *P. audax* may reach 20 mm long (Edwards, 2004).

Anatomy and Physiology

Like other spiders, jumping spiders have eight legs and two body regions, a cephalothorax and an abdomen. Jumping spiders (family Salticidae) are distinguished from other spider families by their characteristic eye pattern, described in the next section. Their namesake jumps are achieved by increasing local hydrostatic pressure on hinge joints in their legs (Parry and Brown, 1959). *Phidippus* requires the provision of drinking water in the lab, and high humidity greatly improves survival (E. M. Jakob and S. M. Long, unpubl. data). However, jumping spiders from arid regions may not require water beyond what is in their prey (N. Morehouse, pers. comm.).

Jumping spiders have two well-developed respiratory systems, comprised of a pair of book lungs and a tracheal system, that allow high levels of aerobic activity (Schmitz and Perry, 2000; Schmitz, 2004). However, they cannot recover quickly from exhaustion and do not return to peak performance even after a 2-day rest (McGinley *et al.*, 2013). The design of cognitive tests relying on movement, such as the speed to complete a maze, should account for potential within-species relationships between size, speed and endurance (e.g. McGinley *et al.*, 2013).

Spiders feed through external digestion. In a lengthy process, venom and digestive fluid are injected into the prey, and then nutrients are sucked out (Foelix, 2014). Many species do well in the lab on only 1–2 feedings per week. Because satiation affects motivation, designing learning trials using food rewards requires creativity.

Perception

The principal and secondary eyes differ in morphology, perceptual capabilities, developmental origins and visual processing pathways to and within the brain (Land, 1985;

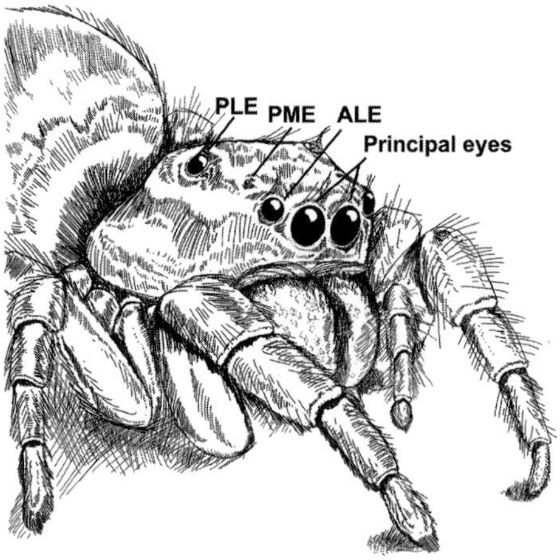

Figure 17.1. The eight eyes of a jumping spider. The principal eyes have small retinas positioned at the back of moveable tubes, inside the spider's cephalothorax. The three secondary eyes (ALE or anterior lateral eyes, PME or posterior medial eyes and PLE or posterior lateral eyes) are excellent motion detectors, especially the large PLE and ALE. The ALE overlap in field of view with the principal eyes. Illustration by S. M. Long.

Land and Nilsson, 2012; Strausfeld, 2012; Figure 17.1). Each of the two principal eyes possesses a tiny boomerang-shaped retina that offers remarkable spatial acuity (reviewed in Harland *et al.*, 2012). The retina's small size gives it a small field of view, but it sits at the back of a moveable tube that can be directed to different areas of the visual field (Land, 1969a). At the elbow of the boomerang is the area of highest spatial acuity, comprised of four layers of retinal cells aligned along the optical axis of the lens (Land, 1969b). The wavelengths of light that jumping spiders can see vary across species, but include UV and green (see Lim and Li, 2006). Some species use spectral filtering to see red (Zurek *et al.*, 2015). Defocusing of light on the different retinal layers has been implicated in depth perception (Nagata *et al.*, 2012).

Up to three pairs of secondary eyes possess flat sheets of green-sensitive retinal cells. Eye-masking techniques allow researchers to study the capabilities of, and interaction between, different eye types (Forster, 1979; Zurek *et al.*, 2010; Spano *et al.*, 2012; Zurek and Nelson, 2012a, b). The secondary eyes mediate responses to object motion, whereas the principal eyes scan objects for spatial detail and spectral properties.

Other senses are also well-developed. With sensory hairs concentrated on the tarsi (Foelix, 2014), jumping spiders use contact chemoreception and sometimes airborne chemical cues to detect the presence of food and mates (Clark *et al.*, 2000; Jackson *et al.*, 2002; Cross and Jackson, 2009; Tedore and Johnsen, 2013; Cross, 2016). Jumping spiders detect substrate-borne vibration, an important component of male courtship displays in many species (e.g. Elias, 2003; Elias *et al.*, 2012). *Phidippus audax* also responds to airborne sound (Shamble *et al.*, 2016). Combining sensory information from different modalities can help reinforce learning in spiders (Skow and Jakob, 2005; VanderSal and Hebets, 2007; Long *et al.*, 2012).

Life Cycle

Male spiders generally undergo fewer moults than females prior to maturity. *Phidippus* spiders are often protandrous, with males maturing earlier than females. Taylor and Peck (1975) report that *P. audax* males mature in 8–9 instars and females in 10, but note that there is variability even within a population, a common phenomenon in spiders. In our study sites in New England, *P. clarus* males mature before the females and disappear from the population months before the females do (Hoefler and Jakob, 2006). In *Phidippus*, the transition to adulthood is marked by a change in behaviour. Juvenile males and females, in our experience, have similar behaviour, foraging for food during the day, and building and reusing silken nests for shelter. As they approach maturity, females increase site fidelity, building and guarding a thick silken nest to shelter their eggs. Adult males, in contrast, do not show site fidelity unless they are guarding a female (Hoefler and Jakob, 2006). It is not unusual to find several *Phidippus* females sharing a nest, as well as 2–3 males guarding the females.

When preparing to moult, spiders become lethargic and their visual responsiveness appears to decline, and they are thus unsuitable for behavioural testing. In our experience, adult males are less motivated to feed than adult females, and extremely gravid females feed very little. While we have kept *Phidippus* in the laboratory for close to a year after they moult to maturity, older spiders (6–8 months past maturity) decline in responsiveness and eventually become unable to grip surfaces well with their tarsi.

Identification of Sexes and Individuals

Jumping spider species vary widely in their coloration and degree of sexual dimorphism. Adult males and females are distinguishable by their reproductive organs, including palps and epigyna (Foelix, 2014). The pedipalps, at the anterior end of the spider next to the mouth, are used by both sexes to manipulate prey. In adult males, they also serve as intromittent organs, and this function is reflected in their complex structure. Female palps are comparatively simple in structure; adult males and females can usually be distinguished with the naked eye. Penultimate males (one moult away from maturity) can also often be sexed, because their palps appear to be swollen. In *Phidippus* species, adult males tend to have more robust anterior legs and smaller abdomens than females.

Ecological Characteristics

Jumping spiders are found in all non-polar ecosystems in a diversity of habitats (Maddison, 2015) and species may be ground-dwelling, arboreal, found under bark, or even in burrows in sand. We focus here on our three *Phidippus* species. Information on range and habitat is from the excellent revision of the genus by Edwards (2004). There are 60 *Phidippus* species distributed from Alaska to Costa Rica, and in the Bahamas, Bermuda and Greater Antilles. *Phidippus audax* is common in fields and open woodlands of the eastern and central USA and southeastern Canada, and has been introduced to southern California and Hawaii. In the northern part of its range, *P. audax* overwinters as large juveniles, often in groups in hibernacula, and matures in the spring. In southern Florida, adults of both sexes can be collected year-round. *Phidippus princeps* is found from New England south to northern Georgia and west to Saskatchewan, Utah, and northern Texas, inhabits old fields and hardwood understorey, and matures in spring. In Massachusetts, we collect large juvenile *P. audax* and *princeps* in late summer, keep them under a long-day light cycle (16:8), and they mature without hibernation during late autumn. *Phidippus clarus* is widespread in southern Canada and the USA except for the desert Southwest. It inhabits old fields and matures in summer.

Various reports and our own observations indicate that *Phidippus* spiders are preyed upon by dragonflies, birds, wasps, lizards and other spiders (e.g. Young and Lockley, 1988). To escape attack, spiders may freeze, run, jump away or move quickly to the bottom side of a leaf.

The hunting behaviour of jumping spiders is often compared to that of cats: they orient to the prey, creep up on it with lowered body postures and then leap. Most jumping spiders are euryphagic, attacking a broad range of arthropod prey of diverse body forms. Salticids, including *Phidippus*, may have innate preferences for particular prey types (Edwards and Jackson, 1993, 1994), but preferences may change depending on experience with prey, availability of the preferred food, the spider's hunger level, prey palatability, and sex or size of the spider. Males prefer smaller prey and are less efficient than females at extracting nutrients (Givens, 1978). When live prey are not available, *P. audax* can also survive by scavenging (Vickers *et al.*, 2014). In contrast to *Phidippus*, some species are more stenophagic (Jackson and Cross, 2011), preferring, for example, ants (Li *et al.*, 1999), other spiders (araneophagy) or blood-filled mosquitoes (Jackson *et al.*, 2005). Note that tests of prey preference need to be thoughtfully designed (see Nelson and Jackson, 2012a, for examples of protocols).

Social Characteristics

Jumping spiders generally tolerate each other only before they disperse from the nest, during courtship and mating and, in some species, when sharing nests or overwintering sites. Given the high risk of cannibalism (e.g. Okuyama, 2007), it is important to keep spiders separated from one another during rearing, and to be alert for it when designing experiments. In studies of conspecific interactions, one might, for example, provide videos of potential partners (Clark and Uetz, 1992) or rivals (McGinley and Taylor, 2016) rather than live animals. In addition, it may be desirable to keep spiders visually isolated, so they do not display to one another from their cages.

State of the Art

A thorough review of work on cognition in the Araneae is beyond the scope of this chapter. Please consult instead recent reviews (Cross and Jackson, 2006; Jackson and Cross, 2011; Jakob *et al.*, 2011; Nelson and Jackson, 2011; Harland *et al.*, 2012;

Japyassú and LaLand, 2017), as well as our compendium of failed methods used in attempts to study spider learning (Jakob and Long, 2016).

A good deal of research on salticid cognition is focused on the salticid subfamily Spartaeinae, particularly the genus *Portia*. In contrast to more typical salticids such as *Phidippus*, many spartaeines routinely prey on other spiders, often invading their webs and drawing them close by making vibrations that mimic an insect caught in the web (Su *et al.*, 2007; Jackson and Cross, 2011; Chang *et al.*, 2017). Some, like *Portia*, resemble debris and even move unlike typical salticids, very slowly and jerkily, and present their own set of challenges for study (Box 17.2). Here we will focus on cognition in more typical salticids, but will also mention particular cognitive skills studied in *Portia*, many of which have not been thoroughly examined in other groups.

There are many ways in which learning may be beneficial in the context of predation, such as improving prey-capture techniques, learning to select some prey and avoid others, and associating other cues with the presence of prey. For example, the attack success of *P. regius* improves with repeated trials (Edwards and Jackson, 1994). *Phidippus princeps* can learn to avoid distasteful milkweed bugs (Skow and Jakob, 2005) and distasteful fireflies (Long *et al.*, 2012) after a few encounters, especially if contextual cues (i.e. background cues presented near the prey) are held constant (Skow and Jakob, 2005). Similarly, *P. princeps* more readily learn to avoid toxic, non-luminescent fireflies if they are next to a flashing LED light simulating a firefly flash, as opposed to an unlit LED (Long *et al.*, 2012). Spiders can learn to avoid toxic prey of a particular colour and then generalize to other prey (Taylor *et al.*, 2016; Raška *et al.*, 2017). With live prey, it can be a challenge to ensure that the spider consistently captures it and receives the reward. A promising workaround is based on the fact that many spiders will readily consume sugar water (Jackson *et al.*, 2001), which can serve as a positive reward (Liedtke and Schneider, 2014). The speed of predatory decisions may also correlate with the aggressiveness of the individual spider (Chang *et al.*, 2017).

Jumping spiders need navigational skills in several contexts. First, some species reuse their silken nests and must find their way back. *Phidippus clarus* can use beacons or landmarks close to a goal to find their nests, and can learn to attend to the colour of a beacon (Hoefler and Jakob, 2006). In *Serveae incana*, beacon use was demonstrated in an elegant virtual reality set-up in which a tethered spider moved through a virtual world (Peckmezian and Taylor, 2015a). Spiders might also benefit by associating particular cues with the presence of prey. *Phidippus princeps* can learn that prey is hidden behind blocks of a particular colour in a T-maze (Jakob *et al.*, 2007). Stalking spiders also need to keep track of a prey's location. *Phidippus* stops frequently to reorient to its target (Hill, 1979), whereas other species routinely follow even more complex detours. For example, the web-invading salticid *Portia* can identify an approach route even among incomplete distractor routes, and even when the route requires looking away from the prey (Tarsitano and Jackson, 1992, 1994, 1997; Tarsitano and Andrew, 1999; Cross and Jackson, 2016). In contrast to *Portia* and other spider-eating species (Cross and Jackson, 2016), *P. audax* are usually unable to reach the prey in even the easiest of the reversed-route detour tests that could be successfully completed by *Portia* (Carducci and Jakob, 2000; Figure 17.2).

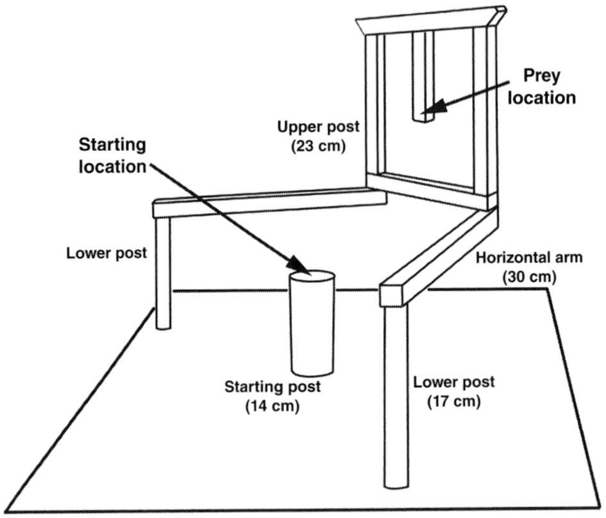

Figure 17.2. A simple detour test that can easily be completed by *Portia fimbriata*, but not by *Phidippus audax*. To reach the prey, the spider must move away from it, so that it is no longer in the line of sight of its principal eyes.
Illustration is reprinted from Carducci and Jakob (2000). Modified from Tarsitano and Jackson (1994), with permission from Elsevier.

Animals may perceive a wide range of stimuli, but may attend to only certain ones – a process called selective attention. Attention may be captured by the features of a particular stimulus. For example, *Evarcha culicivora* specializes in eating mosquitos and can identify even an abstract representation of a mosquito, as long as the image elements form the correct angle (Dolev and Nelson, 2014). Attention can also be modified by experience (Cross and Jackson, 2006). For example, *E. culicivora* primed with odour cues were better at finding cryptic prey than those that were not primed. *Portia labiata* was more likely to find prey after experience with prey of a similar type (Jackson and Li, 2004). Our recently developed spider eye-tracker will help us understand how both stimulus characteristics and priming experiences influence the exploration of a visual scene by the tiny retinas of the principal eyes, coupled with the newly developed ability to record how the brains of living spiders respond to visual stimuli (Menda *et al.*, 2014).

Flexible behaviour may also be apparent in the assessment of mates and rivals. Several species, including *Phidippus*, can discriminate among prospective mates based on size (e.g. Cross *et al.*, 2007; Hoefler, 2007). The duration of contests between male *P. clarus* is primarily driven by self-assessment and secondarily by mutual assessment, and fighting behaviour is influenced by prior experience (Elias *et al.*, 2008; Kasumovic *et al.*, 2010). Some species can assess opponent size by vision alone, as demonstrated by the use of video rivals presented in different sizes (Tedore and Johnsen, 2015; McGinley and Taylor, 2016).

Phidippus spiders exhibit anti-predator behaviour, freezing when they hear airborne wasp sounds (Shamble *et al.*, 2016). The flight initiation distance of *P. clarus* from a predator depends on the spider's body size and hunger level (Stankowich, 2009). Further work on anti-predator behaviour might yield insight into underlying cognitive processes. For example, in *Jacksonoides queenslandicus*, courtship behaviour decreases when spiders are aware that a predator is nearby (Su and Li, 2006).

Salticids present fertile ground for comparative studies of the evolution of cognition, and several labs have attempted to generate standardized cognitive tests. For example, foot shock is an effective aversive stimulus to demonstrate that *P. princeps* learns about contextual cues (Skow, 2007) and that *P. audax* can distinguish between two visual stimuli (Bednarski *et al.*, 2012). Vibration is also effective (Long *et al.*, 2015; Figure 17.3). In other species, researchers carefully assessed the effect of aversive shock on behaviour (Peckmezian and Taylor, 2015b) and used shock in a learned passive place avoidance procedure (Peckmezian and Taylor, 2017). To test trial-and-error problem-solving, researchers developed a confinement problem. Spiders can choose to attempt to escape from a box by either leaping or swimming, and researchers can aid or thwart the spiders after they make their choice (Jackson *et al.*, 2001; Cross and Jackson, 2015). Spiders have also been trained to associate particular colours with an aversive level of heat (Nakamura and Yamashita, 2000; but see Jakob and Long,

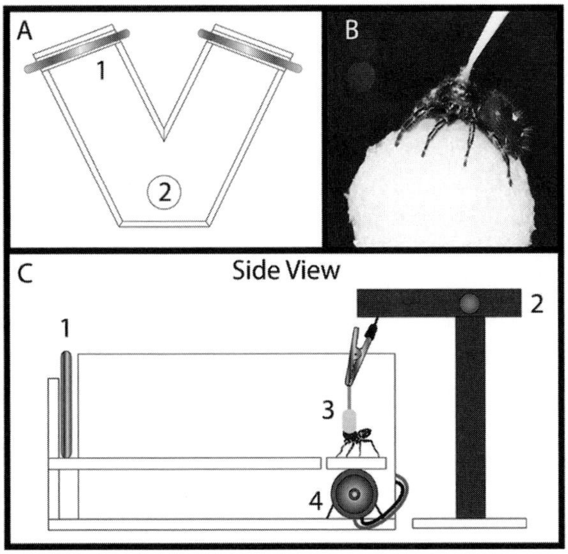

Figure 17.3. An apparatus for aversive conditioning. (A) A choice arena. An iPod is placed at the end of each arm (1) and a spider is introduced into the area with a syringe with its tip cut off, inserted through a hole in the arena floor. (B) Spiders are tethered by a wax and resin 'hat' attached to a small plastic stick. (C) The training arena. The spider views an image on an iPod (1), while tethered to a stand (2) by its hat (3). Its tarsi rest on a platform that is vibrated by a small motor (4). Later, when given a choice between the image paired with the vibration and a novel image, a spider that has learned the association chooses the novel image.
Illustration is reprinted with permission of *Journal of Arachnology*, where it was first published (Long *et al.*, 2015).

2016). An interesting protocol employs expectancy violation: a spider is presented with a scene, then out of the spider's view the scene is either manipulated or not. When the spider sees the scene again, it behaves differently depending on whether the scene is the same as it remembers. Results from this method (e.g. Cross and Jackson, 2017), as well as others (Nelson and Jackson, 2012b), support the hypothesis that at least some salticid species are sensitive to the number of objects.

All for One and One for All

Box 17.1 Natural History Informs Cognitive Experiments: Arthopod Cognition

Cole Gilbert

Determining the cognitive abilities of non-verbal creatures is no trivial undertaking. Tests must be cleverly designed, considering the animal's natural history and imagining its Umwelt. Different creatures require different spatial contexts; some do well in restricted laboratory spaces, or even in confined, partially dissected protocols allowing examination of neural substrates of cognitive function. Others may only reveal their abilities in natural spaces comprising hundreds of square metres. An animal's mode of locomotion, walking, running or flying, may influence its ability to perform particular cognitive functions. Moreover, human subjects can be paid to motivate cognitive performance, but non-human animals require different motivation to perform behaviours that allow probing particular cognitive functions. Escape is easiest to elicit. Feeding can be relatively easy, if one knows what the animal eats in nature. However, courtship, even with male subjects, is often difficult to elicit in the laboratory.

Given those considerations, how do we investigate cognitive functions in arthropods, such as attention, perception, learning and memory, higher reasoning or language? Jumping spiders studied by Beth Jakob's group (this chapter) are relatively slow-moving, highly visual predators. Thus, attention can be tested by presenting multiple prey while the spider is slowly stalking. On the other hand, the tiger beetles we study are fast visual predators that generate a strong optic flow field, in which distractor targets may disappear due to motion blur (Gilbert, 1997). Investigating an arthropod's perceptual world requires understanding its sensory world. Jumping spiders have relatively slow photoreceptors (DeVoe, 1975) and are not bothered by the flickering fluorescent lights that illuminate our labs. However, the photoreceptors of fast-flying insects, such as bees, easily resolve 50–60 Hz flicker, which bothers many individuals.

Researchers rig their experimental room with three banks of lights 120° out of phase (van Praagh, 1972), or work under natural or incandescent light. Perceptual abilities may also be context-dependent. For instance, flying, but not stationary, honeybees perceive magnetic fields (Walker *et al.*, 1989). Most animals are capable of learning and memory. Minimally, they exhibit latent learning when moving about their environment. However, some animals, such as honeybees, are much better for studying these cognitive functions, because of fluctuations in their Umwelt. Bees

(*cont.*)

collect nectar, which varies seasonally as different flowers bloom in different parts of their environment. Thus, bees evolved to learn temporal and spatial patterns of this resource and are excellent experimental animals to probe sophisticated mechanisms of learning and memory, as Randolf Menzel describes (Chapter 3). Higher reasoning can be addressed in some arthropods with experiments carefully tailored to the animal's natural behaviour. Because jumping spiders deliberately stalk prey, we were able to use a two-choice paradigm to demonstrate that they differentiate between shorter and longer paths to prey (Perkins and Gilbert, 2016). Conversely, tiger beetles simply run at their prey, so we used frequency of approach to show that they can also judge prey at closer versus farther distances (Layne *et al.*, 2006). Finally, Karl von Frisch (1967) was able to elucidate the abstract language by which a honeybee communicates the location of nectar sources to her sisters, because honeybees are social. Solitary species would be less-rewarding subjects to probe this cognitive function.

References

DeVoe, R. D. (1975). Ultraviolet and green receptors in principal eyes of jumping spiders. *Journal of General Physiology*, **66**, 193–207.

Gilbert, C. (1997). Visual control of cursorial prey pursuit by tiger beetles (Cicindelidae). *Journal of Comparative Physiology A*, **181**, 217–230.

Layne, J. E., Chen, P. W., and Gilbert, C. (2006). The role of target elevation in prey selection by tiger beetles (Carabidae: *Cicindela* spp.). *Journal of Experimental Biology*, **209**, 4295–4303.

Perkins, M. Q., and Gilbert, C. (2016). Spatial cognition in jumping spiders: assessment of path length to prey and vantage point. *Denver Museum of Nature & Science Reports*, **3**, 92.

van Praagh, J. P. (1972). Towards a contolled-environment room suitable for normal colony life of honeybees 1. Description and general observations. *Journal of Apicultural Research*, **11**, 77–87.

von Frisch, K. (1967). *The dance language and orientation of bees*. Cambridge, MA: Harvard University Press.

Walker, M. M., Baird, D. L., and Bitterman, M. E. (1989). Failure of stationary but not of flying honeybees (*Apis mellifera*) to respond to magnetic field stimuli. *Journal of Comparative Psychology*, **103**, 62–69.

Field Guide

In this section, we will focus primarily on our own experience with *Phidippus* spiders. However, as our spiders are typical of many species in terms of hunting behaviour, prey diversity, nest building, etc., our tips should be easily transferrable.

As with most any study on wild animals, our first challenge in studying *Phidippus* spiders is to find them in numbers. Our species prefer unmown fields with a mixture of flowers and grasses, and as these are ephemeral, we are continually looking for new sites. In addition, distribution is patchy: next to a field with many *Phidippus* might be another field of the same size with the same plant species, but with no spiders. We capture many *P. audax* on human-made structures, but even these are subject to change. One of our best sites, the buttresses of a bridge over a river, was unfortunately colonized by invasive spiders and now has no jumping spiders.

To capture spiders, we use a combination of hand-collecting in small vials (medicine vials or a similar size) or sweep netting. A suction 'pooter' can be used for small individuals. The best weather seems to be sunny and dry, late enough in the day so that the dew has dried, and with little wind. To hand-collect, we move slowly through the field looking for movement. Our spiders are often found at the tops of plants or sitting on stems or leaves. We also look for the white, thick silk of nests in curled-up leaves, in the closed-up flowers of Queen Anne's lace, or in crevices like the space between a guardrail and its post. An artist's paintbrush is useful for poking spiders out of hiding places and into a vial. We also have a good deal of luck using a sweep net through long grass and flowers (see below for a link to a comprehensive video by Wayne Maddison on how to collect jumping spiders).

For field experiments on jumping spiders similar to ours that live in fields, we recommend the deployment of plastic tubes that are enticing for spiders as nest sites – we use black plumbing tubing that comes in rolls at the hardware store, cut into sections of about 5 cm, threaded with string or twist-ties and hung on dowels stuck into the ground. We set tubes out in a grid, in order to track the life history and movements of spiders (Hoefler and Jakob, 2006). Our lab intercepted spiders on the way back to their nests late in the day, and tested whether they recognized the colour of beacons associated with their nests (Hoefler and Jakob, 2006). To run experiments under natural light, it is also possible to use field enclosures. Our lab has used field enclosures with walls of metal flashing but open on top (Baker, 2007), as well as small, closed, clear boxes (Long *et al.*, 2012).

In *Phidippus*, in spite of their large size relative to other jumping spiders, distinguishing among individuals with confidence is quite difficult, even for *P. audax*, which has variable colour patterns (Edwards, 2004). We mark spiders with dots of non-toxic paint on the top of the abdomen (Testor's enamel paint provides a large array of colours), or with bee tags, which are small numbered tags that can be glued to the dorsal surface of the abdomen. Spiders can be marked without anaesthesia by placing them in a large plastic syringe with the tip cut off, covered instead with either netting or a piece of Parafilm stretched over the top. The spider can be captured in a vial, popped into the syringe, and gently pressed against the netting, which in turn can be snipped or pulled away from the spider, to expose only the part to which the mark is applied. We have had bee tags last in the field for over a month. Of course, any such marks are lost during moult, so this method is best used for adults. Care must be taken when marking spiders, as the sealing of either the openings to the book lungs or the spiracles can cause a severe reduction of activity or even death (Schmitz, 2005).

Table 17.1. Key aspects relevant to studying *Phidippus* spiders.

Field guide – materials and skills
Appropriate field sites for collection and study
Collecting gear (nets, vials)
Lab rearing supplies (boxes, crickets or other prey)
Artist's paintbrushes for coaxing spiders out of vials
Access to craft supplies, especially foam core, for building arenas
Access to video presentation equipment as appropriate (iPods, tablets, video projected onto screens)
A laboratory area free from disruptive noise or vibrations
Patience and slow movement

For the sake of controlling experimental conditions, we conduct most of our experiments in the laboratory. We prefer to use field-collected spiders, as they perform better than lab-reared spiders on various behavioural tests; however, behavioural problems can be mitigated with larger cage sizes and the provision of environmental enrichment (Carducci and Jakob, 2000). For larger temperate-zone species, such as *Phidippus*, we use plastic boxes (18 × 13 × 10 cm) with a ventilation hole cut with a Dremel and covered with screening secured with hot glue. Smaller species can be kept in ventilated deli cups. We provide enrichment in the form of green-painted dowels, angled so that the spider can crawl on the underside, a nest tube, and pieces of plastic foliage from the craft store. We provide water in test tubes plugged with cotton. Species from arid regions, such as *Habronattus* from the southwestern USA, can be kept in deli cups without additional water aside from that provided by prey (N. Morehouse, pers. comm.). We feed larger spiders crickets, which are in turn fed dog food and fish flakes, and small spiders an array of prey (see Taylor *et al.*, 2011, for other potential diets).

We have designed a diversity of experimental arenas, from simple boxes or alleys to mazes and arenas with slots for iPods. Our usual method is to make them out of foam core, which is cheap and easy to cut to particular specifications with an Exacto knife. We assemble the arenas with a glue gun or pins. We generally video-record our experiments, keeping spiders in focus, and we discourage them from climbing the cage walls with a thin layer of petroleum jelly; too much and they will incessantly groom their tarsi after they contact it. In other cases, we have covered the wall sides with plastic photocopy transparencies. The smaller the spider, the more readily they climb walls. It is important to consider the colour of the arena and the contrast of any objects with the walls. All three of our *Phidippus* species are preferentially attracted across an open space by a stick painted green rather than white – unsurprisingly, given their natural habitat (Baker *et al.*, 2009).

In arena design, one can take advantage of jumping spiders' propensity to climb objects. For example, the Jackson research group often uses ramps, so that spiders climb from the release point to the top of a ramp where they confront a stimulus, such as their reflection in a mirror (Harland *et al.*, 1999). Alternatively, spiders may have to crawl up out of a starting place into an arena before the test begins (e.g. Tarsitano and Jackson, 1997). *Phidippus* do not startle easily, and we have had success by placing them in a large syringe with the tip cut off, inserting the open end through a hole in the wall or floor of the arena, and then slowly pushing the plunger to introduce the spider into the arena (e.g. Long *et al.*, 2015).

When we design experiments, one of our earliest considerations is whether the stimulus we present to the spiders is alive (e.g. prey or conspecifics), a still model or lure, or a video or animation. With live stimuli, one needs to consider whether only visual information will be available, or whether the spiders will also have access to chemosensory, vibratory and tactile information. Often, the research question demands that the interaction between the spider and the organism be as realistic as possible (e.g. Taylor *et al.*, 2016).

Some questions demand more manipulation. For example, to test whether spiders could learn about cues indicating the location of prey, we had to secure prey in place. However, spiders are well known to be attuned to motion in a variety of contexts (e.g. Clark and Uetz, 1992; Tarsitano and Jackson, 1992). *Phidippus* spiders attend to both global motion (e.g. the movement of a cricket across a video screen; Figure 17.4) and local motion (e.g. the movement of antennae and heads of a running cricket; Bednarski *et al.*, 2012). Thus, in some experiments, we secured crickets in place but allowed for small movements (Jakob *et al.*, 2007). While spiders will attend to non-moving models or lures once they spot them (Jackson and Tarsitano, 1993) – *Phidippus* spiders will even attack a paper silhouette of a cricket – many researchers help draw the attention of a spider to a lure by moving it slightly with a hidden mechanism at the start of a trial (e.g. Tarsitano and Jackson, 1992).

Naturally, videos or still models allow more control over the presentation. Clark and Uetz (1990) were first to show that spiders respond to video and were equally likely to choose a cricket and a live video feed of that cricket; we replicated that experiment in *P. audax* (Bednarski *et al.*, 2012). Of course, potential issues with using video and animation in behavioural experiments have been well-documented (Oliveira *et al.*, 2000; Woo and Rieucau, 2008). Video is tuned to human vision and in particular lacks the UV frequencies that are important to jumping spiders (Lim and Li, 2006). Nonetheless, video allows a degree of manipulation of the moving image that is otherwise impossible, and with

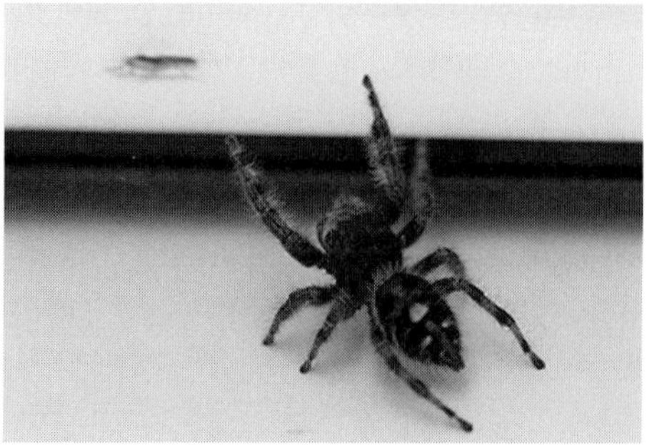

Figure 17.4. A spider orients to a video of a cricket, which it attacked a few seconds later. Photo by E. M. Jakob.

proper controls and caveats it is often the best choice. Recent advances with virtual reality open exciting new possibilities (Peckmezian and Taylor, 2015a).

The location from which video is viewed by the spider is important. For example, many iPods, especially earlier models, were best viewed only from directly in front – if the viewer was slightly off-axis, it meant that the image appeared blurry and strangely coloured. Some tablet computer models have wider viewing angles, as they are designed to be viewed simultaneously by several people. We have successfully presented stimuli on iPods and iPhones, and with video back-projected onto a translucent screen.

While running trials, consider the following. Daylight or full-spectrum light may elicit more natural behaviour, and is necessary when UV is important. Spiders attend better to video displays when the surrounding lights are dimmed. Jumping spiders are extremely attuned to movement, and with their nearly 360° field of view, it is crucial that the experimenter remains still during the experiment. We often monitor an experiment with a live video feed so that the experimenter can remain out of the spider's line of sight. Spiders are also distracted by vibration and loud sounds, such as a slamming door or heavy footsteps. Recently, we have presented tethered spiders with loud wasp sounds while we tracked the movement of their principal eyes with a specialized eye-tracker (Canavesi *et al.*, 2011), and our pilot data suggest that their eye movements increased when hearing the sounds (even a loud sneeze elicits eye movements). Finally, it is important to control chemical cues in silk and faeces left by previous spiders by cleaning arenas between trials. We wipe them down with dilute alcohol or, in the case of plastic or glass arenas, soap and bleach.

In studying learning, we alluded earlier to issues in deciding upon appetitive or aversive stimuli, and discuss these in more detail elsewhere (Jakob *et al.*, 2011; Jakob and Long, 2016). For example, in appetitive conditioning with prey, we have successfully used long periods between trials to allow for long feeding duration (e.g. one trial per day; Jakob *et al.*, 2007). For experiments with live prey, it may be challenging to ensure that spiders consistently capture and receive the reward, an important factor in designing learning experiments. In *Phidippus*, we are thus testing the use of small drops of sugar water, as pioneered by Liedtke and Schneider (2014), which avoids the problem of satiation. For aversive stimuli, it is relatively easy to study how spiders learn to avoid distasteful prey, as *Phidippus* simply drop the prey after tasting it (Skow, 2007), and thus satiation is not an issue. In studying preferences for particular prey, it is also possible to modify the prey itself, such as colouring tiny crickets by offering them coloured water to drink (Taylor *et al.*, 2014). Depending on the question, it is sometimes necessary to use other aversive stimuli that can be paired with, for example, a given location. Electric foot shock has been used both by our lab and others (Skow, 2007; Bednarski *et al.*, 2012; Peckmezian and Taylor, 2015b). We also developed high-frequency vibrations as an aversive stimulus (Long *et al.*, 2015).

As described in the previous section, new techniques are constantly being developed by other researchers for other species, which we are eager to try with *Phidippus*. It is an exciting time to study jumping spider cognition, as we begin to make headway on comparative studies in this diverse taxon.

The Devil Is in the Details

Box 17.2 Detouring by Salticids to Reach Prey

Fiona Cross

Some salticids are known to take detours for reaching their prey (Jackson and Cross, 2011), but there are differences in how this strategy is deployed between 'typical' salticids and salticids from the subfamily Spartaeinae. For example, *Phidippus* is a genus of typical salticids, which often preys on the insects it encounters on herbaceous plants. In this complex environment, *Phidippus* only rarely has a direct path to its prey and, instead, it uses a strategy of first reaching other parts of the plant to reduce its distance to the prey. After reaching one part of the plant, *Phidippus* reorients to the prey and visually inspects the environment, before reaching another part of the plant (Hill, 1979). By breaking its path into multiple short paths, *Phidippus* is highly effective at using detours for prey capture, with each choice of where to reach next on the plant being an instance of planning.

Yet, a capacity to plan may be even more important for the salticid subfamily Spartaeinae, as many of these species prefer eating other spiders (Su *et al.*, 2007) and use strategies to avoid being attacked by their prey. For example, one genus from this subfamily, *Portia*, takes planned detours for reaching a safe vantage point, before capturing its prey (Tarsitano and Jackson, 1997; Jackson *et al.*, 2002), but this capacity is now known to be widespread among spartaeines. In a recent experiment on 15 spartaeine species (Cross and Jackson, 2016), each spider began a trial at the top of a tower, from which it could view two boxes: one containing prey (i.e. lures made from dead spiders) and one containing pieces of dead leaf (side determined at random), but the distance was too far for the spider to reach by leaping. Instead, to reach the prey, the spider had to walk down from the tower and take a pathway. However, advanced planning was necessary, because the prey lures and leaf pieces were moved out of sight after the spider had walked down the tower. To reach the correct pathway, the spider also first had to walk away from the location of the prey, and sometimes it even had to first walk past the incorrect pathway. Yet, individuals from all 15 species chose the correct pathway significantly more often (Cross and Jackson, 2016).

It may be advantageous for typical salticids, such as *Phidippus audax* (Carducci and Jakob, 2000), to rely on multiple short detours, accompanied by accurate reorientation (Hill, 1979), because their prey are usually active and likely to move elsewhere before a long, complex detour can be completed. By contrast, planning a long detour for safe prey capture may be especially useful for spider-eating spartaeines, because their prey, although dangerous, are also more likely to remain in place.

References

Carducci, J. P., and Jakob, E. M. (2000). Rearing environment affects behaviour of jumping spiders. *Animal Behaviour*, **59**, 39–46.

(cont.)

Cross, F. R., and Jackson, R. R. (2016). The execution of planned detours by spider-eating predators. *Journal of the Experimental Analysis of Behavior*, **105**, 194–210.
Hill, D. E. (1979). Orientation by jumping spiders of the genus *Phidippus* (Araneae: Salticidae) during the pursuit of prey. *Behavioral Ecology and Sociobiology*, **5**, 301–322.
Jackson, R. R., and Cross, F. R. (2011). Spider cognition. *Advances in Insect Physiology*, **41**, 115–174.
Jackson, R. R., Pollard, S. D., Li, D., and Fijn, N. (2002). Interpopulation variation in the risk-related decisions of *Portia labiata*, an araneophagic jumping spider (Araneae, Salticidae), during predatory sequences with spitting spiders. *Animal Cognition*, **5**, 215–223.
Su, K. F. Y., Meier, R., Jackson, R. R., Harland, D. P., and Li, D. (2007). Convergent evolution of eye ultrastructure and divergent evolution of vision-mediated predatory behaviour in jumping spiders. *Journal of Evolutionary Biology*, **20**, 1478–1489.
Tarsitano, M. S., and Jackson, R. R. (1997). Araneophagic jumping spiders discriminate between detour routes that do and do not lead to prey. *Animal Behaviour*, **53**, 257–266.

Resources

Websites:

- World Spider Catalog: www.wsc.nmbe.ch/
- How to collect jumping spiders (a video by Wayne Maddison): www.youtube.com/watch?v=oZ1P_3fHtPk
- American Arachnological Society: www.americanarachnology.org

Conferences:

- AAS holds a very informative annual conference.

Spider identification and collection:

- Edwards, G. (2004). *Revision of the jumping spiders of the genus* Phidippus *(Araneae: Salticidae).* Gainesville, FL: Florida Department of Agriculture and Consumer Services.
- Foelix, R. (2014). *Biology of spiders.* New York, NY: Oxford University Press.
- Ubick, D., Paquin, P., Cushing, P. E., and Roth, V. (2009). *Spiders of North America: an identification manual.* American Arachnological Society.

Profile

Elizabeth did her postdoc with the salticid biologist Robert Jackson in New Zealand, but returned to her previous work on group-living spiders for the next decade. However, after mentoring several studies on salticids, she focused on them exclusively. Recently, she worked with many collaborators to develop an eye-tracker to monitor the gaze direction of the principal eyes, a tool that will open questions about cognition.

Skye finished her PhD in Jakob's lab and worked both on eye-tracker development and on perfecting techniques for examining the neuromorphology of spider brains. As a post-doc at the University of Arizona, she studied the neural underpinnings of navigation in amblypygids. She is now a lecturer at UMass Amherst.

Maragret has finished her first PhD year in Jakob's lab using the eye-tracker to study the gaze of female spiders as they view male displays and how attention is controlled by the secondary eyes.

References

Baker, L. (2007). Effect of corridors on the movement behavior of the jumping spider *Phidippus princeps* (Araneae, Salticidae). *Canadian Journal of Zoology*, **85**, 802–808.

Baker, L., Kelty, E. C., and Jakob, E. M. (2009). The effect of visual features on jumping spider movements across gaps. *Journal of Insect Behavior*, **22**, 350–361.

Bednarski, J. V., Taylor, P., and Jakob, E. M. (2012). Optical cues used in predation by jumping spiders, *Phidippus audax* (Araneae, Salticidae). *Animal Behaviour*, **84**, 1221–1227.

Canavesi, C., Long, S., Fantone, D., Jakob, E. M., and Jackson, R. R. (2011). Design of a retinal tracking system for jumping spiders. *Proceedings of SPIE*, **8129**, 8129091–8129098.

Carducci, J. P., and Jakob, E. M. (2000). Rearing environment affects behaviour of jumping spiders. *Animal Behaviour*, **59**, 39–46.

Chang, C. C., Ng, P. J., and Li, D. (2017). Aggressive jumping spiders make quicker decisions for preferred prey but not at the cost of accuracy. *Behavioral Ecology*, **28**, 479–484.

Clark, D. L., and Uetz, G. W. (1990). Video image recognition by the jumping spider, *Maevia inclemens* (Araneae: Salticidae). *Animal Behaviour*, **40**, 884–890.

Clark, D. L., and Uetz, G. W. (1992). Morph-independent mate selection in a dimorphic jumping spider: demonstration of movement bias in female choice using video-controlled courtship behaviour. *Animal Behaviour*, **43**, 247–254.

Clark, R. J., Jackson, R. R., and Cutler, B. (2000). Chemical cues from ants influence predatory behavior in *Habrocestum pulex*, an ant-eating jumping spider (Araneae, Salticidae). *Journal of Arachnology*, **28**, 309–318.

Cross, F. R. (2016). Discrimination of draglines from potential mates by *Evarcha culicivora*, an East African jumping spider. *New Zealand Journal of Zoology*, **43**, 84–95.

Cross, F. R., and Jackson, R. R. (2006). From eight-legged automatons to thinking spiders. In *Diversity of cognition* (pp. 188–215). Kyoto: Kyoto University Academic Press.

Cross, F. R., and Jackson, R. R. (2009). Cross-modality priming of visual and olfactory selective attention by a spider that feeds indirectly on vertebrate blood. *Journal of Experimental Biology*, **212**, 1869–1875.

Cross, F. R., and Jackson, R. R. (2015). Solving a novel confinement problem by spartaeine salticids that are predisposed to solve problems in the context of predation. *Animal Cognition*, **18**, 509–515.

Cross, F. R., and Jackson, R. R. (2016). The execution of planned detours by spider-eating predators. *Journal of the Experimental Analysis of Behavior*, **105**, 194–210.

Cross, F. R., and Jackson, R. R. (2017). Representation of different exact numbers of prey by a spider-eating predator. *Interface Focus*, **7**, 20160035.

Cross, F. R., Jackson, R. R., and Pollard, S. D. (2007). Male and female mate-choice decisions by *Evarcha culicivora*, an East African jumping spider. *Ethology*, **113**, 901–908.

Dolev, Y., and Nelson, X. J. (2014). Innate pattern recognition and categorization in a jumping spider. *PLoS ONE*, **9**(6), e97819.

Edwards, G. B. (2004). *Revision of the jumping spiders of the genus Phidippus (Araneae: Salticidae)*. Gainesville, FL: Department of Agriculture and Consumer Services.

Edwards, G. B., and Jackson, R. R. (1993). Use of prey-specific predatory behaviour by North American jumping spiders (Araneae, Salticidae) of the genus *Phidippus*. *Journal of Zoology London*, **229**, 709–716.

Edwards, G. B., and Jackson, R. R. (1994). The role of experience in the development of predatory behaviour in *Phidippus regius*, a jumping spider (Araneae, Salticidae) from Florida. *New Zealand Journal of Zoology*, **21**, 269–227.

Elias, D. O. (2003). Seismic signals in a courting male jumping spider (Araneae: Salticidae). *Journal of Experimental Biology*, **206**, 4029–4039.

Elias, D. O., Kasumovic, M. M., Punzalan, D., Andrade, M. C. B., and Mason, A. C. (2008). Assessment during aggressive contests between male jumping spiders. *Animal Behaviour*, **76**, 901–910.

Elias, D. O., Maddison, W. P., Peckmezian, C., Girard, M. B., and Mason, A. C. (2012). Orchestrating the score: complex multimodal courtship in the *Habronattus coecatus* group of *Habronattus* jumping spiders (Araneae: Salticidae). *Biological Journal of the Linnean Society*, **105**, 522–547.

Foelix, R. (2014). *Biology of spiders*. New York, NY: Oxford University Press.

Forster, L. M. (1979). Visual mechanisms of hunting behavior in *Trite planiceps*, a jumping spider (Araneae, Salticidae). *New Zealand Journal of Zoology*, **6**, 79–93.

Givens, R. P. (1978). Dimorphic foraging strategies of a salticid spider (*Phidippus audax*). *Ecology*, **59**, 309–321.

Harland, D. P., Jackson, R. R., and Macnab, A. M. (1999). Distances at which jumping spiders (Araneae: Salticidae) distinguish between prey and conspecific rivals. *Journal of Zoology*, **247**, 357–364.

Harland, D. P., Li, D., and Jackson, R. R. (2012). How jumping spiders see the world. In *How animals see the world* (pp. 133–163). Oxford: Oxford University Press.

Hill, D. E. (1979). Orientation by jumping spiders of the genus *Phidippus* (Araneae, Salticidae) during the pursuit of prey. *Behavioral Ecology and Sociobiology*, **5**, 301–322.

Hoefler, C. D. (2007). Male mate choice and size-assortative pairing in a jumping spider, *Phidippus clarus*. *Animal Behaviour*, **73**, 943–954.

Hoefler, C. D., and Jakob, E. M. (2006). Jumping spiders in space: movement patterns, nest site fidelity and the use of beacons. *Animal Behaviour*, **71**, 109–116.

Jackson, R. R., and Cross, F. R. (2011). Spider cognition. *Advances in Insect Physiology*, **41**, 115–174.

Jackson, R. R., and Li, D. Q. (2004). One-encounter search-image formation by araneophagic spiders. *Animal Cognition*, **7**, 247–254.

Jackson, R. R., and Tarsitano, M. S. (1993). Responses of jumping spiders to motionless prey. *Bulletin of the British Arachnological Society*, **9**, 105–109.

Jackson, R. R., Carter, C. M., and Tarsitano, M. S. (2001). Trial-and-error solving of a confinement problem by a jumping spider, *Portia fimbriata*. *Behaviour*, **138**, 1215–1234.

Jackson, R. R., Clark, R. J., and Harland, D. P. (2002). Behavioural and cognitive influences of kairomones on an araneophagic jumping spider. *Behaviour*, **139**, 749–775.

Jackson, R. R., Nelson, X. J., and Sune, G. O. (2005). A spider that feeds indirectly on vertebrate blood by choosing female mosquitoes as prey. *Proceedings of the National Academy of Sciences*, **102**, 15155–15160.

Jakob, E. M., and Long, S. M. (2016). How (not) to train your spider: successful and unsuccessful methods for studying learning. *New Zealand Journal of Zoology*, **43**, 112–126.

Jakob, E. M., Skow, C. D., Popson Haberman, M., and Plourde, A. (2007). Jumping spiders associate food with color cues in a T-maze. *Journal of Arachnology*, **35**, 487–492.

Jakob, E. M., Skow, C. D., and Long, S. M. (2011). Plasticity, learning, and cognition. In *Spider behaviour: flexibility and versatility* (pp. 307–347). Cambridge: Cambridge University Press.

Japyassú, H. F., and Laland, K. N. (2017). Extended spider cognition. *Animal Cognition*, **20**, 375–395.

Kasumovic, M. M., Elias, D. O., Sivalinghem, S., Mason, A. C., and Andrade, M. C. B. (2010). Examination of prior contest experience and the retention of winner and loser effects. *Behavioral Ecology*, **21**, 404–409.

Land, M. F. (1969a). Movements of the retinae of jumping spiders (Salticidae, Dendryphantinae) in relation to visual optics. *Journal of Experimental Biology*, **51**, 471–493.

Land, M. F. (1969b). Structure of the retinae of the principal eyes of jumping spiders (Salticidae: Dendryphantinae) in relation to visual optics. *Journal of Experimental Biology*, **51**, 443–470.

Land, M. F. (1985). The morphology and optics of spider eyes. In *Neurobiology of Arachnids* (pp. 53–78). Berlin: Springer.

Land, M. F., and Nilsson, D. E. (2012). *Animal eyes*. Oxford: Oxford University Press.

Li, D. Q., Jackson, R. R., and Harland, D. P. (1999). Prey-capture techniques and prey preferences of *Aelurillus aeruginosus, A. cognatus*, and *A. kochi*, ant-eating jumping spiders (Araneae: Salticidae) from Israel. *Israel Journal of Zoology*, **45**, 341–359.

Liedtke, J., and Schneider, J. M. (2014). Association and reversal learning abilities in a jumping spider. *Behavioral Processes*, **103**, 192–198.

Lim, M. L. M., and Li, D. Q. (2006). Behavioural evidence of UV sensitivity in jumping spiders (Araneae: Salticidae). *Journal of Comparative Physiology A*, **192**, 871–878.

Long, S. M., Lewis, S., Jean-Louis, L., Ramos, G., Richmond, J., and Jakob, E. M. (2012). Firefly flashing and jumping spider predation. *Animal Behaviour*, **83**, 81–86.

Long, S. M., Leonard, A., Carey, A., and Jakob, E. M. (2015). Vibration as an effective stimulus for aversive conditioning in jumping spiders. *Journal of Arachnology*, **43**, 111–114.

Maddison, W. P. (2015). A phylogenetic classification of jumping spiders (Araneae: Salticidae). *Journal of Arachnology*, **43**, 231–292.

McGinley, R. H., and Taylor, P. W. (2016). Video playback experiments support a role for visual assessment of opponent size in male–male contests of *Servaea incana* jumping spiders. *Behavioral Ecology and Sociobiology*, **70**, 821–829.

McGinley, R. H., Prenter, J., and Taylor, P. W. (2013). Whole-organism performance in a jumping spider, *Servaea incana* (Araneae: Salticidae): links with morphology and between performance traits. *Biological Journal of the Linnean Society*, **110**, 644–657.

Menda, G., Shamble, P. S., Nitzany, E. I., Golden, J. R., and Hoy, R. R. (2014). Visual perception in the brain of a jumping spider. *Current Biology*, **24**, 2580–2585.

Nagata, T., Koyanagi, M., Tsukamoto, H., *et al.* (2012). Depth perception from image defocus in a jumping spider. *Science*, **335**, 469–471.

Nakamura, T., and Yamashita, S. (2000). Learning and discrimination of colored papers in jumping spiders (Araneae, Salticidae). *Journal of Comparative Physiology A*, **186**, 897–901.

Nelson, X. J., and Jackson, R. R. (2011). Flexibility in the foraging strategies of spiders. In *Spider behaviour: flexibility and versatility* (pp. 31–56). Cambridge: Cambridge University Press.

Nelson, X. J., and Jackson, R. R. (2012a). Fine tuning of vision-based prey-choice decisions by a predator that targets malaria vectors. *Journal of Arachnology*, **40**, 23–33.

Nelson, X. J., and Jackson, R. R. (2012b). The role of numerical competence in a specialized predatory strategy of an araneophagic spider. *Animal Cognition*, **15**, 699–710.

Okuyama, T. (2007). Prey of two species of jumping spiders in the field. *Applied Entomology and Zoology*, **42**, 663–668.

Oliveira, R. F., Rosenthal, G. G., Schlupp, I., *et al.* (2000). Considerations on the use of video playbacks as visual stimuli: the Lisbon workshop consensus. *Acta Ethologica*, **3**, 61–65.

Parry, D. A., and Brown, R. H. J. (1959). The jumping mechanism of salticid spiders. *Journal of Experimental Biology*, **36**, 654–662.

Peckmezian, T., and Taylor, P. W. (2015a). A virtual reality paradigm for the study of visually mediated behaviour and cognition in spiders. *Animal Behaviour*, **107**, 87–95.

Peckmezian, T., and Taylor, P. W. (2015b). Electric shock for aversion training of jumping spiders: towards an arachnid model of avoidance learning. *Behavioral Processes*, **113**, 99–104.

Peckmezian, T., and Taylor, P. W. (2017). Place avoidance learning and memory in a jumping spider. *Animal Cognition*, **20**, 275–284.

Raška, J., Štys, P., and Exnerová, A. (2017). How variation in prey aposematic signals affects avoidance learning, generalization and memory of a salticid spider. *Animal Behaviour*, **130**, 107–117.

Schmitz, A. (2004). Metabolic rates during rest and activity in differently tracheated spiders (Arachnida, Araneae): *Pardosa lugubris* (Lycosidae) and *Marpissa muscosa* (Salticidae). *Journal of Comparative Physiology B*, **174**, 519–526.

Schmitz, A. (2005). Spiders on a treadmill: influence of running activity on metabolic rates in *Pardosa lugubris* (Araneae, Lycosidae) and *Marpissa muscosa* (Araneae, Salticidae). *Journal of Experimental Biology*, **208**, 1401–1411.

Schmitz, A., and Perry, S. F. (2000). Respiratory system of arachnids I: morphology of the respiratory system of *Salticus scenicus* and *Euophrys lanigera* (Arachnida, Araneae, Salticidae). *Arthropod Structure and Development*, **29**, 3–12.

Shamble, P. S., Menda, G., Golden, J. R., *et al.* (2016). Airborne acoustic perception by a jumping spider. *Current Biology*, **26**, 2913–2920.

Skow, C. D. (2007). *Jumping spiders and aposematic prey: the role of contextual cues during avoidance learning*. Amherst, MA: University of Massachusetts.

Skow, C. D., and Jakob, E. M. (2005). Jumping spiders attend to context during learned avoidance of aposematic prey. *Behavioral Ecology*, **17**, 34–40.

Spano, L., Long, S. M., and Jakob, E. M. (2012). Secondary eyes mediate the response to looming objects in jumping spiders (*Phidippus audax*, Salticidae). *Biology Letters*, **8**, 949–951.

Stankowich, T. (2009). When predators become prey: flight decisions in jumping spiders. *Behavioral Ecology*, **20**, 318–327.

Strausfeld, N. J. (2012). *Arthropod brains*. Cambridge, MA: Harvard University Press.

Su, K. F. Y., and Li, D. Q. (2006). Female-biased predation risk and its differential effect on the male and female courtship behaviour of jumping spiders. *Animal Behaviour*, **71**, 531–537.

Su, K. F. Y., Meier, R., Jackson, R. R., Harland, D. P., and Li, D. (2007). Convergent evolution of eye ultrastructure and divergent evolution of vision-mediated predatory behaviour in jumping spiders. *Journal of Evolutionary Biology*, **20**, 1478–1489.

Tarsitano, M. S., and Andrew, R. (1999). Scanning and route selection in the jumping spider *Portia labiata*. *Animal Behaviour*, **58**, 255–265.

Tarsitano, M. S., and Jackson, R. R. (1992). Influence of prey movement on the performance of simple detours by jumping spiders. *Behaviour*, **123**, 106–120.

Tarsitano, M. S., and Jackson, R. R. (1994). Jumping spiders make predatory detours requiring movement away from prey. *Behaviour*, **131**, 65–73.

Tarsitano, M. S., and Jackson, R. R. (1997). Araneophagic jumping spiders discriminate between detour routes that do and do not lead to prey. *Animal Behaviour*, **53**, 257–266.

Taylor, B. B., and Peck, W. B. (1975). A comparison of northern and southern forms of *Phidippus audax* (Hentz) (Araneidae, Salticidae). *Journal of Arachnology*, **2**, 89–99.

Taylor, L. A., Clark, D. L., and McGraw, K. J. (2011). Condition dependence of male display coloration in a jumping spider (*Habronattus pyrrithrix*). *Behavioral Ecology and Sociobiology*, **65**, 1133–1146.

Taylor, L. A., Maier, E. B., Byrne, K. J., Amin, Z., and Morehouse, N. I. (2014). Colour use by tiny predators: jumping spiders show colour biases during foraging. *Animal Behaviour*, **90**, 149–157.

Taylor, L. A., Amin, Z., Maier, E. B., Byrne, K. J., and Morehouse, N. I. (2016). Flexible color learning in an invertebrate predator: *Habronattus* jumping spiders can learn to prefer or avoid red during foraging. *Behavioral Ecology*, **27**, 520–529.

Tedore, C., and Johnsen, S. (2013). Pheromones exert top-down effects on visual recognition in the jumping spider *Lyssomanes viridis*. *Journal of Experimental Biology*, **216**, 1744–1756.

Tedore, C. and Johnsen, S. (2015). Visual mutual assessment of size in male *Lyssomanes viridis* jumping spider contests. *Behavioral Ecology*, **26**, 510–518.

VanderSal, N. D., and Hebets, E. A. (2007). Cross-modal effects on learning: a seismic stimulus improves color discrimination learning in a jumping spider. *Journal of Experimental Biology*, **210**, 3689–3695.

Vickers, M. E., Robertson, M. W., Watson, C. R., and Wilcoxen, T. E. (2014). Scavenging throughout the life cycle of the jumping spider, *Phidippus audax* (Hentz) (Araneae: Salticidae). *Journal of Arachnology*, **42**, 277–283.

Woo, K. L., and Rieucau, G. (2008). Considerations in video playback design: using optic flow analysis to examine motion characteristics of live and computer-generated animation sequences. *Behavioral Processes*, **78**, 455–463.

World Spider Catalog (2017). Natural History Museum Bern, online at http://wsc.nmbe.ch, version 18.5 [accessed 21 September 2017].

Young, O. P., and Lockley, T. C. (1988). Dragonfly predation upon *Phidippus audax* (Araneae, Salticidae). *Journal of Arachnology*, **16**, 121–122.

Zurek, D. B., and Nelson, X. J. (2012a). Hyperacute motion detection by the lateral eyes of jumping spiders. *Vision Research*, **66**, 26–30.

Zurek, D. B., and Nelson, X. J. (2012b). Saccadic tracking of targets mediated by the anterior-lateral eyes of jumping spiders. *Journal of Comparative Physiology A*, **198**, 414–417.

Zurek, D. B., Taylor, A. J., Evans, C. S., and Nelson, X. J. (2010). The role of the anterior lateral eyes in the vision-based behaviour of jumping spiders. *Journal of Experimental Biology*, **213**, 2372–2378.

Zurek, D. B., Cronin, T. W., Taylor, L. A., Byrne, K., Sullivan, M. L. G., and Morehouse, N. I. (2015). Spectral filtering enables trichromatic vision in colorful jumping spiders. *Current Biology*, **25**, 403–404.

18 Tortoises – Cold-Blooded Cognition: How to Get a Tortoise Out of Its Shell

Anna Wilkinson and Ewen Glass

Species Description

What Are Chelonia?

Turtles, tortoises and terrapins make up the group Chelonia, but what's the difference between them? Well, it very much depends on where you come from. If you speak American English, then they are all turtles; however, if you speak Australian English, then everything but sea turtles are tortoises. In British English, there are important distinctions, although what these distinctions are based on is debated. Turtles are almost entirely aquatic, terrapins spend a substantial amount of time in the water (and are often found in brackish areas) but also spend time on land, while tortoises are almost entirely land-dwelling. As we are British, we will be using these definitions. Together, tortoises, turtles and terrapins make up the group Chelonia, which comprises 327 species (van Dijk *et al.*, 2014). This chapter will largely focus on tortoises and in particular on the red-footed tortoise, but we will reference the others when relevant.

Distribution and Diet

The red-footed tortoise (*Chelonoidis carbonaria*; formerly *Geochelone carbonaria*) is a land-dwelling chelonian, native to Central and South America. It can be found across large parts of tropical and subtropical South America and has been introduced to some Caribbean islands (van Dijk *et al.*, 2014). This tortoise inhabits a variety of ecosystems, from tropical rainforests and grassy savannas to dry thorny forests (Vinke *et al.*, 2008). This species is omnivorous, but has a high proportion of fruit in its diet (Strong and Fragoso, 2006), although this varies across its range and over seasons (Vinke *et al.*, 2008). These tortoises are highly motivated by food and, as such, make an ideal species to study reptile cognition.

When we claim that the red-footed tortoise is an active species, our reviewers insist that this be put in the context of it being a tortoise; however, if you come and visit the cold-blooded cognition lab in Lincoln, you will see how active they are. The myth of the slow-and-steady tortoise is challenged by capture–release studies, which show that they are capable of travelling up to 85 m per hour (Moskovits, 1985, cited by Strong and Fragoso, 2006).

Anatomy

Red-footed tortoises have an elongated carapace (top of shell) that is generally of a dark base colour with bright yellow or orange areola (central areas in the scute; Figure 18.1). The plastron (base of the shell) is yellowish brown and can have dark pigmentation around the edge of the scutes. The specific colour of the plastron may be an indicator of the origin of the animal (Vinke and Vinke, 2003). The skin on their head and neck is dark, normally grey, but the scales on and around the head can be yellow, orange or red. These markings can be used to individually identify animals (Figure 18.2). Likewise, the scales on the legs are predominantly grey/brown, with large scales being red, orange or yellow.

Males are generally larger than females (Wang *et al.*, 2011), although females are frequently heavier. Size varies across their range. The largest documented red-footed tortoise was a male from the Gran Chaco region of Paraguay, with a carapace length of 59.3 cm and a weight of 28 kg, while in the more northern part of their range they will typically measure 25–30 cm (Vinke *et al.*, 2008). Red-footed tortoises can live up to 50 years in captivity.

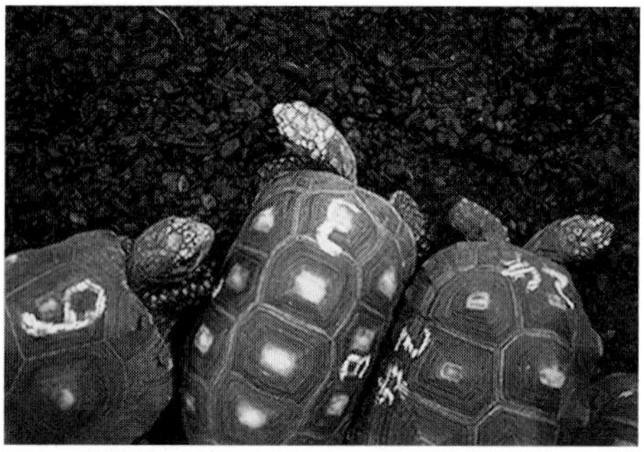

Figure 18.1. The red-footed tortoise.

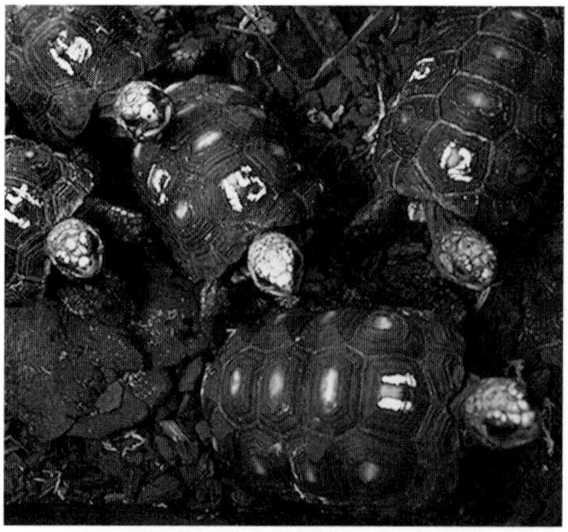

Figure 18.2. Individual variation in markings on head.

They are closely related to the yellow-footed tortoise (*Chelonoidis denticulata*), from which they are difficult to distinguish, as the colour of their feet is not a precise method of doing so. However, morphological differences in shell shape, mostly related to differences in the plastron (Barros *et al.*, 2012), and differences in their frontal nose scales can be used to tell them apart. When adult, yellow foots are generally larger than red foots (Vinke *et al.*, 2008).

Sexual Identification

Prior to adulthood, sexing red-footed tortoises is extremely difficult. We have now given up this task until they reach sexual maturity (10–15 years old, carapace length 18–30 cm). However, you can start to see sex-related differences at around 5–7 years of age (15–20 cm; Vinke *et al.*, 2008). In captivity, sexual maturity is more likely to be based on size rather than age, as animals fed on inappropriate diets grow artificially fast and can reach sexual maturity much faster than they naturally would. This accelerated growth is associated with health complications which can be fatal, including obesity, pyramiding (the raising of scutes during growth, which gives tortoises a hedgehog-like appearance to their shell; Figure 18.3), renal disease and metabolic bone disease (Ritz *et al.*, 2010). Males from most areas in the range have a concave plastron when compared to females (Figure 18.4), and those from more northern areas have a longer, fatter tail (Vinke *et al.*, 2008). The northern tortoises also have a constricted carapace in mature males, making it look like they have a waist (Figure 18.5).

Perception

Chelonia have good colour vision, and colour seems to be a particularly salient cue to red-footed tortoises (maybe because of their fruit-eating habits). There is also evidence of colour preferences in Hermann's tortoises (*Testudo hermanni*; Pellitteri-Rosa *et al.*, 2010) and yellow-footed tortoises (Passos *et al.*, 2014). Furthermore, there is evidence of picture–object recognition in this species (Wilkinson *et al.*, 2013). Red-footed tortoises behave towards a pictorial stimulus as if it is the object that it represents (Wilkinson *et al.*, 2013), and appear to respond similarly to video stimuli (Wilkinson

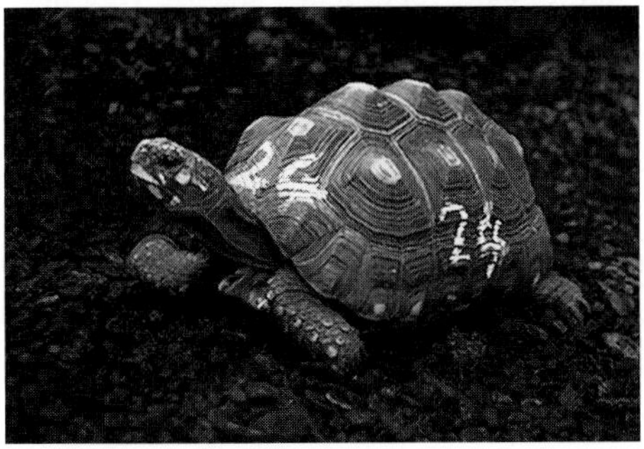

Figure 18.3. Pyramiding can be observed on the carapace of this animal.

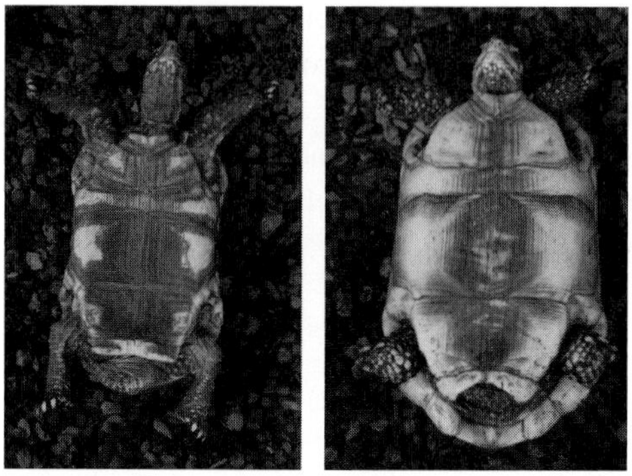

Figure 18.4. (A) The plastron of a male – note the concave plastron and longer tail. (B) The plastron of a female – note the flat plastron and shorter tail.

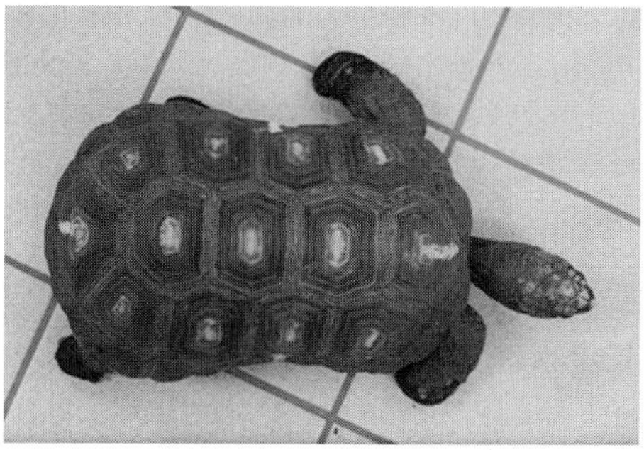

Figure 18.5. Male red-footed tortoise with waist, which is characteristic in some areas of their range.

et al., 2011). When differentially reinforced for doing so, they can learn to discriminate between the two (Wilkinson *et al.*, 2013). This is extremely useful for investigation of complex cognitive processes. Some evidence suggests that Greek tortoises (*Testudo graeca*) may be able to learn to discriminate shapes (Glavaschi and Beaumont, 2014). Little work has directly examined tortoise odour discrimination, but we generally test for it as a confounding variable during our experiments, and see very little evidence of discrimination on this basis (but see Mueller-Paul *et al.*, 2012).

Behavioural Ecology

Red-footed tortoises are considered non-social animals, as they do not live in organized groups or provide parental care. However, they can be observed sharing shelters in areas when environmental conditions are severe. In the Chaco, there are severe fluctuations in weather conditions, and the red-footed tortoises are only able to survive in this environment by seeking shelter. One such appropriate shelter are holes dug by giant armadillos. As these holes are large and relatively rare, several tortoises can be found in them

(Vinke and Vinke, 2003; Noss *et al.*, 2013). Interestingly, when performance on socio-cognitive tasks are compared, little difference is observed (Wilkinson, unpubl. data).

Red-footed tortoises are considered key seed dispersers in their natural environment (Strong and Fragoso, 2006). Most seeds (90 per cent; Wang *et al.*, 2011) pass through the tortoise intact. Males consume more fruit species in their diet than do females (Wang *et al.*, 2011), which is thought to be the result of travelling more in search of females. Further, they can ingest large seeds that are dispersed by a very limited range of dispersers, due to large mammalian extinction (Wang *et al.*, 2011). As a side note, the introduction of giant tortoises (*Aldabrachelys gigantea*) to replace extinct, endemic tortoises has led to the restoration of seed dispersal interactions with an endemic ebony tree (Griffiths *et al.*, 2011). The tortoises do not only ingest and disperse the large seeds, but gut passage also leads to improved seed germination. As they are ectothermic, tortoises are also motivated to visit forest clearings to sunbathe, which is likely to impact substantially on seedling success (John *et al.*, 2016). Our recent work has examined the impact that cognition might have on seed dispersal processes using the red-footed tortoise as a model (John *et al.*, 2016; Soldati *et al.*, 2017).

State of the Art

Chelonia are of particular interest when studying cognition, as recent phylogenetic analyses have placed them as a sister group to the Archosauria (birds and crocodiles; Shaffer *et al.*, 2013). Therefore, the exploration of similarities and differences in performance, using paradigms similar to those used with mammals and birds, is likely to provide insight into the evolution of cognition. Reptiles have traditionally been considered to be sluggish, inert and largely governed by innate drives, with suggestions that their cognitive ability, if it exists at all, is fundamentally different from that of mammals and birds (e.g. Day *et al.*, 1999). As Tinklepaugh (1932) noted, however, 'the physical sluggishness and awkwardness of the turtle may have earned him an undeserved reputation for stupidity'. Indeed, more recent research has started to reveal an impressive suite of cognitive abilities in this group (e.g. LaDage *et al.*, 2012; Kis *et al.*, 2015). However, the body of research in the area remains very small. In this section, we will briefly summarize the state of the field, focusing mainly on the red-footed tortoise but, where pertinent, introducing work with other species.

Spatial Cognition

Efficient navigation through space is likely to be adaptive, as it allows an animal to move between food sources, shelter and other key resources in their environment. Reptiles are particularly interesting in this context, because their brain structures differ from those of mammals and birds in important respects. It has been suggested, on the basis of anatomy, that homologous structures and similar circuity exist (Jacobs and Schenk, 2003; Naumann *et al.*, 2015). However, the behavioural evidence remains unclear.

Red-footed tortoises are able to use a range of different strategies to find a spatial goal. Our work has revealed that the red-footed tortoise is able to master a radial arm maze (Wilkinson *et al.*, 2007). To do this, it must remember multiple different spatial locations within each trial (Mueller-Paul *et al.*, 2012a, b). Under some circumstances, the tortoises appear to use room cues in a cognitive map-like manner (Wilkinson *et al.*, 2007), as the terrapin *Pseudemys scripta* does (López *et al.*, 2000, 2003; see Mueller *et al.*, 2011, for an extensive review). However, if cues are not salient, then the red-footed tortoise also exhibits stereotypic response strategies (Wilkinson *et al.*, 2009; Mueller-Paul *et al.*, 2012a). These response rules can be transferred from a 2D to a 3D environment (Mueller-Paul *et al.*, 2014), but if animals have information about a specific context, then they are more likely to discriminate between them than generalize across (Mueller-Paul *et al.*, 2014). Odour, too, may be used, but only under circumstances when other cues are unavailable (Mueller-Paul *et al.*, 2012a). This finding has been replicated across experiments with our tortoises, and similar observations have been made in other species (Roth and Krochmal, 2015; but see Galeotti *et al.*, 2007).

Social Cognition

Red-footed tortoises are particularly interesting for studies of social cognition as they allow the examination of key hypotheses, which might be more difficult to test in mammals and birds. We have demonstrated that red-footed tortoises respond to the gaze direction of a conspecific (Wilkinson *et al.*, 2010b) and that they respond more to these cues than other similar ones (Wilkinson *et al.*, unpubl. data). We have shown that, in a detour task, red-footed tortoises can learn to get to an otherwise inaccessible goal by observing the behaviour of a conspecific (Wilkinson *et al.*, 2010a). The specific mechanisms underlying this behaviour remain unclear. However, the tortoises did not learn to follow the exact route of the demonstrator, but learned some more general principles of how to solve the task (Wilkinson and Huber, 2012). Tortoises' large shells make it difficult to observe demonstrators' fine-grained movements, and thus use of a bidirectional control or a two-action procedure is tricky.

Red-footed tortoises have also been used to test contagious yawning. There is debate about the cognitive processes that underlie this ability. It has been suggested that contagious yawning is the result of a fixed action pattern, for which the releaser stimulus is the observation of another yawn (Yoon and Tennie, 2010). More high-level interpretations suggest that it may be the result of non-conscious mimicry, emerging through close links between perception and action (Yoon and Tennie, 2010), or the result of empathy, thus requiring the ability to engage in mental state attribution (e.g. Anderson *et al.*, 2004). However, at this point, no research has yet attempted to pull apart these hypotheses. Tortoises are ideal for investigating such questions, as they are able to use social cues but, to our knowledge, there is no evidence of social mimicry, mental state attribution or empathy in this species. After training a red-footed tortoise to yawn on cue (which took approximately 6 months), we presented conspecifics with conditioned yawns, both live and on videos, as well as video-recorded real yawns, along with several control conditions

(Wilkinson *et al.*, 2011). We found no differences across conditions and thus no evidence of contagious yawning. This was the first time that video stimuli were used with tortoises, and we showed that they react to video and real stimuli in a similar way.

Long-Term Memory

Chelonia can remember things for a long time. We have demonstrated that red-footed tortoises can retain a learned spatial discrimination for 3 months (Mueller-Paul *et al.*, 2014) and, even more impressively, they are able to remember the relative reward value of a stimulus for at least 18 months (Soldati *et al.*, 2017). We do not know the limits of their memory, but, in this case, they outlasted the student. Other work with chelonia has found similarly impressive memory retention of food acquisition behaviour for 36 months (Davis and Burghardt, 2007, 2012) and visual discriminations for 3.5 months (Davis and Burghardt, 2012).

All for One and One for All

Box 18.1 Reptile Cognition and Model Species

Gordon M. Burghardt

Anna Wilkinson and Ewen Glass provide some important background information on the biology, ecology and behaviour of their preferred model species, the red-footed tortoise. They then present guidance for testing these animals in captivity in experimental cognition studies. Much of this is useful for people setting out to study reptile cognition in other non-avian reptiles as well. Here, I will provide some general comments and related work on other species, additional sources that might usefully be consulted, and mention a few cautions.

Wilkinson's laboratory has been a leader in revitalizing studies of reptile learning and cognition, thanks to their studies of spatial learning, picture recognition, navigation, gaze following, social learning and other topics, as well as in applying modern technology, such as touch screens, to the field. Wilkinson's recent review (Wilkinson and Huber, 2012) complemented my much earlier review (Burghardt, 1977), but the field has grown so much that there are now numerous additional studies on many species, primarily lizards but also snakes, crocodilians and even the tuatara; and many more are in the pipeline! Studies on environmental enrichment, cognition, personality and controlled deprivation are also having impacts on housing, maintaining, studying and exhibiting captive reptiles (Burghardt, 2013, 2017). Researchers interested in pursuing studies on other species should search archival websites for the most recent studies on an ever-widening list of species. The recognition that there are no class-specific taxonomic differences in learning among vertebrates, as was claimed into the 1960s and beyond, is not new (Burghardt, 1977), but recent research has definitely sealed the case.

Comparative psychology and comparative ethology must also take the 'comparative' label seriously, and thus studies of differences and similarities among related

(cont.)

species are essential, as differences in ecology and behaviour can affect cognitive processes and many other behaviourally relevant traits. Thus, a focus on a few 'model' species can actually deter scientific progress in behaviour, if not in other areas of biology. Without comparative work, it is often premature to make assertions about relative abilities across taxonomic leaps, especially vertebrate orders and classes, and yet that is the goal of many students of comparative cognition.

Reptilian genera with many species provide ample opportunities for such work. Anoline lizards are a prime group receiving much attention across many dimensions, including behaviour, ecology and learning (Losos, 2009; Leal and Powell, 2012). Gartersnakes (*Thamnophis*) are another well-studied group that has the advantage of large litters and laboratory breeding, and in which population differences in life history and behaviour are readily documented (Burghardt and Schwartz, 1999). Even closely related snakes in the same genus may differ in their ability to modify and improve prey capture tactics (Halloy and Burghardt, 1990). As this latter study also illustrates, ontogeny is important, and more rapidly maturing and easily sexed reptiles may offer research opportunities that more slowly maturing and long-lived turtles and tortoises may not. Finally, homoplasy or convergent cognitive processes are also important to study (Burghardt, 1977). One interesting comparison would be between the red-footed tortoise and the terrestrial box turtles (*Terrapene*), which are closely related to the largely aquatic emydid pond turtles in the Americas, also showing social learning (Davis and Burghardt, 2011). Box turtles are easy to keep and show some cognitive prowess (Leighty *et al.*, 2013). Do any of the abilities shown in red-footed tortoises appear in box turtles that have a similar terrestrial lifestyle and diet, although in a more temperate environment? More effort is needed to understand the neural underpinnings of reptilian cognitive feats, and to dispel misconceptions about reptilian brain and cognition, based on inadequate data and outdated models of brain evolution (see Reiter *et al.*, 2017). Brain differences among species of *Anolis* have been documented (Powell and Leal, 2012), which could further such efforts.

Finally, two terminological caveats. Referring to studies of reptiles as cold-blooded can be misleading in several respects. Reptiles are actually poikilothermic or ectothermic, and the term 'cold-blooded' is an archaic term. We know that many reptiles, and not just tropical ones, often are at their behavioural and cognitive best when they are hot. Indeed, many thrive in desert environments, where small mammals are mainly nocturnal to avoid daytime heat. In fact, many of the early studies on reptile learning and cognition found limited learning, because they tested reptiles at temperatures typically used in rodent studies. Documenting these pernicious effects occurred decades ago (Burghardt, 1977; Brattstrom, 1978). Wilkinson and Glass do discuss the temperature they have found best for their species, and elsewhere are clearly mindful of the importance of temperature (Matsubara *et al.*, 2017; see also Clark *et al.*, 2014), but possible confusion remains among psychologists not familiar with reptiles. The second terminological point is referring to a species as 'non-social'. We now know that reptiles are social in many more respects than formally thought (Doody *et al.*,

(*cont.*)

2013). To limit sociality to animals that live in organized groups or have parental care is problematic, as different types and degrees of sociality exist, and their mechanisms can vary greatly. Leyhausen (1965) discussed this at length in terms of 'solitary mammals'. Referring to species as solitary rather than as non-social is preferable. In short, we need to be careful in the labels we use, as they may lead novice researchers and non-herpetologists astray. In any event, cognition and learning in non-avian reptiles is now going mainstream, and I look forward to many future important and exciting findings from the Wilkinson laboratory.

References

Brattstrom, B. H. (1978). Learning studies in lizards. In *Behavior and neurology of lizards* (pp. 173–181). Rockville, MD: National Institute of Mental Health.

Burghardt, G. M. (1977). Learning processes in reptiles. In *The biology of the Reptilia* (pp. 555–681). New York, NY: Academic Press.

Burghardt, G. M. (2013). Environmental enrichment and cognitive complexity in reptiles and amphibians: concepts, review and implications for captive populations. *Applied Animal Behaviour Science*, **147**, 286–298.

Burghardt, G. M. (2017). Keeping reptiles and amphibians as pets: challenges and rewards. *Veterinary Record*, **181**, 447–449.

Burghardt, G. M., and Schwartz, J. M. (1999). Geographic variations on methodological themes in comparative ethology: a natricine snake perspective. In *Geographic variation in behavior: perspectives on evolutionary mechanisms* (pp. 69–94). Oxford: Oxford University Press.

Clark, B. F., Amiel, J. J., Shine, R., Noble, D. W. A., and Whiting, M. J. (2014). Colour discrimination and associative learning in hatchling lizards incubated at 'hot' and 'cold' temperatures. *Behavioral Ecology and Sociobiology*, **68**, 239–247.

Davis, K. M., and Burghardt, G. M. (2011). Turtles (*Pseudemys nelsoni*) learn about visual cues indicating food from experienced turtles. *Journal of Comparative Psychology*, **125**, 404–410.

Doody, J. S., Burghardt, G. M., and Dinets, V. (2013). Breaking the social–nonsocial dichotomy: a role for reptiles in vertebrate social behaviour research? *Ethology*, **119**, 95–103.

Halloy, M., and Burghardt, G. M. (1990). Ontogeny of fish capture and ingestion in four species of garter snakes (*Thamnophis*). *Behaviour*, **112**, 299–318.

Leal, M., and Powell, B. J. (2012). Behavioural flexibility and problem solving in a tropical lizard. *Biology Letters*, **8**, 28–30.

Leighty, K. A., Grand, A. P., Pittman Courte, V. L., Maloney, M A., and Bettinger, T. L. (2013). Relational responding by eastern box turtles (*Terrepene carolina*) in a series of color discrimination tasks. *Journal of Comparative Psychology*, **127**, 256–264.

Leyhausen, P. (1965). The communal organization of solitary mammals. *Symposia of the Zoological Society of London*, **14**, 249–263.

Losos, J. (2009). *Lizards in an evolutionary tree: ecology and adaptive radiation of anoles.* Berkeley, CA: University of California Press.

(*cont.*)

Matsubara, S., Deeming, D. C., and Wilkinson, A. (2017). Cold-blooded cognition: new directions in reptile cognition. *Current Opinion in Behavioral Sciences*, **16**, 126–130.

Powell, B. J., and Leal, M. (2012). Brain evolution across the Puerto Rican anole radiation. *Brain, Behavior and Evolution*, **80**, 170–180.

Reiter, S., Liaw, H.-P., Yamawaki, T. M., Naumann, R. K., and Laurent, G. (2017). On the value of reptilian brains to map the evolution of the hippocampal formation. *Brain, Behavior and Evolution*, **90**, 41–52.

Waters, R. M., Bowers, B. B., and Burghardt, G. M. (2017). Personality and individuality in reptile behavior. In *Personality in non-human animals* (pp. 153–184). New York, NY, Springer.

Wilkinson, A., and Huber, L. (2012). Cold-blooded cognition: reptilian cognitive abilities. In *The Oxford handbook of comparative evolutionary psychology* (pp. 129–143). New York, NY: Oxford University Press.

Field Guide

Captive Care

The consideration of welfare of captive reptiles is essential from both an ethical and a scientific perspective. It is just as important and relevant as it is in birds and mammals, but reptilian needs are often very different from those of endotherms. For a long time, reptiles were considered stoic and unresponsive, and therefore assumed to cope well with captivity. However, as they can be relatively behaviourally inflexible and extremely sensitive to their environment (Warwick *et al.*, 2001), they have poor ability to cope with imperfect captive conditions (Burman *et al.*, 2016). Thus, special care must be taken to ensure adequate housing and care. Very little is known about measuring welfare in chelonia (Burghardt, 2013). However, recent research has revealed that in a novel environment red-footed tortoises take longer to move and have shorter neck lengths than in a familiar one (Moszuti *et al.*, 2017), suggesting that some measures used with mammals and birds may be appropriate for assessing the welfare of the red-footed tortoises. In order to truly test the cognitive capacities of your species, it is essential to ensure that you meet their environmental needs. This is particularly important in the case of reptiles, as they rely on environment for regulation. We will not review all the needs of the red-footed tortoise here, but we include some useful guides below.

Temperature

Reptiles are ectothermic and thus reliant on external heat sources to maintain their body temperature. If they are too cold, then activity is constrained (Brown and Shine, 2002). It is therefore essential to test them in appropriate thermal conditions. Much of the historical work that found reptiles to be 'sluggish and unintelligent creatures' (Yerkes,

Table 18.1. Essential experimental tools required to study tortoises and their function.

Key things to take in mind when testing tortoises
Tortoises can and do generalize, but context exerts a strong influence on behaviour
Red-footed tortoises do not use odour information, unless they do not have access to any other cues
Red-footed tortoises can use social information, so you should test them in isolation
You have to be imaginative when developing social learning tasks for this species, because of their cumbersome shell and lack of dexterity
Red-footed tortoises can remember for a long time. Consider the impacts of previous learning on your experiments

1901, p. 520) likely used inappropriate testing conditions. Bearing this in mind, you need to prepare yourself appropriately for the temperature. Generally we run our animals at ~28°C, which is the recommended baseline temperature for this species. The first test trials that AW conducted took at least 30 minutes, with some of them taking up to 90: it was difficult to concentrate on a tortoise moving (admittedly a little slowly) through a maze at that heat for an hour and a half!

Humidity

Humidity can vary across the red-foot habitat (Vinke *et al.*, 2008). As such, it is important to ensure they have access to areas of varying humidity within their enclosure. We have drier areas near our heat lamps and use a humidifier along with damp caves (long plastic buckets turned on their sides and filled with damp moss) to allow them to choose between a variety of humidities. We do not use extra humidifiers in our test rooms, but for some experiments the tortoises receive a bath before the test (Wilkinson *et al.*, 2007; Soldati *et al.*, in prep.).

Motivation and Rewards

Being cold-blooded, tortoises require substantially less food than a mammal of equivalent size/weight. Therefore, do not reward your tortoise a similar amount to what you would reward a dog, as they will stop working fast. In our first ever tortoise experiment, which was run with a rather small tortoise, we used 8 mm^3 pieces of strawberry. This was rewarding. We now use slightly larger rewards, depending on the experiment and the number of trials we want to run.

Tortoises can distinguish between reward quantity (e.g. 125 mm^3 vs. 27 mm^3 jelly) and quality (preferred mango-flavoured jelly vs. less-preferred apple-flavoured jelly; Soldati *et al.*, 2017). It is therefore important to take this into account when designing your experiments. If taking part in long experiments with substantial amounts of reward, tortoises will not always find the same reward highly motivating. In recent work, we found that tortoises will switch away from a favoured choice if overfed on this food. One way to overcome this problem is to reward them with a variety of foods (Mueller-Paul *et al.*, 2012a; Wilkinson *et al.*, 2013).

Moreover, it is important to consider the appropriate number of trials to run in a day, which may differ wildly from other species. We generally run between 6 and 10 trials per session, and 1–2 sessions per day. However, in experiments where substantial rewards are offered, we reduce the number of trials and will occasionally run one trial per day.

Do not reward tortoises with your fingers. Tortoises have very poor aim when biting food and very strong jaws. Rather, deliver your reward into a feeding bowl or via tweezers. Please note that the use of fruit is only appropriate for some tortoise species. Other tortoises should not eat fruit (even though they like it). Similarly, many species may be highly motivated to work for animal protein. This does not form a major part of the diet for most species, and as such should be avoided in experiments.

Tortoises are frequently overfed in captivity, which can result in growth rates that substantially exceed those of natural populations (Ritz *et al.*, 2010). This is thought to have substantial negative effects on the animals and can potentially lead to pathological consequences (Ritz *et al.*, 2010). Over and above the potential health issues, overfeeding can impact on the validity of the data collected. We believe that this overfeeding plays a major part in the misconception that these animals are unresponsive. It is very important to feed your animal appropriate food types and amounts.

Moreover, rewards other than food can be used during tasks. Being ectothermic, tortoises need to modify their temperature behaviourally. As such, heat *may* be highly motivating. However, we have run a number of experiments with heat as reward, and they have not worked, possibly for two reasons. First, when basking, tortoises absorb heat through their shell, and it is likely to take time for them to feel the warmth. This reduces the contiguity between the action and the perception of the rewards, and as such may make learning extremely hard. Second, it may be that heat is only reinforcing when an animal is in need of it. Our tortoises are always tested within their optimal temperature ranges, and as such may simply not be motivated to learn for heat.

Furthermore, water may be highly motivating. Although many tortoise species are desert-living animals that can survive a substantial amount of time without water, anecdotal reports suggest that they rush out of shelter and bathe in the rain. It is thus possible that water may be an excellent reinforcer for these species.

Materials

Tortoises are very strong; they like to push things and, if they move, they like to push more. This can be problematic when it comes to experimental apparatus, for a number of reasons. Given that tortoises are not very good with glass, for instance, they will push it continually. Therefore, glass and transparent plastic should be avoided in all experimental set-ups and housing areas. If you are using a glass tank, you should cover it with something opaque, so that the tortoises perceive it as a barrier. You also should not test them with an apparatus held together with bits of tape. You need to use thick wood or MDF (if your tortoise requires a humid environment, MDF does not last long), properly drilled or nailed together. Normally, when presenting some discrimination to tortoises, we place a barrier in front of the tortoises (wire mesh) and only release it once it has looked at both stimuli and is facing the centre. When working with a small tortoise, a hamster cage works beautifully. However, any tortoise with a plastron length over about 7 cm will be able to move this fairly easily, so you need to ensure you reinforce it well and make sure that it does not move, as the tortoises will spend their time pushing rather than looking at the stimuli you want them to look at. To get past this, we frequently mount mesh barriers on a frame, and then place them inside runners and slide them in and out. Moreover, tortoises can also be heavy. This makes it very difficult to move them around and position them as you would like – you need to let them come to you, which can take some time.

Finally, tortoises really like feet, particularly if you are wearing brightly coloured shoes. They need no invitation to bite them. We see this frequently with the red-foots, and recent communication with a student working with Aldabran tortoises (Andrin Duerst, pers. comm.) suggests that it does not appear to be a red-foot-specific habit. Brightly coloured shoes (and plastic lab shoe covers) should therefore be avoided, as these are extremely attractive to tortoises and can be accidentally ingested.

Testing Procedures

Tortoises with experimental experience readily habituate to novel environments. However, those that are naïve can take several sessions before they reach criteria. To habituate a tortoise to an arena, we place it in the arena for at least two sessions lasting around 20–30 minutes, and scatter food around the floor. If it readily moves around (Moszuti *et al.*, 2017) and eats the food two sessions in a row, then we consider it habituated. We generally give them only one habituation session a day.

When training tortoises to perform discrimination tasks, we generally use visual stimuli, as they largely use visual information to solve tasks (e.g. Wilkinson *et al.*, 2009). Moreover, it is usually very easy to train a tortoise to approach a specific stimulus. All tortoise species that we have worked with are attracted to brightly coloured objects (not just shoes), so we frequently use colour discriminations for our experiments (e.g. Soldati *et al.*, 2017). Initially, we use a very brief classical conditioning phase in which we present the stimulus close to the tortoises followed by a reward. After 3–5 trials, we move on to shaping through successive approximation. You can train a naïve animal to approach a specific stimulus and avoid another one very rapidly. However, training them to actively touch the target takes much longer (see below). Therefore, we make sure that the stimuli are spatially separate, and use a criterion in which a choice is made, when the tortoise approaches to within 5 cm of the stimulus, with its head oriented towards it.

Tortoises readily develop side biases. If excluding them from the task is not an option, for instance because only few individuals are available, then correction trials can be used. This is a standard procedure in pigeon research. If the tortoise gets a trial incorrect, it receives the same trial repeated again and again, until it makes the correct choice. This can result in some rather time-consuming sessions at the beginning, but it is well worth it.

Tortoises can also be trained to use touchscreens. The touchscreens most commonly used for humans are capacitative, i.e. the touch of a user (with an electrical charge) disrupts the electrostatic field and causes a decrease in capacitance, the point of which is then detected. These monitors require the electrostatic charge of the user to detect a touch, and can be worked by tortoises. However, they only work when touched by certain body parts (i.e. nose, not beak), so their use is not recommended. Instead, we would suggest using resistive or infrared touchscreens. A resistive touchscreen works by detecting a connection between two metallic layers caused by the user touching the screen, which results in electrical flow. Thus, these screens work via pressure, and tortoises are good at pushing things. In contrast, infrared monitors have a frame which creates a grid of invisible (to us) light beams in front of the monitor. When these are interrupted, the sensors can locate the touch point. These are very good for use with animals; however, as the frame is in front of the monitor and is sensitive to any break in the beam, they can frequently be set off by an animal learning near them.

Red-footed tortoises readily learn to use a touchscreen. We trained them using an auto-shaping procedure followed by ~30 trials of shaping. In collaboration with Masaki Tomonaga, AW has just started similar training with sulcata tortoises (*Centrochelys sulcata*), which need substantially more habituation to the equipment. This may be the result of them being comparatively more naïve to experiments; however, they do readily approach other novel stimuli. These animals are being trained outside, and there is a lot of reflection from the screen which we believe impacts their performance. To get around this problem, we are training the tortoises to approach a specific printed stimulus on paper, which will then be presented on screen. An alternative approach (one that has been successfully used with a number of species) is to put a photograph of food on the screen, and train them to approach and touch.

Wild vs. Lab

Box 18.2 Where the Wild Things Are: A Naturalistic Approach to Studying Cognition in Chelonians

Timothy C. Roth II and Aaron R. Krochmal

This chapter provides suggestions for testing chelonian cognition in the laboratory. Here, we consider the applicability of these ideas for fieldwork. Laboratory and field studies of cognition share several common elements. As in the lab, understanding animal motivation is critical in the field to provide the proper context for interpreting behaviours. The natural environment provides motivation in the form of selection pressures (e.g. predation risk, risk of starvation). Often, these factors are more extreme than would be allowed in the lab, enhancing the relevance of field studies by providing naturalistic levels of motivation. Similarly, as in the lab, knowing the

(cont.)

natural history of the focal species (e.g. optimal temperature, diet) is critical to provide ecological contexts for designing experiments and interpreting results. However, field studies of cognition present several unique challenges:

- fieldwork often precludes direct control over environmental (e.g. temperature, moisture) and individual variables (e.g. reproductive status, body condition);
- the relevant temporal and spatial scales are large, making detailed observations difficult;
- repeated measures on a specific individual may not always be possible, as recapture may not be predictable; and
- wild animals are not habituated to human interaction, so handling effects have the potential to bias behaviours, potentially confounding the study.

Each challenge can, however, serve as a marked advantage, providing unique insight into aspects of Chelonian cognition:

- while some aspects of field studies preclude control, they also present a more naturalistic view to how, why and under what conditions aspects of cognition manifest. For example, there is no need to train animals in the field, as natural selection has already 'trained' them. By limiting study to the natural behaviours of the animals, the ecological factors that influence cognitive decisions emerge;
- the large temporal and spatial scales inherent in field studies can provide broad insight into large-scale phenomena, including the relevance of cognition to population dynamics, the role of multispecies interactions in the development and expression of cognition, the responses to multiple stimuli and population-level aspects of cognition (e.g. local adaptation, cultural/social learning and ontogenetic effects);
- although individuals may not be easily recaptured, between-subjects designs can benefit greatly by working with the larger sample sizes that an entire population can provide; and
- by limiting the handling and disruption of individuals, the natural quality of the observed behaviour is more likely to be retained.

We use these challenges to investigate the role of cognition in navigation in Eastern painted turtles (*Chrysemys picta*; e.g. Roth and Krochmal, 2015a, b, 2016). Wild turtles move unabated over large areas within their natural environment, so we use radiotelemetry to collect highly accurate spatial positions (± 2 m) every 15 minutes to determine their detailed movement patterns. Telemetry allows us to collect repeated data on a single individual from a distance, without disturbing its behaviour, and to do so over multiple years. Without such unbiased, intensive data collection we could not know the precision with which the turtles navigate, their use of spatial memory, the ontogeny of their critical leaning period or the possibility that they use a cognitive map.

(*cont.*)

References

Roth, T. C., and Krochmal, A. R. (2015a). Cognition-centered conservation as a means of advancing integrative animal behavior. *Current Opinion in Behavioral Sciences*, **6**, 1–6.

Roth, T. C., and Krochmal, A. R. (2015b). The role of age-specific learning and experience for turtles navigating a changing landscape. *Current Biology*, **25**, 333–337.

Roth, T. C., and Krochmal, A. R. (2016). Pharmacological evidence is consistent with a prominent role of spatial memory in complex navigation. *Proceedings of the Royal Society of London B: Biological Sciences*, **283**, 20152548.

Resources

There is not too much information to go on.

- The Edition Chimaira Chelonian Library has some very good books that cover a number of tortoise species.
- In terms of red-footed tortoises, the one to read is the following: Vinke, S., Vetter, H., Vinke, T., and Vetter, S. (2008). *South American tortoises: Chelonoidis carbonaria, Chelonoidis denticulata and Chelonoidis chelensis.* Frankfurt: Edition Chimaira.
- To learn more about reptile welfare visit: www.cold-bloodedcare.com
- Good websites to help with tortoise husbandry include: www.tortoisetrust.org/ and www.britishcheloniagroup.org.uk/

Profile

Who wouldn't want to study reptiles? Anna, 15 years ago. Little was known about their cognitive abilities and *a lot* instead about apes'. After graduating, Anna studied wild gibbons in Thailand and realized that her real passion was the lab side of animal cognition, so she moved to work at a zoo. When she began her PhD, she got herself a pet red-footed tortoise called Moses and he became the key to the next phase of her career. After a lecture on rats in mazes, Geoff Hall and Anna (and a game undergraduate, Hui-Minn Chan) tested Moses with success (Wilkinson *et al.*, 2007)! For her postdoc, Anna presented this work to Ludwig Huber, whose excitement equalled her own. Together with Geoff, she started the cold-blooded cognition lab. So *now* when she asks the initial question, it requires no answer beyond an exclamation mark: who wouldn't want to study reptiles?!

References

Anderson, J. R., Myowa-Yamakoshi, M., and Matsuzawa, T. (2004). Contagious yawning in chimpanzees. *Proceedings of the Royal Society of London B: Biological Sciences*, **271**, 468–470.

Barros, M. S., Silva, A. G., and Ferreira Junior, P. D. (2012). Morphological variations and sexual dimorphism in *Chelonoidis carbonaria* (Spix, 1824) and *Chelonoidis denticulata* (Linnaeus, 1766) (Testudinidae). *Brazilian Journal of Biology*, **72**, 153–161.

Brown, G. P., and Shine, R. (2002). Influence of weather conditions on activity of tropical snakes. *Austral Ecology*, **27**, 596–605.

Burghardt, G. M. (2013). Environmental enrichment and cognitive complexity in reptiles and amphibians: concepts, review, and implications for captive populations. *Applied Animal Behavior Science*, **147**, 286–298.

Burman, O. H. P., Collins L. M., Hoehfurtner T., Whitehead M., and Wilkinson, A. (2016). Cold-blooded care: understanding reptile care and implications for their welfare. *Testudo*, **8**, 83–86.

Davis, K. M., and Burghardt, G. M. (2007). Training and long-term memory of a novel food acquisition task in a turtle (*Pseudemys nelsoni*). *Behavioural Processes*, **75**, 225–230.

Davis, K. M., and Burghardt, G. M. (2012). Long-term retention of visual tasks by two species of emydid turtles, *Pseudemys nelsoni* and *Trachemys scripta*. *Journal of Comparative Psychology*, **126**, 213.

Day, L. B., Crews, D., and Wilczynski, W. (1999). Spatial and reversal learning in congeneric lizards with different foraging strategies. *Animal Behaviour*, **57**, 393–407.

Galeotti, P., Sacchi, R., Rosa, D. P., and Fasola, M. (2007). Olfactory discrimination of species, sex, and sexual maturity by the Hermann's tortoise *Testudo hermanni*. *Copeia*, **2007**, 980–985.

Glavaschi, A., and Beaumont, E. S. (2014). The escape behavior of wild Greek tortoises *Testudo graeca* with an emphasis on geometrical shape discrimination. *Basic and Applied Herpetology*, **28**, 21–33.

Griffiths, C. J., Hansen, D. M., Jones, C. G., Zuël, N., and Harris, S. (2011). Resurrecting extinct interactions with extant substitutes. *Current Biology*, **21**, 762–765.

Jacobs, L. F., and Schenk, F. (2003). Unpacking the cognitive map: the parallel map theory of hippocampal function. *Psychological Review*, **110**, 285.

John, E. A., Soldati, F., Burman, O. H., Wilkinson, A., and Pike, T. W. (2016). Plant ecology meets animal cognition: impacts of animal memory on seed dispersal. *Plant Ecology*, **217**, 1441–1456.

Kis, A., Huber, L., and Wilkinson, A. (2015). Social learning by imitation in a reptile (*Pogona vitticeps*). *Animal Cognition*, **18**, 325–331.

LaDage, L. D., Roth, T. C., Cerjanic, A. M., Sinervo, B., and Pravosudov, V. V. (2012). Spatial memory: are lizards really deficient? *Biology Letters*, **8**, 939–941.

López, J. C., Rodriguez, F., Gómez, Y., Vargas, J. P., Broglio, C., and Salas, C. (2000). Place and cue learning in turtles. *Learning and Behavior*, **28**, 360–372.

López, J. C., Vargas, J. P., Gómez, Y., and Salas, C. (2003). Spatial and non-spatial learning in turtles: the role of medial cortex. *Behavioural Brain Research*, **143**, 109–120.

Moszuti, S. A., Wilkinson, A., and Burman, O. H. (2017). Response to novelty as an indicator of reptile welfare. *Applied Animal Behaviour Science*, **193**, 98–103.

Mueller, J. S., Wilkinson, A., and Hall, G. (2011). Spatial cognition in reptiles. In *Reptiles: biology, behavior and conservation*. New York, NY: Nova Science Publishers.

Mueller-Paul, J., Wilkinson, A., Hall, G., and Huber, L. (2012a). Radial-arm-maze behavior of the red-footed tortoise (*Geochelone carbonaria*). *Journal of Comparative Psychology*, **126**, 305.

Mueller-Paul, J., Wilkinson, A., Hall, G., and Huber, L. (2012b). Response-stereotypy in the jewelled lizard (*Timon lepidus*) in a radial-arm maze. *Herpetology Notes*, **5**, 243–246.

Mueller-Paul, J., Wilkinson, A., Aust, U., Steurer, M., Hall, G., and Huber, L. (2014). Touch-screen performance and knowledge transfer in the red-footed tortoise (*Chelonoidis carbonaria*). *Behavioural Processes*, **106**, 187–192.

Naumann, R. K., Ondracek, J. M., Reiter, S., *et al.* (2015). The reptilian brain. *Current Biology*, **25**, 317–321.

Noss, A. J., Soria, F., Deem, S. L., Fiorello, C. V., and Fitzgerald, L. A. (2013). *Chelonoidis carbonaria* (Testudines: Testudinidae) activity patterns and burrow use in the Bolivian Chaco. *South American Journal of Herpetology*, **8**, 19–28.

Passos, L. F., Mello, H. E. S., and Young, R. J. (2014). Enriching tortoises: assessing colour preference. *Journal of Applied Animal Welfare Science*, **17**, 274–281.

Pellitteri-Rosa, D., Sacchi, R., Galeotti, P., Marchesi, M., and Fasola, M. (2010). Do Hermann's tortoises (*Testudo hermanni*) discriminate colours? An experiment with natural and artificial stimuli. *Italian Journal of Zoology*, **77**, 481–491.

Ritz, J., Hammer, C., and Clauss, M. (2010). Body size development of captive and free-ranging Leopard tortoises (*Geochelone pardalis*). *Zoo Biology*, **29**, 517–525.

Roth, T. C., and Krochmal, A. R. (2015). The role of age-specific learning and experience for turtles navigating a changing landscape. *Current Biology*, **25**, 333–337.

Shaffer, H. B., Minx, P., Warren, D. E., *et al.* (2013). The western painted turtle genome, a model for the evolution of extreme physiological adaptations in a slowly evolving lineage. *Genome Biology*, **14**, 28.

Soldati, F., Burman, O. H., John, E. A., Pike, T. W., and Wilkinson, A. (2017). Long-term memory of relative reward values. *Biology Letters*, **13**, 20160853.

Soldati, F., Burman, O. H., John, E. A., Pike, T. W., and Wilkinson, A. (in prep.). How do animals predict cyclical resource availability?

Strong, J. N., and Fragoso, J. (2006). Seed dispersal by *Geochelone carbonaria* and *Geochelone denticulata* in Northwestern Brazil. *Biotropica*, **38**, 683–686.

Tinklepaugh, O. L. (1932). Maze learning of a turtle. *Journal of Comparative Psychology*, **13**, 201.

Van Djik, P. P., Iverson, J. B., Rhodin, A. J., Shaffer, H. B., and Bour, R. (2014). *Turtles of the world, 7th edition: annotated checklist of taxonomy, synonymy, distribution with maps, and conservation status.* Chelonian Research Monographs, No. 5 (pp. 329–479). Lunenburg, MA: Chelonian Research Foundation.

Vinke, T., and Vinke, S. (2003). An unusual survival strategy of the red-footed tortoise *Geochelone carbonaria* in the Chaco Boreal of Paraguay. *Radiata*, **12**, 21–31.

Vinke, S., Vetter, H., Vinke, T., and Vetter, S. (2008). *South American tortoises: Chelonoidis carbonaria, Chelonoidis denticulata and Chelonoidis chelensis.* Frankfurt am Main: Edition Chimaira.

Wang, E., Donatti, C. I., Ferreira, V. L., Raizer, J., and Himmelstein, J. (2011). Food habits and notes on the biology of *Chelonoidis carbonaria* (Spix 1824) (Testudinidae, Chelonia) in the southern Pantanal, Brazil. *South American Journal of Herpetology*, **6**, 11–19.

Warwick, C., Frye, F. L., and Murphy, J. B. (2001). *Health and welfare of captive reptiles.* London: Springer Science and Business Media.

Wilkinson, A., and Huber, L. (2012). *Cold-blooded cognition: reptilian cognitive abilities. The Oxford handbook of comparative evolutionary psychology* (pp. 129–143). New Jersey: Oxford University Press.

Wilkinson, A., Chan, H. M., and Hall, G. (2007). Spatial learning and memory in the tortoise (*Geochelone carbonaria*). *Journal of Comparative Psychology*, **121**, 412.

Wilkinson, A., Coward, S., and Hall, G. (2009). Visual and response-based navigation in the tortoise (*Geochelone carbonaria*). *Animal Cognition*, **12**, 779.

Wilkinson, A., Kuenstner, K., Mueller, J., and Huber, L. (2010a). Social learning in a non-social reptile (*Geochelone carbonaria*). *Biology Letters*, **6**, 614–616.

Wilkinson, A., Mandl, I., Bugnyar, T., and Huber, L. (2010b). Gaze following in the red-footed tortoise (*Geochelone carbonaria*). *Animal Cognition*, **13**, 765–769.

Wilkinson, A., Sebanz, N., Mandl, I., and Huber, L. (2011). No evidence of contagious yawning in the red-footed tortoise *Geochelone carbonaria*. *Current Zoology*, **57**, 477–484.

Wilkinson, A., Mueller-Paul, J., and Huber, L. (2013). Picture–object recognition in the tortoise *Chelonoidis carbonaria*. *Animal Cognition*, **16**, 99–107.

Yerkes, R. M. (1901). The formation of habits in the turtle. *Popular Science Monographs*, **58**, 519–525.

Yoon, J. M., and Tennie, C. (2010). Contagious yawning: a reflection of empathy, mimicry, or contagion? *Animal Behaviour*, **79**, 1–3.

Epilogue

Nereida Bueno-Guerra

From the ground-breaking chicks, dogs and cats solving wooden puzzle boxes out on the verge of a new century (Thorndike, 1898), to salivary dogs (Pavlov, 1910) and superstitious pigeons (Skinner, 1948), we have been able to see in the present book how the field of animal cognition has widely broadened the array of species and cognitive areas to explore. Easy-to-handle species (in terms of economy and convenience) has given way to deep-water whales, nocturnal bats or living fossils such as monotremes, to name a few. Studies on learning and basic reflexes now walk together with experiments about personality, decision-making or innovation. Moreover, through the previous pages it has been clear that the research interest not only accrues to the study of humans by means of non-human animals, but it also expands to the study of those non-human animals per se in an attempt to understand the environmental challenges that shaped cognition throughout evolution. It has also been demonstrated how the advancement of the available technology has fuelled the discipline's potential. Researchers adapt the newest gadgets to overcome the most enrooted problems of the field, such as elusive species (e.g. using GPS and drones to follow animals through water, air and down into the earth), migrations (e.g. through bio-loggers and telemetric devices) and human inability to perceive some sensory information (e.g. using apparatus able to detect magnetic fields or infrasound waves). The advances also extend to computational power, which currently allows us to deal with larger data sets and conduct finer-graded analyses to address our research questions. In this respect, in Box E.1 and Box E.2, Evan MacLean and Richard McElreath, respectively, provide us with two wonderful examples of how this can be achieved. Altogether, the present volume aimed to introduce current animal cognition as the sum of diverse species, multiple cognitive areas, a less anthropocentric perspective and the most modern technology and statistical advances at the service of researchers.

Box E.1 Comparative Methods in the Study of Animal Cognition

Evan L. MacLean

Studies of animal cognition have the potential to yield insights into diverse questions about how and why cognition evolves. One of the most powerful approaches to answering these questions involves the 'comparative method' – the study of variation in traits between species, with the aim of testing evolutionary hypotheses.

(*cont.*)

Comparative methods provide a framework in which variation in traits can be assessed in the context of phylogenetic relationships between taxa. In this box, I highlight common comparative methods, along with examples of the questions they are designed to answer. For a detailed review of these methods, and their application to animal cognition, I direct the reader to MacLean and colleagues (2012) and MacLean and Nunn (2017).

- **Estimating phylogenetic signal**. Measures of *phylogenetic signal* quantify the extent to which trait variation is correlated with the phylogenetic relatedness of species. When cognitive traits exhibit high levels of phylogenetic signal, this suggests that variation in species' phenotypes is closely tied to their evolutionary history. In contrast, cognitive traits characterized by low phylogenetic signal may be more evolutionarily labile.
- **Testing adaptive hypotheses**. Many exciting questions about animal cognition concern the proximate mechanisms and selective pressures that have led to species differences in cognition. In comparative studies, these questions can be addressed in a regression framework by assessing whether particular biological or ecological factors predict species differences in cognition. *Phylogenetic generalized least squares (PGLS)* is a regression model that accounts for the non-independence of species-level data by incorporating a variance–covariance matrix, which reflects evolutionary relationships between species. PGLS provides a flexible framework that can accommodate multiple predictor variables (continuous or discrete) along with an assortment of branch-length transformations to reflect different underlying models of trait evolution (e.g. Ornstein–Uhlenbeck). By accounting for evolutionary relationships between species, PGLS can reduce both type I and type II statistical errors.
- **Ancestral minds**. Although comparative psychologists study living species, many important questions involve inferences about the minds of extinct, ancestral species. Methods for *Ancestral State Estimation* use information about the traits of extant species along with a phylogenetic tree to generate estimates about ancestral states. When using a maximum likelihood approach, these methods can produce trait estimates at the internal nodes of a phylogeny, along with confidence intervals for these estimates.

In sum, comparative methods provide a powerful toolkit for investigating animal cognition in a phylogenetic framework, and will play a central role in future discoveries about the processes of cognitive evolution.

References

MacLean, E. L., and Nunn, C. L. (2017). Phylogenetic approaches for research in comparative cognition. In *APA handbook of comparative psychology: basic concepts, methods, neural*

(*cont.*)

substrate, and behavior (pp. 201–216). Washington, DC: American Psychological Association.

MacLean, E. L., Matthews, L., Hare, B., *et al.* (2012). How does cognition evolve? Phylogenetic comparative psychology. *Animal Cognition*, **15**, 223–238.

Box E.2 Bayesian Data Analysis

Richard McElreath

Inference requires assumptions. To assess the compatibility of different assumptions with evidence, a purely logical approach is to count up all the ways data could occur, according to each set of assumptions. Assumptions with more ways to produce the data are more plausible.

And that's Bayesian data analysis (BDA). A model and specific values of its parameters comprise a set of assumptions. The relative plausibilities of each set of assumptions comprise the *posterior distribution*. Combinations of parameter values with high posterior probability are more consistent with the data. Combined with other procedures, the posterior distribution assists hypothesis testing and prediction (see Gelman *et al.*, 2013; McElreath, 2016).

BDA is much older than the typical tools of introductory statistics, most of which were developed in the early twentieth century. Versions of the Bayesian approach were used in the late 1700s and throughout the nineteenth century. However, in the early twentieth century, influential statisticians such as Sir Ronald Fisher argued that BDA 'must be wholly rejected' (p. 9 of Fisher, 1925; for context, see Zabell, 1989). BDA became increasingly accepted during the second half of the twentieth century. All philosophy aside, it worked (Gelman and Robert, 2013). Beginning in the 1990s, new computational approaches led to a rapid rise in application of Bayesian methods (Fienberg, 2006). BDA has a reputation for being complicated and fancy, but it is often the simplest way to fit a model to data.

BDA helps to solve important problems. For practical scientists, the ability to deal with hierarchical data, measurement uncertainty and the risk of overfitting have been particularly important. Other approaches also address these issues, but BDA does so in a particularly direct and flexible way. *Hierarchical data* contain repeat observations of different units, such as individuals or locations. Models that pool information among these units, while estimating the distribution of these units, are variously known as *hierarchical, mixed, multilevel* and *random effects* models. *Measurement uncertainty* arises from imprecision and missingness. For example, failing to detect a species does not always mean the species is absent, and the dating of fossil remains is highly uncertain under the best circumstances. BDA cannot remove this uncertainty, but it can honestly incorporate it to avoid overconfident conclusions. *Overfitting* occurs when we learn too much from a sample, increasing

(*cont.*)

fit to sample but reducing the accuracy of prediction. All approaches to statistical inference have invented ways to guard against overfitting. BDA makes it easy through the use of prior distributions.

Prior distributions sometimes have a bad reputation – might priors allow rigging models to produce desired results? Priors could be used that way. However, nearly all uses of prior distributions result in more conservative inferences than in their absence, because priors are used to reduce overfitting. Non-Bayesian solutions to overfitting, such as penalized likelihood, are sometimes mathematically identical to the use of prior distributions.

References

Fienberg, S. E. (2006). When did Bayesian inference become 'Bayesian'? *Bayesian Analysis*, **1**, 1–40.

Fisher, R. A. (1925). *Statistical methods for research workers*. Edinburgh: Oliver and Boyd.

Gelman, A., and Robert, C. P. (2013). 'Not only defended but also applied': the perceived absurdity of Bayesian inference. *The American Statistician*, **67**, 1–5.

Gelman, A., Carlin, J. C., Stern, H. S., Dunson, D. B., Vehtari, A., and Rubin, D. B. (2013). *Bayesian data analysis*. London: Chapman & Hall/CRC.

McElreath, R. (2016). *Statistical rethinking: a Bayesian course with examples in R and Stan*. London: Chapman & Hall/CRC.

Zabell, S. (1989). R. A. Fisher on the history of inverse probability. *Statistical Science*, **4**, 247–263.

However, this book aimed not only to become an up-to-date piece of evidence on how to approach species from the most naturalistic and scientific possible point of view, but also to become an invitation to further research. This invitation is made in the form of three D-words: dehumanization, dialogue and diversification.

We use the word *dehumanization* to refer to how contributors have made an effort to introduce their respective animals in a way they excelled for themselves, with no comparison with humans needed. As Uexküll noted, 'we are easily deluded into assuming that the relationship between a foreign subject and the objects in his world exists on the same spatial and temporal plane as our own relations with the objects in our human world' (1934/2010, p. 14). Indeed, imagining the world with a different perspective from the one we daily live in is particularly tough. However, as it was once said, *there is grandeur in this view of life*. Similar to the descriptive reports which became popular during the eighteenth and nineteenth centuries thanks to the observations of naturalists, the previous chapters contained abundant descriptive information about the species that were later put into context with the state of the art in research. Therefore, we hope to have convinced the readers about how fundamental it is to get (and to accompany our data with) this knowledge prior to conducting tests because it may condition the experimental design or the behavioural interpretation.

Because dehumanization is also a method of interspecific respect, we encourage researchers to raise awareness of it within the general public by undertaking or supporting educational initiatives (see Denis Connolly and Anne's 'metaperceptual helmets' or the 3D Parisian Vendôme Square experienced in the eyes of different animals).

It is clear that fostering *dialogue* between groups testing different species has become hugely fruitful throughout the book, as the boxes within the chapters have shown. Surprisingly, we have discovered how an environmental fact was crucial to some species' behaviour but not to a close cousin, as well as how two research groups studying distant species could collaborate in sharing their tricks when approaching their respective testing animals. As in 'The blind men and an elephant' parable, the individualistic study of animal cognition may hinder the understanding of the discipline as a whole. This is also true in nature: it works as the interplay between species and environment and no separate fact accounts for the totality. Therefore, we hope the dialogue exposed in the form of our boxes had encouraged readers to keep an overall perspective in their studies, awakening questions about the potential relations between their data, the environment and other species. We would be more than happy if this book stimulated scientific cooperation, meaning sharing detailed methods (which will help novices to autonomously initiate themselves in this fascinating field and experts to adapt procedures to other species), negative results (which will save precious time and resources for other researchers) and tricks (which will ease the path to others on how to approach a concrete animal). In this sense, we are very grateful to all the contributors for their generosity in sharing their hands-on experience with us. Similarly, we invite future researchers and current specialized journals to join them in disseminating this type of useful information.

Finally, *diversification* refers to broadening the species' testing range. It is clear that reptiles, insects, monotremes and marine animals are still underrepresented in the study of animal cognition, despite the huge potential their study may provide to explore the origins of cognition. These animals posit still unrevealed questions regarding the anatomical structures needed to harbour complex cognitive capacities; whether solitary species can produce through evolution similar cognitive skills as those found in social species; or to what extent neonatal development and habitat have an impact on cognition. While trying to solve these interrogations, we also warn readers to embrace new challenges, which may involve questioning what we understand as 'cognition', as the recent hot debate about the possibility of 'minimal cognition' (Calvo Garzón and Keijzer, 2011), communication (Gagliano *et al.*, 2012) and 'brain-like' command centres in plants (Baluška *et al.*, 2010) has brought to discussion (see Trewavas, 2003; Firn, 2004; Alpi *et al.*, 2007).

In sum, we hope this book encourages an open-minded, inquisitive and rigorous scientific spirit, always in the respectful search of the evolutionary roots of cognition.

References

Alpi, A., Amrhein, N., Bertl, A., *et al.* (2007). Plant neurobiology: no brain, no gain? *Trends in Plant Science*, **12**, 135–136.

Baluška, F., Lev-Yadun, S., and Mancuso, S. (2010). Swarm intelligence in plant roots. *Trends in Ecology & Evolution*, **25**, 682–683.

Calvo Garzón, P., and Keijzer, F. (2011). Plants: Adaptive behavior, root-brains, and minimal cognition. *Adaptive Behavior*, **19**, 155–171.

Firn, R. (2004). Plant intelligence: an alternative point of view. *Annals of Botany*, **93**, 345–351.

Gagliano, M., Renton, M., Duvdevani, N., Timmins, M., and Mancuso, S. (2012). Acoustic and magnetic communication in plants. *Plant Signaling & Behavior*, **7**, 1346–1348.

Pavlov, I. P., and Thompson, W. H. (1910). *The work of the digestive glands*. London: University of California Libraries.

Skinner, B. M. (1948). Superstition in the pigeon. *Journal of Experimental Psychology*, **38**, 168–172.

Thorndike, E. L. (1898). Animal intelligence: an experimental study of the associative processes in animals. *The Psychological Review: Monograph Supplements*, **2**(4), i–109.

Trewavas, A. (2003). Aspects of plant intelligence. *Annals of Botany*, **92**, 1–20.

Uexküll, J. (1934/2010). *A foray into the worlds of animals and humans with a theory of meaning*. Minneapolis, MN: University of Minnesota Press.

Index